To University of Chester
with best wishes

From the authors

John E. Cooper

Margaret E Cooper

Introduction to Veterinary and Comparative Forensic Medicine

Reading maketh a full man; conference a ready man and writing an exact man.

Francis Bacon

The design of a book is the pattern of a reality controlled and shaped by the mind of the writer. This is completely understood about poetry or fiction, but it is too seldom realised about books of fact.

John Steinbeck

Writing a book is an adventure. To begin with, it is a toy and an amusement; then it becomes a mistress, and then it becomes a master, and then a tyrant. The last phase is that just as you are about to be reconciled to your servitude, you kill the monster and fling him out to the public.

Winston Churchill

Introduction to Veterinary and Comparative Forensic Medicine

John E. Cooper, *DTVM, FRCPath, FIBiol, FRCVS*
Diplomate, European College of Veterinary Pathologists

Professor of Veterinary Pathology
The University of the West Indies
St Augustine, Trinidad and Tobago

Margaret E. Cooper, *LLB, FLS*
Solicitor of the Supreme Court

Guest Lecturer
The University of the West Indies
St Augustine, Trinidad and Tobago

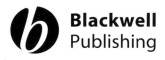

Blackwell
Publishing

Blackwell Publishing editorial offices:
Blackwell Publishing Ltd, 9600 Garsington Road, Oxford OX4 2DQ, UK
Tel: +44 (0)1865 776868
Blackwell Publishing Professional, 2121 State Avenue, Ames, Iowa 50014–8300, USA
Tel: +1 515 292 0140
Blackwell Publishing Asia Pty Ltd, 550 Swanston Street, Carlton, Victoria 3053, Australia
Tel: +61 (0)3 8359 1011

First published 2007 by Blackwell Publishing Ltd

2   2008

ISBN: 978-14051-1101-0

Library of Congress Cataloging-in-Publication Data
Cooper, J. E. (John Eric), 1944–
Introduction to veterinary and comparative forensic medicine / John E. Cooper, Margaret E. Cooper.
p. ; cm.
Includes bibliographical references and index.
ISBN-13: 978-1-4051-1101-0 (hardback : alk. paper)
ISBN-10: 1-4051-1101-1 (hardback : alk. paper)
1. Veterinary forensic medicine.   I. Cooper, Margaret E.   II. Title.
[DNLM: 1. Pathology, Veterinary–legislation & jurisprudence.   2. Expert Testimony.   3. Forensic Medicine. SF
769 C777i 2007]

SF769.47.C66 2007
636.089′4–dc22

2006022478

A catalogue record for this title is available from the British Library

Set in 9¼ on 12 pt Galliards
by SNP Best-set Typesetter Ltd., Hong Kong
Printed and bound in Singapore
by Fabulous Printers Pte Ltd

The publisher's policy is to use permanent paper from mills that operate a sustainable forestry policy, and which has
been manufactured from pulp processed using acid-free and elementary chlorine-free practices. Furthermore, the publisher ensures that the text paper and cover board used have met acceptable environmental accreditation standards.

For further information on Blackwell Publishing, visit our website:
www.BlackwellVet.com

Contents

Dedication

To the memory of Francis and Elizabeth Vowles, for their
encouragement and guidance and in recognition of their
shared concern for social justice

and

To Eric and Dorothy Cooper, for their interest in our joint work and their unchanging
welcome, succour and support

and

To Moses Cooper, born 10 February 2006, when this book was drawing to its conclusion
and who represents the future

Foreword

There can be no doubt that forensic medicine – whether applied to humans alone or to all animals – is becoming increasingly important in this modern, litigious world. The medical/legal interface, both civil or criminal, is becoming increasingly challenging and it is essential that there are practitioners available to the courts who have both the requisite knowledge and experience to perform the examinations in a satisfactory manner and who can also provide evidence to enable the court to reach its verdict.

The application of forensic techniques to the understanding and solving of crimes has been well established for a century or more. Despite this longevity, forensic medicine still continues to develop new specialist areas in response to pressure from the police and the criminal justice system. The speciality of veterinary forensic medicine is now an established, but infant, specialist area. It has been clear for some time that it is essential that it should be provided with a clear, accurate and accepted academic footing on which to develop. This book provides such a footing.

This textbook emphasises the need for a methodical, careful and precise approach to all problems. It accepts that not all practitioners will have all of the precise skills that may eventually be needed in any particular case and it emphasises that the adoption of the correct approach that will allow others – possibly someone with greater specialist skills or maybe simply an expert acting for the defence – to understand and to trust the process by which the information was obtained so that they may form their opinions based on reliable evidence.

Just as forensic medicine covers many disparate areas so too does forensic veterinary practice and all of the relevant subjects from animal welfare to biodiversity and international regulations are carefully and comprehensively considered in this book. The extent and the variation of legislation around the world means that no one book can deal with all legal aspects, and this book relates in the main to the law as currently enacted to England and Wales, but it also deals with the increasingly important, and voluminous, European legislation and with the important international treaties.

The authors have ensured that the book is specifically designed to be practical and they have included useful, focused and reliable advice on the handling of case-work throughout the text. The case histories that are included provide a superb basis for learning and for the understanding of both basic and more advanced forensic concepts. However, the practice of forensic medicine does not stop at the examination of a scene or the examination of the victim or perpetrator and this book recognises these crucial aspects and also deals with report writing and the giving of evidence in court.

This excellent book is entitled *Introduction to Veterinary and Comparative Forensic Medicine*, but it is far more than just an 'Introduction'. It is a thorough and complete overview of this developing speciality and provides both practitioners already working within this field and those seeking to develop a specialist interest and skill in veterinary forensic medicine with a reliable and comprehensive textbook.

Those who choose to practise Veterinary Forensic Medicine must now move their subject forward. They must ensure that current and future practitioners are both skilled and experienced in all the relevant areas of practice. They must insist on the development of professional bodies and they must ensure that the police, the courts and the public insist on that professionalism and expertise.

John and Margaret Cooper have worked tirelessly for veterinary medicine around the world. To bring to one book such experience and expertise is rare

and their joint efforts in writing this book reflect their immense knowledge and enthusiasm for their subject.

Richard Shepherd, BSc, MB BS, FRCPath, DMJ
Senior Lecturer and Head of Department
Forensic Medicine Unit, St. George's Medical
School, London
Past-President
Section of Clinical Forensic & Legal Medicine
The Royal Society of Medicine, London

Authors' Preface

Democracy and human rights are inseparable.

Nelson Mandela

When we first proposed writing a book on forensic medicine, we did so because of our awareness of the necessity for members of the veterinary profession to have readily available information concerning the principles and practice of forensic science and its applicability to work with animals. Below we describe that need, which is now stronger than ever, and then analyse it in more detail in the introductory chapters.

Over the past two years, however, our rationale for producing this book has extended and we believe that the demand for such a text is even more pressing. This is because the term 'forensic' is increasingly being employed in a broader sense than its original meaning of 'relating to the law'. People from diverse scientific backgrounds are regularly referring to the use of 'forensic' methods in their work. For example, the designation is often made use of by those investigating environmental changes, such as oil spills or damage to or destruction of coral reefs. In a similar vein, archaeologists, palaeontologists and historians talk of employing a 'forensic' approach to their excavations or literature searches.

'Forensic' here implies a detailed investigation and collection of evidence, regardless of whether or not there is a specific legal case or enquiry pending. Those involved are effectively applying forensic method, with all its meticulousness and need for proper record-keeping, to their routine activities. In short, the detective work that has always been the hallmark of the forensic scientist is now being applied to a whole spectrum of scientific endeavour, much of which relates to animals, plants or the environment. The pressure for this has come from many quarters, not least the increasing need nowadays to be able to defend one's opinions, judgements and statements if challenged at a later stage. Here the 'forensic' approach offers an ideal paradigm.

In view of these trends, we decided to broaden the scope of this book so as to provide the reader with an introduction to techniques and methods of working that are not only essential when dealing with animals or their derivatives when part of a legal action but which are also 'good practice' in other fields. In so doing, we hope that the book will prove helpful to those in various disciplines, as well as veterinarians, biologists and others who are concerned with captive or free-living animals.

Nevertheless, the main thrust of this volume remains how best to provide sound, reliable and objective evidence for court cases or other legally-based hearings that concern animals or their products. There has been an unprecedented increase in litigation relating to animals over the past few years. Typical cases concern such issues as provenance, age-determination and parentage, causes of death, and health and welfare. Forensic evidence is also often an important component of insurance claims and allegations of professional misconduct.

Forensic veterinary medicine is part of the broader field of comparative forensic medicine (see Chapter

2), a rapidly developing discipline that increasingly involves those who are concerned with captive and free-living animals. New fields of activity are emerging – for example, on account of concern about global pollution, the decline in biodiversity and public demands that action should be taken over illegal and irresponsible damage to the planet.

Another area in which the need for sound forensic evidence from veterinary surgeons (veterinarians) and others is expanding concerns the links between animal abuse, maltreatment of children and domestic violence. It is here that veterinary forensic medicine extends into and overlaps with forensic paediatrics, psychology and sociology. A key need is the recognition by veterinary clinicians of 'non-accidental injuries' in animals, but the issue has far wider implications than this because it requires close contact with other groups, including medical and dental practitioners, social workers, teachers and police officers.

Although forensic medicine as it relates to animals has a ubiquitous role and offers exciting challenges, it is as yet not a *bona fide* subject within the veterinary curriculum and is given little or no recognition as a post-graduate specialism. This lack of status, coupled with a paucity and scattering of literature and data, has tended to hamper the ability of veterinarians to contribute their skills and knowledge. A similar situation applies to other groups who work with animals, where involvement in legal cases is often only a relatively small part of their work and the attaining of forensic expertise is not afforded appropriate attention.

It is clearly important that veterinarians and others who work with animals are aware of the potential of litigation and that they orientate their day-to-day activities accordingly. Increased pressure must be put on professional and regulatory authorities to recognise veterinary and comparative forensic medicine as disciplines in their own right and to provide adequate funding and support for their development.

This book is not meant to be either a veterinary or a legal textbook. It is intended to reflect the interdisciplinary nature of modern forensic medicine and the need for mutual understanding between lawyers and those involved with animals, especially veterinarians. However, some medical or legal subjects are discussed in detail because of their particular importance in 'animal forensics' and the pressure nowadays on lawyers to know more about the medical aspects and on those from a veterinary or biological background to understand better the legal process. In that context, two books published by the Royal Society of Medicine, *Law for Doctors* (Branthwaite and Beresford, 2003) and *Medicine for Lawyers* (Palmer and Wetherill, 2004) are to be welcomed.

We have tried to provide a comprehensive index and we have therein included some American spellings, where appropriate, to help colleagues from that side of the Atlantic to locate information immediately. If the reader does not find what s/he wants in the text – or it is judged insufficient – there are likely to be relevant references listed at the end of the book.

Our main objective in writing this book has been to provide a ready guide to the principles of forensic medicine for veterinarians and others who are involved with animals. In compiling the text we have sought to combine our experience and training as a husband/wife, veterinary pathologist/lawyer. We have travelled widely and have dealt with a broad range of animal species, under diverse circumstances. In view of our experiences living overseas, we have tried in these pages to reach out to poorer parts of the world, especially 'developing' countries (152 were listed by the World Bank in 2005) where facilities for forensic work – and the expertise to go with it – are often in very short supply.

The art and science of forensic medicine have largely emanated from the richer, 'developed', countries and, as a result, many of the techniques now advocated and the precision that is demanded, while relevant to well-organised modern societies, can be totally inappropriate in poorer parts of the world. Therefore, in the text we have endeavoured to cater for the needs of the latter by drawing attention to ways in which the standards of forensic medicine can be maintained or enhanced despite the absence of strong or reliable infrastructure. Good forensic medicine *can* be practised in these places but ingenuity is often required, coupled where appropriate with help from outside.

Our hope is that our book will help those involved in legal and other actions concerning animals to gain access to sound evidence that is both based on good science and obtained using best available practice.

We are of the generation born during the Second World War. Our future – and that of our children – was to be enshrined in the Preamble to the Charter of the United Nations (UN), which came into force on 24th October, 1945:

> *We the peoples of the United Nations,*
> *determined to save succeeding generations from*
> *the scourge of war, which twice in our lifetime*
> *has brought untold sorrow to mankind . . .*
> *reaffirm faith in fundamental human rights, in*
> *the dignity and worth of the human person, in*
> *the equal rights of men and women and of*
> *nations large and small. . . .*

Alas, many of the bold statements made in that Charter have failed to prevent further conflict, genocide, oppression and diverse assaults on human rights. At the time of our writing (2006), real and perceived threats of terrorism have prompted governments to introduce measures that are not only contrary to the UN Charter but incompatible with earlier, sometimes ancient, declarations and agreements relating to the freedom of the individual. An independent judiciary, open courts, access to lawyers and verdicts based on sound evidence are all part of ensuring that human rights are not eroded. Raising the standards of forensic medicine as it relates to animals is but a tiny part of that mosaic but it represents our modest contribution. The reader should be aware, therefore, that our book is not intended to help secure punishment for those who transgress laws and codes relating to animals; nor in what we write do we seek to excuse or exonerate those who are, indeed, guilty of crimes or malpractice. Instead, we wish to ensure that, as far as is humanly possible, courts, tribunals, disciplinary hearings and the like are provided with sound evidence as a basis for deliberation.

John E. Cooper   Margaret E. Cooper
St. Augustine, Trinidad & Tobago,
West Indies, January 2006

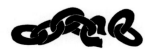

Acknowledgements

Nothing in nature stands alone.

John Hunter

First, we should like to express our gratitude to our friend, Dr. Richard Shepherd, an experienced and highly respected forensic pathologist who has a great interest in veterinary and comparative medicine, for agreeing to write the Foreword to this book and for his enthusiastic and good-humoured encouragement in this and other forensic ventures.

Over the years, many people have catalysed our shared interest in veterinary medicine and the law and the relevance of these two disciplines to the conservation and protection of the natural world. Our early participation in forensic matters was stimulated by Alastair Porter, Registrar of the Royal College of Veterinary Surgeons (RCVS) 1966–1991, Peter Robinson and Michael Chapman. Numerous other veterinary surgeons, biologists, field naturalists and lawyers were involved in those studies or gave us help. Some are mentioned individually, later in these Acknowledgements, or elsewhere in the text. We remember here our friend, Joan Root, naturalist and film-maker, who devoted much of her life to the protection of the wildlife of Kenya and news of whose death reached us as we were completing this part of our book. *Kwa heri, Joan, na Mungu akuibariki.*

JEC owes a great deal to numerous mentors: the training and guidance he received in natural history from Major Maxwell Knight (former MI5 agent, the prototype for 'M' in the James Bond books) and Mr. Gerald Durrell (animal collector extraor-

dinaire and Founder of the Jersey Zoo), in osteology and primatology from Dr. Louis S.B. Leakey and Professor Philip V. Tobias (the internationally recognised Kenyan and South African palaeontologists) and in diagnostic pathology of creatures both great and small from Professor Peer Zwart and Dr. Edward Elkan (arguably 'the father of lower vertebrate pathology').

Our families have always given us support and encouragement. We thank our daughter, Vanessa, and our son, Maxwell, for their interest in all we do and to them both and to Sarah (Hutton) Cooper for commenting on earlier drafts. Part of the text was also reviewed by Diana (Cooper) Dymond. Our parents, to whom we owe so much, are the subject of the Dedication at the beginning of the book.

Writing an interdisciplinary text is never easy and we are therefore indebted to the many people who have assisted us in disparate ways. A number of colleagues and friends have reviewed sections of chapters and appendices or have made helpful comments and criticisms about the book. In this respect we are most grateful to Andrew Adogwa, Sham Bissessar, Gustave Borde, Dane Coombs, Adrian Hailey, Annemarie Phillip-Hosein, Adana Mahase, Howard and Eleanor Nelson, Kristel-Marie Ramnath, Rohini Roopnarine, Ravi Seebaransingh, Verrol Simmons, Rod Suepaul and Cheryl-Ann Wharewood in Trinidad; Donald Broom, Phil Cannings, Simon Chaplin, Martyn Cooke, Neil Forbes, Neville

Gregory, Andrew Greenwood, Mike Hart, Mike Jessop, Martin Lawton, Chris Laurence, Ian McDowall, Fred McKeating, Peter Scott, Holger Schutkowski, Guy Shorrock, Jill Webb and Sean Wensley in the United Kingdom; David Bayvel, Richard Norman and Virginia Williams in New Zealand; Richard Wootton in Australia; Jesús Pérez Jiménez in Spain; Andy Allen and Sharon E. Cregier in Canada; Peter Dawson and Fritz Huchzermeyer in South Africa; Jack Reece in India; and Phil Arkow, Nélio Barros, Michael Fox, Fred Frye and Janet Whaley in the USA. David Watson came to the University of the West Indies from Australia as a volunteer teacher in small animal medicine, not realising that his skills as an editor would be put to immediate good use by the Coopers. We are indebted to him. Madeleine Forsyth, with her combined veterinary and legal qualifications, kindly provided advice at the interface of these disciplines.

Specific guidance on certain aspects was provided by two friends and colleagues, Dr. Steve Bennett, doyen of the veterinary profession in Trinidad and Tobago, and Professor Ram Prabhu. Mr. Emmanuel Walker arranged for us to visit the Forensic Science Laboratory, Port of Spain. The Veterinary Defence Society constructively reviewed certain sections. Mr. Alan Kershaw, Director of the Council for the Registration of Forensic Practitioners (CRFP) advised and gave permission for us to reproduce the CRFP Code of Practice and Mr. Gordon Hockey did likewise in respect of the Guide to Professional Conduct of the RCVS. The Universities Federation for Animal Welfare, through its Chief Executive and Scientific Director, Dr James Kirkwood, authorised the use of the passage from *Animals and the Law* by T. G. Field-Fisher. Chief Superintendent Phil Wilson of the RSPCA gave specific advice on the question of animal abuse and Dr. Roy Rickman, pioneer in tropical medicine, on equipment that can be of use for forensic work in the field.

We are grateful to the librarians and staff of the Hugh Wooding Law School, the Faculty of Medical Sciences (Mount Hope) and the University of the West Indies, all in Trinidad, for their assistance and for permitting us to use their facilities. Particular thanks are owed to Sheree Singh, Ray Ganessingh, Jason Oliver, Brian Castillo and Christian Kalloo for their patience and help on many occasions. As always, we acknowledge the libraries of the Royal College of Veterinary Surgeons, the Department of Veterinary Medicine, University of Cambridge and the Royal Entomological Society, for help with references and their continuing support.

The Case Studies in Appendix D were kindly provided by J. D. Watkins, MRCVS; R. Suepaul, DVM; M. Sugumaran, BVSc; S. Chawla, BVSc & AH and J. F. Reece, BSc, BVSc, MRCVS; and R. Norman, PhD, MACVSc, MRCVS.

Many of the photographs in the book were taken by Margaret Cooper. A number, designated as such, were the work of Richard Spence, our friend, the Medical Photographer at the Faculty of Medical Sciences of the University of the West Indies (UWI). In reproducing portraits of the late Dr Edward Elkan and Major Maxwell Knight, we pay tribute to their families, not only for giving us the pictures but also for their encouragement and hospitality in years gone by. Other kind friends have helped with the artwork. Alësha Naranjit, BSc, leading light in the UWI Biological Society, prepared the line drawings that appear at the end of each chapter. Our friend, colleague and fellow 'Brit' in Trinidad, John Watkins, MRCVS, designed two of the cartoons, provided a contribution to the Appendices and has also given us support in numerous other ways.

We have been given permission to use cartoons by Mahase Calpu and Steve Long that appeared in the Trinidad *Daily Express* and in *Veterinary Times* respectively; we acknowledge this with thanks. We owe a special thanks to Janet Slee and the late David Austin for permission to include in our book four of David's cartoons, which originally appeared in *In Practice*. We intend that their reproduction here should serve as a memorial to David Austin and a tribute to the pleasure that he has given to his veterinary readers over the years.

Avril Patterson-Pierre (University of the West Indies) regularly printed manuscripts and gave cheery assistance in numerous other ways. As with so many books in the past, our family friend, Sally Dowsett, provided much-appreciated ideas and spontaneous help. Ashley Fegan-Earl supplied valuable advice in the early stages of production.

The typing of the manuscript was largely carried out by Deborah Daniel who coped admirably, with humour and enthusiasm, with the vagaries of producing a publication such as this – and, in particular, the idiosyncratic way in which the Coopers usually work. Thank you very much!

The completion of a book is never easy or painless, as Churchill's words at the beginning of our text portray so vividly. It was a pleasure, therefore, to have as our copy-editor Judith Glushanok who worked in partnership with us and on more than one occasion raised our flagging spirits. We are most grateful to her.

One of the most pleasant aspects about working in Trinidad for the University of the West Indies has been to have for our home a colonial-style bungalow with a garden that is full of animal and plant life. Here we have been able to retreat to compile this book, in the company of hummingbirds, iguanas and red anartia butterflies. These reminders of the fragile beauty of our planet, coupled with the kindness of local friends, have made our task far more pleasurable than ever expected. We are grateful.

John and Margaret Cooper
St. Augustine
14th February, 2006

Abbreviations

AVMA   American Veterinary Medical Association
CAWC   Companion Animal Welfare Council
CAWT   Coalition Against Wildlife Trafficking
CITES   Convention on International Trade in Endangered Species of Wild Fauna and Flora
CIWF   Compassion in World Farming
COTES   Control of Trade in Endangered Species
CPD   continuing professional development
CRFP   Council for the Registration of Forensic Practitioners
DEFRA   Department for Environment, Food and Rural Affairs
EBVM   evidence-based veterinary medicine
EU   European Union
FAWC   Farm Animal Welfare Council
GI   gastro-intestinal
GPC   Guide to Professional Conduct (of the RCVS)
HSA   Humane Slaughter Association
ICZN   International Commission on Zoological Nomenclature
IMLU   Independent Medico Legal Units
IUCN   World Conservation Union

MRCVS   Member of the Royal College of Veterinary Surgeons
NAI   non-accidental injury
OIE   Office International des Epizooties
PAW   Partnership for Action against Wildlife Crime
PMI   *post-mortem* interval
RCVS   Royal College of Veterinary Surgeons
RSPB   Royal Society for the Protection of Birds
RSPCA   Royal Society for the Prevention of Cruelty to Animals
SEM   scanning electron-micrograph/micrography
SSC   Species Survival Commission
UFAW   Universities Federation for Animal Welfare
UK   United Kingdom
UN   United Nations
USA   United States of America
USFWS   United States Fish and Wildlife Service
WCA   Wildlife and Countryside Act
WHO   World Health Organization
WSAVA   World Small Animal Veterinary Association
WSPA   World Society for the Protection of Animals

Introduction

CHAPTER 1

What is Forensic Medicine?

Homo homini lupus. (Man is a wolf to man.)

Roman proverb

INTRODUCTION

To many members of the public the term 'forensic medicine' conjures up images of dead bodies, gruesome accidents and painstaking investigation by medical and other scientists, often in unpleasant or macabre circumstances. However, the word forensic, as defined in the Concise Oxford Dictionary, means 'relating to, used in, or connected with a court of law'. The dictionary then defines 'forensic medicine' as 'the applied use of medical knowledge, especially pathology, to the purpose of the law.' Therefore, it encompasses much more than the narrow field of work described above.

The origin of the word forensic is significant. It is derived from the Latin word *forensis* which meant 'public'. This in turn was derived from *forum*, originally a market, later a place of debate – a reminder that forensic work is subject to open discussion and scrutiny, usually in the public arena of court or other legal or quasi-legal proceedings and rarely carried out behind closed doors.

During the last 30 years or so the concept and understanding of the term 'forensic' has broadened, particularly in respect of the following:

- The widespread emphasis in the media and elsewhere on 'forensic science', stressing its multidisciplinary role and the contributions from different areas of science and technology (see later).

- An increasing tendency to encompass within the term 'forensic' various non-legal aspects – as discussed in Chapter 2.

Quite apart from the above, the methods used in conventional forensic work are also largely applicable to situations outside the courts, such as insurance claims, appearances at tribunals, inquiries, environmental impact assessments, Public Service Commissions and the like (see Chapter 2) – or when defending or propounding allegations of professional misconduct or other disciplinary measures.

HISTORY

Human forensic medicine has a long and interesting, but not always distinguished, history. Some of the earliest records of its use came from China (see Chapter 7 and Smith, 1986). Islamic medicine often applied a forensic approach to the investigation of disease and the causes of death (see, for example, Tibi, 2006). The origins and evolution of forensic medicine in Europe were explored and described by Davis (1974) who reminded readers that continental Europe essentially took the lead in medicolegal investigations in the last millennium. Forensic necropsies were performed in Italy and Germany 500 years before they formed part of coroners' inquests in England and Wales. Medical evidence from physicians and surgeons was

3

admitted at trials in England in the 17th and 18th centuries (Ranson, 1996) but it was not until the late 1800s that the many deficiencies in the British system began to be rectified (Forbes, 1981; Lane, 1990) – and then largely as a result of the work of the famous Hunter brothers (Cornelius, 1978).

William Hunter (1783) wrote a seminal essay on the signs of murder in 'bastard' children and his brother John produced lecture notes and essays describing improved methods for dissection and for the diagnosis of disease (Hunter, undated). In March 1781 John Hunter had a humiliating experience in the trial for murder of Captain John Donellan where his cautious views as the medical witness for the defence were ridiculed and essentially over-ridden by the judge, Mr. Justice Buller, and, instead, 'more emphatic, dogmatic and unscientifically-based evidence of the other doctors' (Davis, 1974) held sway. As a result, Donellan was executed. Hunter was badly shaken by this ordeal and told his students: 'A poor devil was lately hanged at Warwick upon no other testimony than that of physical men [physicians] whose first experiments were made on this occasion' (quoted by Moore, 2005). The 'experiments' referred to were poorly performed toxicological studies carried out on dogs by the doctors called by the prosecution, but Hunter was equally disdainful of the inadequate autopsy that they had performed. The hearings and their aftermaths have been re-examined and analysed by a number of authors, including Grove (1943).

The Donellan case prompted much open debate by the press and public (Blanchard, 1781), and concern amongst the medical profession prompted an upsurge of interest in Britain in the practice of forensics. Farr (1788) produced an enlarged, translated version of Fazelius' *Elementa Medicinae Forensis* and other, rather inadequate, volumes followed. It was left to George Edward Male (1779–1845) to write the first sound text on the subject – *Epitome of Juridical or Forensic Medicine for the Use of Medical Men, Coroners and Barristers* (Male, 1816).

On account of his writings and work, Male is usually considered to be the father of medical jurisprudence in Britain. His publications in 1816 and 1818 set the scene for the development of a more scientific approach towards forensic medicine. It is of interest and significance that Male stated in the preface to his first book, '. . . the indignation which has been excited by the perusal of the medical evidence adduced in some recent trials, has induced me to offer [these papers] to the public.'

The most influential medical forensic man in developing the field in the more recent past was undoubtedly Sir Bernard Spilsbury (1877–1947) who first came to public attention during the trial of Dr. H. H. Crippen and soon became a household name in Britain. Spilsbury was involved in most of the highly publicised murder cases in the UK. In Spilsbury's time the medical forensic expert was generally the key person in forensic investigations. He (and it was usually a man!) would not only have been able to speak and to give an opinion with great authority on medical matters but also would have been the link, the conduit, to people from other disciplines, such as chemists who could analyse poisons, fingerprint experts, botanists and soil scientists.

The long-standing role and status of the medical profession in forensic work in the English-speaking world were aptly summarised and lauded by John Harber Phillips, Chief Justice of Victoria, Australia, who wrote, 'These pictures from the past capture, more vividly than any dissertation, the service that medicine has for so long given to the law. A service given fully and freely, with precision of expression and meticulous attention to detail.' (Phillips, 1996).

It is not surprising that the medical profession has been so often associated with crime investigation. The physician needs powers of observation and the ability to assemble the clinical findings with history and background information to construct a whole picture of the patient. It is also small wonder that the fictitious detective Sherlock Holmes was the creation of an eminent medical man, Sir Arthur Conan Doyle, who was strongly influenced by one of his teachers at Edinburgh University (Peschel and Peschel, 1989). Interestingly, the only real-life case in which Conan Doyle was himself involved related to the mutilation of livestock. The man found guilty of this crime was George Edalji, a solicitor, the Anglo-Indian son of a Staffordshire vicar. He served a seven-year prison term, but

Conan Doyle spearheaded the investigations and campaign that led to Edalji's being pardoned. The story has been dramatised in a recent book (Barnes, 2005), worth reading to gain insight into the life and thinking of the man who created the world's most famous detective.

Many medical texts have encouraged their readers, especially students, to adopt a detective's approach to clinical and pathological investigation. The delightful little book *Exotica* (Symmers, 1984) presented some of the author's more unusual cases and described how they were investigated and often solved using ingenuity and lateral thinking.

THE RISE OF FORENSIC SCIENCE

However, the situation has changed considerably over recent decades. No longer is the medical man or woman central to legal investigations: instead, s/he is one of a team. Forensic science has emerged and matured and the medically-trained expert is now just one part of that discipline, as depicted in Figure 1.1.

We speak now of 'forensic scientists' who, in turn, describe themselves as 'forensic chemists', 'forensic botanists' or 'forensic biologists', and so on. An important, albeit poorly proof-read, introduction to the scope and role of contemporary forensic science is provided in the book edited by

P. C. White (2004), published by the Royal Society of Chemistry.

TEACHING AND ACCREDITATION OF FORENSIC SCIENCE

The growth of forensic science has created a need to educate and teach and to ensure that the training offered is of a satisfactory standard and objectively assessed and accredited by an independent body.

In the UK, many universities and colleges have started undergraduate and other programmes covering a range of forensic disciplines and the Forensic Science Society (see Appendix B) has commenced an accreditation service for such courses. Those eligible for accreditation have normally a Bachelor's degree with Honours or a post-graduate qualification such as a taught Master's degree. The scheme was developed to help establish and maintain standards of education in forensic science and it involves major employers and professional interests. Similar accreditation schemes are evolving in some other countries.

The *accreditation* of those who present forensic evidence is proving more contentious (see Chapter 13). The role in this regard of the UK's Council for the Registration of Forensic Practitioners (CRFP) (see Appendix B) is discussed elsewhere in the book.

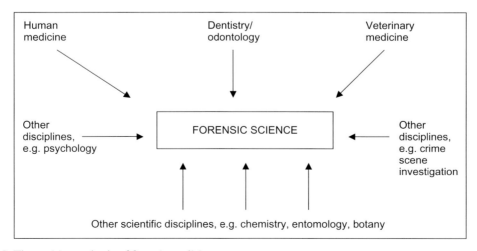

Figure 1.1 The position and role of forensic medicine.

THE CHANGING FORTUNES OF FORENSIC MEDICINE

While forensic science has gained ground, the role and status of human forensic medicine have been challenged. In the UK questions have been asked about the role and competence of 'police surgeons' (forensic physicians), once the backbone of the service, and their ability, as medical practitioners with limited training in forensic matters, to cope with present demands. Forensic pathology has suffered considerably from closure of units and departments, the dismantling of museums (partly a result of concerns over the retention of human tissues – see below and Chapter 7) and a move from official (government/coroner/police) funding towards the use of private pathology services. The recruitment of trainee forensic pathologists has also waned. This is paradoxical because in many countries there is great public interest in forensic pathology, fomented by television and other media (Westwell, 2005) and the increasing demands of society that when a death or accident occurs, there should be no curbs in determining the circumstances and ascertaining where blame or culpability might lie.

At the time of writing (July 2005), the medical profession, including some of those involved in forensic and allied studies, is under attack, especially in the UK. Scandals relating to the retention of human tissues have cast medical pathologists in a bad light and have led to the passage of the Human

Tissue Act 2004 which imposes strict conditions on those working with derivatives of live or dead *Homo sapiens* (see Chapter 6). Individual pathologists have also sometimes fuelled public anxiety – for instance, at the inquest in a high-profile murder case in Kenya, where a forensic pathologist admitted, 'I lied over murder on safari trip.' (Horsnell, 2004).

Confidence in medical witnesses has also been eroded by miscarriages of justice when innocent people, whose children had died under unusual circumstances, were imprisoned following 'misleading and flawed' evidence by a leading experienced paediatrician (General Medical Council Hearing, June 2005), who was subsequently removed from (later restored to) the British Medical Register (see Chapter 12). How this situation might have arisen has been discussed and analysed (Le Fanu, 2005; Hall, 2006), but the damage had been done and the populace was outraged.

Public concern about the efficiency and reliability of the General Medical Council had earlier been shaken in the UK by the arrest and conviction of a supposedly trusted and reliable family physician, Harold Shipman, who probably killed hundreds of patients and had long escaped detection (www.the-shipman-inquiry.org.uk/home.asp). As Michell (2005) pointed out, the repercussions are likely to be considerable and could finish the tradition of self-regulation by the medical (and possibly other?) professions.

This situation has probably not been helped by the actions of many 'western' governments, to deregulate the professions, in the interests of competition, and thereby reduce their influence in society (Watkins *et al.*, 1996; Michell, 2002). Self-regulation has been criticised on the grounds that the professional body serves as both judge and jury and this has prompted the inclusion of more 'lay members' on some disciplinary and ethical committees. Even the term 'profession' has been devalued and is increasingly used by groups of people who are not subject to the constraints of a body which has disciplinary powers.

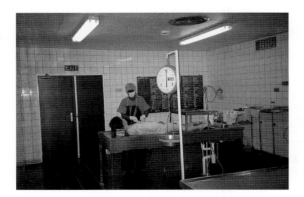

Figure 1.2 Autopsy remains a key part of human forensic medicine but the extent to which medicolegal examinations are carried out varies from country to country.

NEW FIELDS

There are, however, other factors and various public concerns that are helping to mould a new approach

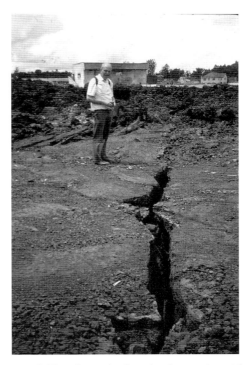

Figure 1.3 The aftermath of a volcanic eruption with extensive lava flow in Central Africa. Natural disasters involve medical forensic specialists.

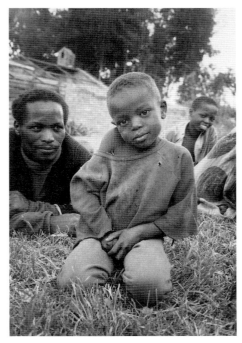

Figure 1.4 A survivor of the Rwandan genocide. Forensic medicine plays an important part in the investigation of disasters, including civil war.

to forensic medicine. These relate particularly to the protection of human rights and to the provision of relief in, and investigation of, disasters. There is some overlap between these two.

Insofar as human rights are concerned, there is increasing disquiet in some countries and groupings, galvanised by the United Nations (UN) and organisations such as Amnesty International (see Appendix B), about the continuing abuse of individuals and communities in many parts of the world (Cox, 2003). Often this has been accompanied by an increase in the use of harsh punishments, aggressive interrogation and detention without trial – sometimes justified on the grounds of 'protecting national security'. The medical profession is playing a leading role in the investigation of such claims – for example, by the clinical examination of those who claim to be victims of torture or who seek asylum because of alleged oppression (Heisler *et al.*, 2003; Shepherd, 2003). An extension of this is

collaboration by doctors and lawyers to provide professional help to those finding themselves in such a position – for example, the Independent Medico Legal Units (IMLU) established in South Africa and Kenya (Olumbe *et al.*, undated).

Disasters can be conveniently divided into those that are:

- Natural, physical – hurricanes, volcanoes, earthquakes, tsunamis.
- Natural, infectious – outbreaks of Ebola, Marburg, avian influenza.
- Anthropogenic (human-induced) – transportation (e.g. aircraft crashes), war, civil unrest, genocide (Blau and Skinner, 2005), torture, terrorism (including the use of biological and chemical agents) (Durrant, 2002).

They can also be categorised according to their scope (international, national or local), rate of onset (sudden or slow) and source (Sprayson, 2006).

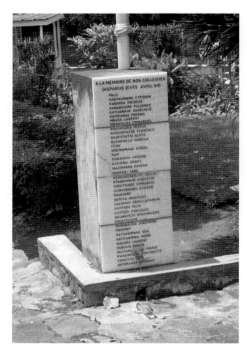

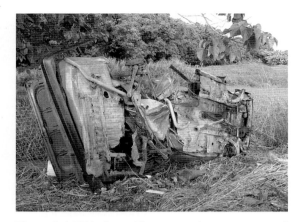

Figure 1.6 Vehicular accidents are an important cause of death and injury and frequently require a forensic medical input.

Figure 1.5 A memorial in Kigali, Rwanda. This lists United Nations personnel who were killed during the genocide.

Enhanced public and inter-governmental concern over disasters has led to a demand for a greater number of appropriately trained and experienced people, to include forensic physicians, pathologists, psychiatrists and paediatricians, often together with anthropologists (Klepinger, 2006), who can respond, investigate and report back to the international community. The medical profession plays an influential part in such disaster relief and reconstruction. Its expanding contribution is reflected by the appearance of many relevant publications and by the launching of a new interdisciplinary Faculty of Conflict and Catastrophe by the Society of Apothecaries of London (see Appendix B), for example.

It is clear that despite changes in the responsibilities and fortunes of human medical forensic experts recently, they still have an indispensable part to play. Fields of forensic science in which the medical profession continues to be active, often taking the lead role, are described in many texts – see, for example, DiMaio and DiMaio (2001); Siegel *et al.*

(2000); and Shepherd (2003). The main categories are listed below.

Clinical and/or post-mortem examination of human victims

- Physical injuries (wounds) including those caused by firearms and explosives, traffic, railway and aircraft injuries.
- Asphyxia.
- Immersion and drowning.
- Heat, cold, electricity.
- Sexual offences.
- Abortion.
- Infant neglect, elder abuse, starvation.
- Torture, armed conflict.
- Disasters – natural and anthropogenic.
- Poisoning.
- Alcoholism.
- Drugs of dependence and abuse.
- Over-dosage of medical drugs.

Post-mortem examination of human victims

As above, plus:

- Unexpected and sudden death.
- Exhumation.
- Identification and aging/dating of human remains.

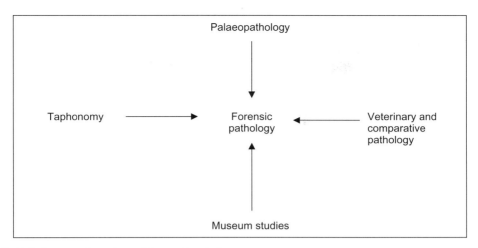

Figure 1.7 Links between forensic medicine and pathology.

INTERDISCIPLINARY LINKS

There are close links between contemporary forensic medicine and various other disciplines. Some of these, in just one area, pathology, are depicted in Figure 1.7.

These and other spheres of shared interest mean that those working in forensic medicine in future will need to collaborate more and to share experiences and skills. Such co-operation is likely to grow as other fields mature, including veterinary and comparative forensics, the subject of this book, and 'environmental forensics' (Morrison, 1999; Murphy and Morrison, 2002), which relates to human health and that of animals, plants and ecosystems (see Chapters 2 and 13).

A very broad spectrum of experts already work closely with medical forensic personnel. They include anthropologists, DNA specialists, drug analysts, entomologists, ballistics experts, fingerprint specialists, fire-scene examiners, collision investigators, document examiners, footwear analysts, fingerprint experts, vehicle examiners, archaeologists, computer specialists, toxicologists and blood-pattern analysts. The roles of some of these are described further elsewhere.

THE REQUIREMENTS

Forensic medical work differs in many ways from routine diagnosis and treatment. As pointed out earlier, the origin of the term 'forensic' provides a constant reminder that forensic work is subject to open debate. The person providing evidence (even if an 'expert') may well be exposed to interrogation, criticism and attempts to discredit (see Chapter 12). Therefore, forensic medicine needs a special approach and not all general practitioners, physicians, surgeons, paediatricians and pathologists may be comfortable with this. The transparent nature of modern forensic science, especially if court appearances are required, means that members of the medical or allied professions likely to participate must be fully prepared, both professionally and psychologically. Even those who do their utmost to steer clear of legal issues may have no choice but to be involved in what is perceived generally to be a very specialised area.

Special Features of Veterinary and Comparative Forensic Medicine

When a dog bites a man that is not news, but when a man bites a dog that is news.

Charles Anderson Dana

In the foregoing chapter, the essence of forensic medicine as it has traditionally related to medico-legal work with humans was discussed. In this chapter the particular features of veterinary and what we define as 'comparative' forensic medicine are described. Essentially the two relate to *animal* forensics – that is, matters of a legal or similar serious nature in which animals play a substantial part.

First, it is important to remember that animals can be involved in legal actions in two distinct ways: they can be either the victim (i.e. the object) of an assault or illegal act, or the instigator (i.e. the subject) where the animal *causes* the incident. This second area, when animals bring about the incident, is, arguably, an area of forensic veterinary medicine as well as forensic human medicine, because any ensuing legal case will probably require expert evidence from a veterinarian and/or others with specialised knowledge. The basic principles of forensic investigation, in relation to meticulous record-keeping, systematic examination and proper treatment of material are the same, regardless of whether the victim is human or not.

THE ANIMAL AS THE VICTIM (THE OBJECT)

Injuries and insults may be inflicted on animals maliciously or accidentally and can embrace a variety of attacks, perversions and mutilations. Examples are given in Table 2.1 (see also Chapters 6 and 7). Arkow and Munro (2006) provide a useful categorisation of assaults on companion animals.

There has been extensive study of some forms of 'human-induced' damage to animals – for example, non-accidental injury caused to dogs and cats (see Chapter 6), the effects of traps, snares and shooting on wildlife (see Chapter 5) and the various factors that can cause injury or death in marine mammals (Read and Murray, 2000).

Death, injury, ill health, pain or distress may result from most of the examples above but the implications usually differ, depending on species and circumstances. There are often parallels with human forensic work: the 'battered pet' syndrome described some years ago (Munro, 1996) led to recognition of links between animal abuse and violence to humans and development of a new discipline (see Chapter 6).

THE ANIMAL AS THE CAUSE (THE SUBJECT)

Injuries provoked by animals include bites from wild and domestic species, trauma, electrocution, stings and hypersensitivity reactions (Strickland, 1991). Animals can infect humans with sundry pathogenic organisms leading to various zoonotic diseases (see later).

Table 2.1 Injuries and other insults that may be inflicted on animals by humans.

Insult	Features	Comments
Physical	Injuries due to trauma, heat, cold, immersion in water, etc.	Often unintentional but can include 'non-accidental injury' (NAI)
Sexual	Attempted copulation Surgical or malicious damage or manipulation to genital organs, castration, ovariectomy, vasectomy, etc.	May be part of sexual abuse or normal veterinary/husbandry practices
Psychological	Deprivation of company or unsuitable social grouping Taunting, teasing or threatening	Sometimes part of normal veterinary or husbandry procedures Can be part of animal abuse

Table 2.2 gives some examples of bites, stings and other non-infectious insults that may be inflicted by animals on humans or other species.

The clinical and *post-mortem* appearances in such cases may be similar or very different: initial lesions are likely to change, if the affected individual survives, because of inflammatory/allergic reactions, contusion, infection or self-inflicted injury.

FORENSIC SIGNIFICANCE OF ANIMAL BITES AND STINGS

Animal bites and stings can be of forensic (legal, insurance, malpractice) significance for various reasons, particularly if they cause:

- Physical damage to humans, other animals or property.
- Toxic damage to humans and other animals.
- Psychological damage to humans, possibly to other animals.
- Infection, with or without clinical disease, in humans and other animals.

Bites and stings from animals can be inflicted inadvertently: a dog may bite a person's hand when the animal is offered an item of food; a farmer can be 'bitten' while restraining a calf because his fingers are in its mouth; an otherwise inoffensive snake may strike at an owner because it is shedding its skin and therefore has impaired vision (Cooper, 1967). Alternatively, bites may be deliberate: the animal bites because it is aggressive or is frightened or feels

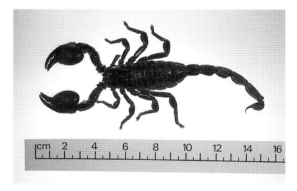

Figure 2.1 An emperor scorpion. Not a very venomous species but liable to elicit fear and psychological effects.

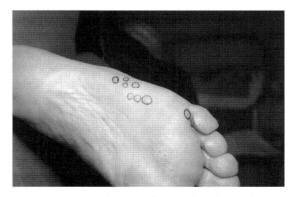

Figure 2.2 Sea urchin wounds, ringed with a marking pen, in the foot of a tourist, several weeks after the incident.

Table 2.2 Bites, stings and other non-infectious insults from animals.

Insult	*Features*	*Comments*
Bite		
From a mammal	Bruising, skin wounds, tooth marks Other lesions may be present if the animal has also scratched (e.g. cat) or kicked/trampled (e.g. horse) Goring by bulls and other ungulates can cause severe internal damage, sometimes death	Appearance of wound depends upon circumstances and species of animal (e.g. a carnivore's teeth tend to tear whereas the flat cheek teeth of a ruminant will grind and crush tissue) (see Chapters 6 and 7)
From a bat	Tooth marks, persistent bleeding if a vampire (*Desmodus* sp.) involved	Bats may transmit infections including rabies, other viruses and trypanosomiasis
From a bird	As for bat but no tooth marks Some species (e.g. parrots) bite, others (e.g. storks) stab, others (e.g. falcons) strike with talons, ratites (e.g. ostriches) kick	Wound appearance very variable Various micro-organisms can be transmitted by bites and scratches
From a snake: • Venomous (e.g. cobra, rattlesnake, fer-de-lance)	Fang marks and lesions depend on snake and type of venom	The bites of all snakes, even those that are non-venomous, can introduce pathogenic organisms, especially bacteria
• Non-venomous (e.g. python)	Tooth marks (not fangs – rows) with local haemorrhage and swelling	See above In exceptional cases ocular damage can ensue (Cooper, 1967) Traumatic asphyxia has been reported following constriction (DiMaio and DiMaio, 2001)
From a lizard (only two significant species of venomous lizard, both *Heloderma* spp.)	Bite marks and local, sometimes systemic, signs	The bites of non-venomous carnivorous lizards can introduce bacteria The saliva of some other 'harmless' lizards may contain toxic chemicals
From a crocodile	Tearing wounds, sometimes dislocation of limbs May cause drowning	Much anecdotal and some scientific documentation (see Fergusson, 2004)
From a fish (e.g. shark)	Ragged bite and tear wounds (especially limbs); can be fatal Drowning possible Death may be due to hypovolaemic shock	Sometimes occur in freshwater, in shallow or coastal reef areas (Williams *et al.*, 1998) but usually in deep sea. Much variation in shark behaviour Other species of fish, e.g. moray eels and barracuda, may also cause damage
From a spider (Arachnida: many species). The black widow *Latrodectus* sp. is probably most notorious)	Erythema and oedema of the skin, often associated with puncture marks	Although most species of spider can bite, few are able to penetrate human or animal skin and only a handful are sufficiently toxic to cause envenomation

(Continued)

Table 2.2 *Continued.*

Insult	Features	Comments
From a tick (Acarina: many species)	Ticks attach to the skin of vertebrates and usually suck blood They can cause blood loss, local tissue damage, skin infection, sometimes paralysis or systemic disease	Ticks take time (days) to engorge Different ticks are found in diverse locations The presence of dead ticks may indicate that the animal has been dipped or sprayed with an insecticide: this can be significant in some legal cases
From a mosquito (Diptera)	Mosquito bites are usually raised and inflamed, pruritic Some species, e.g. *Anopheles* and *Aedes* spp., can transmit serious infectious diseases	Some humans and animals attract mosquitoes and react more severely to bites than do others
From biting flies (e.g. horse flies – Tabanidae, and tsetseflies – Glossinidae)	Often painful bites with local inflammation Some species can transmit infectious agents, including blood-parasites	Many species in different parts of the world Tsetse flies are restricted to Africa
From flies that lay eggs on living tissues (e.g. Old World screw worms, *Chrysomya bezziana*)	Maggot-infested skin wounds, especially around soiled or damaged areas	Infestation of tissues of live animals by dipterous larvae is termed myiasis and is important in forensic terms because it can sometimes be associated with neglect of humans or animals
From a leech (Hirudinea)	Skin wound (usually not initially pruritic), blood loss Sometimes mechanical effects, e.g. obstruction of nares Leeches pierce the skin with their 'teeth' Following feeding the leech drops off but bleeding continues	Leeches tend to attach to certain parts of the body, e.g. nostrils or eyes and this may dictate their effect (Cooper, 1990c)
Sting from a fish (e.g. stingrays – Dasyatidae or scorpion fish – Scorpaenidae)	Venomous spines produce deep painful wounds	Stingray injuries heal poorly because of the venom (Fenner *et al.*, 1989) Other species, e.g. surgeon fishes (Acanthuridae) have sharp spines or bony plates that can cause incisions, but no poison is involved The spines of sea urchins (e.g. the Caribbean species *Diadema antillarum*) can have a similar effect and pieces of spine may remain embedded in the body for years (Symmers, 1984)
From a jellyfish (Scyphozoa) or colonial hydroid (e.g. Portuguese man-of-war, *Physalia physalis*)	Severe acute inflammation (often linear tentacle marks), sometimes systemic shock	Only a few species are dangerous Toxins are injected into the skin and may cause dermatonecrosis and cardiac damage

(Continued)

13

Table 2.2 *Continued.*

Insult	Features	Comments
		Williams *et al.* (1998) described the Pacific box jellyfish *Chironex fleckeri* as the 'world's most dangerous animal'
From a cone shell (Conidae Mollusca)	Acute inflammation, sometimes death	Eight species are considered lethal, others can cause painful stings (Strickland, 1991)
From a stinging coral (e.g. *Millepora* spp. – Anthozoa)	Painful, pruritic sting with local inflammation	Many toxic species, ubiquitous
From a wasp or bee (depends on species)	Anaphylaxis, including laryngeal oedema Systemic (e.g. renal) damage	Well-documented for the honey bee (*Apis mellifera*) and certain species of wasp (e.g. Vespidae)
From a scorpion (depends on species – buthid scorpions are particularly dangerous)	Painful sting with local inflammation Sometimes systemic effects	As with many other species, contact with a scorpion, even if it is not dangerous, may evoke a psychological effect that can complicate diagnosis and treatment
Surface exposure (skin, mucous membrane) to toxic or irritant products	Local inflammation, pain Sometimes systemic effects	Depends on product/species (see below)
– musk glands of certain mammals (e.g. ferret, skunk)	Strong nauseating smell	Smell persists, even on equipment and wrappings (if, say, a dead skunk is submitted for necropsy)
– scent glands of certain reptiles (e.g. *Natrix* snakes)	Also odiferous but less severe	May persist as for skunk, etc.
– parotoid glands of certain amphibians (e.g. *Bufo* toads)	Irritant to mucous membranes, eyes, etc. Can cause fatal systemic lesions	See Case Study 1, Appendix D and Bedford (1974)
– irritants (allergens) from larvae, sometimes other stages, of lepidopterous insects	Pruritus, swelling and inflammation Sometimes conjunctivitis Occasionally systemic signs	Urticating hairs are often responsible (Cooper, 1985a)
– poison (usually formic acid) from certain insects (e.g. *Formica* ants)	Pin-prick pain on skin, more severe on eyes or mucous membranes	May be combined with bites
– irritant haemolymph, e.g. from 'Nairobi eye fly' and other beetles	Marked skin and (especially) ocular pain and tissue damage	Only liberated if the insect is damaged or crushed: therefore swatting should be avoided when a beetle is on the body surface

threatened and tries to defend itself (see Chapter 6). Sometimes a human specifically encourages an animal to bite or sting someone, e.g. by urging a dog to attack, or by holding a ferret, 'pet' rodent or scorpion to the person's skin and taunting or frightening it so that it bites or injects poison.

All animal-inflicted injuries must be differentiated into those that occurred *ante mortem* and those that were caused *post mortem*. The latter are the result of predation, for example, by dogs and feral pigs on land or by fish and crabs in water (Shepherd, 2003; Williams *et al.*, 1998). Much has been published on *post-mortem* scavenging so as to aid differential diagnosis in respect of stranded marine mammals (Read and Murray, 2000). Animals of diverse species may mutilate and devour human bodies after death – either individual corpses, or in vast numbers as occurred after the 1994 genocide in Rwanda, when stray dogs roamed and marauded widely. *Post-mortem* predation is usually characterised by lack of inflammation or other reaction and it tends to be concentrated on exposed, unclothed areas in humans (see also Chapter 7).

Animals can cause damage or disturb humans in many other ways. Examples are given below:

- Physical damage to property, e.g. cattle knocking down fences, baboons destroying crops.
- Noise, e.g. barking dogs, guinea fowl making alarm calls.
- Smell, e.g. from a piggery or poultry house adjacent to residential dwellings.
- Allergens, e.g. sensitivity to animal derivatives, such as feathers, leading to allergic alveolitis (see Appendix C).
- Irrational fears, e.g. of spiders (arachnophobia) or cats (ailurophobia).

Sometimes attacks on humans by wild animals are seasonal (for example, during the breeding season when young are protected) or represent a change in behaviour (for example, attacks by gulls, which in some locations can reach epidemic proportions). Increasingly, in Africa in particular, attacks result from closer contact between humans and wildlife and the ensuing competition for land and resources (see also Chapter 5). It is easy for this situation to be dismissed as irrelevant by those living in industrialised countries, but for millions in rural communities in poorer parts of the world it is an everyday threat to health and livelihood. In Tanzania alone, with a population of only 32 million, there were 563 known deaths and many more injuries from lions over a 15-year period (Packer *et al.*, 2005). Rarely is there proper redress for such incidents.

Any attack or insult inflicted on a human by an animal may be claimed to have affected physical or mental health and attract the attention of personal injury lawyers or 'claims consultants', quite apart from any contraventions of criminal law.

ZOONOSES

Zoonoses are 'those diseases and infections that are naturally transmitted between vertebrate animals and humans' (definition based on World Health Organization [WHO] wording). Examples are given in Table 2.3. They are of considerable importance in forensic medicine. Occurrence or spread of a zoonosis may constitute a criminal act, especially if appropriate risk assessments have not been done (Walsh and Morgan, 2005) and may be grounds for civil action, insurance claims or allegations of veterinary negligence.

Zoonoses can be categorised in various ways but a practical approach, often appropriate to discussion in court, is to divide them into three groups:

(1) Those equally hazardous to humans and animals, e.g. rabies, anthrax.
(2) Those that only rarely or slightly impair animal health in general but which may cause serious disease in humans, e.g. brucellosis, hydatidosis, *Herpesvirus simiae* infection.
(3) Those responsible for serious epizootics (epidemics) in domestic or wild animals but rarely of great significance to humans, e.g. foot-and-mouth disease, Newcastle disease.

Infections that can be serious in both animals and humans may be subclinical in some species under certain circumstances, e.g. chlamydophilosis (ornithosis or psittacosis). This situation can engender much debate in legal cases.

Certain organisms, e.g. *Salmonella* bacteria, may be acquired by humans from various other species – including people! Some apparent zoonoses are acquired from the environment, not from animals, e.g. *Pseudomonas* bacteria contracted from water and soil.

Specific studies have been carried out on zoonotic risks presented by certain wildlife species when they come into contact with humans, e.g. marine mammals (Mazet *et al.*, 2004). There is extensive literature on diseases and organisms transmissible from fish, much of it in the public

Table 2.3 Some examples of zoonoses.

Species	Zoonosis
Farm livestock (cattle, sheep, goats, pigs)	Rabies
	Hydatidosis
	Salmonellosis
	Brucellosis
	Tuberculosis
	Leptospirosis
	Campylobacteriosis
	Anthrax
	Q fever
	Escherichia coli 0157 infection
Dogs	Rabies
	Ringworm
	Toxocariasis
	Leptospirosis
	Streptococcosis
	Leishmaniasis
Cats	Toxoplasmosis
	Pasteurellosis
	Cat-scratch fever
	Ringworm
Rodents	Lymphocytic choriomeningitis (LCM)
	Rat-bite fever
Monkeys and apes	Shigellosis
	Herpesvirus simiae (B virus) infection
Birds	Chlamydophilosis
	Yersiniosis
	Avian influenza
Reptiles	Salmonellosis
	Atypical mycobacteriosis
Fish	*Erysipelothrix insidiosa* infection
	Listeriosis
	Mycobacteriosis

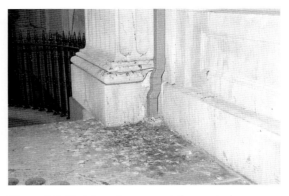

Figure 2.3 Bird droppings present dangers to humans, including slipping accidents and spread of pathogenic organisms.

Of increasing importance in the medical and the legal context are the 'new' zoonoses, some of which are also 'emerging' infections (Gibbs, 2005). These can be divided into two main groups:

(1) Zoonoses associated with novel exposure to unusual animals (e.g. primates, rodents) or animal products (e.g. meat, brain or spinal cord, heart valves). Examples are:
    (a) Ebola virus disease
    (b) Marburg disease
    (c) Spongiform encephalopathies.
(2) Zoonoses associated with immunodeficiency, the latter often due to HIV infection or clinical AIDS, malaria or other infectious diseases, neoplasia, irradiation, chemotherapy or splenectomy. Examples of these are:
    (a) Cryptosporidiosis
    (b) Toxoplasmosis
    (c) Giardiasis
    (d) Listeriosis
    (e) *Rochalimaea* infection
    (f) Atypical mycobacteriosis
    (g) Babesiosis
    (h) Aspergillosis.

Humans may contract zoonoses in various ways but the main routes of infection are:

- Ingestion.
- Inhalation.
- Penetration through mucous membranes or cornea.
- Bites or scratches.

health arena. Bites from some wild animals may be associated with religious or cultural traditions – for example, in Delhi, India, food is put out for macaques each Tuesday (the monkey god's day) and many people are bitten, requiring medical attention (Anon., 2005a). Faeces and other material from wild birds can present health hazards of both an infectious and a physical nature.

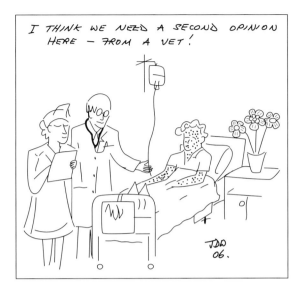

Close contact is often a prerequisite for spread of pathogens and for that reason legal cases concerning zoonoses usually relate to pets or other domesticated species where there is bonding between animal and owner. As Jonathan Swift put it: 'Perhaps we are so fond of one another because our ailments are the same.'

Transmissible spongiform encephalopathies have been recognised for a long time (centuries in the case of ovine scrapie) but have assumed increased importance recently since a 'new' disease, bovine spongiform encephalopathy (BSE), appeared first in the UK and later elsewhere (Wells and Wilesmith, 2004). The nature of BSE and other spongiform encephalopathies and their mode of transmission have stimulated much debate (Doherr, 2003) and there is evidence that new-variant Creutzfeldt-Jakob disease (nv-CJD) in humans may be linked with the consumption of BSE-infected food (European Commission, 2000).

Current thinking is that BSE and related diseases are transmitted by prions (Chesebro, 2003). These agents are extremely difficult to eliminate using standard chemical or physical sterilisation methods. From a forensic point of view, the spongiform encephalopathies present many challenges. Much remains unknown about their origins and pathogenicity and the dose of infectivity, incubation period and isolation of the infective agent are just a few of the critical areas that remain to be elucidated. The link between BSE and nv-CJD in humans is largely circumstantial. Nevertheless, the possible risks need to be recognised and, in any associated legal case, it is essential to involve veterinary and medical specialists with experience of these diseases.

Another recent concern has been the possible spread of methicillin-resistant *Staphylococcus aureus* (MRSA) from domestic animals to humans and *vice versa*. MRSA has been identified in several species, including dogs, horses and cats (Bender *et al.*, 2005; Shaw, 2004). Its control requires collaboration between medical and veterinary professions (Anon., 2005b). How the risk of infection is confronted is important from a legal point of view, even down to hand-washing procedures in veterinary practice (Gregory, 2005).

Collaboration in the study of zoonoses has been facilitated within the European Union by the establishment of Med-Vet-Net, a 'virtual institute' (Belcher and Newell, 2005) that should be of value to those involved in legal and other actions relating to infectious diseases.

BITES

The detection and investigation of wounds are discussed in more detail in Chapters 6 and 7. Here initial mention is made of the most common and potentially litigious form – bites from domestic dogs and cats. Morgan (2004) pointed out that most of the 20,000 patients presenting to British emergency departments with animal bites are children, and the animal usually involved is the (domestic) dog. Some significant features of dog and cat bites are given in Table 2.4 below.

Dog bites have been the subject of much discussion and debate and some research. A useful recent review is in the *European Journal of Companion Animal Practice* of October 2005, where three authors discuss, respectively, why dogs bite (Heath, 2005), dog bites in children (Lakestani *et al.*, 2005) and dog-bite prevention (de Keuster, 2005). Avoidance of cat and dog bites in a veterinary setting – for example, by labelling cages properly and using muzzles – was discussed by Drobatz and Smith (2003). The legal issues can be complex, especially

Table 2.4 Some features of dog and cat bites.

Dog	*Cat*
Much force – crushing injury	Relatively little force but penetrate deeply
Legs and gluteal region most commonly affected in adults; elsewhere in children, including face	Hands most commonly affected, joints frequently involved
Both aerobic and anaerobic bacteria may be introduced	Both aerobic and anaerobic bacteria may be introduced
Predominant organisms include *Staphylococcus intermedius, Pasteurella multocida, P. septica,* and anaerobes, e.g. *Bacteroides, Capnocytophaga canimorsus*	Predominant organisms include *Pasteurella multocida, P. septica,* staphylococci and anaerobes, e.g. *Bacteroides, Capnocytophaga canimorsus, Bartonella henselae* (cause of cat-scratch fever)

when a dog bites a veterinarian (Flemming, 2004).

Other animal species kept in captivity can also transmit pathogenic organisms in bites or by other means (see Table 2.5). Microbes transmitted by bites from wild animals are often similar to those from their domestic relatives – for instance, most large felids, such as tigers and cougars, harbour *P. multocida* – as do pet cats (Morgan, 1999).

Rabies is worthy of particular note. It can be transmitted by any mammal and birds are very occasionally infected. In the UK a bat or an illegally imported/inadequately vaccinated dog or cat is the most likely source; in other parts of the world 'sylvatic' rabies may predominate – for example in areas of southern Africa, where mongooses maintain the virus.

Bites, scratches and injuries are an important consideration when working with free-living, wild species (see Chapter 5).

Animal bites inflicted on humans are, *par excellence*, a field in which medical and veterinary professions should work together (Cooper, 1985b). The respective roles in a potential legal case are illustrated in Table 2.6, in the context of severe injuries to a child inflicted by a Rottweiler dog.

Interestingly, a few weeks after the compilation of the above, simultaneous editorials appeared in the *Veterinary Record* (Alder and Easton, 2005a) and the *British Medical Journal* (Alder and Easton, 2005b), promoting the concept of veterinary/medical collaboration and, in the former, giving as an example co-operative work on dog bites!

Animals also bite one another (see Chapters 5, 6 and 7) and such incidents may be grounds for a criminal or civil action if the victim is someone's property (see Chapter 3). Sometimes bites and injuries occur because of aggression between free-living animals – for instance, dolphins and porpoises (Ross and Wilson, 1996) – and these may need to be differentiated from potentially litigious anthropogenic injuries.

VETERINARY/MEDICAL COLLABORATION

The increasing emphasis on interdisciplinary studies was highlighted in simultaneous issues of the two journals above in November 2005. Topics covered included zoonoses, emerging diseases, antibiotic resistance and bioterrorism. As one of the November editorials put it (Anon., 2005c), 'the two issues give a sense of how doctors and vets are working together.' In legal cases such collaboration can prove very productive.

OTHER HEALTH AND SAFETY MATTERS

Many of the examples given above are part of the spectrum of health and safety that is now given so much emphasis in some countries. Other elements associated indirectly with animals may also attract the attention of the authorities and prompt legal action – for example, exposure of citizens to

Table 2.5 Infections from bites from species other than the dog and cat.

Species	Organism	Comments
Ferret	*Pasteurella multocida* *P. septica* *Salmonella* spp. *Mycobacterium* spp.	A carnivore, therefore oral flora often reflects food items
Rabbit	*P. multocida* *Salmonella* spp.	Rarely bite in captivity
Rat	*Streptobacillus moniliformis* *Salmonella* spp.	Rarely bite in captivity Urine and faeces may be source of infection to humans
Mouse	*S. moniliformis* Lymphocytic choriomeningitis virus (LCM) *Salmonella* spp.	As for rat but more inclined to bite (nip)
Golden (Syrian) hamster	LCM *Salmonella* spp.	Readily bite
Parrots and other birds	*Chlamydophila psittaci* *Salmonella* spp.	Parrots bite with their strong beaks, others peck
Reptiles	*Pseudomonas* *Aeromonas* Other Gram-negative organisms *Salmonella* spp.	Depends upon prey items (carnivores) and oral health of the reptile (Cooper, 1967)
Amphibians	As for reptiles	Rarely bite but organisms may be present in the water or environment
Fish	As for amphibians plus (e.g.) *Listeria* *Edwardsiella* *Erysipelothrix*	Some species bite (see Table 2.2) Otherwise as for amphibians
Invertebrates	*Plasmodium, Trypanosoma* and other protozoa *Salmonella* spp. and other bacteria Various viruses Some metazoan parasites, e.g. *Angiostrongylus cantonensis* (from molluscs)	Some organisms are transmitted mechanically, e.g. salmonellae in the gut of cockroaches In other cases invertebrate serves as a biological host (Cooper, 1986)

Table 2.6 A physician and veterinarian working together in the case of a child bitten by a Rottweiler dog.

Physician	Veterinarian
Examination and clinical care of the child	Restraint and examination of the dog
Swabbing bite wounds for microbiology	Swabbing dog's mouth for microbiology
Examination, description, photographing, possible casting of bite wounds	Examination, description, photographing, possible casting of dog's teeth
Reference to medical literature – case reports	Reference to veterinary literature – studies of oral flora and canine behaviour
Discussion and collation of joint report	

medicinal products or agricultural chemicals, including pesticides (see Chapter 6). The veterinary practice itself may be the source of injury or present a threat to humans for a variety of reasons, in addition to those brought about by direct contact with animals (Irwin, 2005). These can range from allergic reactions to rubber gloves through to exposure to toxic chemicals, including agents used for chemotherapy, and self-inoculation with vaccines containing live organisms or chemicals, especially Freund's adjuvant (Skilton and Thompson, 2005; Windsor *et al.*, 2005).

Increasingly, organisations where people work with animals produce questionnaires for their staff, asking about allergies and other medical matters, so that appropriate precautions can be taken. Many also provide cards or letters for employees, which, in the event of unexplained ill-health, can be presented to a medical practitioner explaining that the person works with animals and may therefore have contracted a zoonosis or encountered allergens or toxic substances.

VETERINARY FORENSIC MEDICINE AS A DISCIPLINE

As Chapter 1 explained, human forensic medicine remains a well-recognised and highly developed speciality despite some changes in its fortunes in recent years. For many decades, members of the medical profession in various countries have been able to undertake training, obtain post-graduate recognition, and find full-time employment in this field. However, there have been few comparable developments in veterinary medicine, and veterinarians who have become involved in forensic work have usually been self-taught or, in a few cases, attained a qualification aimed primarily at those in human medicine.

The absence of specialist training in veterinary forensic medicine is surprising considering that members of the profession have long played an important role as expert witnesses in court cases concerning animals. As legislation relating to animal welfare, conservation and allied subjects increases (see Chapter 3) and society becomes more litigious,

especially in Western countries, the demand for specialists in animal forensics is likely to grow and the gaps in education and training are likely to be gradually filled (see Chapter 13).

Confirmation that veterinary forensic medicine has not yet been recognised as a discipline in its own right is to be found in some of the major international lists of publications. For example, the National Library of Medicine (Bethesda, Maryland, USA) supported by the National Institutes of Health in the USA, has for many years included under its medical subject headings Forensic Anthropology, Forensic Dentistry, Forensic Medicine and Forensic Psychiatry. Even though the National Library publications include veterinary literature, the word 'forensics' does not feature there as such, and the reader wishing to search for publications relevant to that discipline must turn to 'legislation, veterinary'. A similar situation applies in *Index Veterinarius* (published since 1933) and the *Veterinary Bulletin* (1931), both produced by CABI Publishing, UK (see Appendix B), where 'forensics' does not appear but 'legislation' does.

Forensic organisations are often equally guilty of ignoring the veterinary field. For example, the 17th meeting of the International Association of Forensic Sciences in 2005 (www.iafs2005.com) hosted a magnificent programme in Hong Kong covering 27 themes ranging from clinical medicine to victims of torture and genocide. Veterinary forensic work was not mentioned, the nearest topic being 'Forensic Biology'. The American Association of Forensic Sciences (see Appendix B) lists archaeologists, nurses and radiologists amongst 25 specialist groups shown on its 2006 website but veterinarians are not included.

Until recently very little had been published specifically on forensic veterinary medicine although some texts furnished specific information on the provision of evidence in legal cases regarding domestic livestock (see, for example, Dabas and Saxena, 1994).

It is surprising that animals attract little attention in human forensic medical texts, except for cases in which they cause injury or death. For example, the 544-page tome by Schwär *et al.* (1988) contained a handful of allusions to animals (for instance, under 'Bestiality') and only two specific references to non-human species appeared in the index – to the mutilation of bodies by rats and dogs and to attacks by a 'dog, lion, baboon, fish or shark' (sic)! Nearly two decades later, a guide to the essentials of forensic science (White, 2004) did not include 'animal' or 'veterinary' in its eleven-page index, although a section on veterinary forensic science was included in a book produced by two lawyers in the same year (Townley and Ede, 2004).

The increasing prominence of veterinary forensic medicine in the courts and elsewhere was linked closely with the expansion of 'wildlife crime' (see Chapter 5). In the early 1980s, Robinson (1982) wrote of the role that could be played by appropriately motivated and experienced veterinarians in legal cases involving wild birds, and we developed much of our interest and early expertise working with him at that time (Figure 2.4). The importance of this and allied fields of work were then detailed in papers about veterinary forensic medicine directed primarily at members of the profession in Britain (Cooper and Cooper, 1986, 1991, 1997, 1998). Soon after, the UK's Forensic Science Service (see Appendix B) established a unit devoted to analysing animal DNA and at about the same time, numerous small laboratories, in the UK and elsewhere, began to develop and advertise an 'animal forensics' capability.

In the United States of America, the establishment by the United States Fish and Wildlife Service (USFWS) of a wildlife forensic laboratory resulted in provision of a service to wildlife law enforcement bodies and others (Stroud, 1995). At about the same time, Wobeser (1996) published valuable guidance on medicolegal necropsy of wildlife from a Canadian perspective.

Since then the important potential of the veterinarian in conservation cases has been acknowledged (see, for example, PAW, 2005) and an awareness has emerged of the need to have stronger input by the profession in legal cases relating to other fields concerning animals, such as welfare and abuse (Townley and Ede, 2004).

Although veterinary forensic work is similar in many respects to human forensic medicine, the focus is often different; welfare and conservation

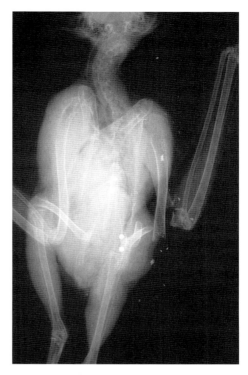

Figure 2.4 An early (1976) case concerning the fatal shooting of a peregrine falcon. Nowadays it is expected that radiographs will be properly labelled, including designation of 'left' and 'right'. At least two views of the bird would be investigated, with careful positioning to facilitate interpretation.

concerns usually predominate animal cases whereas the circumstances of death or incidents relating to drug abuse are more likely to be the focus of human forensic investigation (see Chapter 1).

WHAT IS COMPARATIVE FORENSIC MEDICINE?

If, as was suggested earlier, both 'veterinary' and 'comparative' forensics relate to legal cases and situations involving animals, are they not the same?

In this book we seek to distinguish the two, drawing attention to areas where they overlap but also to aspects that distinguish them. Throughout we have endeavoured to use the term 'veterinary' primarily in its classic sense – that is, relating to the health of domesticated animals (Latin *veterinarius*). It might be said, however, that the remit of the veterinarian has broadened enormously in recent years and now s/he may be consulted on species ranging from stick insects to simian primates. Nevertheless, the focus of the veterinarian's work, whether in practice, academia or research, remains the health and welfare of a handful of domesticated mammals and birds – a situation often reflected in legislation (see Chapter 3).

Forensic cases can, however, involve many species other than those that are domesticated. Wildlife crime alone is an example. Here those involved in obtaining evidence concerning (for instance) the killing or taking of protected species are dealing with wild (as opposed to domestic) animals that can be anything from brotulid fish or birdwing butterflies to herons or howler monkeys. Such species may or may not be the preserve of the veterinarian, in law or in practice. Legal cases concerning wildlife often involve a range of disciplines and certainly not just veterinarians – an important example of both interdisciplinary and 'comparative' forensic work.

Another reason for differentiating comparative forensic medicine is because it is a discipline in its own right. It is a branch of comparative medicine, which is essentially the bridge between studies on humans and other animals. Comparative medicine has long existed *de facto* on account of the earlier eclectic work and the writings of Greek, Roman, Arab and European scholars. The comparative approach is epitomised in Virchow's famous words: 'Between animal and human medicine there is no dividing line – nor should there be. The object is different but the experience obtained contributes the basis of all medicine.' In writing this, Virchow meant *all* animals, not just domestic livestock and familiar household pets.

Comparative medicine has long been recognised as a discipline in the UK. This is illustrated by the many published contributions by medical people to animal pathology, and by the recognition of veterinary surgeons and others working with diverse species by professional bodies like The Royal College of Pathologists and the Royal Society of

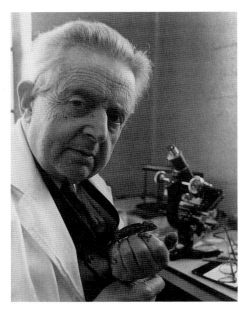

Figure 2.5 Dr. Edward Elkan, with microscope and live chameleon, who applied a forensic approach to his studies on the morbidity and mortality of lower vertebrates.

Medicine (RSM) (which has its own Section of Comparative Medicine). Lord Soulsby of Swaffham Prior recently served as the first qualified veterinarian President of the RSM.

A comparative approach means that one can learn from studies on different species and then apply the findings to taxa where specific information may be limited or lacking. Many biomedical mechanisms are essentially the same in different species. Where differences exist, they usually relate to specific aspects of the biology of the animals in question (Table 2.7). Thus, physiological and pathological changes in organs and tissues of a bird and a reptile diverge because the former is a 'warm-blooded' (endothermic) animal while the latter is 'cold-blooded' (ectothermic). Changes are likely to take place more rapidly in the former, which can maintain its own body temperature, than in the latter, which can only thermoregulate by behavioural means.

In this book, therefore, 'comparative forensic medicine' is defined as:

the discipline concerned with forensic studies on
different vertebrate and invertebrate species of
animals, including humans, and the application of
such work to the provision of scientific information
to assist in judicial and other processes.

How human, veterinary and comparative forensic
medicine relate to one another is depicted in
Figure 2.6.

It can be seen that 'comparative' forensic medicine encompasses areas of both human and

Table 2.7 Biological features of vertebrate and invertebrate animals which are of relevance to comparative forensic medicine.

Taxon	Significant biological features	Relevance to forensic studies
Mammals (Class Mammalia)	'Warm-blooded' (endothermic) Haired Lungs Produce live young Non-nucleated red blood cells Acute inflammatory cell is neutrophil	Predictable physiological and pharmacological responses Hair available for analysis and identification
Birds (Class Aves)	Warm-blooded (endothermic) Feathered Lungs Lay eggs Nucleated red blood cells Acute inflammatory cell is heterophil	Predictable physiological and pharmacological responses Feathers and eggs available for analysis and identification
Reptiles (Class Reptilia)	Cold-blooded (ectothermic) Ectodermal scales Lungs Lay eggs or produce live young Nucleated red blood cells Acute inflammatory cell is heterophil	Physiological and pharmacological responses are temperature-dependent Eggs, scales and shed skin available for analysis and identification
Amphibians (Class Amphibia)	Cold-blooded (ectothermic) Mucous skin Gills or lungs Lay eggs or produce live young Nucleated red blood cells Acute inflammatory cell is heterophil Partial dependence on water	Physiological and pharmacological responses are temperature-dependent Water samples can play a limited role in investigations, especially relating to health
Fish (three classes)	Cold-blooded (ectothermic) Mesodermal scales Gills or (a few species) 'lungs' Lay eggs or produce live young Almost total dependence on water Nucleated red blood cells Acute inflammatory cell is heterophil	Physiological and pharmacological responses are temperature-dependent Water samples can play a major role in investigations, especially relating to health
Invertebrates (many phyla and classes)	Vary greatly Some have tough exoskeletons, others are soft Gills or cutaneous diffusion of oxygen Some are terrestrial, some aquatic Blood cells, when present, are usually amoebocytes	Depends on the taxon Knowledge of the species' biology is vital in forensic investigations Millions of species exist, most still undescribed

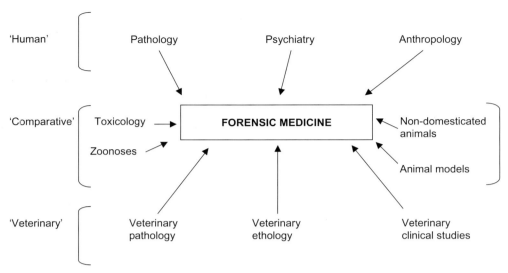

Figure 2.6 The components of forensic medicine.

veterinary work, where the investigative methods used are usually similar. It also includes various topics, e.g. zoonoses, where there is important overlap between those working with humans and animals. Finally, it introduces a broad approach to the Animal Kingdom, rather than focusing solely on the domesticated species and *Homo sapiens*.

ANIMAL MODELS

This implies the use in biomedical research of one species as a prototype for, or representation of, another. Advances in human forensic medicine are often hampered because of legal and ethical constraints on the performance of experimental work using humans. Studies on living people are, increasingly, contested and have to be limited in scope, following strict ethical guidelines. Human cadavers have been used for forensic research in the past – for example, on the effects of trauma (see Chapter 7) – but this too is becoming less accepted. One answer is to use live or dead animals.

The concept that we can learn about human beings by doing research on other animals is ancient. Greek, Roman and Arab scholars observed and manipulated living organisms in a broad-based way, seeking to discover how the vertebrate body

functioned and why disease occurred. The underlying rationale for this was perhaps best encapsulated by Charles Darwin in his book *The Descent of Man*:

> *Man with all his noble qualities, with sympathy that feels for the most debased, with benevolence which extends not only to other men but to the humblest living creature, with his god-like intellect which has penetrated into the movements and constitution of the solar system – with all these exalted powers – still bears in his bodily frame the indelible stamp of his lowly origin.*

The even broader approach of some researchers was reflected in the words, 80 years ago, of Sir Arthur Keith, himself medically-trained but with broad comparative interests, in an obituary of a friend and colleague:

> *For Professor Shattock, as for [John] Hunter, the healing of a wound of a plant and the healing of a wound of a human body were but variations of the same process. The manifestation of malignant growth, whether in animal or vegetable tissues, he investigated as if they were the varying aspects of a single problem.*

The study of the anatomy, pathology and diseases of vertebrate and invertebrate animals has contributed immeasurably to the health and welfare of humans – and indeed to other species. Most educated and informed people accept some such usage, so long as the work is carried out in accordance with the law and codes of practice and follows a proper cost:benefit analysis. In some quarters, however, there remains strong opposition to all research using live animals (see Chapters 3 and 4).

There are two types of animal model that can contribute to forensic medicine – 'natural' and 'induced'. Each will be discussed briefly.

Natural models

Both live and dead animals already serve as natural models in various fields of forensic science. This means that without any intentional (or, in the case of live animals, damaging or painful) manipulation or intervention, such animals can provide answers to questions about pathological and other processes or clarify the circumstances of an incident that is of legal significance.

Sometimes animals serve as natural models or 'sentinels', by default. An example is when animals are present in a building and a fire or other incident occurs. In one such case, large numbers of common starlings were killed in an explosion and their carcases were badly damaged (Figure 2.7).

Forensic examination of these birds, including histological investigation of respiratory tracts, pro-

vided valuable information about the accident and the chemicals that might have caused it. The use of birds as environmental sentinels is not new: many decades ago caged canaries were taken down into coal mines to detect traces of toxic gas dangerous to miners. Smoke inhalation injury is not uncommon in captive birds and presents therapeutic challenges for veterinarians. It and other syndromes can provide information about the environment or specific circumstances relevant to human health – for instance, exposure to 'second-hand smoke' from tobacco (Cray *et al.*, 2005).

Another example of environmental monitoring involving animals concerns anthracosis, the deposition of carbon in the respiratory tract and associated lymph nodes. This is well-documented in humans but also recognised in dogs, cats and other animals that live in urban environments and inhale polluted air (see Chapter 7).

Such animals can serve as sentinels for humans and are therefore valuable in forensic investigation

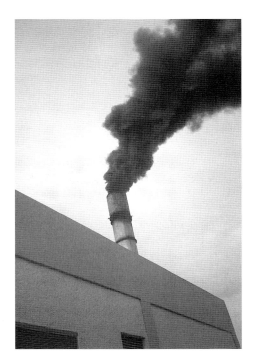

Figure 2.8 Health hazards associated with environmental pollution – in this case, a faulty incinerator – are increasingly a cause of litigation.

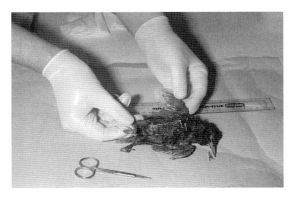

Figure 2.7 One of a number of common starlings killed in an explosion. This figure also appears in colour in the colour plate section.

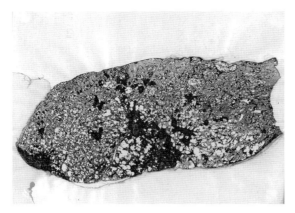

Figure 2.9 Section of the lung of a man who was a coal miner for many years: black deposits of carbon (anthracosis) are present.

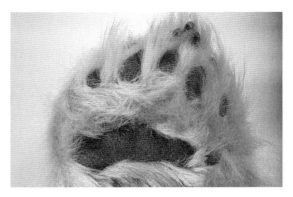

Figure 2.11 The surface of a polar bear's foot showing well-keratinised pads.

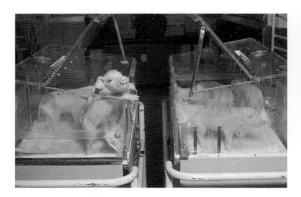

Figure 2.10 Piglets used as natural models to study health problems associated with 'light-for-dates' babies.

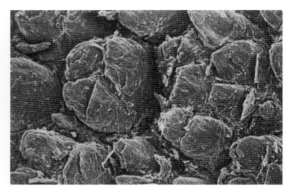

Figure 2.12 A low-power scanning electronmicrogram (SEM) of part of a polar bear's pad, showing the raised papillae that increase the coefficient of friction and thus minimise slipping on ice.

and in research (Breeze and Wheeldon, 1979). The finding of anthracosis in marine mammals (Rawson *et al.*, 1991) suggests that these animals too may be able to provide information relevant to environmental health and applicable to some forensic cases.

Many natural animal models contribute to forensic medicine because their anatomy and physiology provide information applicable to human safety. For instance, piglets have been used to study post-natal development and the particular problems faced by human 'light-for-dates' babies (Figure 2.10).

So-called 'slip and trip hazards' are an important cause of ill-health and death, prompting sick leave, legal investigations and insurance claims. They occur even in veterinary practices (Irwin, 2005).

Studies on the specialised structures of the feet of polar bears (Manning *et al.*, 1985) and bighorn sheep (Manning *et al.*, 1990) have provided insights into why slipping accidents occur and how best to prevent them (Figures 2.11 and 2.12).

The foregoing relates to live animals as natural models. Dead animals have also been used to study mechanisms pertinent to forensic medicine, an example being the use of carrion rather than human cadavers for studying 'faunal succession' associated with decay (Smith, 1986).

Animal bones have long been the subject of research on skeletal damage in forensic medicine (see Chapter 7) and studied by palaeontologists interested in the lives of early humans. The late

Louis Leakey, living and working in East Africa, often tested his hypotheses by exposing animal bones to the types of insult that might have caused *ante-mortem* or *post-mortem* damage to the skeletons of early humans or australopithecines. He also investigated and verified the efficacy of ancient stone implements by fashioning and using them to skin a gazelle or to cut and carve wood.

Induced animal models

Here the animal is *manipulated* in some way beforehand, rather than being studied in its naturally occurring state as outlined above.

It is possible to render an animal more suitable for studies of disease or certain normal and abnormal physiological or metabolic processes by various methods, including:

- Splenectomy or thymectomy to reduce the animal's resistance to infectious agents.
- Administration of a drug to cause specific tissue damage (e.g. destruction of pancreatic islet cells to induce diabetes mellitus).
- Implantation or transplantation of foreign material to elicit a local or systemic reaction.
- Wounding in various ways, in order to study tissue responses.

Many such 'induced' animal models play an important role in medical research and the findings may also be relevant to forensic studies.

Live animals were used routinely to test medical hypotheses in the 18th and 19th centuries. For example, the great John Hunter (1728–93), despite having a strong affinity with his own pet animals, used dogs and other species to investigate the effects of poisons, with a view to applying some of what he learnt to humans.

More recently, animals have been employed for forensic research in a number of fields – for instance, studies on vehicular accidents and shootings, where pigs and dogs (usually anaesthetised) have been used (Adams *et al.*, 1983). A wide range of laboratory species have contributed to research on wounds and wound-healing (Bucknall and Ellis, 1984). Animal models have also played a critical role in our understanding of traumatic brain injury (Finnie

and Blumbergs, 2002). All of the above are very relevant to legal and insurance cases. The use of genetically-modified (GM) animals has created new possibilities for study of disease processes and for the production of antibodies, antigens, hormones, and other substances; some of this work provides information that is also of forensic significance.

The public reaction to the use of live animals in research – and, indeed, whether or not a particular procedure is even permitted in law – differs from country to country (see Chapter 3). As in all forms of 'exploitation' of animals, it attracts strong opposition in some circles (see Chapter 4).

Whatever one's personal views about research on live animals, there can be no doubt that it has contributed substantially to forensic medicine and is likely to continue to do so. There is another positive aspect. Laboratory animals have often provided the template and stimulus for development of standards and guidelines that ultimately benefit other species – the recognition and assessment of pain and distress being an important example (Morton and Griffiths, 1985) (see Chapter 4).

BIOSECURITY

Biosecurity has always involved both the medical and veterinary professions, but in recent years various factors, including public health scares and concerns over international terrorism (Durrant, 2002), have prompted a far greater interdisciplinary approach to the exclusion of unwanted organisms. In legal cases and official enquiries and insurance claims concerning biosecurity, the experts are likely to come from various disciplines but most will have a 'comparative' background and orientation.

THE INTERDISCIPLINARY NATURE OF COMPARATIVE FORENSIC MEDICINE

The broad definition of the term 'comparative forensic medicine' means that it will embrace certain disciplines which are, *sensu stricto*, not constituents of veterinary medicine but whose expertise is relevant to it. A comprehensive review of the many

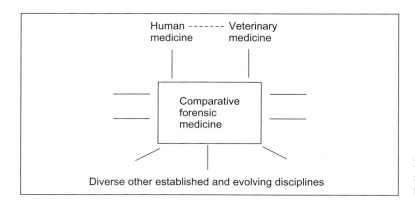

Figure 2.13 Comparative forensic medicine may provide a bridge between disciplines.

specialities that are part of contemporary forensic work is to be found in Townley and Ede (2004).

This expanding role of different scientific specialities in legal and other cases involving animals is reflected by the fact that a number of professional bodies now produce guidance to their members about appearing in court or serving as expert witnesses (see, for example, the Institute of Biology, 2004). Comparative forensic medicine may therefore provide a bridge between human and veterinary medicine and numerous other, non-medical disciplines, as depicted in Figure 2.13.

There are various biological disciplines that can contribute to human and veterinary forensic studies and thus constitute part of the spectrum of comparative forensic medicine (Gunn, 2006). Some examples are discussed briefly below.

Forensic entomology

Forensic entomology is the study of insect fauna and their relationship to legal cases. It is particularly relevant to the determination of time of death where the presence of larvae, especially maggots, can provide unique information. In a broader sense, forensic entomology includes investigation of invertebrates other than insects that may be relevant to a crime scene (see Chapter 7). It is applicable to forensic work involving any species of animal.

Forensic botany

Forensic botany, a subject in itself, is also relevant to veterinary and forensic medicine. DNA technol-

ogy, plant morphology and ecology are important aspects that contribute to forensic investigation. The recognition and identification of pollen, seeds, diatoms, flowers and plant fibres sometimes play a unique part in providing 'trace' evidence in veterinary and comparative studies.

Palaeopathology

This term refers to the study of disease in early human and animal remains (see also Chapter 7) and is a field in which there was a substantial input by veterinarians some decades ago (Baker and Brothwell, 1980; Harcourt, 1971). Palaeopathology is not usually concerned with the law because of the antiquity of the material being examined but, with a broadening of definitions (see below), it can be considered part of the spectrum of modern forensic science. It is particularly important in comparative forensic medicine because of its contributions to our understanding of skeletal pathology (see Chapter 7).

Studies on health and biodiversity

The need for a comparative approach to investigation of diseases of humans and other species has assumed increased importance in recent years and was given additional momentum by the First International Conference on Health and Biodiversity in Galway, Ireland, in August 2005. Many of the papers demonstrated links between emergence of disease and reduction in biodiversity and the need when studying such relationships to employ forensic

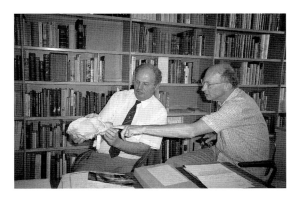

Figure 2.14 A veterinarian and a zoologist discuss the anatomical and pathological features of a gorilla skull.

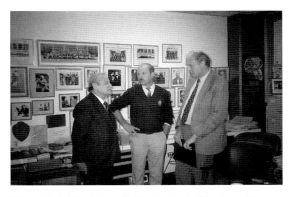

Figure 2.15 Professor Philip Tobias (left), the eminent palaeontologist, discusses the study of bones.

methods. This approach can be considered part of the new field of 'environmental forensics' (Morrison, 1999) and an important contribution to comparative forensic medicine.

THE IMPORTANCE OF COMPARATIVE FORENSIC MEDICINE

Who stands to benefit from the comparative approach to forensic medicine advocated here? The answer is: many people and many disciplines. First and foremost, forensic science as a subject is likely to be strengthened by a comparative approach, and the quality of evidence should thus be improved. Second, those already working in different forensic fields will gain from the input of persons trained and experienced in medicine and biology related to diverse species. Gone will be the days when the local physician or veterinary practitioner is asked to give an opinion on some animal-related topic of which s/he has only very limited knowledge. The courts, police, enforcement agencies and others will have access to people with a truly comprehensive approach to the subject.

A BROADENING OF THE TERM 'FORENSICS'

The foregoing text has concentrated on conventional forensic medicine, viz. that concerned with matters of law.

The traditional restrictiveness of the term 'forensics' is illustrated by reference to standard dictionaries and specialised volumes that define medical and veterinary terms. Thus *Baillière's Comprehensive Veterinary Dictionary* (Blood and Studdert, 1988) gave as a definition of forensic: 'pertaining to or applied in legal proceedings in courts of law' and such restricted usage continues in most human medical texts, such as Dorland's *Illustrated Medical Dictionary* (2000), where the meaning is 'pertaining or applied to legal proceedings'.

However, as pointed out in the Preface, the term 'forensics' is now frequently used in a much broader sense in the general community. Examples of fields of investigation where the term 'forensics' or 'a forensic approach' has been applied in publications, reports, lectures and interviews in recent years include:

- Archaeological 'digs', especially the detailed examination of human artefacts and the investigation of remains of domesticated animals which early humans kept or used.
- Palaeontological research.
- Analysis of the circumstances of death of historical figures, such as Nelson and Napoleon.
- Studies on skeletal lesions in endangered apes, such as the mountain gorilla.
- Investigation of oil spills and associated environmental changes, e.g. coral reef destruction or decline.

- Research on declining species, including the possible role of the fungal disease, chytridiomycosis, as a cause of mortality of amphibians.
- Collection of museum material for DNA studies on, for example, Indian Ocean kestrels and other Mascarene species.

In his Foreword to the fascinating book *Secrets of the Dead* (Miller, 2000), Chambers discusses the broadening of this definition and declared:

> *Using forensic evidence to shed light on history is a new science. So new, in fact, it hasn't yet got a name.*

In the introduction to this text, Miller expands on this concept and says that

> *applying the description 'forensic' to any activity nowadays is to risk an accusation of cliché-mongering. The term is widely abused, so it should be said that in the context of this book, 'forensic' is used in the sense of 'suitable or analogous to pleading in court.'*

There is little doubt that the use and understanding of the term 'forensics' is changing fast, as exemplified in a recent obituary to Robin Cook, former British Foreign Secretary, described as a 'brilliant coruscating debater whose most devastating performances combined lofty ridicule and forensic analysis in equal measure' (Wilson, 2005).

SPECIALISED AREAS OF ANIMAL FORENSICS

Although this book is intended to provide an overall introduction to animal forensics, it should be clear to the reader that the subject is large, covering the whole Animal Kingdom, and that some of its aspects are best dealt with by other experts in their own fields, as well as by veterinarians. Thus, cases relating to whales or dolphins, such as allegations of boat or firearm damage, must involve cetologists and others who have experience of marine mammals. Similarly, investigations relating to reptiles and amphibians should include herpetologists and, where birds of prey are involved, the experts should embrace people with specific knowledge of raptors.

However, even those cases that ultimately require specialist opinion usually start with persons who are present or summoned at the time, who may have only limited knowledge of the species or situation. This is why a *methodical* approach is so essential. Even without specialist knowledge, a veterinarian or similarly qualified individual who is familiar with the legal process can (and, indeed, may *have* to) initiate the all-important first steps, such as securing the crime scene, describing the animal and starting contemporaneous notes (see Chapter 9). Specialists who are then called in can perform their work confident in the knowledge that the preliminaries have been carried out properly. An example would be when a whale or dolphin is found stranded, alive or dead, and 'foul play', such as net-entanglement or a collision with a boat, is suspected. It may be hours before experts arrive, especially if they come from another country, during which time the all-important preliminary investigations must commence.

CONVENTIONAL VETERINARY FORENSIC MEDICINE

The veterinarian has traditionally become involved in a legal case in several ways: as a 'witness of fact', a 'professional witness' or an 'expert witness' (see Chapter 12). A fourth role that may be linked with serving as an expert witness has emerged recently: here the veterinarian is asked to assist an individual or organisation that is prosecuting or defending a case in court and needs technical input.

It cannot be over-emphasised that some knowledge of forensic medicine – and where to obtain necessary information – is important to all veterinarians or others who work with animals, as even the most innocuous situation can become a criminal prosecution, a civil action, a professional disciplinary hearing or an insurance claim (see later) in which that individual may be asked to give evidence. In some fields, e.g. analysis of natural and intentional incidents of infectious disease, the veterinary investigation is likely both to use forensic methods and to be asked to produce a report that may be used in court (McEwan *et al.*, 2006).

What does involvement in conventional veterinary forensic medicine usually entail? Forbes (2004) defined 'forensic veterinarians' as:

> *. . . registered veterinary practitioners who have a particular knowledge and experience of a field of veterinary science, the recovery of forensic samples and, if appropriate, the provision of opinion, preparation of evidence for court or the giving of oral or written evidence based on that opinion.*

Some might disagree with this description, arguing with (for example) the premise that any form of 'registration' is necessary, but the role and responsibilities that Forbes outlines are essentially true for a veterinary expert witness.

There are four main areas in which veterinarians may become involved as an expert witness:

(1) Assessment of welfare (pain, discomfort or distress), including provision of an opinion as to whether an animal may be 'suffering' or has 'suffered' in the past. This is a complex field (see Chapter 5).
(2) Determination of the cause, time and circumstances of death of an animal, together with associated investigations such as recognition and interpretation of changes in tissues, detection of poisons and identification of parasites (see Chapters 7 and 8).
(3) Verification of the origin (provenance) and history of live or dead animals and their derivatives. Some such cases relate to domestic species but others fall into the category of possible 'wildlife crime' (see Chapter 5), where the legal case may rest on whether conservation legislation has been breached. On a global scale, there has been an increased involvement in this field by the veterinary profession, including knowledgeable or experienced practitioners, particularly regarding international legislation, such as the Convention on International Trade in Endangered Species of Wild Fauna and Flora (CITES) (see Chapter 3).
(4) Carrying out clinical examinations and sometimes necropsies when abuse of animals and violence to humans appear to be linked (see Chapter 6).

To these, Forbes (2004) would add:

- Food safety – ranging from welfare at slaughter to meat inspection standards.
- Human welfare – zoonoses and personal injury cases (kicks, bites, etc.).
- Miscellaneous cases relating to liability, negligence, nuisance, fraud, environmental pollution and damage (in the UK and certain other countries) to Crown property, such as Queen Elizabeth's swans.

Negligence is a subject in its own right and is discussed in a clinical context in Chapter 6.

The veterinary profession is playing an increasingly important and recognised role in legal cases and other hearings. Forbes (2004) emphasised that it was no longer true that a local veterinary practitioner appearing as a witness would have his evidence accepted with little disagreement, merely because of his standing in the community: 'nowadays, expert witness work has become a science.' Specialised forensic investigations are likely to be the remit of the pathologist, the toxicologist and other specialists (see relevant chapters in this book), even though the preliminary examination of live or dead animals and instigation of supporting tests will probably long remain the province of the practising veterinarian.

How might a veterinary surgeon become involved in forensic work? There are four main scenarios, as shown in Table 2.8.

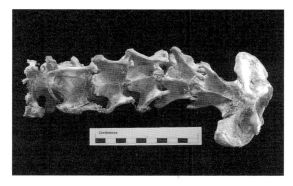

Figure 2.16 A veterinary practitioner should be able to assist when bones of domestic animals are found and need to be identified. (Courtesy of Richard Spence.)

Table 2.8 Categories of involvement in forensic work.

Category	Comments
Occasional participation in cases, routine examination of animals, preparation of reports, sporadic appearance in lower courts	Essentially a 'practitioner' with much day-to-day knowledge but likely to be lacking experience, and possibly confidence, insofar as report writing and court work are concerned
More specialised involvement relating to particular types of case, in-depth examination of animals, frequent preparation of reports, occasional but regular appearance in courts	Has a practical base but regularly exposed to the legal process Perhaps the optimal situation
Full-time forensic work or consultancy	Provides extensive experience of investigation and court work but leaves little or no time for day-to-day contact with the practice of the discipline
Academic forensic work – teaching/writing	An excellent base for the preparation of detailed or specialised reports (library facilities, etc.) May or may not provide opportunities for practice

Forbes (2004) warned of implications for veterinary practices becoming involved in forensic work and in particular:

- The advisability of using permanent staff for forensic duties, because court attendance may be required in 6–18 months' time.
- The need for back-up arrangements for court appearances or urgent forensic investigations; the work can cause disruption and hearings may be cancelled at short notice.
- The importance of avoiding conflicts of interest, as when a client, friend or relative is involved.

Participation in forensic veterinary work can be challenging and enjoyable. But it is not for the overly-cautious or faint-hearted. It can involve distressing incidents relating to the health or well-being of humans and animals and may sometimes even prove hazardous through exposure to physical injury, infectious agents and dangerous animals or humans. Then there are the emotional aspects – not only when giving evidence that may culminate in the loss of someone's liberty or livelihood, but also because many cases involve pain, stress, suffering, clinical disease or death in humans and animals. Moreover, the adversarial nature of criminal and of civil hearings, where the object can be to discredit the other side's expert witness, often

proves a devastating experience to the unprepared (see Chapter 12).

RELATED FIELDS OF ACTIVITY

As emphasised here and in Chapter 1, forensic veterinary investigations and provision of expert opinion can be applicable in criminal legal cases and also in various other circumstances, including:

- Civil actions.
- Inquests.
- Malpractice hearings.
- Insurance claims.
- Industrial disputes.
- Environmental impact assessments.
- Governmental and other enquiries.
- Inspections of pet shops, boarding establishments, zoos, etc.
- Checks on trading standards.

The list is almost endless. In this age of 'transparency', more matters are open to review, contentious items are dealt with by arbitration, and individuals and organisations are inclined to appeal against decisions of governments and private bodies. Consequently, there is often a need for written statements and sometimes verbal evidence, and many other mechanisms involved in a legal action may come into play. In any animal-related matter, veterinarians and others may be asked to appear, or give advice, and they will need to exercise the same skills and cautions that they would use in a court of law.

Some of these aspects are discussed in detail elsewhere in the book but further clarification is given here.

In all types of work where expert advice or opinion is sought, it is vital to ensure that one has clear written instructions *before* starting and a contractual agreement to ensure that a fee is paid.

Civil actions

The civil courts deal with allegations, for example, of negligence, trespass and nuisance. These provide remedies for damage to person or property (see Chapter 3) and must be distinguished from the role of regulatory (professional) bodies (see below). However, 'recklessness' in a case of negligence can result in a charge of misconduct.

Inquests

Inquests into human deaths may have an 'animal' component, as when a dog, shark or crocodile is alleged to have killed the victim. A report from a suitably experienced veterinary pathologist or (e.g.) animal behaviourist may form part of the proceedings in such cases.

Malpractice

The establishment and maintenance of standards has long been a hallmark of professional bodies. An indication of the antiquity of such practices in Europe is to be found in the 'Seal of Clause' of the Royal College of Surgeons of Edinburgh, 1505, where it states:

> *. . . that no manner of person occupy or practise any points of our said craft of surgery . . . unless he be worthy and expert in all points belonging to the said craft, diligently and expertly examined and admitted by the Masters of the said craft and that he know Anatomy and the*

> *nature and complexion of every member of the human body . . . for every man ocht to know the nature and substance of everything that he works or else he is negligent.*

Professional bodies, whether veterinary, medical, dental or otherwise, have an important, but limited, regulatory responsibility. To investigate and enforce their role in maintaining standards, each has a disciplinary committee, for example, the Disciplinary Committee of the Royal College of Veterinary Surgeons (RCVS) in the UK (see Appendix B). To support this role, the RCVS produces a *Guide to Professional Conduct* (GPC) which outlines the responsibilities of veterinary surgeons (veterinarians) towards their patients, the public and professional colleagues. In becoming a Member of the RCVS, and so being admitted to the veterinary profession, graduates make a declaration that his/her 'constant endeavour will be to ensure the welfare of the animals committed to [his/her] care' (see Chapter 4).

The authority of a professional body is usually restricted. In the case of the RCVS, the following is the situation as described in the GPC:

Jurisdiction of the RCVS
Under the Veterinary Surgeons Act 1966 the RCVS has authority to deal with three types of case:

(a) fraudulent registration
(b) criminal convictions
(c) allegations of disgraceful professional conduct

A disciplinary committee can have a judicial status and is therefore expected to follow certain standards. A recent update of the GPC reminded RCVS members of this:

The Disciplinary Committee – revised paragraph 2

(2) The Disciplinary Committee is a properly constituted judicial tribunal and must comply with the Veterinary Surgeons and Veterinary Practitioners (Disciplinary Committee) (Procedure and Evidence) Rules 2004 which provides that 'any charge which may result in a direction by

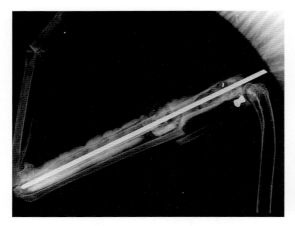

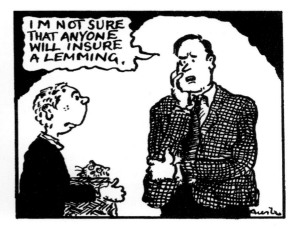

Figure 2.17 Legal and malpractice cases often relate to the quality of veterinary diagnosis and treatment. In this case a shot bird had its wing pinned but an osteitis supervened.

> the Committee that a respondent be removed from the register, shall be proved so that the Committee is satisfied to the highest civil standard of proof, so that it is sure.'

Allegations of professional malpractice are usually based on:

• Breach of the duty of care.
• Failure to practise to the standard expected of a competent veterinarian.
• Consequent damage.

Insurance

Insurance is important in veterinary and other animal work because:

(1) The expert may become involved in cases where an insurance claim is made or disputed and a professional opinion is needed. Relatively little has been published on how a veterinarian should approach an insurance case, but Dabas and Saxena (1994) provided valuable advice on the background to livestock insurance in India, and how necropsies should be performed, emphasising the particular difficulties of such work in remote areas.

(2) In countries where 'pet insurance' is prevalent, legislation dictates how consumers are given advice about insurance and insists on safeguards if things go wrong. For example, new regulations came into force in the UK in 2005 and a few veterinary practices are now 'authorised' to provide advice on insurance by the Financial Services Authority, which is, essentially, a quality-control scheme. King (2005) discussed this in some detail, and, interestingly, emphasised the importance of keeping records ('whatever you do, make sure that there is a paper trail to support your case') – an essential requirement in the practice of forensic veterinary medicine.

(3) Dogs and cats are not the only animals insured for veterinary treatment: policies are available for species as diverse as ponies and parrots. Claims inevitably involve veterinarians and the terms of the policy often need explanation and discussion. For example, equine insurance usually covers different risks:
   (a) 'Perils' (fire, lightning, accidents during transportation)
   (b) 'Mortality' (life-threatening conditions, e.g. colic)
   (c) 'Use' (loss during racing, breeding, etc.)
   (d) The owner's veterinarian has a responsibility to advise him/her to inform the insurance company of any necessary pro-

cedures that need to be undertaken, such as administration of anaesthesia or performance of surgery that may be relevant to the policy.

(4) Insurance companies use experts, including members of the veterinary profession, when drawing up policies and considering claims. Insurance databases are of considerable value. For example, most horses are insured for veterinary medical care in Sweden, and information stored by insurance companies is used to study the occurrence of equine diseases (Penell *et al.*, 2005).

(5) Practising veterinarians are usually themselves insured. The importance of this in the present, highly litigious, society cannot be overemphasised. In the UK the reports, advice and warnings of the Veterinary Defence Society (see Appendix B) are a sombre reminder of the necessity of appropriate insurance. In that country and certain others, it is a professional requirement that veterinary surgeons are adequately insured. These policies usually automatically cover criminal and disciplinary proceedings and human injury but the indemnity limit for clinical negligence will depend upon the circumstances and wishes of the individual veterinarian.

Industrial disputes

These can occasionally involve animals or animal-related concerns, e.g. alleged exposure to zoonoses or allergens, and evidence may be sought from veterinarians or others with appropriate knowledge. For example, it is not uncommon for veterinary surgeons to be consulted about the potential for adverse reactions to agricultural chemicals. A common problem in such cases is that, by the time an inquiry or litigation has started, it is too late to obtain samples because they have been used or destroyed. Expert opinion is then limited to the damage that *might* have been caused.

The production of reports and the provision of expert advice in these cases demand standards that are just as high as conventional, court-orientated, forensic work.

Environmental risk assessments

These are discussed in Chapter 5.

Governmental and other inquiries

In most countries, governments at various levels (central, local, federal, state/provincial) hold inquiries into matters of public concern. Sometimes these anticipate an action being taken but more often they follow an incident that warrants analysis. Essentially an inquiry is an investigation into one or more problem(s) or event(s). It has specific Terms of Reference and may have a special title (in the UK, a 'Royal Commission on . . .'). In most inquiries the public can submit their own views and the Committee or Commissioners may also request submission from organisations or specialists in different fields. Although a Commission of Inquiry is neither a criminal trial nor a civil action to determine liability, the standard rules still apply in relation to collation of material, preparation of reports, production of specimens or 'evidence', when appropriate, and maintenance of high standards of integrity.

Inspections

Inspections have long been a part of enforcing legislation relating to captive animals (see Chapter 3). The inspection and the inspector are usually authorised under national or local legislation. Davies (1989) described the work in the UK of 'the veterinary surgeon as a law enforcement officer' and drew attention to the professional demands of such work. Inspections usually entail the production of reports; these may be available to the public and media, as well as to the persons for whom they were intended. There may be an appeal if, for example, a licence is not granted as a result of an inspection. High standards are expected of an inspector and reports should be based on sound evidence that can be substantiated, supplemented by professional opinion where this is permitted.

Inspections bring with them responsibilities relating to such matters as the health and safety of humans and disease prevention in animals. At the time of writing (January 2006), DEFRA in the UK has introduced 'Biosafety/Security Procedures' for those carrying out inspections of premises and captive wild animals under the Wildlife and Countryside Act. Although aimed at preventing the spread of highly pathogenic avian influenza (HPAI), it is a reminder of the responsibilities and vulnerability of those authorised to carry out inspections on behalf of government or other bodies (Kirk, 2000).

Trading standards

The role of the expert in this respect was discussed by Durnford (2005).

THE POSSIBLE SEQUENCE OF EVENTS

It is not always obvious in advance that a situation will lead to legal or disciplinary action, or to an insurance claim. Sometimes this is apparent from the start, as when an animal is presented by a Police Officer or animal welfare inspector requesting that a detailed examination be carried out. However, this is only the tip of a large iceberg: as Table 2.9 shows, there are various levels at which the possibility of 'legal' action arises and the veterinarian should be suitably prepared.

Ideally, examination of all animals, alive or dead, should be performed in such a way that the chain of custody (see Appendix C and later) and the records retained would prove adequate if a court case were to ensue. Although this is often not realistic in practice, the veterinarian should always consider possible legal/malpractice/insurance implications and adhere as closely as possible to the rules and advice that are likely to minimise the risk of being found wanting. In many instances, subtle clues or a sixth sense will prompt feelings of unease, so that appropriate measures can be introduced, as indicated above.

WORKING WITH OTHER DISCIPLINES

As declared earlier, forensic science is an interdisciplinary subject, *par excellence,* and this will be emphasised repeatedly in this book. Working with people from other backgrounds is often the key to fruitful investigation and production of sound evidence. Such collaboration does not simply happen, however, but needs to be nurtured. In animal forensics, where the support framework available to medical pathologists rarely exists, it is essential to create and foster appropriate contacts.

Examples of disciplines that can directly help the forensic veterinarian are human medicine, dentistry,

Table 2.9 Levels of preparedness.

Situation	Comments
Direct request for a statement for a legal action or other claim	Institute immediately all necessary safeguards, including highest level of record-keeping, chain of custody and retention of evidence
	Explain and discuss with all staff and others to whom samples are likely to be sent
Suggestion or suspicion of possible legal action or other claim	Initiate medium level of record-keeping and chain of custody
	Alert all staff and others (as above)
The veterinarian is uneasy about some aspects of a patient's treatment or progress, or the client's attitude	As above
No apparent likelihood of a legal action or other claim	Existing record-keeping and chain of custody should be adequate

zoology, botany and animal ethology. Archaeologists and palaeontologists are increasingly contributing to our understanding of animal health, both prehistoric and historic (Murphy, E.M., 2005). Veterinary practitioners should forge links with individuals with skills in these and other subjects in the local community. A practising doctor or dentist in the locality may not have, or claim, particular knowledge of forensics but could still give advice or put the veterinarian in touch with someone in their discipline who is more experienced. A secondary school, college or university should be able to provide a biologist and local natural history societies may well harbour persons knowledgeable in botany, entomology, geology and other fields of natural science.

VETERINARY INVOLVEMENT

The veterinary surgeon may be involved in a legal case in a variety of ways. In particular, input may be sought on one or more of the following:

- A clinical examination (see Chapter 6).
- A *post-mortem* examination (see Chapter 7).
- Laboratory investigations (see Chapter 8).
- A site visit (see Chapter 9).
- Viewing radiographs or other images.
- Examining histological sections or electron-micrographs.
- Giving advice based on reading reports or viewing photos or video recordings.

CASES INVOLVING DEATH AND BEREAVEMENT

As in human medicine, a death is often the trigger for an investigation that may lead to a legal case, disagreement over an insurance claim or allegations of professional malpractice. The death of an animal may be of forensic significance on the following grounds:

- Killed illegally – domestic or wild.
- Caused suffering – usually domestic.
- A pet – companionship and emotional connotations.

- An agricultural or working animal – financial value.
- An animal valuable for breeding, racing or hunting – financial value.

In poor communities in the 'developing world', the loss of one animal such as a cow on which a whole family depends for milk, may be disastrous and prompt claims for compensation from government, officials or a neighbour. In some places, the animal's death may even initiate a revenge attack (see Figure 4.9). On the other hand, such incidents may be resolved through negotiations based on a strong community structure.

It is not only when a pet animal dies that there may be profound psychological effects on human beings. Some farmers who had livestock slaughtered in the UK's foot-and-mouth disease outbreak in 2001 committed suicide because they lost animals that had been an integral part of their lives for years. Surprisingly intense feelings can be shown by, for example, those who keep horses, breed guinea pigs, sell tropical fish or tend laboratory animals, even if these enterprises are essentially of a business nature (see also Chapter 4).

The whole question of dealing with the death of animals and its effects on people is not new but has become increasingly complex and has been studied in some detail in recent years (Lagoni *et al.*, 1994). A meeting in London (Anon., 2004) at the Royal Society of Medicine discussed this theme, emphasising the many parallels between bereavement involving humans and animals. The loss of an animal through death is a profound shock to many people, particularly in the western world, and the expert has to be aware of, and sensitive, to this.

The medical profession has recognised for some time a need for experts to be aware of different attitudes, some religious, towards suffering and death and to incorporate these into forensic work. A useful and thoughtful review was provided by Rutty (2001) who emphasised the need for medical pathologists, as part of the forensic team, to be cognisant of the feelings of people of different faiths – and those of none – and to make appropriate adjustments.

The situation with animals is generally different. A religious component is not usually a major consideration with animal death, perhaps in contrast to how live animals are treated (see Chapter 4). However, the need for all involved to be sensitive and aware of the feelings of owners remains the same. Redman (2005) discussed this from the viewpoint of a Christian lay minister with family veterinary connections and drew a number of parallels between the human and animal situation.

This is not to suggest that experts should be sentimental and thus risk the accusation of lack of objectivity in their reports, but being aware of the effect of a death or injury of an animal on its owners is an important prerequisite to being a trusted witness. The 'human-companion animal bond' (HCAB) can be very strong and helps people with diverse health and social needs (Ormerod *et al.*, 2005). This is not a new concept: the value of animals in hospitals and schools was being discussed three decades ago (Cooper, 1976) and Florence Nightingale (1860) stated that 'A small pet is often an excellent companion for the sick, for long chronic cases especially.' This is mentioned again in Chapter 12.

DISASTERS

As pointed out in Chapter 1, human forensic medicine has been boosted recently because of the need for skilled pathologists, physicians and psychiatrists to investigate natural and human-induced disasters.

This applies increasingly to veterinary forensic medicine (Heath, 1999) because domestic animals are also killed or injured in disasters. Endangered species may also be involved. The response to hurricanes in the USA in 2005 vividly drew attention to the role that veterinarians can play in disasters, including provision of human medical care (Clark and Kahler, 2005) (www.fema.gov).

Chemical attacks and bioterrorism could conceivably be directed at animals and agriculture as well as against 'human' targets (Durrant, 2002), so the veterinarian is again likely to be part of any response team (Sprayson, 2006).

Important considerations for anyone involved in disaster work are presented in Chapter 4.

It is important to remember that the role of the veterinary profession in disasters and other emer-

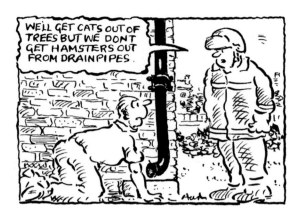

gencies can range from the large-scale and often distressing duties carried out following the 2004 tsunami (Sprayson, 2005; Yarrow, 2005) to more mundane, but no less important, rescue of stranded or displaced animals, both large and small. All such work can have a legal/forensic component.

LEGAL AND ETHICAL CONSIDERATIONS IN COLLABORATIVE WORK

As pointed out earlier, veterinarians may be involved in cases where there are animal and human elements. The most common examples are probably dog-bite incidents or allegations that an individual contracted a zoonosis from recently purchased animals. A less frequent but serious scenario is where there is a dead person and a dead animal, perhaps because someone shoots his family and pet dog or if both humans and animals are killed in an accident. In these circumstances, the veterinary clinician or pathologist is likely to be working alongside medical counterparts.

Sometimes the veterinarian or other expert is asked to examine a human cadaver because of specialised knowledge of, say, injuries inflicted by the horns of ruminants or bites from crocodiles.

In such cases it is important to remember the restrictions in the UK and other countries on how human tissues or organs are handled and stored (see Chapter 7).

Restrictions on the performance of clinical or *post-mortem* procedures on animals by non-veterinarians

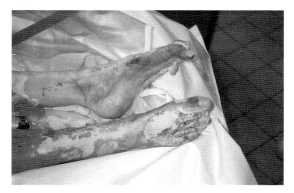

Figure 2.18 The embalmed feet of a person who was killed by a crocodile. The main physical damage was to the arms and the victim probably drowned. The feet illustrate *post-mortem* predation by fish and other aquatic organisms.

can be very strict. In many countries (see Chapter 3) the making of a diagnosis in an animal, alive or dead, is part of the definition of 'veterinary surgery' (i.e. the practice of veterinary medicine). The medically or dentally-trained pathologist or clinician has to be particularly careful about examining and taking samples from an animal, unless requested to do so by a registered veterinary surgeon. Rutty (2004) emphasised the value of radiographing any animal that is found dead with its owner under suspicious circumstances, 'to ensure that it also does not have a projectile within it'; but, alas, neither mentioned the legal implications nor the overall value of involving a veterinarian in such investigations.

The key to a successful outcome must be partnership – each person (medical doctor/veterinarian/others) doing his/her part, with overlap and probable synergy.

THE CONTRIBUTION OF ANIMALS TO OTHER ASPECTS OF FORENSIC WORK

Animals have contributed directly or indirectly to modern forensic science in various ways, quite apart from their role as 'models' in research (see earlier). Some examples are given below.

The important forensic role of invertebrate animals is discussed in Chapters 7 and 9.

Provision of evidence in human cases

Animals are often a significant part of investigations in legal and forensic work relating to humans. A good example was the landmark case in Canada where a pet white cat ('Snowball') provided key evidence – genomic DNA from hair – that implicated a man in a murder (Menotti-Raymond *et al.*, 1997). There are historical literary precedents also. The world's most famous detective, Sherlock Holmes, was largely concerned with 'human' cases but animals did not escape his attention, as witnessed by the following quotation:

> '*Is there any point to which you would wish to draw my attention?*'
> '*To the curious incident of the dog in the night-time.*'
> '*The dog did nothing in the night-time.*'
> '*That was the curious incident,*' remarked Sherlock Holmes.

Use of dogs

Dogs, and sometimes other species, are used in various aspects of crime investigation – for instance, in the following of scent or detection of mines or narcotic drugs. They also play a role in disaster relief.

Cadaver dogs, for example, are trained to locate human bodies after avalanches and other incidents. They detect blood and therefore have to work close to the ground. Amongst their advantages is that they search under adverse conditions (for example, amongst debris following a disaster) and do not seriously disrupt other search techniques.

However, during the course of their work, dogs may themselves be injured or killed, bringing another comparative component to the equation (see Chapter 6).

Assistance animals

Dogs have been used for some years to help those who are blind or deaf. Recently they have begun to provide assistance to, e.g., those prone to epileptiform seizures, and a recent report (WHO, 2005) mentioned the possible role of dogs in protecting women from domestic abuse (see Chapter 6). Although adults have been the main beneficiaries of the use of assistance dogs, there is now increasing interest in providing such help to children.

Other animals, such as farm livestock and horses, may also provide a degree of assistance to humans, particularly in encouraging physical, emotional and social wellbeing. All those interactions raise ethical and legal considerations and there is current interest in the extent to which the welfare of such animals may be compromised – horses used in therapeutic riding programmes (Kaiser *et al.*, 2006), for example.

The human-companion animal bond (HCAB) was mentioned earlier. Where there is a close relationship, death, injury or disease in the animal can have profound effects, often far exceeding the financial consequences (see Chapter 4).

TERMINOLOGY

Even the language of medicine, especially pathology, has allusions to animals – so-called 'zoography' (Allen and Cooper, 1983).

One of its greatest proponents was John Hunter (1728–1793), who investigated a variety of animals in his research and often compared and contrasted tissues and lesions in human patients with those of other species (Turk *et al.*, 2000). In one case, a woman who died of pericarditis in 1757, Hunter described clots covering the heart and pericardium as looking 'as if they had been torn by cats'. In another, he recorded the pericardium of a human patient as being 'covered with a layer of soft coagulated lymph which presents a finely reticulated appearance somewhat resembling that of the interior of the fourth stomach of a calf . . .'

This was comparative medicine *par excellence!*

REQUIREMENTS OF A FORENSIC VETERINARIAN

What makes a good 'forensic veterinarian'? In specialised work, such as interpretation of radiographs or identification of a lesion, the main requirements, other than an ability and willingness to give evidence and to appear in court, are professional skill and integrity. But for the veterinarian who wishes to be involved more extensively in the field of animal forensics, additional talents are desirable.

Chapter 1 drew attention to the link between the medical profession and crime detection and how numerous traits that characterise a good physician also pertain to detective work. The same applies to veterinarians: if participating routinely in forensic work, they need to be skilled observers and, as Celsus said to medical students 300 years ago, 'to know the invisible as well as the visible'. This implies an ability to carry out detailed investigations with an open and inquisitive mind. Although veterinary science, like human medicine, has become increasingly instrumented and automated in recent years, the 'art' of acquiring and retaining clinical acumen remains crucial to being a good diagnostician and thus an able forensic investigator.

In that delightful book *The No. 1 Ladies' Detective Agency* (McCall Smith, 1998), the central figure, Mma Ramotswe, stated that 'detective agencies rely on human intuition and intelligence', with the accurate and pertinent caveat that 'No inventory would ever include those, of course'. This is true of forensic work and it is quite often the intrinsic skills and 'sixth sense' of the investigator rather than technology that solves the problem.

Allusion is increasingly made to the strong links between detective work and diagnostic medicine (Peschel and Peschel, 1989). One of many examples in the animal field is the literature of the Wildlife Conservation Society (WCS) (see Appendix B) where discussion on how the health of animals is studied is entitled *Veterinary Pathologists: Medical Detectives* (WCS, undated).

It is in the investigation of wildlife crime that powers of observation, curiosity and unconventional lateral thinking are most salient (see Chapter 6). To succeed, one needs the eyes and other attributes of a countryman, a field worker or 'nature detective' as Maxwell Knight put it nearly forty years ago (Knight, 1968). Over the years, various pioneers have extolled the virtues of field observation in such areas as the tracking of wildlife and the undertaking of ecological research and it is worth remembering that a century ago Lord Baden-Powell, the founder of the Scout Movement, repeatedly stressed the value of such an approach to training of young people in citizenship and self-reliance. This theme was pursued by Gerald Durrell in his wonderful book *The Amateur Naturalist*

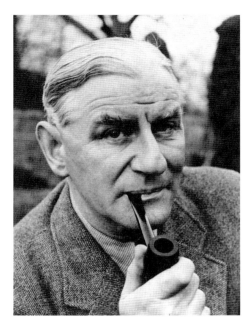

Figure 2.19 Maxwell Knight: the original nature detective.

(Durrell, 1982) when he wrote that one who pursues natural history as a pastime must have a very enquiring mind and, in stressing the importance of not just looking, cited Sherlock Holmes' words, 'You see, but you do not observe'.

CONCLUSION

So what message is enshrined in this long and somewhat labyrinthine chapter? The main points are as follows:

- What can be broadly termed 'animal forensics' is of increasing importance in a blame-orientated and litigious world.
- In legal and other actions concerning animals, the animal is either the victim or the perpetrator. In both cases there is a human/animal component that requires close interdisciplinary collaboration.
- Conventional veterinary forensic medicine, concerned primarily with domesticated animals, is a rapidly evolving discipline.
- A new discipline of 'comparative forensic medicine' is proposed. This caters for studies on many species, not just domestic animals and humans, with appropriate analogy and extrapolation. It provides a bridge between the work of the medical and veterinary professions and some of the many emerging disciplines, especially those that are biology-based, that constitute contemporary forensic science.
- Veterinary and comparative forensic medicine principles can be applied to various quasi-legal situations, such as insurance claims, malpractice suits and environmental impact assessments. The techniques used are also relevant in disaster relief and management of emergencies.
- Those involved in animal forensic work, whether veterinarians or not, need to have a sound background in knowledge of the law, an understanding of the principles involved in legal investigations, a well-honed ability to observe and think logically and an intense spirit of curiosity.

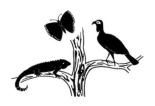

Importance and Application of Animal Law

No man shall exercise any Tyranny or Crueltie towards any bruite Creature which are usuallie kept for man's use.

The Bodie of Liberties. Massachusetts Bay Colony 1641.

He who brings any Eyess-Hawk from beyond the Sea, shall have a Certificate under the Customer's Seal where he lands.

Nelson, W. (1753) *The Laws Concerning Game,* 5th edn. T. Waller, London, UK.

INTRODUCTION

The law relating to animals is a specialised field. Forensic investigations and expert evidence may be used in most areas of animal law and may involve any species of animal. There is also a growing need for forensic investigation and the provision of expert evidence in associated aspects such as veterinary law, health and safety and insurance. The veterinary, wildlife or other expert working in these areas will benefit from an understanding of the animal law and its associated topics.

Legislation relating to animals has ancient origins and, in many civilizations, a variety of species have held particular significance, be it religious, cultural, nutritional or sporting. Some of the earliest laws on the subject were carved in stone. The stone hieroglyphics of the 18th century BC *Codex of Hammurabi* proclaimed it illegal to overwork animals. It was also decreed that a fine should be paid for theft of farm animals and compensation awarded to the owner for the destruction of animals entrusted or hired to another person, although this did not apply in the case of an accident, an act of God or an attack by a lion (King, undated). The Emperor Asoka (King Ashoka) of India issued an edict in 225 BC to protect wildlife and forests and to forbid cruelty to animals. He also provided for the veterinary care of animals and made imported medicinal plants available for this purpose (Dhammika, 1993 and 1994).

Once a species becomes of value, legislation evolves to protect a person's rights in it. Thus, William the Conqueror (William I of England) ordered the *Domesday Book* of 1085–1086 to be compiled as an inventory of farm stock, forests, fishing rights and other assets on which he could levy taxes. Early laws relating to forests and game protected royal hunting interests. Game laws defended landowners' rights to hunt wild animals on their property (Nelson, 1753).

Other early aspects of animal law related primarily to domesticated and other captive animals as property (i.e. goods) such as contract (for example in buying and selling horses) or in licensing or taxing the use of animals (Nelson, 1753). Litigation over the ownership of animals and the damage done by them also features in the early annals of courts. Likewise, present-day legal remedies for damage caused by animals have their origins in the early common law.

The concept that animals need protection from abuse emerged alongside the other philanthropic movements of the 19th century. Nevertheless, the first animal welfare legislation in English is usually attributed to the Massachusetts Bay Company (AWI, 1990; Cooper, 1987). A body of law has since evolved in a range of countries that shows concern for the sentience of domesticated and other captive animals (see Chapter 4). In New Zealand and Britain, particular attention has been given to drawing up new animal welfare legislation that primarily aims to prevent suffering rather than to punish it after the event. A number of countries have a welfare statute under which guidance and codes of practice on welfare are intended to encourage good animal management. Some countries, including Australia, Britain, Canada and New Zealand, have councils (representing the many, disparate points of view on animals) that provide independent advice to the government on aspects of animal welfare.

In the early 20th century, it became more widely recognised that wildlife required legal protection against the extinction of species. Numerous international agreements on the protection of species and land and marine habitat have emerged, culminating in the Convention on Biological Diversity 1992 (CBD). There are also various treaties relating to environmental conditions, such as pollution and climate change (de Klemm and Shine, 1993; Lyster, 1985 and Rees, 2002).

The history of the protection of areas for environmental purposes goes back further, to 1765, when the Main Ridge Reserve of Tobago became the first forest reserve in the Western Hemisphere. It took ten years to convince the British Parliament (then responsible for Tobago) that the island and its plantations depended on these 'woodlands for the protection of the rain' as a water catchment area. The Reserve is still in place today and has even been augmented. Yellowstone National Park in the USA, established in 1872, was the first national park to be set aside for the purpose of combining wildlife conservation with human recreational use. Today, there are many areas designated, with various degrees of legal protection, although they are far from immune to a wide range of threats. Litigation is sometimes used to protect such areas and evidence on all aspects of the site, including animals and plants that are dependent on it may be required in support.

The other area of animal-related legislation that has grown substantially deals with veterinary matters, such as animal health, medicines and the veterinary profession. These have been thoroughly influenced by the extensive law emanating from the European Union (EU).

The insurance of animals, for their value and against liability for the costs of veterinary treatment, has expanded (see Chapter 6) and has led to the need for resolution, often with the help of expert advice or evidence. Other litigation relating to veterinary practice takes the form of disciplinary action for professional misconduct and claims for professional negligence in the treatment, examination or certification of animals. Veterinary or other scientific evidence may also be needed at quasi-legal hearings, such as planning enquiries, particularly when an endangered species is affected (see Chapters 2 and 5).

Since the 1970s, animal law has seen particular growth in, and revision of, the relevant legislation, together with concern for better enforcement, especially, but not exclusively, in the developed world. In other countries, however, animal law has remained fairly static while they grapple with overwhelming problems of poverty and governance. At times, the modernisation of their laws has resulted from outside pressure; for example, for better animal health controls in the face of pandemics, or improved conservation laws in countries where wildlife is a valuable asset in attracting foreign currency through tourism. Responses to EU obligations and international law have had the same effect in Europe and elsewhere.

LITIGATION INVOLVING ANIMALS

The animals likely to be affected by litigation can be categorised as:

- Domesticated species, such as pets, equids or farm livestock.
- Non-domesticated species that are kept in captivity for various purposes, such as conservation, education, display or sport, trade, rehabilitation, captive-breeding or as pets.
- Free-living ('wild') species.

Typical areas of the law relating to animals that give rise to investigations and litigation are:

- Welfare – in respect of domestic (pets and livestock) or other captive animals; farm animal welfare (farm, market, slaughter); the transport of animals.
- Species protection – laws regulating the taking and killing of wild animals and their exploitation.
- The keeping of animals – regulated through licensing.
- Commercial activities – involving pedigree animals; horses and other performance or traction animals, pets and non-domesticated species.
- The illegal movement of animals – smuggling and illegal possession of animals, particularly wildlife; animal health controls.
- Insurance claims – for injuries, death or damage caused by animals or to animals; under veterinary fees policies.
- Civil law claims – trespass, nuisance, negligence, strict liability for animals, malpractice (professional negligence).
- Breach of contract – non-payment of veterinary fees; failure to fulfil the terms of a contract.
- Disciplinary proceedings (professional misconduct).
- Breaches of the medicines legislation.
- Abuse of humans and animals.
- Accidents and occupational health and safety.

Some of these are discussed in more detail in Chapters 2, 4, 5 and 6.

There is considerable crossover between the two lists above in that animals from one category may be subject to a variety of laws. While some law applies to specific species or activities, for example the breeding of dogs, other legislation, such as that on welfare or animal health, may apply to a range of species in different situations. For example, the animal health controls for foot-and-mouth disease can apply not only to farm animals but also to certain valuable species kept in zoological collections. In Britain, the definition of an animal for the purposes of controlling foot-and-mouth extends to all four-footed beasts and all birds and, since the full implications of this became clear, special provi-

sions for animals in zoos have been put in place (http://www.defra.gov.uk/animalh/diseases/fmd/disease/zoo.htm).

The foregoing point also illustrates that it is extremely important, when dealing with any piece of animal legislation, to ascertain precisely to which species or category of animals it applies. The definition section of an Act of Parliament or statutory instrument usually provides this information but it may be subject to further refinement elsewhere in the document, in subsidiary legislation or in case law.

ETHICAL, RELIGIOUS AND CULTURAL ISSUES

There is an extensive literature on the subject of animal ethics, from the philosophical to the scientific and the practical, produced by authors from many backgrounds. A recent text which is worth consultation is *The Ethics of Research Involving Animals* (Nuffield Council, 2005). This is primarily concerned with the issues of animal research but provides much useful information on the key concepts and ideas on how to confront ethical dilemmas relating to animals. Writers in the broadly veterinary field include Broom (2003) and Webster (1994, 2005), amongst many others.

The judicial process is concerned with the law, rather than animal ethics (although some would consider this a matter of debate). Nevertheless, litigation involving animals is often driven by moral persuasion and concerns and the animal welfare legislation (and, to some extent, conservation law) is derived from ethical attitudes. Much passion is generated by issues of animal welfare. Expert witnesses need to be aware of the different viewpoints and their implications, particularly in cases that have been instigated for ethical motives (see Chapters 4 and 5). In England, some suspected offences are investigated and brought to court by animal charities either alone in the form of private prosecutions or in conjunction with the enforcing authorities.

Religious beliefs can also play an important part in animal issues and may be a significant element in animal law, as in the exemptions made for religious slaughter (see Chapter 4) in Western law and the legislation regarding holy animals in India. Further, most of the mainstream religions have some textual or moral references to treating animals kindly.

The Universities Federation for Animal Welfare (UFAW) was one of the first organisations in the West to analyse religious attitudes towards animals and to see how these might be applied to welfare. Two important papers appeared over fifty years ago, by Hume (1951), UFAW's founder, and Smith (1951). Hume's paper was the more philosophical and it is interesting that, amongst other things, he discussed pain and the various ways in which religions view and deal with it. Smith compared different religions and pointed out how often dogma and practice diverge, with the result that animals often suffer, even in an environment where religious teaching stresses the importance of kindness to other creatures. A range of literature on religious attitudes to animals is provided by Epstein (undated).

Sometimes, the cultural importance of a species is taken into consideration in applying the law. For example, in New Zealand, Maori attach cultural significance to certain indigenous birds (see Chapter 7). Many of these are also protected by legislation and considerable efforts are made to accommodate the two approaches to wildlife, its conservation and traditional use. In the Cook Islands, a traditional community-based conservation practice called 'ra'ui' is applied in conjunction with legislative measures to manage sustainable harvesting of natural resources. Anita (2004) has demonstrated, in the context of the Solomon Islands (in the Pacific Ocean), the issues and conflicts that can emerge when sensitive species, such as dolphins, are utilised both traditionally and with a view to developing a sustainable resource for its people. Traditional hunting, culture, religion and commerce had to contend with wildlife protection and animal health and welfare. National and international legislation and standards had to be addressed. The government, and island veterinarians, had to steer a path between the different needs and cultural attitudes of their own citizens as well as external pressures from conservation and marine animal welfare groups.

LEGAL BACKGROUND AND CONCEPTS

Law in the UK

The law that will be discussed is primarily that of England and Wales (for brevity mainly referred to in this chapter as England); nevertheless, some of the ensuing material will be of use in any country, or at least, of relevance to countries with common law legal systems (see below and Chapter 12).

The law and legal systems of Scotland and Northern Ireland are similar but distinct from those of England and Wales. Other countries that derive their legal system from English origins, 'the common law countries', have similar systems and one can often find comparable animal laws on their statute books (see Chapter 12).

Britain is unique in having no written constitution although many constitutional rights derive from law and learned writings from Magna Carta in 1215 to the Human Rights Act 1998. When working overseas, the British person should take into consideration the impact of any relevant provisions of the host country's constitution. For instance, there sometimes is a specific statement that all wildlife belongs to the nation, although, alternatively, this may be found in the wildlife laws.

A number of legal concepts are discussed in Chapter 12, such as the distinction between civil and criminal law, that are also relevant to this Chapter. A few further points are set out below.

Levels of law

There are four main levels at which law is found:

(1) International – global and multilateral treaties.
(2) Regional – treaties and other legislation relating to a part of the world.
(3) National – the law of individual nations; in countries with a federal constitution there are two tiers, federal (or national) government level and state level (see Chapter 12).
(4) Local – byelaws made by city or other district authorities.

There are many international treaties relating to conservation whereas animal health and welfare legislation and veterinary law occur at regional or national level. The conservation and environment Conventions have informative websites that also provide copies of the relevant documentation. Treaties are implemented by the countries that join them through national legislation. Highly influential examples of regional legislation are the European Union and the Council of Europe (see below). The main body of animal law is made at the national level. In federal countries, there may be animal law at both levels. At the state level there may be considerable variation in the law on a particular subject. In order to encourage uniformity between states the federal government of Australia has produced model animal welfare codes which the individual states may use (http://www.daff.gov.au/animal-welfare). National legislation may be available on the Internet and the US Library of Congress provides a useful portal to the law of many countries that might otherwise be difficult to find at http://www.loc.gov/law/guide/about.html.

European legislation

Legislation on animals has been produced by both the European Union (EU) and the Council of Europe (CoE). The European Community (the legislative 'pillar', or section, of the EU) has produced a large body of 'regulations' and 'directives' relating to animal health, farm animal welfare, research animals, wildlife conservation and the international trade in endangered species. These form part of the law of the individual countries, either directly (if the law originated in regulations) or (if derived from directives) through national legislative or administrative measures. The Member States can be subjected to penalties for failure to implement directives. The relevant legislation is available on Europa, the European Union website (http://europa.eu.int/eur-lex/lex/en/repert/index.htm) (see Appendix B).

Details of the implementation in Britain of European animal and conservation law is to be found on the Department for Environment, Food and Rural Affairs (DEFRA) website (http://www.defra.gov.uk/animalh/animindx.htm) (both for agricultural animals and wildlife). The Joint Nature Conservation Committee (JNCC) website (http://www.jncc.gov.uk/page-1359) also provides information on the implementation of European law in the conservation field. General information on the EU is available on http://europa.eu.int/index_en.htm.

The Council of Europe has drawn up a number of Conventions on farm animal welfare, research animals, conservation and pets. These Conventions were made before the existence of EU legislation on the subject and some apply to many more countries. Parties to the Conventions have an obligation to implement the provisions but there are no legal sanctions to force them to do so. These documents are available on the Council of Europe website (www.coe.int).

Terminology relating to animals

There are many words used to describe animals and they can be grouped as follows:

- Their common name (for which non-scientific language is used). For, example, cat, horse, lion, falcon, iguana.
- Their scientific name, the binomial system given in Appendix F, for example *Falco peregrinus* for the peregrine falcon.
- In legislation, the common name is normally used for domesticated animals. Some words occur, such as 'equids', which can apply to non-domesticated species. Non-domesticated species are normally identified in endangered species legislation by both common name and scientific name; the latter usually designated to be the definitive version. In some countries, a main language and a vernacular name may be used.
- Adjectives used to describe animals, such as wild, free-living, non-domesticated, indigenous, endemic, introduced, feral, exotic, captive, domestic, domesticated, companion, pet, agricultural, exhibition, sporting, working, traction, research are, at times, used very loosely. For example, it is common (and, to many, scientifically correct) to refer to animals in a zoological collection as 'wild' animals because of the origin of their species, despite the particular specimens being patently captive. It is important that such terms are chosen with care, fully defined and used precisely in forensic work and

also when preparing reports and giving evidence. A list of commonly used adjectives is given in Cooper (1987).

- Adjectives correctly applied in a legal context may not necessarily accord with scientific definitions or in common parlance. Thus, the Convention on the Conservation of Migratory Species applies to species that fit its stated definition of a migratory species, although this may not be in accordance with the scientific criteria used to classify a species as migratory.

It must be emphasised that precision in the use of these terms is essential in legal interpretation and in forensic work. An expert should carefully and clearly define such terms and explain their implication when they are used in a report or in court. It is also important to clarify different usages, anticipate possible conflicts between disciplines and to find a way to avoid ambiguity and confusion.

LITERATURE AND SOURCES OF INFORMATION

There is a considerable literature on animal law covering most of the topics listed above. These tend to relate to countries that have strong legislation in this field. Individual books and papers are mentioned below and, as appropriate, in the text.

In countries with codified law, for example in continental Europe, published versions of the codes are often available in bookshops. There are also standard lawyer's encyclopaedias that are available in good libraries that are useful for in-depth study. They provide the actual legislation, both primary and secondary (see Chapter 12) and definitive accounts of the law on many subjects. For English law these are *Halsbury's Laws of England, Halsbury's Statutes* and *Halsbury's Statutory Instruments*. Volume 2 of *Halsbury's Laws of England* deals with many aspects of the law of animals. With their up-dating service, the three Halsbury's series provide the most authoritative and accessible current account of the English law and its sources that is available in print. New legislation, cases and literature can also be monitored in the *Current Law*

Monthly Digest. A dedicated law library will also hold the many series of case reports, as well as learned books and journals.

Most countries publish their legislation through their government printer. Printed reports of parliamentary proceedings (often called 'Hansard' in Commonwealth countries) and parliamentary websites provide information on the progress of legislation in the making. Government ministries, universities and libraries kept by the judiciary normally have sets of legislation and case reports, although these are not usually available for general public access. In countries with few resources, these may be the only collections.

In some countries Government departments and other websites provide information within the scope of their responsibilities. In England, because DEFRA is responsible for both agriculture and the environment, much of the information about animal legislation is to be found there. The law and administration relating to the Convention on the International Trade in Endangered Species of Wild Fauna and Flora (CITES) is available on the DEFRA, UK CITES, Europa and CITES Convention websites. The Home Office (the UK ministry of the interior) is responsible for animals used in research (see Chapter 4). In the USA, two main sources of information on animal law are the United States Department of Agriculture, its Animal and Plant Health Service and the Fish and Wildlife Service websites. Similar information sources are to be found for Canada, Australia and New Zealand and other countries.

Legislation is also available on the Internet in some countries and a useful starting point is the Library of Congress portal mentioned above. In the UK, online versions of legislation are provided by the Her Majesty's Stationery Office, now part of the Office of Public Service Information (http://www.opsi.gov.uk/) although this goes back only to 1988 for England (http://www.opsi.gov.uk/legislation/about_legislation.htm). Government reports, consultations, and other documents of contemporary importance are often available on the appropriate ministry's website. Legislation and other government publications are also supplied in printed form by The Stationery Office (TSO) (http://www.tso.co.uk/).

Sometimes published or private compilations of animal, conservation or environmental law may be found, especially where it is difficult to locate the legislation or when an organisation has a special interest in it. The IUCN (World Conservation Union, see Appendix B) has published books on the subject of environmental and conservation law. Other IUCN publications have included surveys of environmental legislation as part of regional or national studies carried out with a view to developing better environmental management (http://www.iucn.org/bookstore/). The IUCN Library also provides a searchable catalogue on http://www.iucn.org/bookstore/IUCN-library.htm.

Books, articles and other literature are an important source of information on, and discussion of, animal law. They vary from broad overviews to specialised studies, from commentaries in antiquarian literature to modern books, and from theses to practical guides. Compilations of the English animal law are provided by Palmer (2001) on animals; by Lorton (2000) on wildlife and countryside and Parkes and Thornley (1997) on game and on deer (Parkes and Thornley, 2000). There are also books on the law of horses (Gilligan, 2002; Mackenzie, 2001). Rees (2002) provides a fusion of conservation and environmental law with ecology that is likely to be valuable to the expert who has to understand the interaction of these fields. There are numerous books on wildlife law. Lyster (1985) and de Klemm and Shine (1993) examine the international conservation conventions and Sands (2003) covers the broader context of international environmental law as a whole.

CITES is the global convention that most gives rise to litigation and Wijnstekers (2005) gives a thorough interpretation of the convention and the resolutions that have amended and adapted it over the years. The IUCN (see above) has produced many books aimed at the development and application of international environmental treaties. The websites of CITES and the other conservation and environmental conventions are reliable sources of the relevant legal and other documents. Radford (2001) has written a thorough treatise on animal welfare law and the RSPCA (1999) produced a concise summary of the animal welfare law at that time. North (1972) examined the

Animals Act and liability for damage done by animals.

There are older guides to the animal-related law that, while in need of updating, still provide an overview of the sort of legislation that applies to animals on a broader basis than some of the more specialised books (Cooper, 1987; Field-Fisher, 1964). There are a number of books on USA animal law (AWI, 1990; Bean and Rowland, 1997; Curnett, 2000; Favre and Loring, 1983; Wilson, J.F. 1988). Blood (1985) dealt with Australian animal law; there are books on horse law in French and, in a number of countries (for example, Brazil, France, Germany, India, Portugal), it is possible to find books that reproduce their conservation laws.

Material produced by specialist organisations often provides valuable information on the relevant law, recent changes and judicial decisions that other publications may not report in such detail. For example, in Britain, there are publications on birds (RSPB, 1998) on badgers (NFBG, 2000) on bats (BCT, undated) and on animal welfare (RSPCA, 1999). Such bodies may also be a good source of guides or codes of conduct, for example BASC (2001). Other animal organisations, particularly those relating to horses, dogs, birds of prey and racing pigeons, where the animals are valuable and there has been a history of legislation and litigation, are also a good source of information. The TRAFFIC Bulletin publishes regular reports from many parts of the world of prosecutions for violation of CITES legislation (http://www.traffic.org/publications/index.html#bulletin).

One thing common to the use of any material on law in any country, including this book and all other sources, is that the user must ensure that s/he has also acquired the most recent and accurate version of legislation and other forms of law, including secondary legislation, amendments and judicial decisions.

ANIMAL LAW

English law (and that of many other countries) recognises only natural or legal persons as having rights and duties (see Chapter 12). Consequently, the law treats animals as if they are property or goods. The EU has recognised that animals are sentient beings and, to a limited extent, undertaken to have regard for their welfare needs in the Protocol on Protection and Welfare of Animals annexed to the Treaty of Amsterdam (EU, 1997a,b). There have been attempts to provide a special legal status for the great apes, but at present this amounts only to recognition in some countries that they should not be used in scientific research, or only with special justification.

Animals are considered in English law (and in other common law countries or those based on Roman law) to be either 'domestic' (or 'domesticated') in Latin, *domitae* (or *mansuetae*) *naturae*, or 'wild' (*ferae naturae*, of a wild nature) since the classification is derived from Roman law. Domesticated animals and captive 'wild' animals are treated as the property of their owner (see below). Free-living wild animals are considered to belong to no one unless and until they have been 'reduced into captivity'. Consequently, landowners have very limited (but ancient and complex) rights over animals on their land. A further exception is the right of the Crown, by virtue of the Royal Prerogative, to swans swimming in open waters (that have not been claimed by anyone) and to 'fishes royal' found in local waters (Cooper, 1987). The latter has implications for the occasional findings of whales, dolphins, porpoises and sturgeon. Under a long-standing agreement, the Natural History Museum, London, exercises this right as part of a stranding scheme and has a relevant database, http://www.nhm.ac.uk/research-curation/projects/strandings/index.html. This historical approach to the ownership of wild animals does not necessarily apply in all countries since some have legislation that specifically provides that all wildlife belongs to the nation.

Responsibility for keeping animals

Since, in England, domesticated or captive animals are considered in law to be the property of the owner, the latter has rights and responsibilities in respect of the animal in the same way as any goods. For example, an owner can buy and sell animals under the normal sale of goods law and a person can be prosecuted for stealing an animal.

Breach of contract can occur in many circumstances, and give rise to a claim for damages. Litigation on the sale of animals has a long history and continues today, particularly in the case of the most valuable, such as racehorses (Gilligan, 2002; Mackenzie, 2001; Palmer, 2001). Expert evidence may be required on a variety of aspects, such as the fitness of an animal (Krenger and Straub, 2002), the pre-purchase examination, its identification (either as an individual or a species) or its value (see Chapter 6).

There have always been responsibilities attached to the keeping of animals. The law of tort (part of the civil law, see Chapter 12) has created liabilities, and provided remedies, for damage caused by or to animals. Civil law liability can arise on the grounds of trespass to land, trespass by animals, trespass to the person, nuisance and negligence. In addition, the Animals Act 1971, which codified the previous common law, deals with what is known as 'strict liability' for injury and damage caused by dangerous animals. This means that the person claiming compensation does not have to prove fault or negligence as in the other kinds of tort just mentioned. The provisions of the Animals Act 1971 are complex and the aspects relating to strict liability for damage caused by domesticated species was examined in detail on appeal to the House of Lords in *Mirvahedy v. Henley and another* [2003] UKHL 16. Other common law countries (those that have legislation derived from English law, see Chapter 12) have similar torts. In other jurisdictions, it is necessary to look in the civil code for provisions on damage caused by animals.

Forensic experts are often used in civil law claims. Evidence may be required regarding the nature of the damage, identification of an animal or showing whether or not the animal caused the damage, normal or aberrant behaviour, quantum of damage, sound levels in a nuisance case; in veterinary cases, assessing the standard of surgery or other work or gauging the nature and level of damage in a road accident.

Regulation of animals kept in captivity

The keeping of domesticated (and, in most cases, non-domesticated) animals was originally very little regulated. Some countries have controls on dogs, either for licensing or as dangerous dogs. The latter may give rise to litigation on points such as the identification of the species or whether the animal should be put down. Control over the keeping of non-domesticated animals had developed piecemeal in Britain since the 1970s, as the need for legislation was perceived. Elsewhere in the world, regulation varies from strict and covering most species to non-existent or only instigated under external pressures.

A variety of Acts in force at January 2006 in England and Wales regulate riding establishments, boarding kennels for cats and dogs, dog-breeding facilities and guard dog kennels. Zoos, dangerous wild animals, circuses and performing animals, pet shops and the use of animals in scientific research are also regulated (Figure 3.1 and 3.2).

As a general principle, such establishments must be licensed and inspected. The licence may be subject to conditions and, in some cases, standards have been established for these activities. Some of these are a requirement of the statute, others are voluntary codes. Much of this British legislation is due to be replaced by uniform provisions, together with codes of good practice, in the new Animal Welfare Act 2006 for England and Wales and by separate animal health and welfare legislation for Scotland, thereby integrating the regulation of animal keeping with the welfare law (http://www.defra.gov.uk/animalh/welfare/bill/index.htm). Coverage will extend to horses at livery and animal sanctuaries. The new provisions will be in line with countries such as Australia and New Zealand that have a Welfare Act and codes of practice to cover many forms of animal keeping.

The zoo and research animal licensing systems already have well-established, separate legislation and codes of practice and standards and will not be changed (http://www.defra.gov.uk/wildlife-countryside/gwd/zoo.htm and http://scienceandresearch.homeoffice.gov.uk/animal-research/legislation/).

The national legislation in these fields is derived from European Community law and therefore similar levels of regulation of such establishments are to be found in other EU countries. Many other countries have research and zoo (Cooper, 2003a) legislation; in some of these there are high standards but in others controls may be scant, collections having old-fashioned facilities and poor management (Figure 3.3).

Ethical codes can be helpful to those aiming to improve the standards of science and conditions of animals. The codes can be used to supplement existing official requirements and/or they can be applied in situations where there is no legislation but it is wished to meet standards accepted elsewhere. Well-established codes and guidance may also be useful to experts as a benchmark.

Experts may be needed to provide evidence when there is a breach of the law, either as to licensing or in relation to the standards or codes of practice or welfare. Welfare codes, in English law, do not as

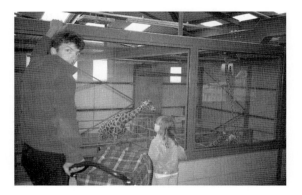

Figure 3.1 Zoos in the European Union and elsewhere are subject to strict laws and standards and must contribute to conservation and education.

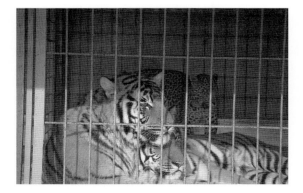

Figure 3.2 A circus tiger in its travelling quarters.

normal workplace activities, such as protection of staff and visitors from hazards.

Implications for the forensic expert are that an expert opinion may be required when there are questions of compliance with licensing requirements relating to the premises or to endangered species. It may also be needed in cases involving liability for accidents and injuries or allegations of ill-treatment. Compliance with provisions on taking sick and injured animals and returning them to the wild may call for evidence of behaviour and identification of species (see Chapter 5) and DNA evidence relating to captive-breeding. In addition, assessment of whether a bird is fit for return to the wild or should be kept in captivity is often provided by a veterinary surgeon with appropriate experience or alternatively by a biologist or bird keeper if behaviour is the criterion.

Theft is not uncommon and proving the identity of a stolen animal may need expert evidence. The keeping of certain species of birds of prey calls for the registration and ringing (banding) of some species (see Chapter 6) and evidence may be required to support prosecutions when there are breaches of these requirements. Some of these birds are valuable and are in demand for captive-breeding. There are not infrequent cases of smuggling and illegal taking from the wild and expert evidence may be needed to show genetic relationships between parent and offspring or to prove that young were not bred from an illegally-taken bird, especially if records are not adequate. Many of these situations relate in general to the keeping of wildlife. While these examples are based on English law, experts would find comparable situations in many jurisdictions.

Animal welfare

Animal welfare has a very high priority and profile in the United Kingdom and a number of other countries. There has been legislation on the subject in Britain since the 19th century and constant efforts have continued to refine, expand and improve it ever since. Various other countries, such as some European countries, Australia, Canada, New Zealand and the USA, have comparable legislation, active promotion of animal welfare and

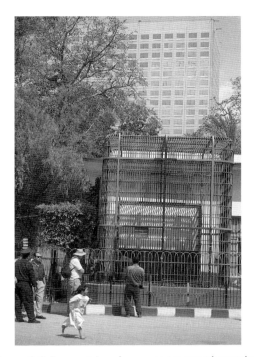

Figure 3.3 In countries where zoos are not adequately regulated, animal accommodation may remain old-fashioned.

such have legal force but failure to comply with the code may be used as supporting evidence in prosecuting an offence under the welfare law. There are experienced inspectors amongst the veterinary profession (Davies, 1989) from environmental health and trading standards departments and zoo inspectors. People with such experience may also be a useful source of expert evidence.

Wildlife rescue centres are usually run by dedicated people, often on a voluntary, charitable basis. In some countries, these are subject to legal controls and wildlife rehabilitators have to undergo training and be licensed. While there is no specific legislation in England to regulate these centres, they might in future be affected by forthcoming provisions on animal sanctuaries in the proposed animal welfare law. Nevertheless, they have to operate within a wide range of other laws (Cooper, 2003b), as do other establishments. This includes liability for damage caused by animals, wildlife legislation, animal health, general welfare, animal health and veterinary treatment, together with enforcement of the relevant legislation. Involvement with animals and animal issues in these countries can be difficult and, at times, dangerous (see Chapter 5).

Many parts of the world do not share the passion of the British for animal welfare and, while a number of countries have laws on the subject, many others may not give the matter significant attention. Similarly, animal welfare organisations tend to be much less powerful and less well-funded than in the UK. Organisations and individuals from outside make considerable efforts (through legislative and other means) to improve the welfare and conservation situations in such countries but to establish sustainable reforms requires patience and persistence together with a good insight and understanding of local conditions. Experts invited to give evidence on animal welfare (or other issues) in a different jurisdiction should bear this in mind, together with the impact of local cultural and religious attitudes.

Animal welfare legislation often includes offences of causing cruelty or unnecessary suffering as well as specific provisions relating to matters such as poisoning, animal fighting, the inhumane use of traps or the welfare of farmed animals. There is variation in the extent of welfare provision in different countries from scant, to laws left over from the colonial era, to the modern laws of, say, Australia and New Zealand that include codes of practice for a wide range of situations in which animals are kept. In England and Wales (and, in the future, in Scotland and Northern Ireland) new legislation (the Animal Welfare Act mentioned above) on the welfare of domesticated and other captive animals is imminent. This will maintain the existing offence of causing unnecessary suffering but new provisions will impose a duty upon a person to take reasonable care to ensure that the needs of any animal for which he or she is responsible are met according to good practice. The licensing of most animal establishments will be brought under the proposed Act (see above) and the restrictions on young people owning animals will be tightened. Enforcement powers and penalties will be strengthened.

The new legislation over-rides previous judicial decisions that free-living animals coming under temporary restraint were not protected by the welfare legislation. One such case, *Steel v. Rogers (1912)*, meant that no action could be taken against people who damaged a beached whale while it was still alive. This problem still exists in many countries (although the new English animal welfare legislation seeks to close the loophole) and is well illustrated by a newspaper cartoon relating to a 2004 whale stranding in Trinidad.

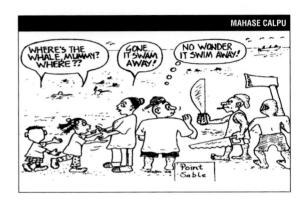

The farm animal legislation instigated in Britain in 1968 made specific provision for the welfare of farm animals, including the use of codes of practice. Other legislation deals with the welfare of farm animals at markets, at slaughter and while they are being transported. Much of this implements EU directives on the subject and is consequently similar to the laws of other EU countries (http://www.defra.gov.uk/animalh/welfare/farmed/index.htm).

Animal welfare offences include the neglect and mistreatment of animals. Some involve acts of deliberate cruelty and others occur because the owner or keeper cannot cope. While it is important to have welfare laws that prevent animal suffering, the cost in terms of human distress when a case is brought on unsound grounds must not be forgotten.

Many cases are ultimately based on an assessment of unnecessary suffering, which is likely to call for expert opinion and evidence. Under the forthcoming English legislation, litigation is likely to require expert evidence in respect of both the detailed definition of 'unnecessary suffering' (see Chapter 4) and the new provision imposing a duty on the person responsible for an animal to take reasonable care of it according to good practice.

As the new legislation is used and tested by the authorities and interested bodies, much expert evidence will be required to aid the courts in their interpretation and decisions.

Wildlife conservation

Most countries have wildlife conservation legislation (see also Chapter 5). This normally provides protection for endangered species and for their habitat. It may also regulate exploitative uses of protected species and areas. Hunting may either be regulated or banned altogether, as in Kenya. Legislation varies from old-fashioned hunting controls (Trinidad and Tobago, Kenya and others) to a modern approach that encompasses the management and use of natural resources, allowing for the authorisation of a range of sustainable practices (Uganda). Many countries have legislation that is supplemented by secondary legislation (usually in the form of statutory instruments, see Chapter 12) or the equivalent (e.g. USA Code of Federal Regulations) that provides detailed rules. In countries with federal constitutions, much of the wildlife legislation is covered by laws of the states while only certain aspects are dealt with at federal level (see Chapter 12).

The legislation usually also provides for species conservation, protected area management (national parks, game reserves, etc.) by a parks service, the management of forests and flora, and the marine environment. This is normally contained in a range of laws that are readily identified. This legislation is usually the responsibility of the environment ministry of a government but, in some jurisdictions, wildlife responsibilities still fall under forest management, and marine mammals may fall within the domain of the fisheries legislation and department, as in some Caribbean countries. Other countries, as in East and Central Africa, have a dedicated wildlife authority or game department.

In Britain, the Wildlife and Countryside Act (WCA) deals with species and habitat protection and also implements the requirements of EC habitat and species protection required by the EU Directives on Habitats and on Birds. The WCA protects all wild birds and provides some protection for other species (mammals, reptiles, amphibians, invertebrates and plants that are listed). Close seasons and hunting controls are provided in separate legislation for deer, seals and other game and there is an Act specifically for the protection of badgers. Restrictions on hunting methods include a law forbidding hunting with dogs.

The provisions of the wildlife law are dealt with in some detail in Cooper (1987), Holden (1998); Lorton (2000); Palmer (2001); Parkes and Thornley (1997); and PAW (2005) (http://www.defra.gov.uk/paw/publications/law/appendf.htm).

The WCA is unusual in that it permits any person to take of sick and injured protected species for the purpose of tending and caring for them until they are fit to return to the wild. Severely injured specimens may be killed if they are beyond recovery. In other countries, for example Canada and the USA, such activities would have to be carried out under permit or by some authorised person or organisation and wildlife rehabilitators have to be trained and licensed (Figure 3.4).

Rehabilitation is carried out within the context of other laws, notably those on welfare and veterinary attention. Thus, while the Veterinary Surgeons Act 1966 (VSA) allows any person to carry out first aid in an emergency and an owner to give minor medical attention, any higher level of treatment must be provided by a veterinarian. Some procedures may be carried out by veterinary nurses or students under various levels of supervision. Schedule 4 listed birds, particularly certain birds of

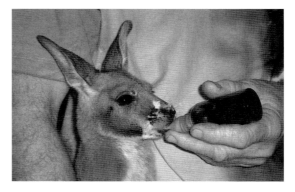

Figure 3.4 Kangaroo rehabilitation in Australia must be carried out under permit.

prey, must be appropriately ringed (banded, see Chapter 4) and registered while held in captivity. This provision applies even if the birds have been taken from the wild for rehabilitation, although there is an exception for veterinary surgeons who may keep such birds without ringing and registration for up to six weeks while undergoing treatment. The legal aspects of wildlife rehabilitation have been covered above by Cooper (2003b).

The wildlife legislation of each country reflects its particular needs (see Chapter 5) but typical wildlife provisions can include:

- Prohibition of killing, taking or injuring protected species.
- Prohibition of taking, disturbing or destroying eggs, nests or shelters of protected species.
- The possession of protected species and derivatives.
- Prohibition of disturbance during the breeding season (Figure 3.5).
- Controls on in-country trade.
- Controls on international trade.
- Controls on the introduction to the wild of alien species other than those that are already established.
- Controls on the use of traps, snares and poison.
- Controls on hunting methods.
- Authorisation of the use of protected species for certain purposes, such as scientific research, education, captive-breeding and sustainable use.
- Authorisation for the control of protected species that damage crops, fisheries and other property or pose a risk to public health.
- Enforcement powers, offences, penalties.
- Protective legislation for individual species, such as the bald eagle in the USA, badgers in Britain and the Philippine eagle in the Philippines.

Implications for the forensic expert

Effective enforcement of wildlife legislation is essential to protect species and habitat that is at risk. Countries vary greatly in the levels of enforcement, depending on the resources available, government policy and priorities, public attitudes and the quality of wildlife legislation. Cases range from small-scale

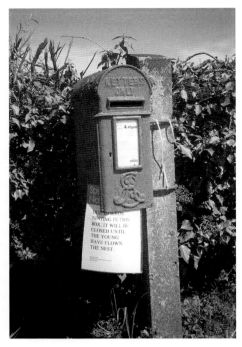

Figure 3.5 A rural mailbox in England is closed while it is in use by nesting birds. By law nests must not be taken, damaged or destroyed while in use.

trapping or poisoning, to complex, dangerous and costly investigations leading to the prosecution of serious criminal activity (see Chapter 5). When enforcement is undertaken, expert advice and evidence is often required. Veterinary and other specialists may be involved in accompanying the police in the execution of search warrants (see Chapter 9). They may be used to examine or identify species and to ring, tag or microchip animals that are likely to be used as evidence.

In England, the wildlife legislation has been extensively litigated over the years. This is due not only to prosecutions taken by the enforcing authorities, Police and Crown Prosecution Service (CPS), Customs and DEFRA but also due to prosecutions initiated by charities such as the RSPB, RSPCA and NFBG (see Appendix B), either by way of private prosecution or in conjunction with the usual enforcement bodies. Many of these prosecutions have used experts, both to give evidence and to assist with the investigation of suspected wildlife crimes. Typical cases are reported by organisations, on the Internet or in their publications such as the RSPB's *Legal Eagle*, the NFBG's *Badger News* and on the website of the Partnership against Wildlife Crime (PAW, see Appendix B) (http://www.defra.gov.uk/paw/prosecutions/default.htm).

The major wildlife and animal charities in Britain tend to be well funded and some of their monies may be donated or earmarked for enforcement of wildlife and other animal protection legislation. Such bodies tend to be passionate about their cause and their partisan approach may not fit easily with the expert witness's duty of giving objective and impartial evidence to the court (see Chapter 12). While some experts act only for either the defence or prosecution/complainant, or for a particular body, other experts may find that their skills are also in demand from the other side. There is no reason why an expert with appropriate skills should not cross the divide, and many do so. That this may help someone in need of support or be in the interests of justice, may not necessarily be understood or appreciated by people or organisations that are strongly partisan. Equally, the expert may have, on occasion, to be able to withstand inappropriate pressures from a dedicated organisation and to advise objectively. Some guidance can be drawn from the strong emphasis now placed in civil law cases upon the expert's objectivity (see Chapter 12).

Trade in protected species

There are extensive controls on trade in endangered species both under national wildlife law and under the legislation on CITES.

National wildlife laws normally restrict the in-country sale of protected species. In some countries, the provisions or their enforcement may be less than adequate. Even countries that have good trade controls cannot totally prevent illegal trading but successful prosecutions, publicity and public education and co-operation amongst enforcers and interested organisations and individuals have a positive effect. The results of such a policy can be seen in the publications and websites of organisations involved in the protection of wildlife, for example, in the RSPB's *Legal Eagle* and *Bird Crime* (http://www.rspb.org.uk/policy/wildbirdslaw/rspb_publications.asp), and the Bulletins of PAW

(http://www.defra.gov.uk/paw/prosecutions/default.htm).

A wide variety of expert evidence has always played an important part in enforcement of wildlife laws. Veterinarians are able to provide opinions on matters such as time and cause of death or injury, identification, breeding condition, welfare or, perhaps based on findings such as parasites or stomach contents (see Chapter 8), provenance.

The CITES Convention (http://www.cites.org/) regulates the international movement (whether for trade or not) of the species to which this treaty applies. Although the provisions of the Convention have to be implemented by each of the 169 Parties (as at February 2006) through their national laws, there is a worldwide system of import and export permits issued by the CITES Management Authority for the relevant country. Any international movement of the species or their 'derivatives' that are listed in Appendices I, II or III to CITES requires permits. These are issued by the national CITES Management Authority subject to the advice of the country's CITES Scientific Authority. These are listed on the CITES website and Management Authorities are usually to be found in the government department that deals with wildlife or the environment.

The key points of the CITES legislation are:

- The CITES Convention requires the Parties (member nations) to implement the Convention's obligations and to provide enforcement measures, such as offences and penalties.
- The species covered by CITES are listed in Annex I, II, III to the Convention.
- A permit is required for live animals, carcases and any derivative of the animal, including biological samples.
- CITES Appendix I specimens that have been captive-bred and individually identified may be traded as if they were Appendix II species.
- Countries are permitted to have national CITES legislation that is stricter than the Convention provisions, consequently there is variation between different countries as to the species listed and the level of protection.
- EC Regulations on CITES directly implement CITES (without the need for national laws) in all EU countries. Annexes A, B, C and D apply to

more species and accord higher levels of protection than do the CITES Appendices. The Annexes are useful in that they give both the EU and the Convention status of CITES species. They also provide the common names in English (and the document is also available in other EU languages) as well as the definitive scientific names. The EU legislation is accessible on the internet at http://www.europa.eu.int/comm/environment/cites/legislation_en.htm.

- CITES species that have entered the EU legally or been acquired legally within the EU may thereafter be moved around EU countries without further authorisation. It is, however, necessary to be able to prove their legal provenance, i.e. that an animal was captive-bred or was taken from the wild or imported under licence.

- The EU law on CITES is enforced by Member States through national law. In England, The Control of Trade in Endangered Species (Enforcement) Regulations 1997 (COTES) (as amended) and the Customs and Excise Management Act 1979 provide the enforcement powers, offences and penalties (http://www.ukcites.gov.uk/default.asp).

The Convention is interpreted in detail by Wijnstekers (2005) and there is extensive information on CITES and its implementation on the Convention website, the website of the EU, of DEFRA, the Joint National Council for Conservation (the UK Scientific Authority) and the UK CITES website. Other countries, such as the USA, also have websites on the subject. Prosecutions take place in many countries and a large amount of illegal material is confiscated. The organisation TRAFFIC (http://www.traffic.org/) investigates, monitors and reports on all aspects of illegal wildlife trade and each issue of its Bulletin lists prosecutions for a wide variety of offences, CITES species and countries (http://www.traffic.org/publications/index.html#bulletin) (Figure 3.6).

The relevance to the forensic expert

There is an extensive illegal trade in CITES (and other endangered) species (see Chapter 5). In value, it is second only to the smuggling of people and drugs and may be combined with other illicit activities. All manner of live animals, trophies and other derivatives of CITES specimens, such as traditional medicines and powdered rhino horn, are smuggled. Snakes and CITES species may be used to disguise or carry drugs or to deter officials from inspecting consignments. There are warehouses full of CITES items that have been seized by Customs around the world and live animals are regularly confiscated (see Chapter 5).

Investigations and prosecutions involving CITES specimens call for experts in species identification, using both gross and DNA techniques, in taxidermy, in veterinary and biological aspects such as health, welfare, public health, behaviour, populations and

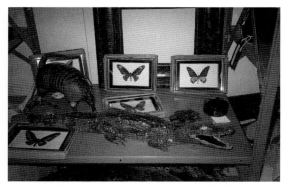

Figure 3.6 International trade in derivatives of CITES species is subject to control and illegal items are frequently confiscated.

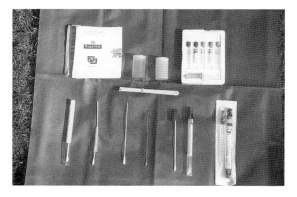

Figure 3.7 The international movement of samples taken from CITES-listed species require CITES, and, in some circumstances, animal health permits.

species, in trade levels, routes and practices. The forensic expert may need to import parts or samples taken from CITES species (for example hair, feathers, skin or blood) in order to examine or produce evidence for a prosecution. The movement of these derivatives is also subject to CITES permits.

Allowance must be made for the time required to obtain CITES animal health or other permits and for the fact that some countries, such as India, are reluctant to permit samples to be processed overseas. A fast-track procedure for time-sensitive biological and diagnostic samples has been agreed although not all countries may have put the procedure in place (Figure 3.7).

CITES prosecutions will often include offences under other legislation. Offences involving general animal welfare, welfare during transportation and animal health requirements often occur when smuggling CITES species, and food hygiene regulations may be broken when selling illegal wild meat (see Chapter 5).

An interesting interaction of laws occurred in 2004 when a fisherman in Wales caught a sturgeon in his nets. He brought it to shore and found out that it was a sturgeon and as such, a 'royal fish' to which the Crown is entitled under the Royal Prerogative. He obtained permission of Buckingham Palace to keep the animal and do with it as he wished. He put it on sale in the market. He was then informed that this was illegal without a permit as the fish was a CITES specimen under the EC Regulations for Annex A species (most sturgeon are Annex A, including the common sturgeon). Meanwhile, the sturgeon was stolen and the police became involved in investigating the theft. Eventually the sturgeon was recovered and given to the Natural History Museum, which coveted it for their collections and is, in fact, the normal beneficiary of 'fish royal' (http://news.bbc.co.uk/1/hi/wales/3776003.stm).

International movement

There is extensive animal health legislation that provides powers to manage outbreaks of disease in animals. It also controls the importation and exportation of animals through veterinary health checks, certification, and licences with the aim of reducing the introduction of disease into a country from outside.

Most countries in the world have legal or administrative procedures that protect animal health since major outbreaks, as in the case of avian influenza, attract international attention and demand for action. The OIE (World Organisation for Animal Health) (see Appendix B) manages the international animal health information system, based on reports of the occurrence of 'notifiable' diseases and the harmonisation of animal health measures and standards (http://www.oie.int/eng/info/en_info.htm). The European Union has extensive legislation on animal health. Offences that may occur are false certification, lack of permits, failure to check animals and documentation, or other breaches of the required procedures.

In-country disease control

There is a duty to report any suspected cases of diseases that are designated in the animal health legislation as a 'notifiable' disease (http://www.defra.gov.uk/animalh/diseases/notifiable/index.htm). The relevant ministry has powers to investigate the outbreak and instigate measures to control it, including the isolation of animals or premises and to impose controls on the movement of animals, people and traffic. Particular offences that may occur are the failure to report a suspected outbreak or breach of the movement controls.

Veterinarians carry heavy responsibilities for accurate and truthful health certification and the checking of documents and consignments (see Chapters 2 and 6). Delays and the mistiming of documentation can lead to heavy financial loss for the importer or exporter. Faulty (not necessarily fraudulent) certificates and documentation can also result in the rejection of animals on arrival at their destination and considerable financial loss. It is still not always recognised that the importation of species that are both listed on CITES and subject to the animal health importation controls require permits from authorities that are usually in two separate ministries or departments. These problems can result in investigations, prosecutions and civil law claims for compensation in which experts may then be required to give evidence.

VETERINARY LAW

Most countries have legislation that regulates veterinary surgeons (veterinarians). Many have strong legislation and a professional body that exercises an extensive control over its members (see Chapter 2). A typical Veterinary Surgeons Act in any country regulates the profession by providing for a supervisory board, council or chamber. This will oversee the management of the profession and the right to practise as a veterinary surgeon (veterinarian), including the registration of duly qualified applicants, the provision of guidance for their conduct and the investigation of unprofessional behaviour.

Conversely, some countries have no more professional organisation than an Act, a veterinary board and registration procedures (which may or may not be active) and may lack a code of conduct or fail to act on the misuse of the appellation 'veterinary surgeon' or its equivalent. Some countries may not have legislation at all. Professional indemnity insurance may not be used or, where the insurance market is not well developed, may be unavailable. A veterinary surgeon accustomed to a strict professional regime who intends to work or give evidence in respect of a less well-organised system may encounter a variety of shortcomings. Further, different attitudes to animals and veterinary practice and a possible lack of awareness of standards required elsewhere may have an influence on a foreign expert's opinion or at least upon how it is presented and how it is received by the litigants and the court.

Normally, registration is required in order to practise in a given country, however limited the general professional regulation may be. Sometimes there is a facility to register but an additional procedure and fee if the veterinarian is actually to engage in private practice, rather than teaching or research. Veterinary surgeons who hold degrees from certain Commonwealth and EU veterinary schools, may have an automatic right of registration in the UK as an MRCVS. If there is no such right to registration, applicants usually have to pass an examination before being accepted. There is some reciprocity for MsRCVS seeking to practise in Commonwealth countries. Registration is unlikely to be required if a veterinary surgeon goes overseas to examine material or to give expert evidence in court, although it may be wise to get an assurance on this from the local lawyer. Veterinary surgeons may be able to obtain cover on their own professional indemnity insurance if they are acting as an expert overseas as an adjunct of their home veterinary practice. However, if the expert is permanently based abroad and the work arises from this, cover may be a problem if it is not obtainable locally.

Veterinary legislation should (but sometimes fails to) lay down clearly what constitutes veterinary practice – the procedure, the animals concerned and who may perform veterinary tasks. Some countries permit veterinary nurses, technicians and others to carry out a limited range of veterinary procedures such as injections, removal of sutures and maintenance of anaesthesia. In many countries, a code of professional conduct supplements the legislation. This can range from basic requirements of loyalty to the profession and restraints on advertising to extensive supervision, standards for practices, relations with clients and colleagues, animal welfare and disciplinary procedures.

Offences under the veterinary legislation are unusual in Britain but may arise there or elsewhere in the EU if foreign veterinarians with an automatic right to register fail to realise that formal registration procedures are a requisite. Likewise, misuse of the title of 'veterinary surgeon' (or 'veterinarian' or 'veterinary doctor') is rare in Britain but may be common in countries where a fully qualified veterinary service is not available in rural and remote areas. Hearings that frequently involve expert veterinary evidence are cases that are brought before a disciplinary committee of the profession. In Britain, disciplinary measures are taken by The Royal College of Veterinary Surgeons in respect of matters such as fraudulent registration, criminal convictions that render a veterinary surgeon unfit to practise and disgraceful conduct in a professional respect. The last category may relate to issues such as animal welfare, the veterinary surgeon's relations with clients, false certification or personal conduct. Situations that have been examined in the disciplinary process (including preliminary enquiries, etc.) are reported on the RCVS website (see Appendix B) and in annual reports; they indicate the scope of complaints and the attitude of the Disciplinary Committee of the RCVS.

It is unusual for disciplinary cases to involve questions of professional negligence (malpractice) because the client has an appropriate remedy of compensation in the courts. However, in recent years professional bodies have started to consider cases of severe negligence as a disciplinary matter. It was held in February 2006 (in the case involving Sir Roy Meadow which was then subsequently reversed on appeal on the issue of witness indemnity) that only a court may refer the conduct of experts to their professional bodies to consider whether the quality of their evidence amounted to professional misconduct (see Chapter 12).

Professional negligence, where the veterinarian (as with any professional) performs below the standard expected of veterinarians of that standing, is a matter of civil law and a complainant must sue in the civil courts for compensation. The principles of professional negligence i.e. the failure to practise to a well-recognised standard of a reasonably competent member of the profession concerned (*Bolam v Friern Hospital Management Committee (1957)*) have been established in the course of extensive litigation in relation to a variety of professions.

Clients are often confused by the distinction between negligence and professional misconduct. A dissatisfied, distressed or disgruntled client may make a complaint whether it appears justified or not (see Chapter 6). The GPC (RCVS, 2000 and http://www.rcvs.org.uk/Templates/Internal. asp?NodeID=89642) has, however, a bearing on professional negligence cases because it demonstrates the standards that are expected of a veterinary surgeon practising within the jurisdiction.

Experts are frequently used in hearings involving veterinarians. Either side in a disciplinary, breach of contract or negligence claim may need supporting expert evidence on a wide range of issues, including veterinary treatment, animal health and welfare, certification, practice standards and assessment of the quality of veterinary services. Human occupational health and safety and other aspects of running a practice can also give rise to litigation and require an expert opinion. New areas of expertise and activity may come under consideration, for example the field of telemedicine, raising questions about liability that may not be immediately answerable (Brahams, 1995).

The medicines legislation is also a source of veterinary responsibilities. These include:

- The right to possess, supply and administer medicinal products.
- The prescription, supply and administration of medicinal products; dosage and withdrawal periods; use of data sheets.
- The choice of medicinal product and use of the cascade, used when approved drugs are not available for the species or the condition.
- Clinical judgement and informed consent.

The levels of compliance and enforcement of the medicinal product legislation vary extensively between different countries. Prosecution arises from the illegal possession and use and abuse of drugs. The veterinarian in practice may also have to deal with claims of negligence in relation to the selection, prescription and administration of medicinal products and issues of lack of informed consent.

ENFORCEMENT POWERS, OFFENCES AND PENALTIES

It has often been said that animal law (as with any other law), is of little real value unless it is effectively enforced. Each piece of legislation is supported by powers of implementation and enforcement. This depends to some extend on the will of the authority but also on the adequacy of the powers provided in the legislation. Efforts to improve legislation, especially relating to animal welfare and conservation, have focused on stronger enforcement powers and tougher penalties as well as better substantive law.

The Partnership against Wildlife Crime (see Chapter 5 and Appendix B) has facilitated collaboration amongst enforcing authorities and other individuals and bodies interested in wildlife. This has produced a concerted voice and has helped to achieve improvements in the legislation and in enforcement. Meetings of PAW provide a forum for the discussion of both achievement and problems involved in enforcement, and an opportunity for exchange of information and expertise. PAW has a Working Group on DNA and other forensic techniques; other Groups are active in public education and improvements in the law (http://www.defra. gov.uk/paw/pack/default.htm).

Enforcement powers include rights of entry and powers of arrest in the investigation of crimes, as well as the range of penalties that include not only fines and imprisonment but also confiscation of equipment and disqualification from keeping animals. Other bodies may also exercise enforcement powers, for example the Customs authority may prosecute offences involving illegal entry of animals under COTES and under Customs regulations; likewise, smuggling may involve a breach of the animal health importation legislation. Further, an individual may bring a private prosecution and this is sometimes used by the animal welfare and wildlife charities when they decide to take action themselves or if the Crown Prosecution Service declines to undertake a prosecution.

Enforcement powers are usually vested in the police, the Minister responsible for the legislation, for example, in Britain, DEFRA in the case of the wildlife legislation and animal health and welfare and the Home Office for research animals. DEFRA collaborates with other enforcement authorities and it also has Wildlife Inspectors who assist in checking compliance (see Chapter 5).

INVESTIGATION OF SUSPECTED OFFENCES

Experts may be involved in law enforcement, in the identification and collection of evidence, or in assisting the police or other enforcing authority at crime scenes to assess evidence *in situ*. In such situations, in Britain, they will be acting under the Police and Criminal Evidence Act 1984 Code B 2005 on searching premises and seizing property. Veterinary surgeons, biologists and other experts such as taxonomists may be used to identify animals (live or dead), to make assessments of the condition and behaviour of confiscated animals and in handling them or applying identification marks or microchips.

CONCLUSION

Animal law and its related topics create many situations that call for the skills of the expert witness, whether from the veterinary and other scientific disciplines or from practical skills and arts. Evidence may relate to animals, humans and property or to abstract matters such as statistics and probability. Evidence on treatment, management, behaviour, suffering, wounding, poisoning, trapping, death, species identification, may enable a court to come to a conclusion. Whether a case arises from an offence, a claim for breach of contract, for compensation or to stop a nuisance, to establish an insurance claim or valuation, in a tribunal or alternative dispute resolution or in a disciplinary action, expert evidence is frequently required. The role of the expert witness in animal law cases is an important aspect of the administration of justice and the protection of humans, animals and the environment but it is also a difficult and demanding one.

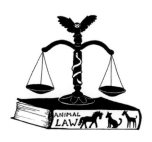

Particular Types of Case

Animal Welfare

Surely we ought to show them [animals] great kindness and gentleness for many reasons, but, above all, because they are of the same origin as ourselves.

St. Chrysostom

Concern for the welfare of animals has long been a feature of many societies (Broom, 2003). Some of the world's major religions, such as Buddhism and Hinduism, preach respect for living things and advocate the principle of *ahimsa* – not harming. In both the Bible and the Koran there are instructions that animals should be treated kindly: examples in the Old Testament include injunctions not to overload animals (Deuteronomy XXII, 4) and for young animals to be with their mother for at least seven days (Leviticus XXII, 27). One Islamic Hadith recounts that a woman was punished after death because she had confined a cat without giving it food or drink 'nor had she left it free to eat the creatures of the earth.'

Over the past 200 years, there has been a growth of interest in, and concern for, the welfare of animals and in sections of some societies this has reached a level that at times borders on irrationality, even extremism, which may actually cause animals more harm and suffering (see later).

In countries such as the UK, cases relating to animal welfare are often the primary occupation of veterinarians who are actively involved in legal work or find themselves called to give evidence. However, welfare cases can be amongst the most difficult to resolve because of the complexity of the subject and the intricacies of many definitions relating to welfare. These issues are discussed, but in most cases not resolved, in the succeeding pages.

DEFINITIONS

What is animal welfare? As indicated above, it is not easy to define and this presents impediments in legal and other hearings. One scientific explanation that is widely used is that 'the welfare of an individual animal is its state as regards its attempt to cope with its environment, with attempts to cope including the functioning of body repair systems, immunological defences, the physiological stress response and a variety of behavioural responses' (Broom, 1996). In practical terms this means that one must accept that a normal healthy animal may be exposed to various stressors such as heat, cold, exertion or disease and in most cases will respond and adapt to them in a variety of ways (see below). Once the stressors become too great, however, the animal's ability to cope may be reduced or inadequate. There are then physiological, behavioural and sometimes pathological changes in the animal and clinical signs of pain, distress or ill-health may follow. It is at this stage that the animal's welfare is compromised.

The term 'cruelty' presents even more difficulties in terms of definition. The Oxford Dictionary gives one meaning as 'indifference to another's suffering.' Often the word implies an *intentional* attitude (in other words, that cruelty is a state of mind as well as an action or omission) but in law cruelty may or may not involve awareness of the physical or mental harm that is being inflicted. The legal definitions of cruelty vary widely from one jurisdiction to another and often encompass the public's perception that the maltreatment must be intentional to warrant court action. As a result, those considering prosecuting can be reluctant to bring charges except in the most egregious cases and the courts may be disinclined to convict. Figures from the Royal Society for the Prevention of Cruelty to Animals (RSPCA) in the UK (see later) help to substantiate this. Similar figures exist in the US where, for example, the Massachusetts Society for Prevention of Cruelty to animals (SPCA) was able to bring charges only against 0.335% of 80,000 investigations of alleged cruelty and neglect over a 20-year period (Arluke & Luke, 1997). Consequently, new categories of animal maltreatment have been proposed; the term 'abuse' is sometimes preferred over 'cruelty', modelling similar changes in the child protection field. 'Abuse' then defines a state of maltreatment without the implication that any intent was involved (see Chapter 6).

Perhaps the most effective definition of 'cruelty' is in a veterinary medical dictionary (Blood and Studdert, 1988) in which the word is given as 'the infliction of pain or distress unnecessarily.' This wisely cautions the reader that 'the definition of unnecessary varies between countries and from time to time in one country. Determination of the prevailing standard of cruelty can only be decided by the courts.'

PAIN

Pain has been defined by the International Association for the Study of Pain (IASP) (see Appendix B) as 'the unpleasant sensory and/or emotional experience associated with actual or potential tissue damage' (Hellebrekers, 2000). Broom (2001) used the word 'aversive' rather than 'unpleasant', arguing that the former was easier to identify and assess in animals.

The deep-seated significance of pain was recognised 2000 years ago by Plato, who described it as 'an emotion that dulls in the brain'. In the 1960s a seminal work appeared, drawing parallels between pain in humans and animals and emphasising the

need to address pain and its consequences (Keele and Smith, 1962). More recently, Broom (2001) emphasised that 'pain is clearly an important part of welfare' (see later).

Pain, which can be acute or chronic, is complex in terms of its physiology, psychology and evolution and has spawned investigation and research involving scientists and others from many disciplines. This is not the place to discuss the various philosophies, hypotheses and proven facts. Useful references to pain include Iggo (1984), Short and van Poznak (1992), Wall and Melzack (1994) and Rutherford (2002).

Pain has evolved and is both functional and adaptive – in other words, it is generally beneficial (Broom, 2001). The 'pain system' probably exists in all vertebrates and, in part, in invertebrates (see later – Sentience, p. 73).

Recognition of pain is not easy and yet can be a crucial consideration in a legal case where cruelty is alleged. The main methods are based on changes in:

- Behaviour.
- Physiology.

Insofar as behaviour is concerned, earlier studies were often very focused, concentrating on laboratory animals. The tail-flick response has been used for several decades to indicate pain in rats (Dubner, 1994). However, as Broom (2001, 2003) pointed out, behavioural patterns differ between species and even within a species at certain times. These are probably survival strategies. African antelopes attacked by a hyaena rarely vocalise, nor do sheep attacked by dogs; a monkey giving birth is generally silent. Cats in a stressful environment or in pain may 'sham sleep' and many species play dead or manifest tonic immobility and display stereotypies – repetitive movements – which may also indicate pain, stress or distress (Mason and Rushen, 2006). To these variables can be added breed and individual differences; there is, for example, often a marked variability in how dogs respond to spinal pain.

Physiological changes in pain may include increases in plasma values of adrenaline, noradrenaline, cortisol or adrenocorticotropic hormone (ACTH), an increase in heart rate and changes in systolic, diastolic and mean arterial blood pressure.

Pain assessment scales are in standard use for laboratory animals in some parts of the world. Similar scales have been used to assess pain in domesticated animals but are not always reliable (Holton *et al.*, 1998). More reliable methods, for acute or chronic pain, are being developed for dogs (Holton *et al.*, 2001).

One approach that is increasingly finding favour is to see if clinical signs or behavioural changes that are assumed to be due to pain are reduced or disappear following the use of an analgesic. This can be self-selected, as shown by studies using the analgesic agent carprofen in lame broiler chickens (Danbury *et al.*, 2000).

Post-mortem examination (see Chapter 7) and supporting laboratory tests (see Chapter 8) can help in assessing whether an animal was likely to have been in pain when it was alive. Gross lesions, e.g. neoplasms, may be found to be pressing on the peripheral or central nervous system. Histopathological examination of ulcerating wounds may confirm damage to nerves and of fractures can provide information on the extent of bone damage and healing (Butterworth *et al.*, 1987).

STRESS

Stress is a frequently used word that is rarely properly defined. Some lay definitions are very broad – for example:

Any physical or psychological condition that tends to disrupt normal functions of the body or mind.

(*Melloni's Medical Dictionary*, 2002)

Our scientific understanding and interpretation of stress are still largely based on Hans Selye's seminal work of the 1930s (Selye, 1950) and this can provide a useful background to those who are unfamiliar with terminology – for example, the difference between *stressors*, that impinge on the animal, and *stress* that can thereby result. This progression is depicted in Figure 4.1.

Selye discussed stressors and described how humans and other species could respond to and finally be overcome by these as part of the General Adaptation Syndrome (GAS). The stages of GAS were, he said, as follows:

* Alarm reaction (AR).
* Stage of resistance (SR).
* Stage of exhaustion (SE).

When an animal reaches the stage of exhaustion, profound and deleterious changes can take place, including the development of pathological lesions, such as gastric ulceration and alterations to the immune system.

Selye's concepts still provide a basis for an understanding of stress. However, it is argued by some that they are too imprecise (Broom and Johnson, 1993) and succeeding decades have seen changes in how stress is perceived. This is particularly the case amongst the public, for whom the word has a very

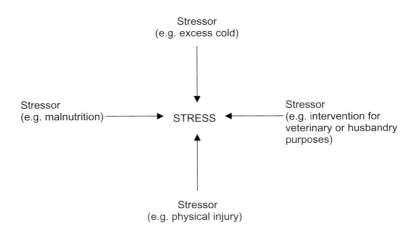

Figure 4.1 The relationship between stressors and stress.

amorphous meaning, encompassing even daily irritations and challenges (although it is worth mentioning that 'informational stress' may be a distinct clinical syndrome – see Restian, 1990).

There has been a substantial increase in scientific thinking about stress: a useful summary of developments in the three decades subsequent to Selye's book was provided by Moberg (1985) and updated fifteen years later by Moberg and Mench (2000). In particular, it is now recognised that environmental stressors may predispose humans and animals to a variety of pathological changes – for example, the various biochemical, histological and infectious lesions that can occur in cattle that are exposed to heat in the tropics (Suliman *et al.*, 1989; Hansen, 1990; see also Chapter 6).

One thing is certain. Any bid to eliminate stress in humans and animals is not, *per se*, well-founded. Stressors and stress have for long been part of a living organism's existence and the mechanisms serve a protective role. Selye himself (1974) stated that an absence of stress occurs only after death! In legal cases, therefore, care must be taken not to assume that stressors are inevitably deleterious or that clinical stress is automatically a bad sign. Nevertheless, stress and animal welfare can be closely linked, as emphasised by Wiepkema and Koolhaas (1993).

OTHER TERMS

Many other words are used in the context of welfare. Some form part of legislation in certain countries, others do not. 'Starvation', 'inanition' and 'neglect' are defined in Chapters 6 and 7 and their detection, clinically or *post mortem*, is outlined there.

The term 'fear' also appears in legislation and might therefore be relevant in forensic cases. Detection and assessment of fear can appear to be relatively straightforward – when, for example, an animal cowers, whimpers or takes evasive action – but fear in animals, as in humans, can manifest itself in other ways. For example, tonic immobility (a catatonic-like state, induced by gentle physical restraint, considered by some to be an anti-predator response) in domesticated poultry is now accepted

as a measure of 'fearfulness' and has elicited considerable study (Mills and Nicol, 1990) that may be relevant to how birds are kept and handled.

The word 'shock' is used in everyday parlance to describe the reaction of humans to bad news or a traumatic incident. The origin of the word and its connotations were ably recounted by Rutty (2004). The various usages, while possibly important, have no proper place in animal welfare terminology and the word 'shock' is best reserved for those circulatory changes that can follow haemorrhage, infection, endotoxaemia, anaphylaxis and certain other insults (Michell, 1985) (see Appendix C).

The word 'suffering' presents particular problems in a legal context, not least because it has broad usage. A simple (Oxford) dictionary definition of 'undergoing or being subject to pain, loss, damage, etc.' is not helped by the alternative explanation of 'tolerating' as the latter could be taken to imply that suffering is not severe. Ultimately it is the court that must decide, based on statute, precedent or reasoned argument.

The main tenet of English and Scottish welfare legislation has in the past been to determine whether or not an animal has undergone 'unnecessary suffering'. The term implies that some suffering may be necessary, e.g. pain during assisted-delivery of a calf, or the treatment of piglets by irritant injection for iron-deficiency anaemia.

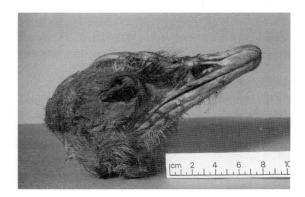

Figure 4.2 The head of a young captive ostrich that was killed by a blow to the head. The question here was 'Did the bird suffer?' This figure also appears in colour in the colour plate section.

ASSESSMENT OF WELFARE

How can animal welfare be assessed? What is cruelty? Is it possible to measure and to grade pain and distress in animals? These and other questions have taxed some people for centuries, as the words of St. Chrysostom, at the beginning of this chapter, remind us. It was not, however, only religious persons who pondered such matters. The great British humanist, Jeremy Bentham, put it succinctly when he said:

> *The day may come when the rest of animal creation may acquire those rights which never could have been withheld from them but by the hand of tyranny. . . . The question is not can they reason? nor, can they talk? but, can they suffer?*

The assessment of welfare (good or bad) has been assisted greatly in recent years as a result of sound science and the appearance of a number of scholarly, but sensitive, publications. Perhaps the best reference material for non-specialists who are involved in forensic work and need to know about current thinking concerning welfare is the UFAW (Universities Federation for Animal Welfare) series (see, for example, Young, 2003 and Gregory, 2004).

Methods of assessing welfare – and, as a corollary, of attempting to determine whether 'cruelty' may have occurred – are at present usually based upon:

- Behaviour.
- Disease.
- Physiological values.
- Immunological parameters.
- Production (e.g. of eggs or milk).
- Response to treatment.
- A combination of the above.

Practical approaches to assessing welfare have been accompanied by more 'scientific', sometimes esoteric, methods. An important landmark was the publication by Morton and Griffiths (1985) which put forward guidelines for the recognition of pain, distress and discomfort in laboratory animals and advocated a simple scoring system for different species. This paper was not only important in its own right but also paved the way for more in-depth research and publications (see, for example, Broom and Johnson, 1993) which led to the introduction

of less subjective methods of assessing welfare in other animals. These have included quantification of changes in tissues that are associated with pain or distress – for example, in all species, the measuring of length, breadth and depth of wounds.

In some cases specific methods have found favour; in horses with chronic foundered feet, for instance, by calculating the position and displacement of the pedal bone using a prepared specimen or model demonstrating this with a Strasser's plastic sheet (Florence and Reilly, 2003). Such approaches make it easier to explain to a court that the animal had lesions that are associated with (e.g.) pain. However, they do not necessarily help in determining whether their presence warrants a charge of 'cruelty' or, indeed, whether the animal's welfare was significantly compromised.

Even in domesticated animals, which have been associated with the human race for thousands of years, what constitutes 'unnecessary suffering' (see earlier and Chapter 3) can be extremely difficult to define. A Friesian (Holstein) cow on a dairy farm in North America may well show signs suggestive of suffering if it is deprived of water for four days but a short-horned zebu in East Africa, accustomed to surviving in semi-arid areas, will readily tolerate 7–10 days without drinking. The situation can be far more complex when dealing with wildlife or captive 'exotic' species (Cooper and Williams, 1995).

Old-age brings its own challenges and geriatric pets are presented in increasing numbers at veterinary clinics with a variety of disorders that affect their quality of life and survival. Some of these can include chronic pain – arthritis, for example – and such cases may attract attention from those who want to suggest that the animal is suffering and thereby cruelty is being caused. The onus is on the clinician, with the aid of second opinions as necessary, to perform a proper assessment and to calculate as far as is possible how the welfare of the animal is compromised through either not being treated or because it is being kept alive.

An assessment of whether suffering occurred is generally even less easy when the animal is dead. The pathologist can use a number of the same criteria as would a clinician but behavioural studies are clearly impossible and many of the other methods listed on the previous page cannot be employed. On the other hand, the pathologist may be able to demonstrate, *post mortem*, lesions that are unequivocally associated with pain or discomfort, such as the stretching of meninges over nerve roots or chronic skin lesions (see also earlier).

As was stated earlier, whether or not an animal has suffered 'unnecessarily' has for nearly 100 years been the key point in English (1911) and Scottish (1912) law (see Chapter 3). The expert should confine him/herself to the animal by sticking to the facts of objective observation and documented investigation and findings and be wary of assessing whether suffering was or was not 'necessary'. The latter judgement can relate to circumstances of

which the expert is not aware and is therefore best left to the court.

The expert in a welfare case may have to be cautious in answers to questions. The answer 'It depends . . .' may well appear hackneyed – and can elicit an impatient retort from a lawyer during cross-examination – but is sometimes a wise response.

ATTITUDES TO ANIMAL WELFARE

How people perceive and respond to animals varies greatly. Kellert (1979, 1988) summarised as follows the spectrum of attitudes that Americans (citizens of the USA) have to animals:

- Humanistic.
- Naturalistic.
- Moralistic.
- Ecologistic.
- Aesthetic.
- Scientific.
- Utilitarian.
- Dominionistic.
- Negativistic.
- Neutralistic.

Although these terms appear self-explanatory, the distinction between them is often imprecise. Attitudes shown towards animals can be more simply divided into three main categories (see Table 4.1).

Awareness of these three broader categories can help those involved in a legal case to understand the

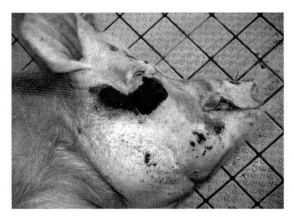

Figure 4.3 The head of a sow that died following a week's recumbency. Skin lesions, that became infected, are apparent. This figure also appears in colour in the colour plate section. (Courtesy of Richard Spence.)

Table 4.1 Three key categories of public attitudes towards animals.

Protectionist	*Stewardship*	*Utilisation*
Animals are seen as fellow beings, often 'companions', worthy of full protection under the law. They may only be kept in captivity under very special circumstances and should only rarely be killed or exploited. Welfare is all-important.	Animals are seen as an integral part of biodiversity worthy of a degree of protection under the law. However, they may be killed, taken into captivity or used under controlled (humane) circumstances. Humans have a responsibility for them.	Animals are seen as just one component of the world, not warranting special protection. They are freely available to be used, taken into captivity or killed in the wild. Welfare is of little or no importance.

different ways in which members of the public may perceive and treat animals. The distinctions are not clear-cut and are discussed in a little more detail below.

To the *protectionist*, virtually all species are worthy of legal protection that helps to ensure their long-term survival and good welfare. Animals have 'rights' and deserve a legal status: great apes may even merit the same privileges as human beings. Having said that, 'speciesism' is often a feature of such views and a charismatic mammal or bird may be deemed more worthy of protection than, for example, the rat in the sewer, the frog in the drain or the mosquito in the forest. Particular types of animal usage or exploitation may also attract undue attention and concern: the use of animals in research, for example, often elicits far more campaigning and demands for action than does the plight of fish caught at sea that are either drowned in a gill net or left to suffocate on the trawler deck. The different categories of animal use (companionship, research, etc.) are linked to 'situational ethics' where animal suffering may be justified in one situation but not in another (Fox, 2001).

Stewards are broader in their approach and it is less easy to classify such people. They recognise the importance of animals and the need both to treat them humanely and to conserve them in the wild. At the same time, however, responsible killing (for human good, or because they are pests) is accepted, as is the keeping of animals in captivity for conservation, education or research so long at this is done humanely.

Those who are proponents of *utilisation* do not consider that animals have any particular features that make them specially worthy of protection. In the eyes of such people, there are no ethical issues associated with killing for food, for sport or because animals are pests. Likewise, animals may be brought into captivity without any need to impose strict rules on, for example, cage sizes or trapping methods.

Within each of these three groups there is much variation and views may be influenced by peer pressure and by the media. Thus, amongst protectionists there are some people who consider it unacceptable to keep birds in captivity, while others argue that if the birds are domesticated, like

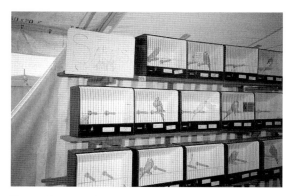

Figure 4.4 Birds being offered for sale in the UK in 'show cages'. While not illegal *per se*, this practice may constitute a de facto offence if the birds cannot fully stretch their wings in all directions.

canaries, they are better adapted to a life of captivity and so do not present an ethical dilemma.

In recent years, especially in North America, the term 'guardian' has often been introduced, as an alternative to 'owner', to describe the relationship between animals and their owners. Although the former would appear to reflect a more caring responsible approach to animals, it is controversial and in 2005 the American Veterinary Medical Association (AVMA) revised its original position and opposed any change in terminology, including the use of the word 'guardian'. This decision was discussed with cases from North America, by Jack (2005).

THE INVESTIGATION OF WELFARE CASES

Welfare investigations always require the following:

- Accurate information about the circumstances of the alleged offence (a 'history'), preferably in writing, with photographic/video documentation (see Chapter 10). This should include details of the relevant legislation.
- Prior discussion with those involved in initiating the investigation or in bringing charges.
- Correct identification of the species and individual animals involved.

- A site visit – to the location where the offence is alleged to have occurred or the premises where (for example) the live animals can be viewed or the dead animals/species can be examined (see Chapter 9).
- Consultation with specialists who may be able to help confirm whether or not welfare has been compromised. For example, in the investigation of suspect fractures in poultry, an experienced avian clinician or trained assistant can use palpation to assess damage (Wilkins *et al.*, 2004) and a pathologist can provide information on pathological lesions.
- A willingness to work with people from other disciplines, including behaviourists, biologists, animal welfarists and those with different opinions about (for example) field sports or the keeping of animals in captivity.

Those who are involved must appreciate that animal welfare cases present many dilemmas, not least of all in how to define terms and to explain the concepts to a magistrate, judge or jury – who then must relate what they have heard to the charge and the legislation under which it is being brought.

PERSONNEL

The field of animal welfare is a complex one. Those involved in studying or promoting animal welfare range from academics (ethologists, neurologists, physiologists), who are interested in the effects of pain or stress in animals, through psychologists, criminologists and sociologists, who attempt to unravel the mechanisms by which human beings become abusive to their fellow living creatures, to ordinary people, in most countries of the world, who believe that animals should be treated in a fair and humane manner.

The veterinary profession was originally established in order to diagnose, treat and control diseases of domesticated animals but in countries such as the UK welfare has become an integral part of its responsibilities. A paper about veterinary students' attitudes towards animal welfare (Paul and Podberscek, 2000) emphasised this when it stated in its opening paragraph that 'Concern for the welfare of animals is central to the role of the practising veterinarian.' The authors go on to remind their readers that when veterinary graduates are admitted to the RCVS, each person pledges that his/her 'constant endeavour will be to ensure the welfare of the animals committed to [his/her] care'.

In recent years the introduction in some countries of post-graduate training in animal welfare (usually linked with law and ethics) means that some veterinarians have received specialised training in the field; the other corollary, however, is that non-veterinarians who hold a similar 'specialist' qualification may command a comparable reputation in court or elsewhere.

METHODS USED IN WELFARE INVESTIGATIONS

- Scene of crime visit.
- Collection and identification of specimens, including physical evidence (e.g. traps, guns) and samples from live and dead animals and the environment for laboratory tests (see below).
- Clinical examination of live animals.
- *Post-mortem* examination of dead animals and derivatives.
- Laboratory investigations.

LEGAL ASPECTS

Many countries have legislation that prohibits cruelty to animals (see Chapter 3). In some the legislation is strictly enforced, in others it is not. Definitions of 'cruelty', 'welfare' and other terms differ. Whether cruelty is even detected depends very much on the willingness of members of the public to report alleged abuses and whether or not there are persons in society who are specifically authorised to investigate animal welfare.

In many respects the UK provides a useful example. It was one of the first countries in the world to introduce modern legislation to protect animals and continues to enact statutes that, while allowing for the reasonable use of animals for agriculture, pleasure or research, emphasise the need for a proper cost:benefit analysis so that these animals are not exploited unnecessarily. Even in the UK however, where the populace is generally very supportive of consideration and 'kindness' to animals, there is a substantial amount of animal cruelty.

The most reliable data are probably those produced by the Royal Society for the Prevention of Cruelty to Animals (RSPCA) which has been in existence for over 100 years, and, while not having specific legal powers, is seen by many as the guardian of national animal welfare. The various reports of the RSPCA give some indication as to the likely extent of animal welfare abuses. For example, in 2003, 928 people in England and Wales were prosecuted for animal welfare offences. Of these, 541 had failed to provide veterinary treatment for their animals; 326 had not provided adequate food or water; 129 had failed to provide suitable living conditions; 93 people were convicted of committing deliberate acts of violence against an animal. These prosecutions were out of over 100,000 reports of suspected animal abuse and neglect. During 2003, the RSPCA received over 1,000,000 telephone calls about animals, rescued 11,800 and collected 182,000. Of the prosecution cases, dogs were most frequently involved, followed by cats and then horses. Two years later the RSPCA reported that over a one-year period (June 2004–May 2005), its inspectors investigated 109,985 complaints of alleged cruelty. In addition, the RSPCA's 'welfare inspection forms' (completed by inspectors each time they visit a home, farm or animal-holding establishment) revealed that of 1,043,982 animals seen, concerns were raised about 63,732, a 78% increase on the previous year (Anon., 2005d).

Increasingly there is a more global approach to animal welfare, trying to bring in codes of practice and commitments by governments, even where little or no legislation is available and where there are laws but no effective enforcement and prosecution. The thrust for this has been provided largely by two bodies, the Office International des Epizooties (OIE) and the World Society for the Protection of Animals (WSPA) (see Appendix B). Bayvel (2005a,b) provided a useful perspective, drawing attention to new considerations relating to international trade and the expanding role of the former in respect of animal welfare (Bayvel *et al.*, 2005).

The OIE's new integrated approach was debated at its Annual General Session in Paris in May 2005, a useful summary of which was published by Clark (2005). Amongst other things, OIE agreed to international guidelines to safeguard the welfare of animals being transported by road and by sea, and to give increased protection to animals before slaughter for human consumption and those culled as part of disease control. The OIE guidelines are advisory and do not have legal status. Nevertheless, together with regulations that do carry the weight of the law (e.g. those in the EU), they could be cited in legal, insurance or malpractice hearings where animal welfare is relevant.

HUMAN–ANIMAL RELATIONSHIPS

The close relationship that can exist between humans and animals has long been recognised (see also Chapter 2). Such a relationship is not confined to wealthier countries and can be strongly influenced by religious and cultural attitudes. Affinity with one's animals may be a feature of situations where livestock is kept for commercial or research purposes, such as farming, but it is particularly pronounced in the 'pet' (companionship) situation.

Sometimes, however, the relationship is one marked by aggression or neglect on the part of the human, as a consequence of which an animal suffers and may die. An association in some people between cruelty to animals and the committing of crime was observed many decades ago (Hellman and Blackman, 1966; Rigdon and Tapia, 1977; Tapia, 1971; Wax and Haddox, 1974). Current thinking about links between animal abuse, child abuse and domestic violence is discussed in Chapter 6 and there are numerous papers relevant to this theme listed in the References (see, for example, Arkow, 1992, 1994; Ascione and Arkow, 1999; Kellert and Felthous, 1985; Munro and Thrusfield, 2001a–d). The important role of the veterinary profession in recognising and preventing family violence is discussed in a new book (Arkow and Munro, 2006).

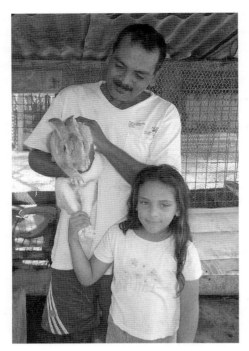

Figure 4.5 A girl who is fond of her rabbits, even though they are being kept for sale as food.

RELIGIOUS INFLUENCES

Animals have long played a part in religious ceremony and tradition (Broom, 2003). The sacrifice of animals played an important part in early Judaeo-Christian-Islamic religious observance and persists in, for example, the insistence to this day on certain methods of slaughter by practising Jews and Moslems. It should be pointed out, however, that some modern animal welfarists and philosophers see the Judaeo-Christian approach, based on the belief that humans alone were made in the image of God, as putting animals in the position of merely performing a utilitarian function.

In other religions the situation may be very different but can still be of relevance to legislation and, as a corollary, to the practice of forensic medicine. Hindus, for example, consider cows (female cattle) to be sacred and there are laws in parts of India that protect these animals and impose penalties on those who intentionally harm or kill them (see Chapter 3). The taboo against euthanasing terminally-ill cattle is based on the notion that to violate the principle of *ahimsa* is to make oneself spiritually impure. Thus cattle in some locations may be considered holy but can suffer because compassionate killing is prohibited by law (see later).

Faith-healing is mentioned in Chapter 6.

RITUAL AND SUPERSTITIOUS BELIEFS

Animals also play a part in other philosophies and in certain cases, e.g. various occult and Satanic rituals, may be subjected to various types of abuse or bizarre methods of slaughter in furtherance of these beliefs. In the USA some of these rituals have received constitutionally-sanctioned protection on the grounds that they constitute freedom of religion (Arkow, pers. comm.).

EXTREMISTS

There are various types of animal 'extremists' – that is, people whose concern (or alleged concern) for animals prompts them to commit aggressive, physically violent, acts. In many such cases the perpetrator is willing to break the law – either actively, for example by breaking into premises or attacking people, or passively, for instance, by staging a 'sit-in' or blocking traffic.

A particularly bizarre example of the fanaticism shown by some animal extremists – with a forensic connotation – relates to a six-year campaign by lobbyists to close down a (laboratory) guinea pig breeding unit in Staffordshire, UK. The owners of the unit were not only intimidated and threatened but in October 2004 the body of one of the family, an 82-year-old woman, was taken from her grave as part of the group's campaign.

The actions of extremists are of relevance to veterinary and comparative forensic work for the following reasons:

- The usual justification for such actions is that it is the *rights* of animals, in respect of their welfare (sometimes conservation), that is of prime importance – rather than their wellbeing *per se*, and that this cause supersedes responsibility for the law and for the rights of other people.

- The actions of extremists often include the release ('liberation') of animals, which can bring in its wake questions and concerns about the welfare of the released animals and the effect of the release on other species and the environment.

Paradoxically, the efforts of extremists can be to lower standards of animal welfare, as in the UK where some pharmaceutical companies, tired of intimidation by 'anti-vivisectionists', have started to do their animal research in countries where the threats from extremists are less but so also is legal protection for laboratory animals.

In the USA, violent action by extremists is commonly termed 'domestic terrorism' (Nolen, 2003) and has led to the inclusion of a provision in the Public Health Security and Bioterrorism Preparedness and Response Act of 2002 that allows those found guilty of such offences to be fined or imprisoned. This and comparable moves elsewhere will open up new challenges (and in some cases raise dilemmas) for veterinarians and others who are called to give evidence.

VALUE OF ANIMALS

The value of animals can be looked at in three ways:

(1) Their worth in human terms because of (e.g.) the pleasure or companionship that they provide, their emotional value and related psychological health benefits (see Chapter 2).
(2) Their compensatory value, if, for instance, the animal is stolen or killed.
(3) Their intrinsic worth, as living, sentient, creatures.

There is much debate about these 'values' and this is relevant to legal and insurance cases. The American Veterinary Medical Association (see Appendix B) has taken a strong stand over this (Kahler and Clark, 2005). In 2005, the AVMA introduced a revised position that, while recognising that some animals have value to their owners that may exceed the animal's market price, stated

that any extension of available remedies beyond economic damages would be inappropriate and ultimately not benefit animals.

REQUIREMENTS OF THE EXPERT

The welfare of animals can be an emotive subject and those likely to be involved in legal or other actions relating to animal welfare need to be aware of this. They themselves must be prepared to be objective and impartial, when serving as experts or providing evidence. They will have to deal with people as well as animals, and those involved may range from distraught owners of animals to pressure groups with a strong, sometimes an unyielding, agenda.

As emphasised earlier, the veterinary profession has traditionally played an important part in animal welfare and alleged abuse/cruelty cases and is still assumed by many to provide the best opinion on whether or not an animal has suffered. In some animal welfare cases, however, even if the veterinary surgeon is the key witness, the defence or the prosecution may call others who have expertise in relevant fields – for example, animal behaviour or nutrition.

JUSTIFICATION FOR PROMOTING THE WELFARE OF ANIMALS

Sentience is the key to current thinking (Wensley, 2005). If an organism can be demonstrated to feel (i.e. subjectively experience) and be affected by adverse stimuli, then its welfare is important, whether it be a humpback whale, a humming-bird or a halibut. Where uncertainty exists as to whether a given species is sentient, it should be given the benefit of the doubt.

The main classes of vertebrates are all, to a greater or lesser extent, responsive to pain and in many countries such animals receive protection under relevant legislation (see Chapter 3). Fish have attracted considerable interest in recent years: there is evidence that they have cognitive abilities and possess the necessary mechanisms to enable them to suffer pain and distress (for a succinct analysis, see Hue,

2005). The same seems true of the other two classes of ectothermic vertebrates – the Amphibia and the Reptilia (see References and Further Reading).

The particular features of ectothermic animals (reptiles, amphibians, fish and invertebrates) (see Chapter 2) that make them difficult subjects for euthanasia (Cooper *et al.*, 1989a; Zwart *et al.*, 1989) (see later) are also relevant to pain.

Interestingly, it is possible that pain may be a 'greater problem' in animals with less good cognitive ability (Broom, 2001). The rationale here is that coping with adversity, including pain, may require sophisticated rationalising ability (Sommerville and Broom, 1998). Pain in 'lower' (ectothermic) vertebrates may, therefore, be of considerably more significance than has hitherto been realised.

The situation regarding invertebrates is more equivocal but there is increasing evidence (based on, for example, behavioural studies and indications of endorphin production following tissue damage) that some metazoan invertebrates, such as molluscs, may not only respond to painful stimuli but be able to perceive them (Cooper, 2001). Two relevant references are Kavaliers (1989) and Sherwin (2001). To suggest that invertebrate animals may be sentient is not new – as Shakespeare put it in *Measure for Measure*:

> ... the poor beetle that we tread upon,
> In corp'ral sufferance finds a pang as great
> As when a giant dies.

Pain and the capacity to experience it are not the sole concern when assessing the welfare of animals. Fear and anxiety are emotional reactions that may need to be considered in a legal hearing. So also are non-pain-associated physiological responses to (e.g.) food- and water-deprivation, extremes of temperature, excessive noise, exposure to light, dark or abnormal photoperiods, social deprivation, extreme physical restraint and overcrowding (see Chapter 6).

PRACTICAL ASPECTS

A legalistic approach to animal welfare was outlined earlier and this is discussed in more detail in Chapter 3. In the past, in Britain, for example, the focus has been on preventing cruelty (beating, kicking, torturing, etc.). In recent years a more positive approach has begun to emerge, with emphasis on the promotion of good welfare in the animal. Often this has used as its framework concepts known as 'The Five Freedoms'. These were developed originally in the UK, by its Farm Animal Welfare Council (FAWC) in order to provide guidelines on how farm livestock should be kept. They continue to provide a basis for the assessment of welfare, together with the actions necessary to safeguard it within the constraints of an efficient livestock industry (FAWC, 2001).

The Five Freedoms and how they can best be ensured are listed below:

(1) **Freedom from hunger and thirst** – by ready access to fresh (potable) water and a diet to maintain full health and vigour.
(2) **Freedom from discomfort** – by providing an adequate environment including shelter and a comfortable resting area.
(3) **Freedom from pain, injury or disease** – by prevention or rapid diagnosis and treatment.
(4) **Freedom to express normal behaviour** – by providing sufficient space, proper facilities and, where appropriate, company of the animal's own kind.
(5) **Freedom from fear and distress** – by ensuring conditions and treatment to avoid mental suffering.

Slight modifications may be made to these Freedoms to accommodate different species of animal and the variable environments in which they are kept but the Freedoms generally serve as goals towards which animal owners and handlers should strive. They may provide the basis for legislation and codes of practice (see Chapter 3). In practice, the Freedoms usually prove to be constructive and functional in terms of promoting better standards of husbandry but are often not easily applied to the judicial process.

FARM ANIMALS

The welfare of farm animals may be compromised on the farm, in the market, during transportation

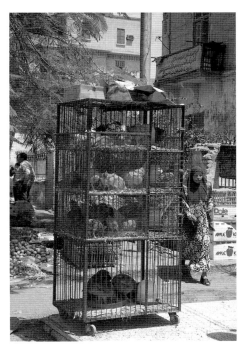

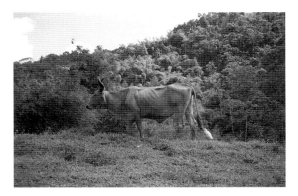

Figure 4.7 Welfare may be compromised even if animals appear to be 'free-range'. This cow, on a Caribbean island, is tethered and vulnerable to the sun or heavy rain.

Figure 4.6 In many parts of the world the welfare of livestock is not a priority: a street scene in Egypt. This figure also appears in colour in the colour plate section.

and at slaughter (Fraser and Broom, 1990). Transportation and slaughter are discussed in more detail later in this chapter and elsewhere in the book.

The use of the Five Freedoms in providing a basis for assessing the welfare of animals on the farm is referred to above.

Methods of husbandry differ greatly and each can be accompanied by its own spectrum of welfare concerns (see also Chapter 6). Free-range poultry, for example, may appear to lead a more 'natural' life than do their housed counterparts but the former are vulnerable to specific threats to their health or welfare, such as parasites, hypothermia and predation (Moberly *et al.*, 2004). Laying hens that are housed in free-range and barn systems, while no longer exposed to the restrictions of movement presented by battery cages, sustain injuries, including bone fractures, which have implications for welfare (Wilkins *et al.*, 2004).

Anyone involved in legal cases concerning livestock should be aware of the various, sometimes conflicting, trends in thinking about how these animals should be managed. For example, at the same time as the EU is moving towards a ban (by 2012) on the keeping of poultry in battery cages, the use of intensive methods of husbandry, including the 'zero grazing' of milk cows, is becoming increasingly prevalent in East and Central Africa.

The carrying out of 'mutilations' on farm animals – beak-trimming in poultry, for instance (Glatz, 2005) – is contentious, and may be grounds for legal action.

Campaigns against companies that produce 'fast food' have become more frequent in recent years, the argument of protestors usually being that they do not take sufficient action to promote the welfare of animals that are destined to be used in their products. Civil actions relating to such activities will necessitate expert opinion.

There is vast literature on the welfare of farm animals. Reference should be made to peer-reviewed papers, textbooks, the legislation itself and the publications of pressure groups, especially those with a constructive approach to the subject, e.g. Compassion in World Farming (CIWF) (see Appendix B). Much of the overall toll of suffering amongst livestock probably relates not to the altercation about intensive versus extensive management but to the quality of stockmanship and the attention that is paid to individual animals – in the detection of lameness in dairy cattle, for example

(Blowey, 2005). These are issues on which an experienced veterinary clinician can and should offer sound advice.

WELFARE OF WILDLIFE

The welfare of wildlife presents legalistic and practical problems because:

- In many countries free-living wild animals are not afforded the same legal protection as are their domesticated counterparts (see Chapters 3 and 5).
- Injury, pain, infectious disease and presumed suffering are everyday occurrences in wild animals, especially associated with predation, drought and other climatic extremes – and are argued by some to be part of Darwinian 'survival of the fittest'.
- Largely on account of the second point above, assessment of welfare is often not easy (Kirkwood *et al.*, 1994).
- There are dilemmas in wildlife work as to how to balance the welfare of the individual animal (e.g. an injured mountain gorilla in Rwanda) against the interests of the group or species as a whole. These and other considerations when working with wildlife were discussed by Cooper and Cooper (2001).

The debate about the welfare of wild animals has been fuelled recently in the UK by the decision of Parliament to ban the hunting of foxes and other species with dogs – pastimes ('sports' – see below) that had been practised for centuries and considered by many to be part of British rural tradition. Before and after abolition there was public and scientific discussion as to the extent to which animals that were chased and killed 'suffered' and how this rated in comparison with, say, their being shot and injured (Fox *et al.*, 2005) or dying from inanition or infectious disease. It has also introduced into forensic work the need for a wildlife pathologist to be able to recognise bites and other injuries that have been inflicted by dogs rather than by other species (PAW, 2005). In any discussion of welfare of wildlife, it is important that the expert witness is objective and concentrates on the animal(s) in question, rather than straying into politics or being swayed by personal points of view. S/he should be cognisant of relevant research and publications on the welfare of wildlife, which is often widely scattered in the literature.

ANIMALS IN SPORT

Animals have been used in 'sport' for centuries, as evidenced by the large numbers and variety (along with uncounted human beings) that were taken to Imperial Rome for combat two thousand years ago and the subsequent persistence in Europe, until relatively recently, of such activities as bear-baiting.

Some sports involving animals still exist and are legal but this depends upon the country and its legislation. In the USA, for example, cock-fighting is banned in every state except Louisiana and New Mexico. Activities that come under the broad heading of 'sport' range from those that are essentially non-invasive, such as horse-racing, to others that involve killing, such as the shooting of deer, other mammals or game birds.

Assessment of welfare of animals used for sporting purposes has to take into account their lifestyle and other factors. For example, a working ferret in the Netherlands that is kept for rabbit and rat control is likely to be housed out-of-doors and even in a cold winter will be well protected by its dense coat. In contrast, a pet ferret accustomed to living in a warm house in the USA would probably be adversely affected if exposed to low temperatures as a result of its being placed in a hutch in the garden (or yard). Such a move might well be construed as 'cruelty'.

Sports that involve the use of animals for racing are usually governed by strict rules concerning health and welfare. In any alleged offence regarding such animals the relevant rules and regulatory bodies should be contacted at the start of the investigations – for example in the UK, the National Greyhound Racing Club (NGRC) (see Appendix B).

Equestrian sports have been in existence for centuries. Many possible welfare issues associated with horses are effectively covered by law or codes of practice. New practices, however, are likely to present legal challenges – endurance riding, for example, which can result in exhaustion, dehydration, electrolyte imbalances, heat stroke and exertional myopathies.

Involvement in activities such as cock-fighting can be grounds for a prosecution in countries, states or provinces where the practice has been banned. The veterinarian or other expert witness may be asked to examine live or dead animals or their remains (e.g. feathers, beaks, spurs) (see Figure 8.9).

Dog-fighting is still practised in many parts of the world and in some countries it is legal. Certain types of wound, sustained by particular breeds or varieties of dog, may be suspicious of such activities and prompt very careful evaluation (see Chapter 6).

In any legal case relating to animal fighting the expert should visit the location where the fighting is alleged to have taken place – the 'crime scene' (see Chapter 9).

Some 'sports' may involve more than one species of animal – for example, badger-baiting, which is still practised illegally in some parts of Britain. Dogs, especially terriers, are used in the baiting and both they and the badger can sustain severe injuries. In a recent case (Badger Trust, 2005) a man found guilty of badger-baiting was ordered to pay £6000 costs, to complete 180 hours of community punishment and was banned for life from keeping terriers. Interestingly, it was reported that a 'specialist vet' had been called to confirm that the dogs' injuries were caused by a badger.

ANIMALS IN ENTERTAINMENT

Animals are also often used in films and television, less frequently in the theatre. In so doing they may be exposed to stressors, pain or discomfort. Fatalities may even occur. The legal and (some) practical aspects of such exploitation were reviewed by Cooper and Cooper (1981).

In some countries live animals may be an important part of cultural tradition, presenting its own legal and ethical dilemmas – the use of snakes in tribal dances in East Africa, for example (Cooper and Cooper, 1996).

'EXOTIC' ANIMALS IN CAPTIVITY

Although 'exotic' (non-domesticated) animals have for long been kept in captivity, in private hands, by naturalists and hobbyists, in recent years a whole range of vertebrate and invertebrate species has become popular with the public at large. The special needs of many of them mean that their welfare can be compromised and this has led in some countries to calls for their confinement in captivity to be banned or strictly controlled. Concern in the UK prompted inclusion of questions about non-domesticated species in a pet census carried out by the Blue Cross (see Appendix B) and the issue was extensively addressed in a report by the country's Companion Animal Welfare Council (CAWC, 2003).

Assessment of the welfare of captive 'exotic' species presents many difficulties. Often little is known of the natural history and biological requirements of these animals. The Five Freedoms are generally applicable – to captive birds, for instance (Cooper, 2002). Ectothermic animals should either be kept within their known preferred optimum temperature zone (POTZ) or be offered a choice by the provision of a gradient (Cooper and Williams, 1995).

ZOO ANIMALS

Animals have been kept in captivity for display for many centuries (Mench and Kreger, 1996). The emphasis was usually on entertainment but slowly changed to encompass scientific study (Cooper, 1981). More recently conservation and education have begun to play a greater part in zoo animal philosophy and practice.

In many countries there is no specific legislation covering zoos but the situation is changing, in part due to the concern of the public and because of lobbying by pressure groups. In the EU, for instance, the Zoos Directive is now applicable to 25 countries (see Chapter 3).

The Five Freedoms provide a useful basis for promoting the welfare of zoo animals and have been used in some legislation (see Chapter 3) and

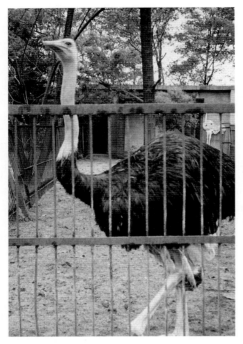

Figure 4.8 An ostrich in a zoo in China. The bird has a damaged, infected, leg. The welfare of animals in zoos is increasingly of concern to the public.

for legally enforceable codes of practice – for example, for zoo standards in the UK (DEFRA, 2004). An important step here was the production by DEFRA, in 2005, of a chapter for the *Zoos Forum Handbook* (DEFRA, 2003 and continuing) entitled 'Animal Welfare and its Assessment in Zoos'. This includes useful sections on behavioural and physiological indicators of welfare, clinical and pathological signs, the role of staff, education and staff training and the recommendations for the development of specific welfare codes.

Welfare considerations in zoos range from how the animals are kept, including behavioural aspects (Carlstead, 1996), to the problem of disposal of surplus stock (Graham, 1996).

AQUARIA

Many aquatic species are kept in captivity. They include fish, crustaceans and molluscs. Large

numbers are maintained for display (in public aquaria or zoos), many for pleasure (fish-keeping), some for scientific research (laboratories) and substantial numbers for food production (fish farms). The welfare of these animals can be easily compromised by poor management. Often the aquatic environment is the primary cause of any problem and water quality tests become a key part of determining why such species are dying or failing to thrive. Such investigations provide useful evidence in legal cases where it is alleged that animals are 'suffering'.

Aquatic species are challenging. Their management is often specialised and complex (Nash, 1991). They are an example of where, in any legal case, disputed insurance claim or allegation of professional malpractice, access to appropriate specialist advice is likely to be essential.

CIRCUSES

The welfare of animals in circuses is often criticised and sometimes is the subject of legal action (see Chapter 3). In some countries, such as Austria and Singapore, the use of live animals in circuses is banned. In others, the animals may be subject to legal controls while in the circus itself but cannot be properly protected when on temporary sites, such as winter quarters.

WILDLIFE CASUALTIES

Sick, injured and displaced wild animals are also covered in Chapter 5. Attention to such wildlife 'casualties' can be conveniently divided into three stages – rescue, rehabilitation and release. Each of these presents ethical and legal dilemmas (Cooper, 1990b; Cooper and Cooper, 2006; Mullineaux *et al.*, 2003).

Concern by animal welfare organisations or enforcement agencies as to how casualties are looked after, or the circumstances in which they return to the wild, may prompt investigation that can lead to legal action. The care and rehabilitation of certain animals is specialised and poorly understood – marine mammals, for instance (Maniere *et al.*,

2004). In any enquiries, investigations or legal actions relating to such species, expert advice must be sought.

In most countries, it is conservation laws that are of the greatest relevance to casualties (see Chapter 3). However, the fact that sick or injured wild species are held in captivity may mean that animal welfare legislation is also applicable. In some countries, such as the UK, the introduction of voluntary codes of practice for rehabilitators has played an important role in encouraging higher standards of care (Cooper, 1996a).

BREEDING ESTABLISHMENTS

Breeding establishments may cater for domesticated species (e.g. farm animals, pets, puppy farms) or captive wildlife (e.g. crocodiles, birds of prey, endangered species). They can be the source of many concerns about welfare, ranging from routine aspects, such as how the animals are housed and fed, to less immediately apparent matters such as the production (usually as a result of in-breeding) of animals with developmental abnormalities (see Chapter 6).

ANIMAL SANCTUARIES

These are discussed in more detail in Chapter 5. They can be the subject of enquiry or legal action on various grounds – conservation (see Chapter 5), welfare or nuisance.

SHELTERS

Shelters are refuges for unwanted, abandoned or stray animals. They provide a home but can themselves generate problems in terms of welfare. For example, disease control can be inadequate, possibly because of the costs involved. The release of animals may be illegal *per se* or, if carried out without proper planning, be viewed as 'abandonment' (see Chapter 3). Release may also lead to civil action because of the damage or disturbance that the liberated animals may cause. Abandonment is a

major international problem and diverse species may be involved – dogs, cats and pet rabbits in countries such as the UK, horses, donkeys, camels, cattle and buffalo elsewhere.

In the USA and some other countries 'shelter medicine' is taught and practised at veterinary schools (see, for example, Lacroix, 2004a). This provides good training for students but may itself raise legal and ethical questions, some relevant to welfare and therefore possibly of forensic importance.

HOARDING OF ANIMALS

This is, perhaps, a form of extremism. A person starts with apparently good intentions – that of 'rescuing' animals – but this develops to a stage at which excessive numbers are being kept, often under unsatisfactory conditions. Suffering, sometimes neglect (see Chapter 6), may result. Many believe that such persons need counselling and help rather than prosecution, but some cases do reach the courts and expert advice is then sought.

HUMANITARIAN ASSISTANCE FOR ANIMALS

The concern of many people, especially but not exclusively in richer countries, about the welfare of animals can prompt them to take action in various ways. Some may assist existing organisations at home or abroad (see also Disasters below). Others feel moved to take in animals themselves (see earlier – Wildlife casualties, Animal sanctuaries and Shelters). While the intentions of most people involved in such work are good, financial and other considerations can mean that the welfare of animals that they are trying to help is compromised. It may in some cases lead to 'hoarding' (see above).

EMERGENCIES

Emergency treatment of animals can sometimes compromise welfare (see Chapter 6).

DISASTERS

As was pointed out in Chapter 2, disaster management and relief increasingly involve veterinarians (Sprayson, 2006). Domesticated animals are likely to be killed or injured in the incident and sometimes wildlife, including endangered species, is affected. There may be both welfare and conservation implications. The former were discussed in some detail by Kearney (2003).

Anyone involved in disaster work, whether or not there is a forensic component, should be aware that:

- The situation is usually an unexpected emergency and therefore optimal planning is not always possible.
- Working conditions are likely at best to be basic, at worst horrific.
- If the disaster is the result of human activity, the site may be a crime scene – and police investigations are likely to take priority over the rescue of animals.
- Close collaboration is vital with others at the scene, particularly those coordinating it – often the emergency services – and with the medical profession if both humans and animals are affected. A chain of custody should be instigated for anything removed from the site, even if there is no immediate indication that legal proceedings will follow.
- Record-keeping will, as always, be of great importance, even though the circumstances for collecting information may be difficult. Photographs and tape recordings are often the best solution.
- A report of the incident should always be produced, even if this is not formally requested or required for legal or investigative purposes. In view of the growing relevance of disaster relief, the report should draw attention to mistakes made and lessons learned.

ANIMALS IN EDUCATION

Animals have for long played a part in teaching. The benefits to young people of contact with live animals were outlined by Cooper (1986). However, scientific studies on animals, alive or dead in schools, may prove to be contentious and in certain cases amount to 'experimentation'. The replacement under such circumstances of live animals by audio-visual educational material (Cooper and Cooper, 1988) has been widely promoted.

LABORATORY ANIMALS

The use of animals in research brings with it many dilemmas in terms of how to balance scientific and medical needs with an obligation to treat the animals as humanely as possible. This is a contentious subject and has led to legislation in many (not all) countries, the establishment of institutional animal care and use committees, the formulation of guidelines and codes of practice, the training of specialist animal technicians, laboratory animal scientists and veterinarians – and continued, often acrimonious, debate coupled with varying types of action, by concerned groups and individuals.

A valuable recent publication on the ethics of research involving animals, which includes a comprehensive index, a glossary and an excellent list of references and further reading, conveniently given as footnotes, is the report by the Nuffield Council (2005). The law is not usually concerned with ethics, *per se*, but how legislation is used and interpreted often stems from, or leads to, ethical concerns. They are also relevant to such matters as professional disciplinary hearings. This Report contains much of legal significance that could be applicable in forensic work.

The UK has had legislation to regulate experiments on animals since 1876 (see Chapter 3) and arguably provides the greatest degree of protection in the world for such animals. The system is governed by the Animals (Scientific Procedures) Act 1986 and is operated by an Inspectorate (all members of which have a medical or veterinary qualification), employed by the Home Office (the UK's Ministry of Internal Affairs). The Inspectors are expected to ensure compliance with the Act so as to keep animal use to a minimum, causing the least possible suffering to the smallest number of animals, the principles here being the '3 Rs' of replacement, reduction and refinement. According to the Inspectorate's report of 21 November, 2005, in 2004 inspectors made 2682 visits to laboratories around the UK, the majority of them unannounced.

Legal cases relating to animals are rare, partly because of strict controls in the UK and other countries on the use and care of such animals. However, as stressed elsewhere, the use of animals in research evokes strong feelings and sometimes direct action. The veterinary surgeon, biologist or animal welfare officer is likely to become involved in debate and may be asked to provide evidence on related matters, such as the pros and cons of carrying out a particular study or whether a research laboratory should be established at a given location.

Forensic work itself brings with it legal and ethical issues relating to the use of animals (see Chapter 2). Some toxicological and microbiological tests that may need to be used in forensic investigations depend upon the performance of tests on live rodents or other species. Even sample-taking – for instance, from free-living wild animals in 'wildlife crime' investigations – may necessitate capture, restraint, chemical immobilisation and surgery. The emphasis here should be on non-interventional or minimally-invasive techniques (Cooper, 1998b; Cooper and Cooper, 2001). Investigators should be encouraged whenever possible to adopt such methods: an example is the utilisation of the 'non-destructive' technique of buccal-swab sampling rather than collecting tissues, developed by French researchers, to obtain DNA from amphibians (Pidancier *et al.*, 2003). Interestingly, there are parallels but, for different reasons, in human forensic work – for example, in the use of minimally-invasive sampling of hair from children to detect drugs associated with abuse (Boroda and Gray, 2005).

EUTHANASIA, CULLING, KILLING, EXTERMINATING, SLAUGHTER

The killing of animals, whether intentional or accidental, frequently results in legal proceedings or the asking of questions that are relevant to insurance claims or assessment of professional competence. It is also often the cause of misunderstanding, loss of trust and distress (see Chapter 2).

Terminology is important: 'euthanasia' (Greek: *good death*) means humane killing; 'culling' usually implies that a perceived surplus is killed, as in the culling of deer; 'killing' is self-explanatory but the word is sometimes considered to have a callousness about it which can upset owners of animals or sensitive members of the public. For that reason other, usually euphemistic, terms are commonly applied – for example, stating that animals were 'sacrificed', or 'put down' or 'put to sleep'. Care must be taken over all of these, as confusion can occur, occasionally with tragic consequences. For example, 'putting a horse down' in Britain will mean killing it but in the USA may imply anaesthetising the animal!

Sometimes animals are deliberately exterminated – for example, for purposes of disease control (ranging from rodent-borne plague to avian influenza). It is also used to eradicate alien wildlife species and feral domesticated animals. Such 'exterminations' often disrupt ecosystems, disturb the public, raise questions relating to welfare and can sometimes, usually in richer parts of the world, prompt a criminal or civil action. In poorer countries animals that are perceived as 'pests' are often hunted and killed indiscriminately. An example (Ross Cooper, pers. comm.) is the African giant rat which, despite its agricultural importance, its biologically interesting matriarchal social structure and its value to humans when (for example) trained in detecting mines, is still widely persecuted by 'slash and burn' and other destructive practices.

The term 'slaughter', in its proper sense, usually refers to livestock being killed for meat but is a term that is also employed, perhaps unjustly, when animals (or humans) are killed on a large scale with little apparent regard for welfare or aesthetics.

The killing of animals can have legal consequences for many reasons, of which probably the most important in the context of this book is the intentional or accidental killing of a domesticated or live animal as a criminal act. How an animal is killed is also significant: failure to do so humanely (or apparently so) may lead to allegations or charges of cruelty to animals or may even be a *de facto* offence – if, for example, slaughterhouse regulations are breached. Emergency slaughter is sometimes

Table 4.2 Some methods of killing.

Type	Method	Species	Comments
Chemical	Overdose of pentobarbital or other injectable anaesthetic agent	All vertebrates	Fastest if given intravenously Other routes can be used Carcase will contain drug and is not suitable for subsequent consumption by humans or animals
	Overdose of isoflurane or halothane by inhalation	All vertebrates, many invertebrates	Induction may be prolonged in some species, e.g. chelonians
	Controlled inhalation of carbon dioxide	Certain vertebrates and invertebrates	Controversial May not be humane See 2005 correspondence in the journal *Laboratory Animals*
	Overdose of certain agents (e.g. benzocaine)	Certain amphibians, most fish, some invertebrates	Absorbed through skin or gills
Physical	Concussion (striking head with hard object or striking animal's head on a surface)	Certain vertebrates	Requires skill and confidence to be performed accurately Should be followed by exsanguination if animal is only concussed, not dead
	Stunning with captive bolt followed by exsanguination	Certain vertebrates	Positioning of stunner needs training and skill Dangers – a firearm
	Destruction of brain with free bullet	Certain vertebrates	As above
	Electrocution	Certain vertebrates	Only humane if electrodes are applied correctly and the correct current is used (see, for example, Giles and Simmons, 1975)
	Hypothermia	Certain vertebrates and invertebrates	Rapid, whole-body, 'snap' freezing probably acceptable for small animals (weighing less than 20 g)

needed on welfare or human safety grounds and this can present legal and practical problems. In some countries the situation is covered by law and the EU is introducing new rules (Regulation [EC] Number 852/2004), prompted mainly by public health concerns but which raise questions about the welfare of animals that are not covered by these Regulations.

Mass euthanasia of animals is sometimes necessary on account of disease control measures. The subject is well documented insofar as some farm livestock are concerned but the choice of a humane method of culling other species remains

problematic, prompting publications on, for example, the killing of poultry (Kingston *et al.*, 2005) and of invertebrates in 'butterfly houses' (Cooper, 1990c,d, 2001).

There are numerous guidelines for the euthanasia of individual animals, largely produced by veterinary and welfare bodies, and most of these are regularly updated in the light of new knowledge or thinking. The expert who may be consulted should be sure to have access to up-to-date versions. They cover most species – companion animals, livestock, wildlife, zoo and laboratory animals. The (UK-based) Humane Slaughter Association (HSA) (see

Appendix B) provides sound, practical, advice and is worth contacting for professional guidance over legal cases that relate to the killing of animals.

The slaughter of livestock is often controversial because of religious convictions and other factors. In India, for example, cows and some bulls are considered sacred and in certain (mainly northern) states it is illegal to kill them. In urban areas, in particular, this causes welfare problems (road accidents if they wander, choking on ingested plastic bags, untreated wounds and diseases) and presents dilemmas for the authorities and animal welfarists alike (Anon., 2005f). Often such problems have a 'forensic' component (see Appendix D), especially if the straying animals cause damage or are attacked by non-Hindus who resent their presence on their land.

Humane killing implies death with little or no awareness on the part of the animal. This does not necessarily mean that death is rapid: an animal given an overdose of an anaesthetic agent may take minutes or hours to die but so long as it is unconscious throughout, undergoes a humane death. A rapid death has much to commend it, in terms of the animal's not being aware of what is happening but aesthetics (and public sensitivities) may have to be taken into account. For example, the most humane way of killing a badly injured bird on the roadside may be to run over it in a car or to hit its head against a wall and thus despatch it instantly. Many people, though, would prefer to see the bird put in a box and taken to a veterinary surgeon to be killed with an anaesthetic agent, thus probably prolonging its pain and stress.

Ectothermic animals present particular challenges insofar as euthanasia is concerned, because of their ability to withstand hypoxia (Cooper, 1987; Cooper *et al.*, 1989a; Zwart *et al.*, 1989). Awareness of the resilience of some species was recognised long ago: in a letter to Edward Jenner, dated March 29, 1778, John Hunter stated that:

> *Frogs live an amazing while after they are dead, as also all animals of their tribe.*
>
> Cornelius and Harding Rains, 1976

It may be helpful for readers who are involved in cases, especially those persons without a veterinary background, to have some reference material concerning methods of killing animals, their efficacy, safety and welfare implications. These are given in Table 4.2.

TRANSPORTATION OF ANIMALS

The movement of animals can present many practical and legal challenges. The effects of transportation are discussed in more detail in Chapter 6. Farm animals may travel long distances but even short periods of movement can have significant effects on an animal's physiology and well-being.

INTERNATIONAL AND CULTURAL CONSIDERATIONS

Although the importance of animal welfare is increasingly being promoted on a 'global' scale

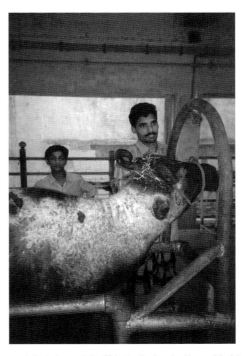

Figure 4.9 A (water) buffalo in India, badly scalded in a revenge attack. This figure also appears in colour in the colour plate section.

(see earlier), there remain wide national variations in how animals are treated and the extent to which the authorities recognise infringements of the law. This can present a challenge to anyone who is called to give advice or present evidence in a country or jurisdiction other than his/her own.

An expert's opinion may change if the circumstances of the alleged offence are different from what was expected and this is often the case when giving advice in other countries or cultures. For example, to slaughter a goat without pre-stunning would be totally unacceptable and probably illegal in most Western European countries but the method is standard practice in the Middle East and large areas of Africa – sometimes for religious reasons, sometimes because of lack of resources for stunning equipment (Cooper, 1995a). Under such circumstances, whether or not a particular animal is considered to have 'suffered' might, therefore, have to be related to specific issues, such as the sharpness of the knife or quality of pre-slaughter handling, rather than the method of killing *per se*.

SOME CONCLUSIONS

Throughout this chapter the increasing importance of animal welfare in a legal/forensic context has been highlighted. Equally, however, attention has been drawn to the difficulties such cases can present in terms of proving innocence or guilt. In preparing the chapter, we sought the advice of numerous colleagues and, almost without exception, they underlined this latter point. In particular, Virginia Williams in New Zealand exhorted us to underscore in our text that a major problem for veterinarians (and others) who are dealing with a welfare case is 'the lack of a clear objective definition of the subject'. This in turn makes it difficult for a court to adjudicate – and for experts to relate their findings and opinions to what is apposite to the law, in contrast to the strong feelings and sentiments of those who are involved. The subject continues to evolve and veterinarians, in particular, who are likely to contribute to judicial, disciplinary or other hearings, need to be aware of current deliberations and dissensions if their evidence is to be of optimal value to those who must arbitrate.

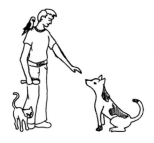

Conservation and Wildlife Crime

There is grandeur in this view of life . . . having been originally breathed by the Creator. . . .
whilst this planet has gone cycling on according to the fixed law of gravity, from so simple a
beginning endless forms most beautiful and most wonderful have been and are being evolved.

Charles Darwin

What is wildlife? According to the dictionary, it is 'animals and plants that are not domesticated, tame or cultivated.' There remains confusion, however. A wild animal is, by definition, of a species that has not been domesticated. Therefore, a lion is a wild animal whereas a pet cat is domesticated. The lion, however, can either be in captivity or be 'free-living'. In the USA the term 'free-ranging' is increasingly being used but this has, in Europe, a different meaning, viz. animals such as deer or ducks that are free to roam but return to the paddock or their housing at the end of the day. These and other terms are explained more precisely in Appendix C.

Throughout this book the term 'domesticated' is used as defined by Mason (1984), viz. an animal that breeds under human control, provides a product or service useful to humans, is tame and has been selected away from the wild type. In contrast, 'domestic' implies that an animal lives in or around human habitation.

The vast majority of the world's animals, both vertebrate and invertebrate, are free-living. This means, for example, that approximately 20,000 species of fish, 4000 mammals, 9000 birds and 6000 reptiles are non-domesticated (Wilson, O.E., 1988). Only a handful have been taken into captivity and become domesticated.

The number of species of wild animals on earth is constantly being augmented as discoveries are made. The International Commission on Zoological Nomenclature (see Appendix F) has governed the naming of new species, through its Code, since 1961, and in 2005 announced the launch of an on-line registration system, ZooBank, to monitor and collate this. The ICZN estimated that a further 20,000 species were likely to be named in 2005 and attributed this to a) the development of DNA techniques that now enable scientists to detect genetic differences between apparently identical animals – orang-utans, for example, and b) the opening-up of terrain, especially forest (but probably also including the marine environment), where thousands of previously undescribed animals, mainly invertebrates, exist.

In this chapter, in keeping with the title of the book, the definition of wildlife will be narrowed to animals – both vertebrate and invertebrate. Plants will be mentioned but not in detail. Nevertheless, they can be a major component in wildlife crime cases. In some instances theft and illegal exportation of plants are the salient features but often the situation is more complex involving, for example, medicinal plants (Hamilton, 2004). Some knowledge of botany and of where to obtain information (herbaria, research institutes, etc.) (Coyle, 2004; PAW, 2005) is usually of value to anyone who is involved in wildlife forensics. As stressed elsewhere, forensics relating to conservation is, *par excellence,*

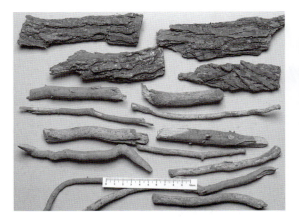

Figure 5.1 Various roots and bark used as traditional medicines in East Africa. (Courtesy of Richard Spence.)

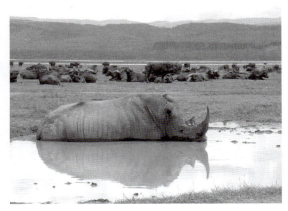

Figure 5.2 Wildlife crime often concerns large, rare species, such as this white rhinoceros.

the field where a broad knowledge of natural history is of inestimable advantage.

There are categories of animals that might be considered to be 'wildlife' but which do not fall into the strict definition. The best examples are domesticated animals such as cats or ferrets, that have returned to the wild or a semi-wild situation either of their own volition or because they have been rejected by owners. These are 'feral' animals and present particular legal problems.

WILDLIFE CRIME

What is 'wildlife crime'? Surprisingly few publications define it, but the meaning, while slightly ambiguous (see below), is largely self-explanatory (Bradley, 1996). Wildlife crime describes activities that threaten wildlife (animals, plants, their habitats) and which usually constitute an offence under national, regional or international law (see Chapter 3). Early, still useful, introductions to the subject were the article about animal smuggling in the National Geographic over twenty years ago (Grove and Raymer, 1981) and the booklet *Inside Wildlife Crime* (Anon, undated) produced by Carlton Television in the UK following a programme on the same subject in 1994. The practicalities of identifying and combating wildlife crime were discussed more recently in the publication by PAW (2005) – see later.

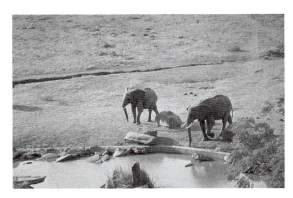

Figure 5.3 Wild animals are particularly susceptible to poaching when under pressure for other reasons – these elephants during a drought in Kenya, for example. This figure also appears in colour in the colour plate section.

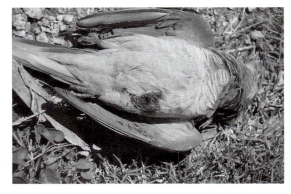

Figure 5.4 A parakeet, one of a number found dead, believed shot, in Uruguay. This figure also appears in colour in the colour plate section.

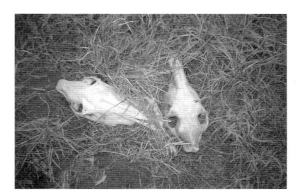

Figure 5.5 Two skulls, from an unidentified equid species, in Kenya. Are they from a zebra or a donkey? Is there a conservation or animal welfare implication? This figure also appears in colour in the colour plate section.

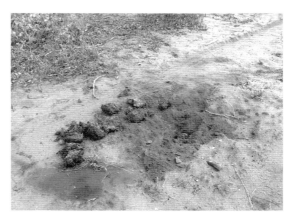

Figure 5.7 Examination of faeces, urine and prints can help in determining when elephant damage occurred.

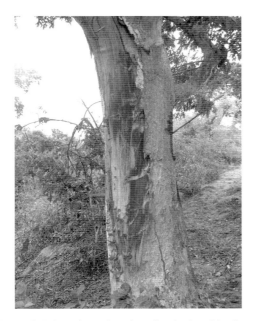

Figure 5.6 A track on the edge of agricultural land habitually used by elephants. This tree has been stripped of bark.

The definition above excludes the converse situation (see also Chapter 2) where wild animals damage property (Figure 5.6) or kill villagers and in some societies may even be punished for it. This and many other examples also could be termed 'wildlife crime' – the ambiguity referred to above – but is not the meaning followed in this book.

Wildlife crime includes:

- The taking (including killing), alive or dead, of protected wild animals or plants, without appropriate authority.
- Unlawful persecution and killing of protected species because of human/animal conflict over land or resources.
- Killing or causing injury to protected species by physical means (e.g. clearing forest) or in other ways (e.g. discharging pesticides into rivers).
- Causing disturbance to specially protected species, their nests or habitats (see Wildlife and Countryside Act – Chapter 3).
- The possession of protected wildlife (animals or plants) or their derivatives, without appropriate authority.
- The importation, exportation or sale of protected wildlife, without appropriate authority.
- Offences relating to (e.g.) how and where protected wild animals are kept in captivity (see Chapter 3).

Cruelty to wild animals may or may not come under the heading of 'wildlife crime'. In many countries welfare legislation relates primarily to animals in captivity (see Chapter 3). However, a wild animal taken into captivity may be subject to such controls. Also, assaults on free-living animals occur and may even form part of a pattern of abuse (see Chapter 6).

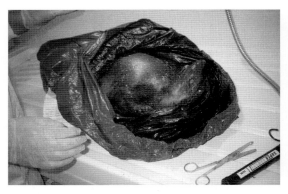

Figure 5.8 A badger, submitted for necropsy to ascertain how it died. There are numerous maggots on the skin and these may assist in determining the *post-mortem* interval (PMI). This figure also appears in colour in the colour plate section.

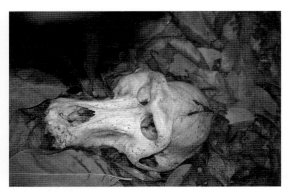

Figure 5.9 Estimation of the time of death is often important. Did this baboon die three months ago, during an organized cull, or was it killed illegally before or after that period?

A useful guide to the use of forensic and other specialist techniques in the investigation of wildlife crime is the publication, available on the Internet (see Appendix B), *Wildlife Crime: A Guide to the Use of Forensic and Specialist Techniques in the Investigation of Wildlife Crime* published by the (British) Department for Environment, Food and Rural Affairs (DEFRA) on behalf of the Partnership for Action Against Wildlife Crime (PAW, 2005). Dealing primarily with the situation in the UK, it provides background to the subject and then covers such fields as scenes of crime examinations, questioned documents, firearms, DNA-profiling, specimen identification, poisoning and pesticide analysis, forensic veterinary pathology, taxidermy, health and safety and laboratory procedures. Although there are useful Appendices (list of contacts, undertaking retention of property, and a laboratory checklist), the publication lacks an index and unfortunately provides no references.

The introductory chapter points out that the investigation of any offence connected with wildlife typically revolves around four questions:

(1) What is the identity of the specimen in question?
(2) What is its provenance?
(3) What was the cause of death or injury?
(4) Can a suspect be connected to a wildlife crime scene?

Contravention of legislation aimed at conserving animals, plants and their habitats has become a subject of great importance. The illicit field of wildlife crime is highly lucrative (Stroud and Adrian, 1996; Wobeser, 1996) and, when linked with other activities, such as drug smuggling, has assumed international significance. The latest disturbing development, highlighted by the International Fund for Animal Welfare (IFAW, 2005), is that 'vast quantities' of live animals and wildlife products are now being traded illegally on the Internet.

The growth of wildlife crime has led to involvement of the veterinary profession (Forbes, 2004; Stroud, 1998; Wobeser, 1996) and others (Adrian, 1992) particularly when the offences relate to international legislation such as CITES, which covers the trade in endangered species (see Chapter 3).

A similar trend is seen, however, on a regional level – for example, within the EU, now comprising 25 countries – where free movement of many products, including those of animal origin, has opened doors to illegal activities and prompted a more concerted approach to their correct identification and recognition.

The enforcement of conservation law is complicated by the international nature of wildlife crime. A species may be protected in one country but legally killed or taken in another. Morphologically similar taxa may be deliberately misrepresented to evade regulation, or the provenance of individuals falsified as, for example, wild-caught sulphur-crested cockatoos which are illegally exported and sold outside Australia as locally captive-bred birds. Live or dead specimens may be smuggled from a developing country to North America or Western Europe – or *vice versa*. Sometimes, a rich and a poor nation share a common border over which rare species migrate – perhaps highly valued on one side, yet persecuted on the other.

Wild animals may be afforded protection under one legal system but denied it under a second. Even within economic and political groupings, such as the EU, individual states' legislation may differ. In many countries law enforcement is poor and facilities for investigation of suspected infringements can be rudimentary (see later).

TYPES OF WILDLIFE INVESTIGATION

The field is vast and the scope international. Forensic cases in which we have been involved have ranged from the investigation of circumstances of death of free-living mountain gorillas in Central Africa to the assessment of 'suffering' in captive insects in Britain. However, these are but a tiny part of the expanding world of wildlife forensics. People from many disciplines are now bringing forensic method (sometimes, not always, culminating in legal action) into work extending from the protection of coral reefs to the identification of previously unknown arachnids.

An example of the extent of wildlife crime, even in Britain which has a long history of public concern for animals and their habitats, is to be found in the reports of the Royal Society for the Protection of Birds (RSPB). In their publication *Bird Crime, 2004* (RSPB, 2005) the Society lists offences against wild bird legislation during the previous year and provides case studies. In 2004, 481 incidents were reported to the RSPB and these covered:

- Shooting and destruction of protected birds.
- Taking and sale of protected birds (including illegal possession).
- Poisoning.
- Illegal importation and exportation.
- Egg-collecting.
- Sale of eggs.
- Photography and disturbance of (specially) protected species.

It should be noted that the term 'wild bird' in England, Wales and Scotland, as used in the Wildlife and Countryside Act 1981, was expanded

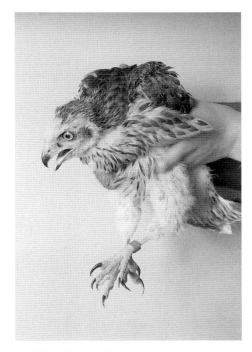

Figure 5.10 A live, confiscated, goshawk.

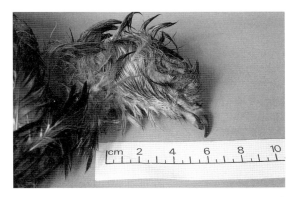

Figure 5.11 Birds of prey are often the subject of a legal case. Correct species identification is important.

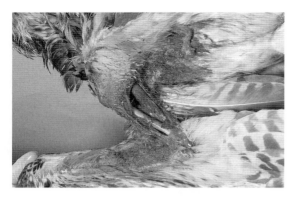

Figure 5.12 A fatal fracture in an osprey. Such lesions require careful investigation and description before a report is produced for the court.

in 2004 to cover all European birds. The legislation applies to such species both in the wild (free-living) and in captivity (Cooper, 1987) (see Chapter 3).

In contrast to the RSPCA (see Chapter 4), the RSPB generally no longer carries out its own prosecutions. Instead, it assists the police (and other organisations) in the investigation and prosecution of offences. All incidents reported are recorded on the Species Protection Database, which is registered with the Data Protection Registrar for the prevention and detection of wildlife crime and the apprehension and prosecution of offenders.

THE INVESTIGATION OF WILDLIFE CRIME

Wildlife crime investigations always require the following:

- Accurate information about the circumstances of the alleged offence (a 'history'), preferably in writing. This should include details of the relevant legislation (Cannings, 2000).
- Prior discussion with those involved in initiating the investigation or in bringing charges.
- Correct identification of the species involved – although it may be wise to avoid specific identification until later (PAW, 2005).
- A site visit – to the location where the offence is alleged to have occurred or the premises where (for example) the live animals can be viewed or the dead animals/specimens can be examined.
- Proper collection, transportation, storage and submission of evidence.
- Collection and evaluation of trace evidence.
- Careful documentation and record-keeping, including appropriate photographic records, leading to production of a report.
- (If the matter proceeds) preparation for, and appearance in, court.

The identification of species of animal and of other relevant evidence, e.g. ectoparasites, carrion beetles, animals and plants in the gastro-intestinal (GI) tract (see Chapter 8) may need an input from people from a wide range of backgrounds – biologists, naturalists, bird-ringers (bird-banders), pest control officers, botanists, staff of museums or zoos.

In all wildlife work it is important to be able to work with other people (see later) including those with different opinions about (for example) field sports or the keeping of animals in captivity.

Depending on the circumstances, the investigator may also need:

- Knowledge of, and empathy with, wildlife in general.
- In-depth knowledge of the taxon (taxa) involved. Wildlife crime can involve animals or plants (or both) and the first of these can include anything from crustaceans to chimpanzees. Even identification may be a key part of a forensic investigation and this can encompass morphological studies, examination of hair (see, for example, Yates, 1999) or DNA analysis (Branicki and Kupiec, 1999; Wolf *et al.*, 1999; Wolfes *et al.*, 1991).
- Some understanding of the principles of specialised techniques, such as microbiology, toxicology and DNA studies, that are likely to be used in wildlife cases (see later).

A good illustration of how complex wildlife crime investigations can be – and the breadth of expertise often needed – was provided by Simpson *et al.* (2006). Their studies into the death of a (protected) Eurasian otter in the UK involved techniques that ranged from both microscopical and DNA examination of hair, to necropsy of an otter

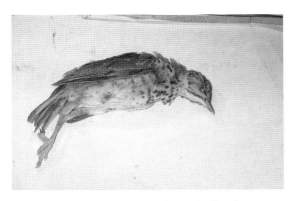

Figure 5.13 A thrush that was found dead under mysterious circumstances. Careful examination revealed talon marks, indicating that it had been killed by a hawk.

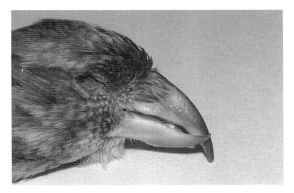

Figure 5.15 The appearance of the beak of this crossbill could be mistaken for an abnormality, perhaps associated with its being in captivity, but is, in fact, normal for the species.

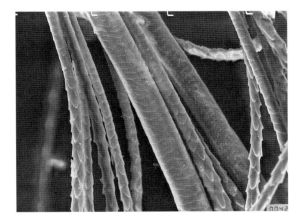

Figure 5.14 Scanning electronmicroscopy (SEM) can often be used to identify hair. These are from a polecat ferret.

and laboratory investigation of the remains of a fish in its stomach.

PERSONNEL

As stressed earlier, forensic wildlife work can involve field workers, naturalists, ecologists, entomologists, botanists, veterinarians, comparative pathologists, molecular biologists, toxicologists, medical or veterinary photographers, ballistics experts, police, Customs officers and representatives of regulatory bodies. There are often close links with those working in human medicine, agriculture, conservation and zoological parks, as well as the pet-owning public and local authorities.

There may be legal considerations (see also later). For example, in the UK only a registered veterinary surgeon may carry out certain procedures. Therefore, when a specimen of blood has to be taken from an animal for DNA-testing, a veterinarian carries out the sampling – but is accompanied by a Wildlife Inspector (see later).

Partly on account of the different disciplines involved and particularly because forensic wildlife work has only recently become so important, cohesion is sometimes lacking. Opportunities for individuals who are active in the field to meet and exchange ideas have been few. Extrapolation of ideas and techniques from other areas of forensic science is possible and sometimes proves successful, but the subject needs to develop its own momentum and attain greater credibility.

An enormous amount of 'detective' work is needed when investigating incidents concerning wildlife or the environment. The need for specialist advice on such issues as health and pathology in wildlife cases has been emphasised by the appearance of papers on the subject in veterinary and other journals, the establishment by the United States Fish and Wildlife Service (USFWS) of a national forensic laboratory, the introduction in the UK of an animal (especially wildlife) component into the work of both the Forensic Science Service (see Appendix B) and the Laboratory of the Government Chemist, and by enhanced interest in the subject by veterinarians and biologists on both sides of the Atlantic, in Australasia and elsewhere.

METHODS USED IN WILDLIFE CRIME INVESTIGATIONS

- Scene of crime visit and assessment.
- Investigative interviews.
- Collection and identification of specimens, including derivatives and specimens for laboratory testing.
- Clinical examination of live animals.
- *Post-mortem* examination of dead animals.
- Correct storage and despatch of specimens for laboratory testing.
- Laboratory investigations.
- Production of report(s).

These aspects are discussed later in this chapter or elsewhere in the book.

The holding of evidence can present difficulties in wildlife cases as it may include live animals and these will need to be properly housed and provided with adequate care (see later).

REQUIREMENTS OF THE INVESTIGATION

Throughout, as in all fields of forensic science, it is vital that investigations of alleged wildlife crime are meticulous, that detailed records are kept and that

a proper 'chain of custody (evidence)' is maintained for each item, to minimise the risk of loss or substitution, and to prove the provenance and veracity of specimens or exhibits (see Chapters 10 and 11). As in all forensic work, the chain should be as short as possible and not include anyone who is unwilling to appear in court.

Wildlife crime investigation requires strict adherence to protocols and high standards of quality control. Health and safety are important (see other chapters); wildlife cases may present additional dangers, e.g. zoonoses and poisons, to those who handle or examine material and precautions, including the use of personal protective equipment, must be taken (PAW, 2005). Hazards presented by live and dead animals are discussed in Chapter 2. To them should be added physical injuries (e.g. from rough terrain, poorly-designed aviaries) or assault by keepers of animals, activists, poachers or others. A risk-assessment is a legal requirement in some countries (see Chapter 3). In the UK, Wildlife Inspectors are issued with a letter that can be presented to the Inspector's medical practitioner, explaining that as a result of his/her duties s/he may come into contact with zoonoses or other health hazards (see also Chapter 2).

CAPTIVE WILDLIFE

Captive wildlife presents its own legal challenges, relating to both species' conservation and welfare (see also Chapter 4). There is not always a clear-cut distinction between captive and free-living wild animals because of movement in both directions (Figure 5.16).

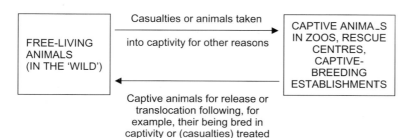

Figure 5.16 The distinction between captive and free-living wild animals may not always be clear.

ZOOLOGICAL COLLECTIONS

Notwithstanding the points above, zoos present their own particular problems insofar as the law is concerned. Some of the difficulties relate to welfare (see Chapter 4), others to species conservation – and therefore sometimes form part of the spectrum of wildlife crime.

Over the decades there have been substantial changes in how zoos are perceived, especially in the richer, industrialised countries (Mench and Kreger, 1996). No longer is it acceptable for them to house animals primarily for entertainment. Modern zoological collections are expected to contribute to conservation, education and research – principles enshrined in, for example, the UK's Zoo Licensing Act (DEFRA, 2004) and in the EU's Zoos Directive (see Chapter 3).

Zoos are of importance from a 'forensic' point of view because they may be at the centre of allegations or of criminal charges relating to:

- The health or welfare of an animal.
- Whether an animal has been imported legally.
- Health and safety of the public or employees.
- Infringements of any licence conditions.
- Insurance.
- Professional behaviour of veterinarians or others who work at or visit the collection.
- Zoos may be targets of attack by individuals (e.g. assaults on animals, bestiality) or groups of terrorists (spread of infectious agents or toxic substances) (Walcott, 2004).

CENTRES FOR WILDLIFE CASUALTIES/ANIMAL SANCTUARIES

The care of sick, injured, orphaned and displaced wildlife is practised in many parts of the world, especially the richer, usually industrialised, countries. It presents many challenges – both logistical and in terms of animal welfare (see Chapter 4) (Cooper and Cooper, 2006; Mullineaux *et al.* 2003). Wildlife casualties are also sometimes the focus of investigation or legal action because of believed contravention of conservation or welfare legislation.

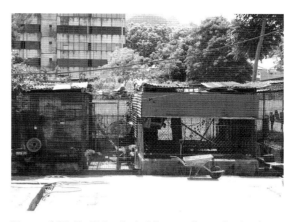

Figure 5.17 Facilities for holding confiscated animals are often sub-standard. This figure also appears in colour in the colour plate section.

Well-meaning individuals and organisations may establish 'sanctuaries' for the care of wild animals (see also Chapter 4). Concern has been expressed over the activities of some such 'rescue' organisations. In the USA, for example, there are claims that while many groups are dedicated to their work and adhere to legal and ethical obligations, a few are taking advantage of the public (Anon, 2005f).

BREEDING PROGRAMMES

Breeding establishments are usually for the production of domesticated animals (e.g. dogs) but in the context of this chapter include captive-breeding units for wildlife, including threatened species. There may be both welfare (Chapter 4) and conservation considerations.

CONFISCATIONS

Confiscated wild animals and those being held as evidence present particular problems. They may spend many months, even years, away from their 'owner' (keeper) before the problem is resolved or the case comes to court. Sometimes they are in the care of agencies with little or no experience of keeping wild animals. Often, especially in poorer

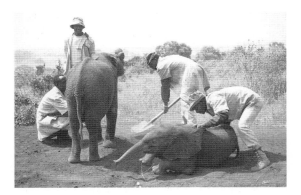

Figure 5.18 Young orphaned animals are tended at an elephant sanctuary in East Africa This figure also appears in colour in the colour plate section.

countries, facilities for holding seizures either do not exist or are inadequate. Even in the UK there have been many allegations that confiscated animals have suffered or died needlessly while being held. Investigation of such claims usually involves veterinarians.

An option that is being used increasingly in the UK at present, in instances where there is little risk that the live animal will be removed, is to leave it with the suspect pending the outcome of the case. A legally binding undertaking is signed, declaring that the animal will not be disposed of in any way.

Disposal of live animals following a case can present even more problems. In some instances, if the accused is found not guilty or the case is not proven, they can be returned to their keeper. Under different circumstances other arrangements have to be made and the main options are then:

- Return to the wild.
- Retention in captivity in a zoo or private hands.
- Euthanasia.

Each of these presents its own problems and may have legal implications. Similar dilemmas face those who have to deal with other 'unwanted' animals, such as stock that remains when a zoological collection has to be closed or the owner of a private collection dies (Graham, 1996).

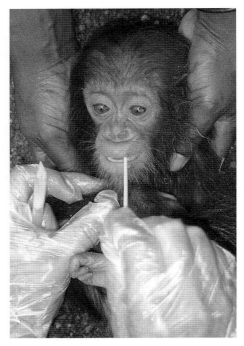

Figure 5.19 A young chimpanzee, orphaned and in need of veterinary attention, because its mother was killed in Central Africa. This figure also appears in colour in the colour plate section.

RELEASES AND INTRODUCTIONS/REINTRODUCTIONS

This is too vast a subject for this book but it is relevant to the law (see Chapter 3) and sometimes to forensic-type investigations. Animals ranging from squirrels and mongooses to cinnabar moth caterpillars and coccinellid beetles have been introduced intentionally into countries where they were not indigenous (see, for example, Lever, 1977). Others, such as species of bird, rodent, lizard and fish have established themselves accidentally. Sometimes the results have been devastating in terms of the effect on local species and habitats, either directly (competition, predation) or indirectly (introduction of infectious diseases or pathogenic organisms). Increasingly the deliberate release of 'foreign' animals and plants is seen as part of wildlife crime.

BUSHMEAT

Bushmeat, sometimes called 'wild meat' (in the Caribbean, for example) can be defined as 'wild animals killed for food' and the species involved can range from grasshoppers to guinea fowl and gorillas (Cooper, 1995b). Its origins go back to early humans, when hunter-gatherers harvested animals from the wild. Millions of people in South America, Africa and Asia continue to depend upon bushmeat, as either an essential source of animal protein or as an important cultural addition at weddings, baptisms or funerals. A continuum exists between this type of harvest and contemporary hunting practices in European cultures.

In recent years, however, bushmeat has become big business and instead of relatively small numbers of animals being taken, sold and eaten at a local level, millions of tonnes of meat and other products are being exported all over the world. A useful summary of the situation is to be found in ZSL (2002).

Why is the trade in bushmeat important? The answer is, for many reasons and these include:

- Depletion of populations of wild animals, sometimes with resulting increases in other species and changes in vegetation (Rapport *et al.*, 1998).
- Contravention of legislation, both national and international (e.g. CITES).
- Spread of diseases of humans and animals and probable role in the appearance of emerging infections.
- Socio-economic effects, especially on local communities – for example, loss of biodiversity affecting health and profound changes in revenue-earning capacity.

There is much international concern about bushmeat and the detection, prevention and control of the trade are an important aspect of countering wildlife crime. However, it is not a clear-cut situation. In many African countries law enforcement is weak, making policies of selective hunting unreliable or impossible (Rowcliffe *et al.*, 2004). Some argue that relatively wealthy people in developed countries want to stop those in poorer parts of the world from benefiting from utilisation of their own wildlife (Cooper, 1995b) and there may be considerations under the Convention on Biodiversity (see Chapter 3). Certain organisations, such as the British and Irish Association of Zoos and Aquariums (BIAZA) (see Appendix B), while campaigning against the growth of the bushmeat trade, also provide education and support for the development of *in situ* alternatives.

The investigation of the bushmeat trade brings with it its own challenges. Such work can be dangerous, especially when the trade is tied up with other interests such as logging, drug-dealing, training of mercenaries or political opportunism.

Examination of bushmeat may involve a veterinary pathologist (see Chapter 7). Questions that are likely to be asked relate to the species of animal, its age, sex and provenance and its health status. The pathologist may also be asked to 'match' carcases (or parts thereof) where more than one animal has been butchered (Stroud and Adrian, 1996).

One approach to strengthening the existing conservation legislation relating to the killing or taking of wild animals for bushmeat is to use public health legislation. In Kenya, for example, the Meat Control Act requires that all meat be inspected and certified safe for consumption before being offered to the public. The Kenya Veterinary Association issued a statement on 14 September 2005 warning that those eating game meat, including animals killed by vehicles, risked contracting zoonotic diseases such as anthrax. Such an approach need not be restricted to poorer, 'developing' countries, however. EU Regulations came into force in 2006, relating to possible human health risks from handling and consuming game species (Coburn *et al.*, 2005). While aimed at protecting humans rather than controlling the taking of wild game, these Regulations could help to monitor the trade in Europe.

PEST SPECIES

Not all species of wildlife are protected and some are only protected at certain times or to a limited degree (Cooper, 1987) (see Chapter 3).

Some species are considered in law to be 'pests' and as such may either be excluded from protected lists or be in a category whereby they can be killed or taken under permit. Such is the case in the UK where, for example, cormorants, goosanders and other species may be killed under licence in order to prevent damage to fisheries. In such cases, there may be debate as to what constitutes 'damage' and whether alternative methods might have been used.

Introduced, naturalised and feral populations may be significant targets of human exploitation, as for example mallard and mallard hybrid duck populations that have established themselves in New Zealand. Casualties in non-target protected species may be a source of community conflict – for example, in New South Wales, Australia, where traditional seasonal waterfowling was banned.

IDENTIFICATION OF ANIMALS OR THEIR PRODUCTS IN FORENSIC CASES

There is always a need in wildlife crime investigations for accurate identification of animal products or derivatives (PAW, 2005). Sometimes the product is immediately recognisable as coming from a particular taxon of animals, e.g. snakeskin, deer antlers, bird eggs. Often, however, it is not so straightforward as, for example, when blood, bile or other body products are seized.

Differentiation of carcases and derivatives of domesticated animals is discussed in Chapter 7.

Identification of whole animals or their parts is facilitated if a whole range of photographs is taken. This is particularly true of problematic species, such as marine mammals, especially if they are autolysed, badly bloated or predated. Fish usually decompose very quickly after death (see Chapter 7). Photography should be accompanied by morphometrics and the collection of gross specimens (which can range from the whole animal to, for example, the head of a whale) and the selection of tissues for DNA and other studies.

Some methods of identifying animal products are given in Table 5.1. Further information about these, including gel diffusion and DNA techniques, is to be found elsewhere in this book or in various papers (e.g. Lawton and Sutton, 1982; Fain and Le May, 1995). It should not be assumed that only one method can be used to identify derivatives of animals. Often in a court case it strengthens the argument if a number of techniques have been applied. For example, in the case of shahtoosh (the wool of the Tibetan antelope), both microscopic and DNA techniques can be used (PAW, 2005).

Taxonomy is the key to identification (see earlier). If a species has not been properly classified and catalogued, material cannot be related to it. The decline in number in recent years of taxonomists and the closing or re-organising of museums has made access to knowledgeable people and properly curated type-material difficult. These problems are being addressed by a number of scientific and professional bodies, including the Linnean Society of London (see Appendix B).

Plant identification is an integral part of many wildlife crime investigations but is only mentioned briefly here because the emphasis of this book is on animal forensics. However, plants may be part of 'animal' evidence: for instance, vegetation found on a mammal's coat or within its gastro-intestinal tract may need to be identified. In the UK those needing help have access to the Royal Botanic Gardens, Kew (PAW, 2005) but in most countries of the world there are herbaria or relevant university departments that can assist.

RINGS, BANDS, TAGS

Marking that can assist in the identification of animals is discussed in Chapter 6. A variety of methods is used and each has advantages and disadvantages.

The presence of a ring or tag can have legal significance. It may help to confirm the identity of animals, e.g. sheep in a market. Certain types of ring (band) on birds provide some support for a claim that the bird is legally held in captivity. In countries such as the UK, rings or cable ties are placed on a leg of a bird as part of a registration process. Closed rings of an appropriate size can be fitted on captive-bred young birds while their legs

Table 5.1 Identification of animal products.

Method	Applicability	Comments
Gross examination	Some animal skins, horns, bones, eggs, feathers, wings, elytra, etc. of invertebrates, some tissues and meats Depends upon characteristic markings, often with comparison with known reference material	Cheap, applicable in countries and circumstances where more sophisticated techniques are impossible
Microscopical examination (hand lens, dissecting/light microscope)	Hairs, feathers, scales, pieces of bone or eggshell, invertebrates, some tissues and meats	As above Microscopy is always wise initially, regardless of what other tests are planned
Scanning electronmicroscopy (SEM)	Some of the above	Detailed SEM can reveal important taxonomic features
Electrophoresis including gel diffusion	Some tissues, including meats	Species identification
Karyotyping	Various tissues Many species: species identification, sexing, detection of chromosomal abnormalities	Determination of species and sex requires knowledge of normal chromosome patterns
DNA techniques (various)	Blood, saliva, other body fluids or tissues Identification of species and individuals, parentage, sexing	Samples for identification must be handled and stored well; to prevent damage and contamination. Polymerase chain reaction (PCR) permits forensic identification of tiny, less-than-optimal, samples

and feet are still small and, as the nestling gets larger, the ring becomes a fixture. The presence of closed rings may be a requirement in law if, for example, birds are to be sold (see Chapter 3).

Although, on the face of it, the marking systems above would appear to be foolproof, this is not the case. Those wishing to pass a bird off as 'legal' sometimes go to great lengths to make it appear so. A number of methods have been devised by criminals to put rings on birds so that they appear to be legally in captivity. Some of the techniques employed have been documented by, or for reasons of security are retained in the files of, bodies such as the Royal Society for the Protection of Birds (RSPB) in the UK, the United States Fish and Wildlife Service (USFWS) and the Canadian Wildlife Service (see Appendix B).

Veterinarians may be asked to examine birds and to give an opinion as to whether a ring might have

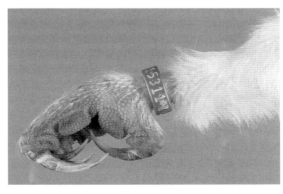

Figure 5.20 A closed ring on the leg of a captive-bred snowy owl.

been applied unlawfully. Often the best person initially for this task is an experienced aviculturist (bird-keeper) and in the UK such people are often used – generally senior members of the British Bird

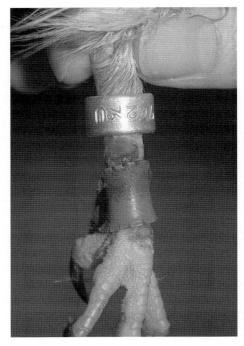

Figure 5.21 A closed ring on the leg of a kestrel, in juxtaposition to a leather jess. Between and beneath the two is an ulcerated area of skin.

Council (see Appendix B) – usually in collaboration with a veterinarian who can give an opinion on foot or leg injuries.

PREDATION

Many wild animals are killed or injured by predators and it is important to be able to differentiate this situation from human-induced wildlife crime or instances when, for example, a domesticated dog, cat or ferret is responsible. It may not be easy. Some predators, such as the fox, can be responsible for mass killings of, for example, free-range poultry (Moberly *et al.*, 2004) or nesting seabirds. Under such circumstances detective work, including detection of fox tracks (Ennion and Tinbergen, 1967) may be needed to determine the sequence of events. Tooth, beak or claw/talon marks may assist in determining which predator killed the animal

(Figure 5.13) (see also Chapters 2, 6 and 7). So also may the scene of the killing – a sparrow-hawk, for example, will often stand on its prey and scatter feathers. Foxes and certain other species cache their food and sometimes the circumstances of such activities may elicit suspicion that a crime has been committed – for instance, when certain species of shrike establish a 'larder' by impaling their dead prey on thorns.

Tracks, spoor and other signs have long been used by naturalists and hunters to follow animals and to determine what may have happened in a particular incident. Numerous texts are available – in Africa, for example, Stuart and Stuart (1994) and Walker (1996) – but no amount of reading equates with practical training from an experienced person in the field.

Post-mortem scavenging needs to be distinguished from *ante-mortem* predation (See Chapter 2).

Some predatory species are very emotive – for example, wolves in North America where controversy over control arises because of the different attitudes towards them of farmers, conservationists and welfarists.

FIREARMS AND UNEXPLODED ORDNANCE

This important topic is discussed in more detail in Chapter 7. Most firearm injuries to wildlife are caused by shotguns, airguns or rifles. Firearms have been described as 'one of the major causes of death and debilitation in wildlife' (PAW, 2005). In some parts of the world free-living animals may be injured or killed by landmines, hand grenades or explosions in munitions dumps – all usually a consequence of civil disturbance or war.

The presence of shot, pellets, bullets or metallic fragments in the body of a wild animal does not necessarily mean that they were responsible for death. They may instead be:

- Residual, from a previous, non-fatal, shooting or similar incident.
- Within the GI tract, having been ingested with prey items (carnivorous mammals, birds and

reptiles); this can sometimes lead to plumbism (lead toxicosis).

- Inflicted *post mortem* – for example, by someone who has killed an animal by some other means and seeks to cover his/her tracks by shooting the carcase to suggest that the animal died of ballistic injuries.

These three scenarios can be detected and differentiated by an experienced wildlife pathologist, using gross necropsy techniques supported by radiography, histology or other relevant tests (see Chapter 7).

Shot animals are sometimes used as poisoned bait for other species (PAW, 2005).

A significant body of literature on human military and civil firearms injuries provides guidance for the scientific examination of ballistic wounds in animals (Beyer, 1962; Pavlettic, 1986a,b). However, the huge diversity of wildlife species and their special anatomical characteristics may require significant conjecture for interpretation of necropsy findings.

Mounted (taxidermy) specimens may also need to be examined for evidence of shot, pellets or bullets. Care must be taken not to confuse pieces of wire used in the taxidermy process for metallic objects of ballistic origin. If a mounted specimen is valuable, or there are concerns about claims for damages if it is dismembered, an endoscope can be used to locate and to remove metal objects (Brearley *et al.*, 1991).

OTHER WEAPONS

Non-ballistic weapons are used to kill or to maim wildlife in many parts of the world. Even in North America, arrows (fired with a conventional bow or crossbow) are used to kill deer and other species. In poorer parts of the world arrows, spears and catapults may be standard means of taking animals, usually for food but sometimes for other illegal purposes, such as the killing of protected adult animals so that their young can be captured (see earlier).

The characteristic features of arrow and spear wounds are discussed in Chapter 7.

TRAPS, NETS AND SNARES

The catching of wild animals is not, *per se*, illegal. Large numbers of different species are trapped because they are pests, or for food or as part of scientific study.

Trapping may prompt legal action for a variety of reasons:

- Trapping can be a *de facto* offence, always or at certain times of year or in that particular location.

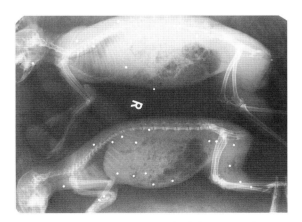

Figure 5.22 Rabbits containing lead shot. Were these animals shot when alive or after death?

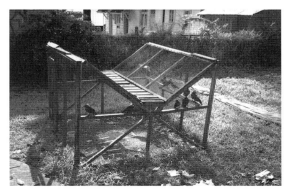

Figure 5.23 A trap for Indian house crows, which are classified as pest species in Tanzania.

- The trap being used may be of an illegal type – perhaps because the use of live bait on the trap mechanism is considered 'cruel'.
- The trapping and trap are legal but the operator is not using the equipment properly or not checking it at regular intervals, or is setting the trap to catch non-target (protected) species.

Traps, nets and snares can cause injury, stress and pain, even if properly used. Trauma is usually characterised by 'patterned injuries' (also shown in vehicular and other damage). Traps may cause crushing lesions; nets and snares cause strangulation or impairment to blood flow (see also Chapters 6 and 7). A trapped animal may succumb to hyperthermia, hypothermia or 'exposure'. It may be predated by another species. Sometimes a decoy animal is intentionally injured. Some such injuries are described and depicted in PAW (2005).

Other trapping methods can also have adverse effects on animals. 'Bird lime' and other sticky materials can prevent a bird from leaving a perch or branch and may damage the integument, eyes and beak.

Pitfall traps can cause falling injuries and may impale animals if stakes are placed in the bottom (often standard when trapping animals for meat). Drowning may occur if pit traps become flooded or if a research worker fails to protect or check his invertebrate traps regularly. Any trapped animal can

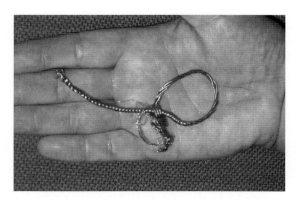

Figure 5.24 Part of a snare, made of braided wire, from Rwanda. This was set to catch small antelope but inadvertently trapped a young mountain gorilla, necessitating amputation of two of its digits. This figure also appears in colour in the colour plate section.

(will) be stressed and, if left long enough, is likely to succumb to dehydration, starvation or death.

Quite apart from legal controls on trapping methods, there are in many countries codes of practice that have been established voluntarily by non-governmental organisations (NGOs) (see, for example, BASC, 2001).

ROAD-TRAFFIC (VEHICULAR) ACCIDENTS

'Collision investigation' is a recognised forensic speciality and while it usually implies conventional traffic accidents involving humans and vehicles, animals are often affected. The effects are discussed in more detail in Chapter 7.

Wild animals are a common cause of collisions. They may be injured or killed themselves but they can also be directly responsible for accidents to humans and damage to vehicles. Injured wildlife may harm those who try to help them. The species involved tend to be the larger mammals, such as deer in Europe and North America, buffalo or gazelle in Africa and kangaroos in Australia. Donkeys and camels, which often sleep on warm roads at night, take their toll in many developing countries.

Some indication of the significance of animal–vehicle collisions is provided by figures from the UK (Langbein *et al.*, 2004) where the annual toll of deer involved in such accidents is 40,000. There are many hundreds of human injuries and some fatalities (at least ten in 2004). As a result of concerns, the Deer Collisions Project has been set up to assess the situation and to seek remedies.

Many wild animals are injured or killed by traffic, even if they do not themselves cause damage. Reptiles and amphibians are amongst those that are particularly vulnerable (Ashley and Robinson, 1996).

OTHER BLUNT TRAUMA

Wild animals may strike buildings, wires or aerials, especially if the weather is bad or if lights cause confusion (see Chapter 6). Novel landscape features such as large-scale wind farms have the potential to inflict significant losses due to collision. 'Bird-strikes' involving aircraft have long attracted interest and research, primarily on account of the dangers to humans and the costs that such encounters incur. Aircraft, including helicopters, can have adverse effects on wild animals, especially flocks of birds and those that are breeding (Grubb and Bowerman, 1997).

'Natural' causes of injury or death include exposure to rain, hail, snow or lightning.

All of the above may necessitate an input by a veterinary pathologist (see Chapter 7). The investigation of birdstrikes includes studies of feathers in order to identify the species responsible (PAW, 2005).

THE RANGE OF HUMAN-INDUCED INJURY IN WILDLIFE

Humans may injure or kill wildlife in a variety of ways – sometimes intentionally, sometimes by neglect, sometimes by accident. The task of the pathologist is not to apportion blame (that is usually the responsibility of a court) but to decide whether or not the injuries or death were likely to have been human-induced (anthropogenic) or caused by other species or events (see Appendix D). Thus, for example, if carcases of protected birds are reported, the investigator needs to initiate:

- A crime scene visit and assessment.
- Specialist examination of the dead birds and their tissues.
- Involvement of other experts, e.g. ornithologists, as necessary.

Much has been published on certain taxa. For example, Read and Murray (2000) documented anthropogenic trauma in small cetaceans (dolphins, porpoises) and listed entanglement in gill nets, purse seines, ropes and lines, gunshot, vessel collisions and blast-induced trauma. They provided valuable information on how to differentiate and diagnose such incidents. They re-stated that entanglement in fishing gear is the most common human-induced cause of mortality in small cetaceans (see also Kuiken *et al.*, 1994) and emphasised that

'the physical evidence associated with entanglement is specific to each combination of cetacean and fishing gear.' A more general review of the effects of non-infectious insults on wildlife, including trauma, electrocution, burning, drowning, hypothermia and hyperthermia, was provided by Cooper (Cooper, J.E., 1996a).

Specialised knowledge can be very important in wildlife cases and sometimes it is the field naturalist, gamekeeper or hunter who can offer the best practical advice. For example, in the UK the investigation of alleged offences against badgers (see Chapter 3) can involve determining whether 1) a hole in the ground is that of a badger, fox or certain other species, 2) an apparent blockage by soil or other material is human-induced or 'natural'.

POISONING OF WILDLIFE

This is an important subject, which is discussed in detail in numerous books and publications (see References). Its importance in wildlife forensic work is described in PAW (2005) and poisoning also features later in this book (see Chapters 6, 7 and 8).

Wildlife (including invertebrates) are susceptible to a wide range of poisoning (Stroud *et al.*, 1999) – both natural (e.g. botulism) and anthropogenic (e.g. misuse of pesticides). Acute poisoning cases are usually more likely to be detected by the public or others because animals are found dead or dying. Toxic substances may be ingested, inhaled (e.g. gases) or pass through the skin. Susceptibility can depend upon the species involved, e.g. there may be ready absorption of certain chemicals through the thin, mucous, skin of frogs. Insects, such as bees, are susceptible to many toxic substances and, by virtue of their social behaviour, may spread the poison to others.

Chronic toxicosis may have profound effects in the ecosystem, especially if the material enters the food chain and accumulates in predator species, as happened with chlorinated hydrocarbons in birds of prey in North America and Europe in the 1950s and 1960s (for background, see Cooper, J.E., 2002). Some toxic substances may be immunosuppressive and thus predispose wildlife to infectious disease – polychlorinated biphenyls (PCBs) in porpoises, for example (Jepson *et al.*, 2005). Petroleum-based chemicals can kill animals by toxicity as well as by having an adverse effect on pelage and thermoregulation (see later).

Poisoned wildlife may attract predators which may be secondarily affected. Equally, wildlife may ingest toxic substances from domesticated livestock that have been poisoned accidentally, euthanased or contain drugs – such as diclofenac which is now recognised as the cause of decline of *Gyps* vultures in Asia (Oaks *et al.*, 2004).

In any investigation of suspected poisoning in wildlife an important component is investigation of local conditions that might be relevant, e.g. use of chemicals for agricultural purposes, effluent from factories. Collection of evidence must be carried out proficiently (see Chapters 8 and 11) with attention to the health and safety considerations of handling, sometimes inhaling, toxic material. In different countries there may be systems for investigating suspected poisoning of free-living animals – the Wildlife Incident Investigation Scheme (WIIS) in the UK, for example (PAW, 2005).

Ionising radiation, radio-active fallout and radio-frequency exposure can have a 'toxic' effect on wildlife (and, indeed, on domesticated species and humans – see Chapter 6).

OTHER PHYSICAL FACTORS

Electrocution, drowning and exposure to high or low temperatures or irradiation, all relevant to wildlife, are discussed in Chapter 6. To them should be added seismic investigations, which are alleged to be one of many stressors that can induce stranding of marine mammals and therefore may prompt the instigation of a legal injunction by conservation bodies.

ENVIRONMENTAL (RISK) ASSESSMENTS

The evaluation of environmental impact when land-use is to be changed is a standard, often a legal, requirement in certain countries (Levins,

1998). Elsewhere it may be carried out on a voluntary basis.

Environmental assessment studies are not part of conventional forensic work but are discussed briefly in this chapter because they fall under the general heading of 'inquiries' (see Chapter 2), where expert opinion is likely to be sought. They can be contentious, especially when they challenge business interests or deal with controversial subjects such as the effects of genetically-modified (GM) organisms on the environment and on other species (Hilbeck and Andow, 2005). Assignment of liability may be an outcome of environmental assessment (Levins, 1998).

An environmental assessment study may incorporate comprehensive surveys of habitat, animals and plants and an analysis, nowadays often involving computer modelling, of the effects that the proposed developments are likely to have. Sometimes, however, a limited assessment is feasible. For example, if the building of a road across an area of marshland is proposed and there is no statutory requirement for a full environmental impact assessment, a decision may be made to carry out only a restricted investigation – for instance, into the likely effects of the development on the status of a rare amphibian, or the possible dangers to travellers from mosquitoes that harbour dengue fever virus.

Advice given as part of environmental assessment should be as professional and evidence-based as in a court case. However, this may not always be the case; Levins (1998), in discussing the rationale behind assessment, stated that in today's world 'control over the measurement of environmental impact is contested territory'.

ENVIRONMENTAL FORENSICS

This is a relatively new discipline and a good example of how the term 'forensics' is increasingly being applied to new situations (see Chapter 2). Environmental forensic science is particularly concerned with contamination of ecosystems by, for example, oil and other petroleum hydrocarbons (Morrison, 1999). The science depends largely upon such techniques as 'chemical fingerprinting' of polluted water, soil, sediments and air. This can include measurement of different chemicals and isotopes. These investigations can be backed up by aerial photogrammetry, statistical analysis and contaminant modelling (Murphy and Morrison, 2002). Environmental forensics overlaps with a number of other disciplines and, in view of growing concerns about 'ecosystem health' (Rapport *et al.*, 1998) is likely to be of increasing importance in the years to come. It can be argued that it is part of 'comparative forensic medicine'.

An example of 'chemical fingerprinting' that is very relevant to animal work concerns oiling incidents. From time to time seabirds are found in substantial numbers with external and internal petroleum oil damage but no obvious origin, such as a damaged tanker, for the oil. Residues on feathers can be 'fingerprinted' in order to identify the fractions present and thus help to pinpoint the source. Sometimes the oil is seeping from a sunken wreck; on other occasions it can be traced to illegal bilge-washing. Organisations that can provide advice on this and other examples of 'chronic oiling' include the Oiled Wildlife Care Network, University of California, Davis, USA (www.owcn.org) and the International Fund for Animal Welfare (www.ifaw.org) (see Appendix B).

Environmental forensics is a truly interdisciplinary subject. It involves, for example, chemists, hydrologists, geologists and global information systems (GIS) specialists. Pollution monitoring using plants, especially lichens (Richardson, 1992) is well established and provides the basis for all-important long-term studies. Palaeoecologists

are increasingly involved in the planning and management of terrestrial landscapes (see, for example, Alexander, 2005) and micropalaeontologists, such as those studying foraminiferal seafloor assemblages (Sen Gupta, 1999), may provide comparable data on the marine environment. People from these disciplines mirror their counterparts in palaeopathology (see Chapters 2 and 7) in contributing usefully to contemporary forensic investigations.

PROCEDURES FOR INVESTIGATION

In some countries, those investigating wildlife crime may have access to the advice, experience and assistance of such people as (in the UK) Forensic Science Managers, Scenes of Crime Officers (see Chapter 9) and official agencies such as the Forensic Science Service (FSS) (see Appendix B). The value of such support has been strongly emphasised (PAW, 2005). Such a situation does not necessarily prevail, however, and those involved in wildlife crime investigation, especially (but not only) in poorer parts of the world may well have to take on a whole range of tasks and then seek advice as appropriate.

Sophisticated, often expensive, laboratory investigations are sometimes a hallmark of wildlife crime investigations. The use of scanning electronmicrography (SEM) to identify birds' eggs (Mikhailov, 1997) and the measurement of stable isotopes in elephant hair to document migration patterns and diet changes (Cerling *et al.*, 2006) are two examples. However, simple, field techniques may be sufficient. When a dolphin was reported to be stranded and then 'went missing' at a coastal location in Trinidad, blood was found on a nearby wooden chopping-board. Smears of the blood, stained with a rapid dye (see Chapter 8 and Appendix E), revealed red blood cells that were anucleate, not nucleated as would be expected if the board had been used, as claimed, to cut up fish (Figure 9.17).

The movement of wildlife samples from one country to another can be daunting, because of bureaucracy, compounded by the fact that some

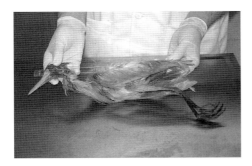

Figure 5.25 An egret that died following oiling in a major tanker disaster.

specimens may themselves require CITES permits (Cooper, 1995c) (see Chapter 3).

RECORD-KEEPING

In the investigation of wildlife crime, as in all fields of forensic medicine, records are vital (see also Chapter 10). Depending on the species, it may be necessary and wise to combine forensic records (clinical, *post-mortem*, laboratory) with the collection of biological data – for example, in marine mammal incidents, where the compilation of a 'stranding report' is routine.

REFERENCE MATERIAL AND DATABASES

Access to reference material and baseline data is of great importance in wildlife forensic work (PAW, 2005). Little relevant information may be available for some species but this situation is changing. Museums serve as an excellent resource and often their staff are highly skilled in both theory (e.g. taxonomy) and practice (e.g. prosection).

REFERENCE COLLECTIONS

Dedicated reference specimens and collections can be of great value in forensic work. In the USA and Australia the term 'voucher specimen' is used (see, for example, Griffiths and Bates, 2002) while the word 'archival' is usually applied to stored laboratory material.

Although a few museums are devoted to human forensic medicine, there are very few collections that relate specifically to animal forensics. This means that there is only limited material available for teaching (see Chapter 13) and for reference in court cases. The situation has improved in recent years with the development of electronic communication, whereby images of specimens or parts thereof can be sent all over the world (see Chapter 10). Nevertheless, depositories of original material that can be handled and even sampled are of great potential value.

Collections relating to wildlife crime are being established. The USFWS has a growing assemblage of reference material at its National Fish and Wildlife Forensics Laboratory in Oregon, USA (see Appendix B). Smaller official or private collections exist in the UK, New Zealand and Australia, and probably elsewhere. It could be argued, especially in view of the legal obstacles to moving specimens (see Chapter 3 and Cooper, 1995c), that each country or region should have a forensic reference collection of its own. This is certainly the aim in Trinidad and Tobago in the West Indies, where plans for such a development are currently (2005) under discussion.

A leaf could be taken out of the book of some zoological societies and conservation bodies where the establishment of reference collections has been standard for many years. The rationale has been discussed by a number of authors, amongst them Bailey *et al.* (1997), Cooper and Jones (1986), Cooper *et al.* (1998), Amato and Lehn (2002), Munson (2002) and Ryder (2002). Davis (1987) emphasised the value of 'comparative collections' for use by zoo-archaeologists and Gippoliti (2005) stressed the vital role of historical museums in documenting biodiversity.

Various criteria are important in the establishment and maintenance of reference collections and these are listed below:

- Legal acquisition of all material.
- Meticulous provenancing of all specimens (essential in order to validate forensic results that are to be used in criminal case-work).
- Proper cataloguing, including unique reference numbers, and reliable labelling of specimens.
- Well-publicised information on how specimens can be studied or used.
- Strict adherence to national and international laws when material is sent overseas.

A progression of this is the establishment of gene banks where micro-organisms, plant seeds and frozen embryos can be stored. The Kew Millennium Seed Bank is one example, the Frozen Ark, a joint initiative between the (UK) Natural History Museum, the Zoological Society of London and Nottingham University, another. Such gene banks are very relevant to those involved in the investigation of wildlife crime.

MOUNTED (TAXIDERMY) SPECIMENS AND COLLECTIONS OF DEAD ANIMALS

Taxidermy (the art of preparing, preserving and mounting the skin of animals) has a long and often distinguished history. Professional taxidermists are responsible people with an interest in natural history, conservation and education – for example, members of the Guild of Taxidermists in Britain. Such people only accept specimens that have been legally obtained, they keep proper records and they have an enforceable code of practice.

In contrast, there are, probably throughout the world, people who practise taxidermy or who prepare bones, horns, antlers or similar specimens who do not adhere to the law and by their actions contribute to the overall incidence of wildlife crime. Under the same broad heading one can include those who mount ('set') butterflies or other insects. Most entomologists who do so are professional, interested in the science of the invertebrates, but some less-scrupulous people obtain their material illegally and prepare it hurriedly, often poorly, usually to sell to tourists as household displays.

Mounted specimens present many challenges (PAW, 2005). The origin (provenance) of the specimen is important, as is its cause of death. Ascertaining its history, including age (when it was collected), may be necessary. Under New Zealand legislation, for example, specimens of protected native wildlife taken prior to 1962 can be owned and traded without permit.

Investigation of mounted material, whether vertebrate or invertebrate, requires the input of specialists. A professional taxidermist can provide evidence on how an animal has been prepared and the materials (e.g. wires, artificial eyes) used. So also can a *bona fide* entomologist: there are different ways of setting insects and a variety of pins of different size and make can be employed. The showcases and cabinets in which mounted material is kept may provide important clues, including good-quality fingerprints (PAW, 2005).

Other disciplines can, however, be involved. A pathologist may be asked to radiograph and examine a dead or stuffed animal, for instance.

Many *post-mortem* and laboratory tests that are applicable to a fresh carcase can also be applied to a mounted specimen or a study skin – hair or feather investigation, for example. Portions of skin and other tissues can be rehydrated and examined histologically.

An ornithologist or herpetologist may need to give an opinion on the species, age or sex of the specimen.

The preparation ('blowing') of birds' eggs is a specialised way of preserving animal derivatives for a collection. Some egg-collectors (oologists) do so legally (nowadays usually for scientific purposes) but there are others who flout the relevant laws (PAW, 2005). This is a complex field that may involve veterinarians and others in such tasks as examination of live or dead birds for evidence of reproductive activity (see Chapter 7), laboratory investigation of eggs and forensic studies on egg-collecting equipment and notebooks. Museum collections provide useful reference material.

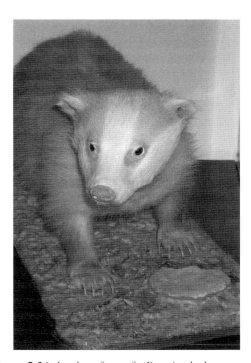

Figure 5.26 A colour form of a Eurasian badger, mounted legally for exhibition by a professional taxidermist. This figure also appears in colour in the colour plate section.

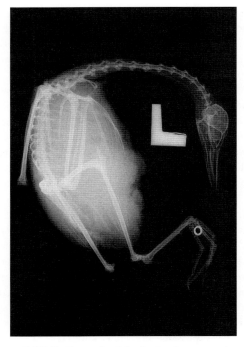

Figure 5.27 Radiograph of the body of a rare grebe retrieved from a freezer. Some portions are missing, suggesting that a 'study skin' had previously been prepared.

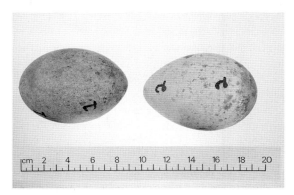

Figure 5.28 Eggs submitted for forensic laboratory investigation.

DNA TECHNOLOGY

The development of DNA and other molecular techniques has revolutionised the investigation of wildlife crime. It has permitted the detection and differentiation of substances from different species,

e.g. bones of tigers, gall bladders of bears. It has also allowed investigation into imported materials, thus assisting Customs officials and those who are charged with enforcing CITES. Databases of DNA are being established which can assist in enforcement – for instance, the UK badger DNA bank (Anon, 2005g).

In addition to all this, DNA studies provide a better understanding of genetic diversity and the conservation of endangered animal species (Zhang *et al.*, 2002) and have been used to differentiate hybrids from pure breeds, e.g. wolves and dogs (Boyd *et al.*, 2001). The use of the polymerase chain reaction (PCR) permits forensic identification of tiny, less-than-optimal, samples – as shown by Wan and Fang (2003) in their work on the forensic identification of tiger species (see also Chapter 7).

Although plants fall outside the remit of this book, it is worth mentioning that DNA technology, using micro-satellite markers, can also be used to genotype trees – the red cedar (*Thuja plicata*), for example – in order to detect stolen wood (White *et al.*, 2000).

DNA technology is discussed in more detail in Chapter 8.

SAMPLES AND DATA

In a paper presented to the American Association of Zoo Veterinarians in 2002, Rideout (2002) of the San Diego Zoo recommended the following basic rules for the establishment of a 'bio-materials archive' that could serve both the conservation and research communities:

- Freeze samples at −70°C.
- Follow specimen-handling and sample-labelling guidelines.
- Use an adequate volume of formalin for fixed tissues, and limit fixation time to less than 72 hours.
- Consider collecting selected duplicate samples in absolute (100%) ethanol for molecular diagnostics when freezing is not practicable.
- Whenever possible, send duplicate samples to central repositories, such as Species Survival Programme (SSP) archives and, for example, San Diego Zoo's frozen zoo.

- When investigating health problems of unknown aetiology, consider archiving unconventional samples such as ocular fluid, *post-mortem* lung smears, whole blood, yolk samples from eggs or chicks, stomach and intestinal content, urine, hair, bone, food and water samples.
- Maintain an inventory of your archives in a computerised database, with appropriate back-up.

These basic rules are also applicable to forensic work.

In practical terms, what should be saved? Below is a list of material that should, ideally, be collected from the carcases of all wildlife species.

Gross specimens

- Hair/feather/scales.
- Pectoral muscle
  - in alcohol for DNA
  - frozen for toxicology.
- Brain – frozen.
- Liver – frozen.
- Kidney – frozen.
- Reproductive organs (gonads) – frozen.
- Body fat.
- Whole skin, if practicable.
- Skeleton/selected bones, where practicable.

Specimens in fixative or frozen

- Lung, liver, kidney (LLK).
- Any abnormalities.
- Others as necessary.

In formalin for histology (see Chapter 8)

- Blood/skin – in ethanol and frozen for DNA studies.

Morphometrics

Morphometric data from wild animals are important (see also Chapter 7) and can be crucial to a forensic case. They should include the following weights (masses):

- Whole body.
- Liver.
- Heart.

- Brain, if available.
- Other organs, if time permits.

Plus

Standard measurements – depends on taxon (see Chapter 7).

Advice must be sought from specialists when measuring and sampling certain species – for example, marine mammals (Dierauf and Gulland, 2001).

USE OF LABORATORIES AND SPECIALIST ADVICE

The investigation of wildlife crime cannot usually be carried out by one individual, organisation or government body alone. Specialist advice is needed. Larger institutions such as the USFWS Laboratory (see earlier) can undertake a wide range of investigations; others may be more limited in scope.

Examples of techniques that may be needed in the detection and investigation of wildlife crime are given in Table 5.2.

How specimens and other evidence are submitted from the field to the laboratory can be critical to the success of a case (PAW, 2005) (see Chapter 8).

SAMPLING OF LIVE WILD ANIMALS

In a legal case it may be necessary to take samples from live wild animals for specific forensic purposes, diagnosis, health monitoring or even a combination of these. Two non-invasive examples that may be relevant to forensic work are the examination of faeces for parasites, for food contents or for corticosteroids and the testing of urine for toxins or abnormal metabolites. Some studies may necessitate intervention, e.g. the sampling of blood or of internal organs.

As a general rule, non-invasive or minimally-invasive methods should be used for wildlife, whether these animals are captive or free-living (Cooper, 1998b) – for example, buccal swabs can be used for DNA analysis in amphibians, rather

Table 5.2 Techniques in wildlife crime investigation.

Category	*Examples*	*Comments*
Identification and morphological studies	Species determination using bones, skins, hair, feathers, scales and derivatives	Involves gross, microscopical and DNA-based techniques
Pathology	*Post-mortem* examination of whole carcases, organs and tissues from dead animals – and samples from live animals (see below)	Can include various supporting tests, e.g. radiology and other scanning techniques (see Chapter 7) and laboratory investigations (see Chapter 8)
Clinical work	Examination and sampling of live animals	Supporting tests as above – and others (see Chapter 6)
DNA technology	Species, sex and parentage determination; other investigations as above	A very important component of most investigations
Crime investigation	Studies on ballistics, chemical assay, soil analysis, fingerprints, tyre marks, etc., etc.	'Standard' investigations, usually involving police and specialists
Crime scene studies	As above in the field, plus other investigations	See Chapter 9

than killing animals in order to remove blood or organs (Pidancier *et al.*, 2003) (see Chapter 4).

Even if there is no question of killing or making a significant intervention, care must be taken. If an accident occurs and an animal is injured or dies, there may be legal consequences. If this happens when examining captive wild animals, the owner may demand compensation. The incident needs to be fully documented and a full report produced. If the animal dies, a necropsy must be performed. In the UK, DEFRA has issued strict guidelines concerning such unexpected incidents for its Wildlife Inspectors, including arrangements for compensation.

When free-living or captive wildlife has to be marked for identification, best practice should be followed – in the interest of the welfare of the animal(s) and also to minimise the risk of claims for compensation or legal action. For example, methods for inserting microchip transponders should follow WSAVA, IUCN/SSC or other recognised guidelines (see Chapter 6). Record-keeping is essential.

Relevant legislation must always be followed – for example, if a veterinary input is needed (see Chapter 3). This may be the situation when wildlife must be captured and handled for enforcement purposes

– for instance, in areas of Africa where rhinos may be immobilised (darted), ear-notched, have transponders (microchips) implanted, radio transmitters inserted and possibly even dehorned.

PRACTICAL ASPECTS OF WILDLIFE WORK

The basic tenets of wildlife crime investigation are given in PAW (2005). Reference should also be made to earlier reports in the UK (Department of the Environment, 1996, 1997, 1998, 2004) and corresponding publications in other countries.

Writing from the USA, Stroud (1998) provided a useful summary of the role of the veterinarian in wildlife forensics. He drew attention to the need to be familiar with the relevant law and reminded the reader that s/he might well be involved in assisting at a wildlife crime scene investigation (see Chapter 9). Stroud emphasised the need to participate in the latter with care, and sensitivity and awareness of the importance of careful examination. He further pointed out that, when working with wildlife, there could be considerable media and public official attention: the veterinarian or other wildlife crime investigator would need to be aware of this and take appropriate action (protests may also ensue if the public feels strongly about an issue: see also Chapter 4).

Stroud discussed forensic necropsy in some detail, with particular reference to determining the cause, manner and mechanism of death of wild animals, the collection and preservation of trace evidence (such as contamination on the surface of the carcase or bullet), the determination of time of death and the importance of documenting observations. Stroud listed as 'pathology of forensic significance' gunshot wounds (which are generally more prevalent in some countries, such as the USA, than in others) and wildlife poisoning. Many of the points above were also made by Wobeser (1996) and in PAW (2005). The former emphasised the paucity of published data on wildlife forensic medicine, especially pathology, and pointed out that extrapolation from work on humans might be necessary.

The investigation of wildlife crime is not, essentially, very different from any other type of forensic work. However, it can involve a whole range of techniques (see Table 5.2), often under field conditions (see later and Chapter 9). Methods that are used in more conventional forensic studies can often be applied – for instance, the casting of footprints and tyre marks – which are as applicable when investigating poaching in a game reserve in Swaziland as they are in a homicide investigation in Sweden. Wildlife crime may also involve the use of equipment such as knives, pliers or climbing irons, all of which may need to be investigated (PAW, 2005).

Fingerprint analysis may be necessary: this and other standard forensic methods should be carried out by experienced personnel (see also Chapter 9). Some prints will be out-of-doors and it may be necessary to protect items from rain in order to increase the chances of detection. Even if an object is not a good medium for fingerprints, e.g. a bird's egg or a reptile's skin, its container (cabinet, plastic bag) or associated equipment may yield them.

DNA technology plays an essential part in many wildlife cases (PAW, 2005). It is discussed in more detail in Chapter 8. The collection of samples for DNA analysis may be part of the duties of a veterinarian or wildlife inspector (see later).

The wildlife crime scene is likely to be in the field

and this can present particular challenges, as emphasised in Chapter 9. The concept is increasingly being recognised, however, as typified by the recent (2005) case involving the killing of a brown bear in the French Pyrenees, which prompted a magistrate and his lawyer to visit the location and reconstruct the crime scene (Penketh, 2005).

Collaboration is a key part of investigation of wildlife crime but, even in countries with a good track record, things can go wrong. The (British) Royal Society for the Protection of Birds (RSPB) recently (Anon., 2005i) expressed its disappointment over the handling of a case by the police and/or Crown Prosecution Service (CPS). The RSPB particularly lamented the failure to consult appropriate agencies and the inconsistent use of 'public interest criteria'. The subject is never free of controversy!

SPECIALISED EQUIPMENT

Because wildlife crime often involves fieldwork, much of the equipment listed in Appendix E is relevant. One advantage of having naturalists involved in wildlife crime investigations is that they often already have relevant equipment that they use, for example, for bird-watching, and which can readily be adapted to forensic studies. Examples include waterproof and submersible cameras and cases, night-vision kits, monitoring devices and handheld radios.

Some investigations involve captive animals (in a sanctuary, zoo or an aviary which then constitutes a wildlife crime scene) and here specialised kits may need to be assembled, especially if live animals have to be handled and examined. Items to be taken to the scene are likely to include gloves, nets, bags, capture and restraining devices, binoculars, reference texts, avian ring (leg-band) pliers and remover, film pots or similar to contain rings (bands), a magnifying glass, scales or balance and (veterinarian's) standard clinical kit. Occasionally during handling an animal becomes injured, sick or stressed (see earlier): appropriate emergency therapy may be needed and the incident must be documented and reported.

ENFORCEMENT OF WILDLIFE LEGISLATION

The extent and success of enforcement varies greatly from country to country. Often the poorer countries, which so often have the greatest number and variety of wild animals, are the ones least able to combat wildlife crime. Richer nations, on the other hand, may have an extensive system of investigation and access to both personnel and equipment that enable cases to be followed through as necessary.

In the United Kingdom the enforcement of wildlife legislation is carried out by the Department for Environment, Food and Rural Affairs (DEFRA) (see Appendix B). The full-time staff of the Department is supplemented by Part-Time Wildlife Inspectors. These Inspectors serve as consultants to DEFRA and join its panel as experts in their own fields, not as representatives of any organisation or body. They are involved in site visits and inspections at the request of the Department. Inspectors come from varied backgrounds but each will have experience or training in some field that is relevant to wildlife law enforcement – for example, identification of birds or reptiles, rehabilitation of wildlife, veterinary medicine, taxidermy, identification of wild plants. The work is carried out at the request of the Department and the letter from the Department to the Inspector serves as a 'letter of authority'.

The Department, through its Chief Wildlife Inspector, provides the individual Inspector with written advice, guidance and information as necessary and he or one of his team is available seven days a week for guidance. Wildlife Inspectors are issued with an identity card, notebook, Handbook, microchip reader, documents, books, etc. all of which remain the property of DEFRA. Wildlife Inspectors operate under a strict Code of Practice and this covers such aspects of their work and responsibilities as authorisation procedures, timing of inspections, health and safety issues, contact during inspections, reporting arrangements, security and confidentiality and situations where there may be conflicts of interest.

A development in the UK that has helped to involve organisations and individuals in wildlife law enforcement is the establishment of the Partnership for Action against Wildlife Crime (PAW) (see Appendix B). PAW is a multi-agency body that has within its membership representatives of organisations ranging from large conservation bodies to small consultancies, all with an interest in combating wildlife crime by raising awareness and promoting effective enforcement. Much of PAW's work is carried out by its Working Groups. One of these is the Forensic Working Group (FWG), whose objective is to assist in tackling wildlife crime through the promotion, development and measured review of forensic methods. In its early days, FWG tended to concentrate on DNA techniques, but in recent years has begun to encompass 'forensics' in its correct, broader, sense. A culmination of this was the production of the publication *Wildlife Crime: A Guide to the Use of Forensic and Specialist Techniques in the Investigation of Wildlife Crime* (PAW, 2005), referred to earlier in this chapter.

Another feature in the UK (and, increasingly, in other countries) is the establishment of police Wildlife Crime Officers (WCOs). The majority of British police forces now have at least one WCO who can respond to reports of breaches of conservation legislation. In 2005 there are over 700 WCOs in all, of which at least 145 are on a full-time basis.

DEFRA announced on 2 February 2006 that the UK Government is to join the 'US-led' Coalition Against Wildlife Trafficking (CAWT), with a view to strengthening the work of the latter, especially in Asia.

In smaller, especially poorer, countries it may not be easy to emulate the systems outlined above but it should be possible to involve the community. In Trinidad and Tobago, for example, there is a network of Honorary Game Wardens who provide support to full-time officers of the Forestry Division. Such people receive training in techniques that include collecting evidence, record-keeping and production of statements (Figure 9.18).

Education plays an important part in the enforcement of wildlife legislation. It is an ongoing, continuous activity that must go hand-in-hand with more proscriptive methods. Some educational programmes are focused on individual species or taxa that, although protected by law, are persecuted because they either are, or are perceived to be, a danger to humans, livestock or crops.

An educational programme has to be informative as well as authoritative. An excellent example is in South Africa where (as in many other countries) eagles are often shot or trapped because they are believed regularly to kill lambs. The Raptor Conservation Group of the Endangered Wildlife Trust has produced educational literature *Innocent until Proven Guilty*, in both English and Afrikaans. This not only draws attention to the fact that domesticated dogs, jackals and caracals are more likely to predate lambs in southern Africa but, with the aid of photographs and drawings, illustrates the features of killing and predation by these and other species (including eagles). It also gives guidelines as to how to distinguish lambs that were stillborn or died soon after as opposed to those that have survived for a few hours or longer – for example, the presence of soft 'slippers' on the hooves and the presence or absence of a blood clot in the umbilicus. More detail is provided in papers by Roberts (1986) and (earlier work in Australia) by Rowley (1970).

INTERNATIONAL CONSIDERATIONS

Although the detection and investigation of wildlife crime is, perhaps, the most international of all fields of animal forensics, it cannot be assumed that countries contribute equally. As is stressed elsewhere, poorer ('Third World') countries are often at a disadvantage because they lack finance or facilities or are limited in their ability adequately to enforce legislation (see below). Sometimes countries are not signatories to international conventions or treaties or have failed to ratify them. This latter situation does not only apply to the smaller, less well-off, states, however; the failure of the USA – at present the world's richest and most powerful nation and a Permanent Member of the UN – to sign the Kyoto Agreement and certain other treaties is a cause of concern to those who want to see a fully global approach to environmental law and ethics.

At a more grassroots level, it is worth noting that it was not until 2005 that Britain police forces started to log wildlife crime incidents. Prior to this, there had been no obligation to record reports received unless the allegation was pursued and proceeded to the laying of charges. Further, in the same year (2005), the UK's National Criminal Intelligence Service stated that 'the penalties and relatively low priority attached to wildlife crime are unlikely to be any deterrent to the serious organised criminal'. These deficiencies are beginning to be addressed, however: the Police Wildlife Crime Officers (WCO) Network, which provides a focus for collaboration and enforcement in the UK, was strengthened by the launch on 22 April 2002 of the National Wildlife Crime Intelligence Unit (NWCIU).

Enforcing wildlife legislation often presents challenges. The reasons are complex – political, financial, corruption. Sometimes external pressure can be helpful but at times it is counter-productive, especially in countries where 'losing face' is considered shameful or embarrassing. At times other non-conservation factors can play a part – for example, following the announcement of the outbreak of severe acute respiratory syndrome (SARS) in China when there were over 9000 prosecutions for infringement of wildlife legislation in the space of only nine days. The possible use of public health legislation, coupled with education, to reduce the consumption of bushmeat was mentioned earlier.

At the time of writing, many governments are contemplating how best to counter wildlife crime. In the UK, for example, there are proposals from DEFRA that include prohibition of keeping of:

- CITES specimens that have been acquired unlawfully or are of certain threatened CITES species.
- All dead tiger specimens, their parts and derivatives.
- All bear bile, paws or gall bladders.
- All unworked rhino horns, apart from antique specimens on licensed hunting trophies.
- All specimens made from the hair of the Tibetan antelope.

Whether these or similar proposals will become law is as yet not certain but the message is clear. The determination of governments, non-governmental organisations (NGOs) and many members of the public to tackle wildlife crime means that the need for professional advice and expert opinion on conservation issues will markedly increase – a point that is alluded to again in Chapter 13.

In the long term, each country or region should consider establishing its own wildlife crime investigation laboratory. It is far preferable, for political as well as legal and practical reasons, that these are in-country rather than thousands of kilometres away in a 'developed' country. Sometimes sophisticated facilities and techniques are not required: thus, identification of parts of a South American rodent may be possible on the basis of its gross morphology, such as how many toes it has on its feet, and whether or not these bear claws, rather than having to submit material for DNA studies.

Combating wildlife crime is not easy. Many of the offences take place a long way from towns and cities where enforcement agencies are usually based. Poor countries face particular problems; they must either try to deal with the problem themselves or seek the help of outsiders. Some countries are reluctant to do the latter. Bringing in experts and expertise can be very expensive and to a new, young nation, proud of its independence, may be considered humiliating. This in turn may be compounded by the fact that wildlife crime is lucrative. As a result, wildlife enforcement in that country further falters and the situation spirals. The resulting situation can have international repercussions: thus in June 2005, at a meeting in Geneva, Traffic International reported that ivory was being openly sold in many African countries, in contravention of CITES.

In addition to all this, some rural people in poorer parts of the world see little merit in protecting what appear still to be widespread species of wildlife, especially while there are so many pressing human needs. This point was illustrated graphically in a report in the *Trinidad Guardian* (Jarrette, 2005) entitled 'Pelican fever'. A man was arrested for killing protected wild birds but his fellow villagers complained that pelicans are common, chickens are expensive and added for good measure (in West Indian dialect) 'Curry pelican does eat nice!'

The situation in some regions is compounded by war and social unrest, meaning that the wildlife cannot be given as much attention as richer countries and conservation bodies might like. It also often leads to poaching because people have become impoverished and/or weapons are more readily available.

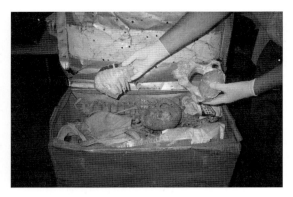

Figure 5.29 A bizarre link between forensic science and osteology. A box of bones of the rare mountain gorilla, that survived the 1994 Rwanda civil war but the metal trunk was used for target practice by the rebels.

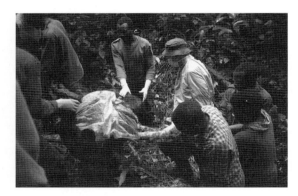

Figure 5.30 One of four mountain gorillas, found dead under mysterious circumstances in Uganda. This figure also appears in colour in the colour plate section.

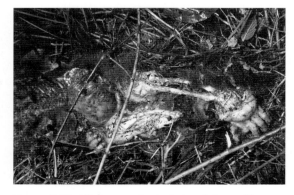

Figure 5.31 All that remained of one of the gorillas – bones, connective tissue and skin. This figure also appears in colour in the colour plate section.

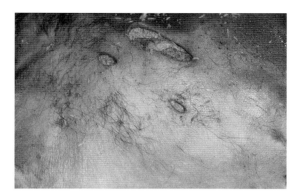

Figure 5.32 Skull wounds in one of the gorillas. The lesions are characteristic of metal arrows, commonly used by local poachers. Live maggots are present. This figure also appears in colour in the colour plate section.

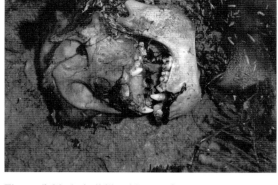

Figure 5.33 A skull like this one, from a mountain gorilla, should be transported back for detailed examination at a secure home base.

There is no clear-cut answer to these problems but closer collaboration between richer and poorer countries, with the two working as partners, is one way forward. The richer nations can provide training and advice. They can offer equipment, such as global information systems (GIS) and digital cameras that will allow better detection of wildlife crime and the possibility of sending electronic data overseas for analysis rather than flying in expensive personnel. The poorer countries can assist by making reference material available to wealthier countries and by providing facilities for training programmes and conferences.

PRACTICAL CONSIDERATIONS IN INTERNATIONAL INVESTIGATIONS

Anyone who is involved in international forensics must ensure that all those with whom s/he works are familiar with the particular needs, sometimes difficulties, of dealing with other countries. Globalisation may be the order of the day but many people still think in terms of their own country (a town, a village!). Using a lawyer or laboratory that cannot easily cope with various time zones, dissimilar English (or perhaps a different language) is not wise. Little things matter in legal cases and the batch of documents that takes eight weeks to travel between England and Venezuela because the posting (mailing) has been entrusted to a junior secretary who has not weighed or stamped the bundle correctly, is at best an embarrassment, at worst a disaster.

Working overseas on wildlife cases can be stimulating, frustrating, or a combination of the two. Some general guidance to those who may be involved on an international basis in forensic work is to be found in Chapter 9 and Appendix E.

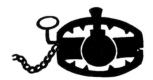

Methodology

CHAPTER 6

Clinical Work

The wounds that cannot be seen are more painful than those that can be treated by a doctor.
Nelson Mandela

Cure the disease and kill the patient.

Francis Bacon

Whenever forensic investigations are to be carried out, the approach must be one of careful preparation. Very rarely in such work is speed of the essence; on the contrary, often the best-performed studies are when planning has been exhaustive, including the use of protocols and the drawing up of precautions in the event of unexpected circumstances.

The clinical examination of live animals is no exception to this. Occasionally there may, indeed, be an emergency, necessitating rapid action, when an animal is acutely unwell or injured and suffering severe pain or distress. These events are rare but will usually involve the most readily available clinician, who may or may not have forensic experience, rather than the more specialised veterinarian who later is to examine the animal as an 'expert'.

PREPARATION FOR EXAMINATION

Preparations for clinical examination follow very closely the guidelines laid down in Chapter 7 (Pathology and *Post-mortem* Examinations) and Chapter 9 (Site Visits, Fieldwork and Collection of Evidence). In each instance as much background information as possible should be obtained including the history of the animal and basic facts as to

its ownership (see below), the circumstances of the case and the questions that are being asked.

TAKING INSTRUCTIONS

The request for clinical examination of an animal may come from the owner, in which case the circumstances are no different from those that pertain in everyday veterinary practice. Difficulties can arise, however, when instructions are received from an individual or a body other than the owner, and this situation is discussed in more detail in Chapter 7.

HISTORY

In all investigations – clinical, *post-mortem*, laboratory – as full a history as possible is desirable. Often in forensic work such a comprehensive history is not available because the animal when found or seized has clinical signs or is dead, and there may or may not be an owner or keeper who can provide background information.

Even if history is available, it may not be correct and can even be fabricated, so the clinician has to perform an examination on an animal without knowing the true background.

The general guidance is as follows:

- Always try to obtain a history before embarking on clinical, *post-mortem* or laboratory investigations – however, brief, inadequate or unreliable this may be.
- Heed the history where appropriate but do not rely upon it.
- When you have the opportunity to take a history yourself, do so.

Be sure to acquire as much information as possible (see below) and try to verify this.

Important features of a good history include:

- Correct dates and times of incidents or findings: it can make a lot of difference as to whether an animal was found sick or dead early in the morning or later in the day.
- The circumstances regarding the animals, how many were involved, the social grouping, accommodation, diet, etc.
- Other circumstances – e.g. the people involved.
- Photographs or drawings.

PERSONNEL AND CIRCUMSTANCES

Clinical examination of a forensic case is based on the same tenets as routine clinical examination of a sick or injured animal. For legal reasons, the work should be carried out by a veterinary surgeon (veterinarian) who must be registered as such in the country where the examination is being performed (see Chapter 12). However, other personnel may be involved, either in a supporting role (e.g. a veterinary nurse [UK] or a veterinary technician [USA]) or because in order to answer the questions that are being posed, some aspects of the examination require input from a person from another discipline. Thus, an animal behaviourist (ethologist) may contribute significantly to ascertaining whether an animal shows any signs of psychological disorders which may be relevant to the case.

Forbes (1998) provided a useful summary of clinical examination of an avian forensic case and much of what he wrote is relevant to clinical work

in general. He emphasised that very often it is the practising veterinarian who is most likely to be asked to examine an animal clinically and to provide written or oral evidence. In some respects this is a similar situation to that which pertains in human forensic work, where the police surgeon/forensic physician (UK) or forensic medical examiner (USA) plays a key part. Nevertheless, it must be remembered that there is an increasing need to involve specialists in all aspects of forensic work and clinical examination is no exception. Therefore the general practitioner may well be needed to carry out an initial examination (usually because of the circumstances – s/he is available at that time) but if a case is complex, there is merit in involving colleagues of other more specialised disciplines, e.g. neurologist or orthopaedic specialist.

Forbes pointed out that clinical cases may require examination for 'forensic reasons' under different circumstances, of which three of the most common scenarios are as follows:

(1) A law enforcement officer or agency requests a clinician's presence at a predetermined place and time, often without any prior information being made available about the impending investigation. This usually involves a search warrant and the circumstances are usually not satisfactory for a full and detailed clinical assessment. However, it is still advisable to perform a limited examination and to take contemporaneous notes.

(2) An animal for clinical examination may be presented at a normal veterinary practice or clinic by a law enforcement officer or agency with the request that an examination is carried out because of a likely legal action.

(3) There is a request for a clinical examination by the owner of an animal – for example, of a newly purchased horse which subsequently turns into a legal action against the breeder or supplier.

To Forbes' list can be added a situation that is not, *per se*, a forensic one but which might lead later to a claim against the veterinarian. This is the clinical examination of an animal prior to purchase – a time-honoured part of the veterinarian's work but now so often potentially litigious. This is discussed later.

Prior to the clinical examination of an animal, the question has to be asked 'Who should be involved?' In any thorough examination, especially if samples are taken, a chain of custody is created and as a general rule, it is best if the number of persons in that chain is kept to a minimum. Nevertheless, this general rule should not outweigh the benefit of having adequate assistance with the clinical examination and access to professional and support staff who can deal both with the animal and with the samples. Contemporaneous notes must be made at the time of the initial examination and it is better to record everything that is observed even if some of the inferences from observations or clinical examinations subsequently prove to be incorrect. The whole question of record-keeping and notes is discussed in more detail in Chapter 10.

IDENTIFICATION OF THE ANIMAL

Correct identification of the individual animal is a key part of clinical examination. The animal should be identified with regard to its species (using scientific as well as common name), breed or variety where appropriate, sex (male, female, entire or neutered), age, weight (body mass), at least one measurement and any special markings. Some of these aspects are discussed, with particular reference to wildlife, by PAW (2005). It is often helpful to use a form that bears an outline of an animal (usually left and right views, sometimes dorsal and ventral) and to use this to indicate any specific markings that may be important in recognition or which is relevant to the case. Specific methods of identification, complementary to the points made above, are listed in Table 6.1. Some animals may already be marked. Others may need marking as part of the forensic investigation in order to be able to recognise and refer to them later. In the case of the latter, the procedure used should be as minimally interventional and non-invasive as possible – coloured 'split' plastic rings for birds are an example (Figure 6.1).

The implantation of a microchip is, arguably, the best way to provide a permanent and safe way of identifying an individual animal. It has much to

commend it from a legal/forensic perspective. It is not, however, without its drawbacks and dangers (see, for example, www.lansdown-vets.co.uk/info-ref-1.htm). Various guidelines exist, for example, those issued by the World Small Animal Veterinary Association website (www.wsava.org/microchp.htm).

Veterinarians can sometimes identify an individual animal because they recognise a lesion or surgical wound. Birds of prey, for example, may have a characteristic 'footprint' following surgery for pododermatitis (Cooper, 2002). Korbel and Sturm (2005)

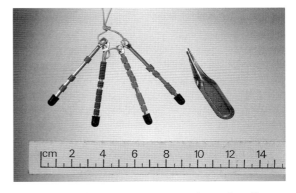

Figure 6.1 Coloured plastic rings, with metal applicator. Such rings are ideal for temporarily marking confiscated birds. This figure also appears in colour in the colour plate section.

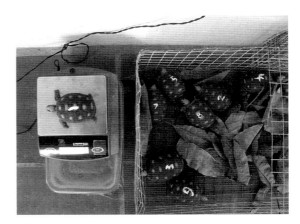

Figure 6.2 A group of red-footed tortoises, seized because they had been imported illegally. They are marked temporarily with white paint.

119

Table 6.1 Methods of identification of individual animals.

Method	Suitable for	Comments
Rings (bands)	Birds, some mammals	Different types – plastic/metal, closed/open (see Gosler, 2004)
Tags	Birds (wings) Mammals (ears, flippers)	Cause short-lived pain when applied
Tattooing	Mammals, sometimes others	Standard techniques and sites can be used Irreversible
Clipping of digits or fins	Reptiles, amphibians and fish	Not recommended – deleterious, painful (see, for example, Van Gelder and Strijbosch, 1996)
Clipping of hair	Mammals	Rapidly regrows but useful temporarily System (pattern) can be used to distinguish animals in a group Use with caution in animals being shown or exhibited
Paints or dyes	Birds, some other species	Use with caution – may increase vulnerability to predation Some dyes, e.g. picric acid are dangerous to handle
Freeze-branding	Mammals	Permanent
Transponders (microchips)	All species	The microchips have to be located, using an appropriate reader Two main types – ISO and Trovan – with significant technical differences that make them incompatible Site of insertion depends upon the species In birds care must be taken to avoid the cranial pectoral muscles, because of possible haemorrhage
Drawings of the animal's markings	All species	A traditional but still very effective, non-invasive method of identification May form part of an animal's 'passport'
Photographs of markings	All species	As above
DNA techniques	All species	Requires tissue samples Usually only applicable to very valuable animals and certain wildlife

described the identification of various birds using a digital scanning ophthalmoscopy technique.

IDENTIFICATION OF SPECIMENS

It is not only the whole animal that needs to be identified. The forensic consultant may be asked to examine skeletons, bones, skulls, horns, antlers, teeth, tusks (ivory), feathers, reptile skins (entire and sloughed), hair and feathers, eggs of birds and reptiles and a variety of plants (Davis, 1987; PAW,

2005). This aspect is discussed in more detail in Chapters 5 and 7.

METHODS OF EXAMINATION

It is not possible in this book to discuss in detail the clinical examination of all types of animals. The general rule is that the animal, regardless of species, should initially undergo a full basic clinical examination, similar to that performed during a (diagnostic) normal veterinary investigation. This means

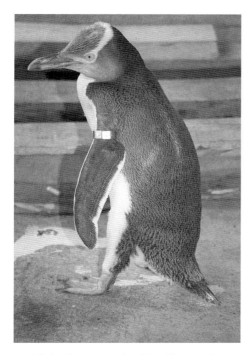

Figure 6.3 A wing tag used to identify a captive penguin.

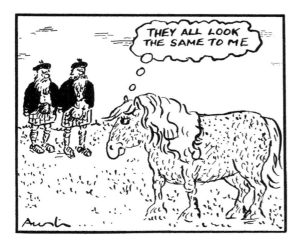

that the animal is examined systemically, even though there may be an obvious presenting wound or lesion of probable importance. The initial examination should include the use of standard aids such as auscultation, percussion and palpation. Equipment should be available *before* the examination begins and the choice may be influenced by the

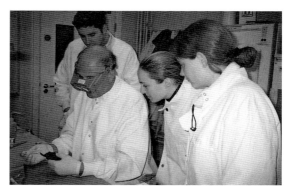

Figure 6.4 A dissecting loupe is used for detailed investigation of a captive 'tarantula' spider that died unexpectedly.

history or allegation. For example, if a domesticated dog is said to have chased and attacked, or bitten, a sheep or a pet rabbit, dental instruments should be on hand (and appropriate containers ready) so that hairs and small pieces of tissue can be taken.

Clinical examination of domesticated animals is fully covered in standard veterinary texts and will not be repeated here. A valuable series on small animals, including 'exotics' is *Kirk's Current Veterinary Therapy . . . Small Animal Practice* (see, for example, Bonagura, 1995).

Clinical examination of non-domesticated species can be more problematic but there is an increasing volume of literature relating to this (see References and Appendix B – Journals). In the UK most practices have access to the BSAVA Manual series, which deal with a whole range of domesticated species and disciplines as well as 'exotic' pets. Standard techniques for handling, weighing and taking of blood are also to be found in standard texts for biologists and field workers – for example, for amphibians in the volume edited by Heyer *et al.* (1994).

In the USA the term 'work-up' is used, especially in avian medicine, to imply a thorough but focused investigation of an animal, performed in order to obtain as much important clinical information as possible in a relatively short time. The basic forensic examination can be considered a version of this.

Use of a clinical record sheet is essential and, like the necropsy sheet (see Chapter 7), is often best compiled specially for the forensic case rather than

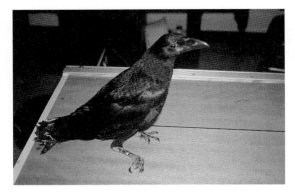

Figure 6.5 A raven with an angulated leg. In a legal case questions would be asked about the age of the injury, its possible causes and whether more might have been done to rectify the damage.

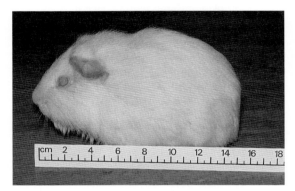

Figure 6.6 Live clinical cases should be photographed. The pictures will need to be produced in court.

relying upon a standard clinical form which may or may not permit answers to be given to specific questions of forensic importance.

The examination, describing and interpreting of lesions is discussed in detail in Chapter 7. Descriptions for forensic purposes need to be as accurate as possible (they may be checked by someone else). Measurements are important and some 'scoring' system is recommended when there is a need to quantify. Colour codes are useful and can also be used to help describe faeces, urine, etc. Objectivity is enhanced if reference can be made to colours on a chart (such as those used by purveyors of paint). The *consistency* of, say, faeces can be difficult to describe in an unambiguous way. Use should be made of the grading systems (usually 1–5, liquid–

solid) advocated by some of the nutritional companies. Photographs always help but should be used in conjunction with description.

WEIGHING AND MEASURING

Both the clinician and the pathologist who are involved in forensic work should heed the words of Stephen Hales, nearly three hundred years ago:

> . . . *the most likely way, therefore, to get any insight into the nature of those parts of creation which seem to come within our observation must . . . be to number, weigh and measure.*

The two parameters which are of greatest potential value and usually amongst the easiest to determine are weight (mass) and one or more body measurements. It is important that both are recorded: many veterinary surgeons will weigh a patient or a carcase for *post-mortem* examination but fail to record any measurement. This markedly reduces the value of the data since a certain weight (mass) may represent a fat small specimen or an undernourished large one. Measurements may also provide additional information, for example the sex of certain species. The weighing and measuring of dead animals is discussed in some detail in Chapter 7. Here the emphasis is on live animals. Recommended methods of measuring are given in Table 6.2.

If accurate weights and measurements are to be taken, appropriate equipment will be required.

Weighing

A balance or scales will be needed. A cloth bag or similar can be used to restrain small 'exotic' species.

Measurements

These must be carried out properly: 'guestimates' are unreliable (McLean *et al.*, 2003). Plastic rules and/or tape and/or vernier (sliding) callipers may be needed (see Chapter 7). It is wise to have a selection since some are more suited to certain species than others. Plastic or glass tubes and strong plastic

Table 6.2 Measuring of live animals.

Group	Method	Comments
Mammals	Either (a) crown–rump (CR) length or (b) snout to base of tail, plus, where appropriate length of tail Specific measuring techniques apply to some species, e.g. marine mammals and bats	The tail may be truncated – for example, because of an injury – and therefore a whole body length, including tail, can be unreliable
Birds	Carpal length	A specially made metal rule with a raised stop is recommended If a reliable carpal length proves impossible because of moulting, feather damage or pinioning, a tarsal length should be recorded
Reptiles	Snout–vent (SV) and vent-to-tail (VT) lengths	A whole body length is to be discouraged because of the possibility of tail damage (see above) Care must be taken when straightening (putting the animal into a plastic tube will assist)
Amphibians	Tail-less species (frogs and toads) – snout–vent length (SVL) Tailed species (newts and salamanders and tadpoles) – as reptiles	A rule with stop is advisable Care as above
Fish	Various methods used If in doubt, in legal cases, measure SV and VT	Different techniques are used by aquaculturists and ichthyologists (see literature)
Invertebrates	Vary, depending upon the species Molluscs, for example, are usually measured in two planes – height and breadth Butterflies may have their wingspan measured	Consult specialist texts Use high-quality sliding callipers

sheets facilitate 'straightening' elongated specimens, such as snakes and certain invertebrates.

If photographs are to be taken, a non-reflecting (non-glare) metric (cm or metre) scale should be available to place by the specimen.

Methods

Weighing is usually straightforward but, if the animal bears any extraneous items such as collars, hoods, bells, splints, plaster casts or dressings, care must be taken to ensure that either (a) these are removed, or (b) allowance is made for them in any calculations. It is also wise to record if, for example, a bird has a crop full of food or a snake has a prey item in its stomach, because these will give erroneous figures. While it is acceptable for an aquatic or amphibious species to be wet when weighed, care should be taken to reduce the amount of water to a minimum. When weighing small animals in the field using a spring balance, the wind can give erroneous results. This can be minimised by either folding the bag so as to reduce the surface area or carrying out the weighing in a bucket (without touching the sides).

Measurements can present dilemmas since different methods are used for different species. Mammalogists, for example, use a number of procedures for taxa ranging from bats to bottle-nosed dolphins (Lundrigan, 1996). Table 6.2 provides initial guidelines for those involved in forensic work with vertebrates or invertebrates.

The veterinarian is often surprised by the wealth of data on morphometrics of wild mammals, birds and other animals, some of them based on museum material, some on capture and measurements of live animals. Such data are not restricted to the richer part of the world: there is, for example, extensive published information on the biometrics of birds throughout the Greater Caribbean Basin (Arendt *et al.*, 2004).

CONDITION

Defining and assessing 'condition' is not easy. An experienced veterinarian (or stockman, or animal welfare inspector) is able to say 'The sheep was in poor condition', on the basis of observation and clinical examination, but a precise meaning of 'body condition' is rarely given. In domesticated species it can usually be equated with how well-nourished an animal is – whether or not its ribs are prominent, fullness of muscle, presence of fat – for instance, but such an assessment can be very subjective. It is preferable in such cases – and certainly makes cross-examination easier in court – to use a condition score. A number of these have been devised, with descriptive pictures, for most domesticated mammals and suitable methods are referred to in the literature.

The definition and determination of 'condition' in non-domesticated species can present particular difficulties. 'Condition' is an ambiguous term because it is commonly used both as an indicator of an animal as a whole and also parts of the body (e.g. 'condition of the plumage'). In few wild animals has the assessment of condition been properly studied, an exception being fish (Weatherley and Gill, 1987). Examples of how condition is assessed by biologists will be given, relating to birds and land tortoises respectively. In birds, condition has been defined as 'some qualitative assessment (which may be determined quantitatively) of the bird that has a direct bearing on its fitness' (Gosler, 2004). Methods used in birds that are discussed by Gosler include:

- Relative mass – the mass (weight) relative to the size of the bird. Often called 'condition' or 'condition index' but this method can be misleading.
- Fat reserves – subcutaneous, internal (*post mortem* or during laparoscopy) or using total body electrical conductivity (TOBEC). The former can be misleading; the latter is expensive, cumbersome and not necessarily better than using non-destructive fat 'scoring' methods.
- Muscle protein – assessment and scoring of pectoral muscles, or recording their shape using fine wire or dental alginate.
- Physiological analysis – usually of blood.
- Moult and plumage – age and condition of feathers, including ptilochronology.
- Parasites – numbers and species.
- Biopsy techniques, permitting tissues to be examined or isotopes to be measured.

Gosler also referred to asymmetry, pointing out that fluctuating asymmetry (FA) can be used as an indicator of condition, but warning of bias because most observers are themselves asymmetrical (left- or right-handed).

Land tortoises (chelonians) present particular problems in terms of assessing 'condition' because of the presence of a protective, often hard, carapace and plastron. Methods of measuring body mass condition were reviewed and discussed by Hailey (2000) and by Willemser and Hailey (2002). They concluded that the easiest method was to calculate the mass of the tortoise in relation to its size, a concept that was originally devised by Jackson (1980). Hailey and colleagues used a condition index (CI), based on log (M/M1), where M is the observed mass and M1 is the mass as predicted from the animal's length. They applied this method to both free-living and captive (European) *Testudo* species and as a result produced a programme (www.ahailey.f9.co.uk/cond.htm) that reliably calculates body mass condition of these species so long as the tortoise is of carapace length 100 mm or more.

A condition score is valuable but in its absence, evidence of increase in weight of an animal following its being put on a normal feeding regime can prove a useful measure in court or in a written statement, as evidence of malnutrition (see later).

FITNESS

This is another term that has different meanings for different people and disciplines. To biologists it indicates how well an animal can survive based on, for example, fat or protein, how well the animal can resist diseases, or its ability to attract a mate (Gosler, 2004). Veterinarians tend to use the word in terms of clinical health and 'fitness' for a specific purpose, e.g. horse-racing (see later).

AGE DETERMINATION

The aging of animals can be very important – as part of identification, in disputes over purchase and 'soundness', sometimes in cases relating to the adequacy of veterinary treatment.

Few methods of aging are entirely reliable: even the time-honoured techniques based on dentition of domesticated mammals have come under scrutiny in recent years, see for example, Cocquyt *et al.*, 2005. Nevertheless, they are often still the basis for assessment (Dabas and Saxena, 1994).

Some techniques that can be used for age determination are listed in Table 6.3.

As will be apparent from the Table, reliable methods of telling the exact age of a live animal (e.g. that an Exmoor pony is eight, as opposed to seven years old) are few. There are so many variables relating to the biology and history of the individual animals. Some useful references exist – mainly to domesticated animals (see standard veterinary and animal husbandry texts) but also a few wild species, e.g. primates (Erwin and Hof, 2002). Age estimations at death based on *post-mortem* remains (see Chapter 7) – as well as species identification and sexing (see below) – have been much refined by the research of zoo-archaeologists (Davis, 1987).

What is not so difficult is to put an animal into an age group or age band. The most familiar of these is determining whether a mammal (e.g. a dog) is a puppy or an adult, on the basis of whether or not it still has deciduous teeth. As always, care must be taken with wild animals: cetaceans, for instance, may have no teeth or only permanent dentition. Some non-domesticated species, especially birds, can be divided into three age groups – adult,

Table 6.3 Some methods of aging live and dead vertebrate animals.

Methods	Species	Comments
External appearance including secondary sexual characteristics	Many	Much variation
History, behaviour	Many	Evidence of parturition, egg-laying and reproductive activity may distinguish adults
Specific age-related external features, such as rings on horns	Ungulates especially bovids Reptiles (shields)	See literature
Specific age-related internal features, such as 'growth rings' in cortices of long bones, sometimes the number of corpora lutea on ovaries	Mammals, birds, reptiles (bone), other species (ovaries)	See literature
Dentition	Mammals, especially equids, ruminants and cetaceans	May make use of eruption patterns or (probably more reliable) microscopical examination of teeth
Stage of metamorphosis	Amphibians, some fish	See literature
Pelage	Some mammals, some birds	Hair and feathers can be indicative of age group

sub-adult and juveniles – usually by analysis of the feathers, eyes or feet. Likewise, young birds can usually be roughly classified as nestlings or fledglings, on the basis of their plumage development.

GENDER DETERMINATION (SEXING)

This is covered in Chapter 7.

DESCRIPTION OF LESIONS

This is discussed in more detail in Chapter 7.

Care must be taken during examination of a live or dead animal to record and describe accurately any lesions that are present, even if they may appear to be of no immediate relevance to a case. Often they provide information, the importance of which is not appreciated until later, perhaps during court proceedings. For example, a farmer who claims that a veterinary surgeon killed a valuable dairy cow during a calving may himself have damaged the animal earlier, by attempting to deliver the calf himself. Evidence of this may be found in, for example, bruising of the vulva. A proper examination and description of lesions may permit differentiation of injuries that occurred before the veterinarian was involved and those that took place during his intervention.

One way of recording the shape and size of a lesion and to monitor change over a period of time or following treatment is to use a transparent plastic sheet that can be applied to the surface of the organ or tissue. A felt pen traces the shape of the lesion and the plastic sheet with its outline is then retained for comparison on the next occasion. Such records can be of great value in legal cases, where clear descriptions and explanations will have to be given to a magistrate, a judge and possibly to a lay jury.

The aging of bruises and other lesions is discussed in Chapter 7.

VETERINARY CERTIFICATION

Veterinary certificates, which usually testify to the health of an animal or animals, are important documents. The accuracy of the certificate, reflected in its wording, can make a great deal of difference to the fate of an animal, to disease control and to the professional status of the person who signed it (Cooper, T., 2005). In most countries of the world great weight is laid upon accurate and truthful certification. In some, such as the UK, the penalties (legal and/or professional) for falsely completing a certificate, as far as making incorrect claims, errors or omissions are concerned, are substantial. In other countries, regrettably, such high standards may not apply and it is not unusual for a veterinarian to be asked or told to sign a certificate for an animal which s/he has not seen or to include wording – for example, relating to 'freedom from disease' – that cannot be substantiated.

Wilson (2005) discussed the principles of certification (see also below) and concluded her lecture, which was directed at British veterinarians, by stating that one should remember: (1) 'your MRCVS is worth more than losing a single client, however important', and (2) 'you will be put in jeopardy if you negligently or falsely sign certificates.'

Some indication of the importance of certification can be gleaned from the Guide to Professional Conduct (GPC) of the RCVS where the basic principles of certification are summarised:

(1) The *twelve principles of certification (see annexes)* were drafted by RCVS, BVA and MAFF (now DEFRA) and adopted by the Federation of Veterinarians of Europe. Eight of the twelve principles are included in the EU Directive 96/93/EC. Their purpose is to provide the foundation of certification for all those who draft or prepare, use or sign veterinary certificates even though at the present time veterinary surgeons may be presented with their certificates which do not conform to all of them.

(2) In framing obligations which veterinary surgeons must fulfill under day-to-day working conditions, the RCVS has taken into account not only the Twelve Principles of Certification but also relevant UK law including the Trade Descriptions Act 1968 (as amended) which specifies the defences open to the signatory of a certificate or equivalent document if he or

she is challenged and also the fact that veterinary surgeons may be presented with certificates which do not conform to all of the Twelve Principles.

(3) Given that veterinary surgeons' professional reputations and livelihoods may be at sake if their signatures on certificates are open to challenge and that they may be presented with certificates that do not conform to all of the Twelve Principles of Certification, the RCVS strongly advises veterinary surgeons as follows:

(4) **CAUTION** Before signing any certificate veterinary surgeons must:
   (a) scrutinise the document whatever its title
   (b) be clear as to whom they are responsible in exercising their authority when they sign the document

(5) **CLARITY** Scrutinising the document includes:
   (a) reading and understanding any explanatory supporting material
   (b) checking carefully for any ambiguity which should be clarified with whoever has issued the certificate

(6) Age, colour, sex, marking and breed may also be used.

(7) The owner's name must always be inserted. (In the case for example of litters of unsold puppies this will be the name of the breeder or the seller).

(8) Where microchipping or tattooing has been applied it should be referred to in any certificate or identification.

The GPC goes on to emphasise:

Medical Certification for Export of Live Animals and Animal Products and Casualty Slaughter Certificates

(1) The simple act of signing their names on documents has a great potential for error for veterinary surgeons. A certificate is a 'written statement of fact made with authority', the authority in this case coming from the veterinary surgeon's professional status.

(2) Some documents (for example, forms, declarations, insurance claims, witness statements and self-certification documents) may involve the same level of responsibility even if they do not bear the name of 'certificate'. If the facts are incorrect or misleading, the professional integrity of the veterinary surgeon is called into question. Cases coming before the [RCVS] Disciplinary Committee may arise from allegations of false certification.

(3) There are three hazards for the veterinary surgeon when 'certifying' in the wider sense:
   (a) **Negligence**: A breach of the duty owed to a relevant party with consequent damage. Negligence may arise from a failure to disclose all of the material facts or supplying incorrect information. The consequence may be civil court proceedings.
   (b) **Criminal Offences**: Criminal offences may be committed under trade descriptions legislation, legislation controlling animal exports and by aiding and abetting a third party. They may include fraud or knowingly or recklessly supplying false information. Any conviction brought to the notice of the RCVS may be considered in relation to the fitness of the veterinary surgeon to practise.
   (c) **Professional Misconduct**: Even if no criminal charges are brought, an aggrieved party or enforcement authority may make a formal complaint to the RCVS. If the complaint is judged to be justified, penalties may follow.

SPECIAL CONSIDERATIONS OF THE FORENSIC CASE

Examination of the forensic case brings with it some extra considerations that may not be part of normal clinical investigation. Laurence and Newman (2000) discussed this in some detail and the Rules below largely reflect their advice as well as that of the authors of the book. Record-keeping should be meticulous and contemporaneous notes are essential (hard copies and/or computerised). Investigations or tests may be carried out which would not form part of a normal standard clinical examination: samples should therefore always be taken (see later and Chapter 8). There are few published texts dealing specifically with forensic clinical examination other than that of the dog and horse. However, information is becoming available on some species, including certain exotic animals and wildlife: see, for example, the papers dealing with the clinical examination of the forensic avian case by Cooper and Cooper (1986, 1991) and by Forbes (1998).

RULES

Any veterinary surgeon may be requested to carry out a clinical examination of an animal that might be the subject of a legal case. Under such circumstances the veterinarian, who may well not have any specialist post-graduate training, must do his or her best. Some general rules are as follows:

- Carry out as full and methodical an examination as possible in the time available and with the equipment that is available.
- Although the examination should initially be general, pay particular attention to any organ systems or parts of the body which may be particularly relevant to the case.
- Depending upon species, certain structures may be particularly relevant to a forensic case. Thus, for example, when examining a bird, the preen gland, important in waterproofing of plumage, should be located and, if present, examined and a comment made on its appearance and whether or not it is functioning. A brood patch may be found in a bird that is incubating eggs. The teeth and scent glands of rodents should always be examined, as should the horns or antlers (they need to be distinguished!) of ruminants and the pouch of marsupials.

- The animal's body temperature should be recorded in °C. It is not acceptable to state that the temperature was 'normal' or 'within normal limits' (Laurence and Newman, 2000).
- If time, facilities or the veterinarian's lack of experience of the species in question limits a full examination, this should be stated in the report. It is preferable at an early stage to admit that certain examinations were not carried out (or feasible) rather than for this to come to light during cross-examination in a court case or similar hearing.
- As in all aspects of forensic examinations, detailed contemporaneous notes should be made together with, as appropriate, tape recordings and photographs.

HOSPITALISATION

When an animal that is the subject of a legal case has to be hospitalised or retained for some other reason, the veterinarian should ensure that it is kept in a secure place where it cannot be moved or interfered with by any person. The cage or enclosure should be locked and careful custody ensured for the keys. Distinguishing marks or means of identification should be noted so as to minimise the risk of mixing the animal with others or a suggestion in a court case that transposition may have occurred. When a batch of animals is involved, it is wise to mark them individually since each or any one of them may form the subject of a legal action and then accurate identification will be essential. There are various ways of marking animals (see Table 6.1).

If an animal dies while being hospitalised or, in the case of a wild animal, while retained in captivity, the details should be recorded and appropriate investigations carried out immediately. This may entail a *post-mortem* examination and this is an instance where it is wise to have the necropsy performed by someone with appropriate specialist skills rather than the veterinary clinician who is responsible for the case.

High standards of care are essential and should be coupled with strict adherence to relevant rules or regulations regarding health and safety.

RECORD-KEEPING

As in other fields of forensic medicine, contemporaneous, usually handwritten, notes of clinical findings are important and these can be supplemented with tape recordings or computerised records (see Chapter 10). In the case of the latter, the files should be kept secure, using an appropriate password and any alterations to them subsequently recorded.

Laboratory results arising from tests on clinical cases should be attached to the paper records for the case and/or added to the electronic files. The reference numbers must match (see Chapter 8).

The clinician may want to use his/her own clinical record sheets or may be asked to use a standard format – for example, the pro-forma issued by the RSPCA in England for the 'Veterinary Examination of RSPCA Equine Welfare Cases' (Laurence and Newman, 2000). The British Veterinary Association (see Appendix B) produces a range of certificates for different purposes, including the exportation of dogs, cats and small mammals.

SUPPORTING INVESTIGATIONS

Clinical examination alone is usually only one part of forensic investigation. It can be linked with:

* Haematology.
* Clinical chemistry.

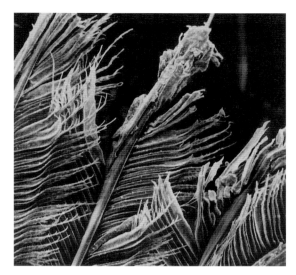

Figure 6.8 Scanning electronmicrograph (SEM) examination of a feather from the kite in Figure 6.7 reveals damage to barbs and barbules that is characteristic of gunshot damage.

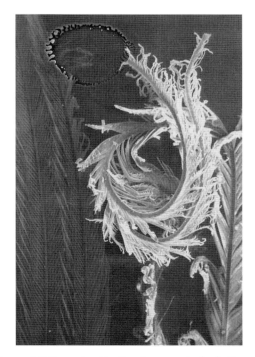

Figure 6.9 In contrast to the above, part of a feather that has been damaged by fire (burning and high temperature).

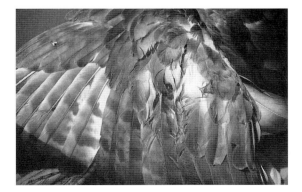

Figure 6.7 A black kite with a wing injury. Blood is present and feathers are damaged.

- Parasitology.
- Microbiology.
- Histology.
- Cytology.
- Electronmicroscopy.
- Radiology.
- Other imaging, e.g. magnetic resonance (MRI), computerised tomography (CT) scan.

MRI is increasingly being used for valuable animals, e.g. in the diagnosis of lameness in horses (Murray and Mair, 2005) and is likely to play an important role in legal cases in future.

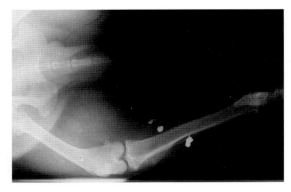

Figure 6.10 The leg of a dog that was shot, but not killed, by a gun. (Courtesy J. D. Watkins.)

RADIOGRAPHY AND RADIOLOGY

Radiography (X-raying) is extensively used in forensic work (Brogdon, 1998). In veterinary and comparative studies it serves a variety of purposes:

- As an adjunct to clinical examination of animals, whether victims or alleged assailants (see Chapter 2) to detect injuries, presence of bullets, lead shot, teeth, etc.
- As part of clinical examination of humans where a forensic investigation is in progress, e.g. fractures, long-standing changes such as spondylosis, detection of bullets, etc. as above.
- As part of *post-mortem* examination of animals (or humans) – as of selected organs or tissues – see Chapter 7.
- To assess nutritional/metabolic status, e.g. abdominal body fat in mammals, bone density in reptiles.
- To investigate non-animal/non-human material, e.g. to detect metallic fragments in foodstuffs or water samples.

Radiography must be used with care. X-rays are dangerous and excessive or unwarranted exposure to them may itself be grounds for legal action (see later).

Digital radiography is increasingly used in veterinary practice and permits manipulation and enhancement so as to produce high-resolution images. However, these may not always be admissible as evidence (see Chapter 10).

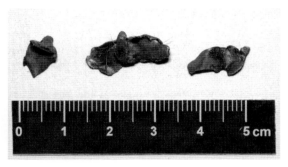

Figure 6.11 Copper-sheathed bullets, removed surgically from the leg above. (Courtesy J. D. Watkins.)

OTHER IMAGING TECHNIQUES

Other methods that can play a part in animal forensic work include:

- Ultrasonography.
- MRI.
- CT.
- Doppler.
- Endoscopy.

None of these can be discussed in detail, but the investigator/expert should be aware of their existence and be prepared to consider their use by an appropriately qualified person. This applies particularly to ultrasonography, where any permanent record of the examination could be impossible to interpret without expert advice.

SAMPLES FOR LABORATORY ANALYSIS

Sampling is discussed in more detail in Chapters 7 and 8 but is also mentioned here because many forensic samples, including those that would be classified as 'trace evidence', come from live animals (see Table 6.4).

All samples, regardless of their identity or destination, must be handled with care and packed correctly (PAW, 2005).

Table 6.4 Samples from live animals.

Sample	Investigations	Comments
Faeces/vomitus, regurgitated material, pellets (birds of prey)	Parasitology Microbiology Chemical tests (e.g. for fat) Toxicology	Readily available
Blood (or haemolymph)	Haematology Clinical chemistry Parasitology Serology DNA technology	Limited investigations can be performed on the haemolymph of invertebrates
Urine	Toxicology Microbiology Clinical chemistry Cytology	An important part of sampling for evidence of 'doping' of racehorses and greyhounds
Pus	Microbiology Cytology	Pus may be liquid or (e.g. reptiles) caseous Pus-like material from any species should be sampled and examined Both aerobic and anaerobic cultures are advisable
Semen	Direct microscopy	Important in alleged bestiality cases Also to investigate infertility (stallions, bulls, etc.)
Tissues (biopsies, scrapings, washings, brushings, etc.)	Histology (histopathology and histochemistry) Scanning electronmicroscopy Transmission electronmicroscopy Cytology Chemical analysis Toxicology Immunological tests (e.g. for detecting snake or scorpion venom) Radiography(plus/minus whole carcase) DNA technology	A whole range of investigations that are not only applicable to diagnostic veterinary work but also to forensic matters, such as alleged trauma, poisoning or spread of zoonoses
Hair, feathers, scales	Low-power examination with hand lens Various other procedures as above	Important samples because they may be shed naturally (trace evidence) or can be obtained readily, using minimally invasive techniques

REPORTING

In routine diagnostic work, the issuing of a prompt report, be it only preliminary, is most important. Clients and practising veterinarians are anxious to have some information as soon as possible – in the interest of the patient and sometimes to reassure themselves (that the animal's problem was not their fault or that the diagnosis was correct). In forensic work, however, the situation is different and there is merit in *not* issuing any report (and certainly not a verbal statement) until one is sure that the findings are correct and that a preliminary announcement is not going to complicate issues. The Swahili maxim *Haraka, hakara, haina baraka* (too much haste is not a blessing) is often very sound counsel in forensic reporting, even though police and others may push for information long before it can reasonably be supplied (see also Chapter 7). Sometimes a preliminary statement of findings can be useful or necessary – for example, to confirm to owners that an animal did, indeed, have a chronic hepatic disease and was not poisoned – but other aspects need not and should not be discussed.

EUTHANASIA

Sometimes it may be necessary or desirable to euthanase (to 'kill humanely', in simple English) an animal (see also Chapter 4). There are usually two reasons for this:

(1) Humanitarian – the animal is suffering excessively.
(2) Practicalities – if, for example, several hundred fish are sick and believed to have been poisoned, examination of a small number of dead animals may provide vital information. However, before embarking on killing animals that may be part of a legal case, the following must be considered:
    (a) Is permission to euthanase required from the owner, the police, the court or others?
    (b) Can euthanasia be carried out humanely under the circumstances that often prevail at a crime scene away from a veterinary clinic and possibly under the watchful eye of owner or neighbours?

Killing an animal often presents practical and ethical challenges (see, for example, Mullan, 2006). This is particularly so when euthanasia is requested, or deemed necessary, without the owner's consent. The relevant part of the (UK) RCVS Guide to Professional Conduct provides useful guidelines:

Euthanasia

(1) Euthanasia is not, in law, an act of veterinary surgery, and may be carried out by anyone provided that it is carried out humanely. No veterinary surgeon is obliged to kill a healthy animal unless required to do so under statutory powers as part of their conditions of employment. Veterinary surgeons do, however, have the privilege of being able to relieve an animal's suffering in this way in appropriate cases.

(2) From time to time veterinary surgeons may face difficulties. For example, an owner may want to have a perfectly healthy or treatable animal destroyed, or an owner may wish to keep an animal alive in circumstances where euthanasia would be the kindest course of action. The veterinary surgeon's primary obligation is to relieve the suffering of an animal but account must be taken not only of the animal's condition but also the owner's wishes and circumstances. It should be recognised that clients are capable of making informed and conscientious decisions concerning the future of their animals. Thus the client is an important contributor to the decision. To refuse an owner's request for euthanasia, therefore, may add to the owner's distress and could be deleterious to the welfare of the animal.

(3) Just as relevant are a veterinary surgeon's concerns about an owner's refusal to consent to euthanasia where an animal's immediate welfare is compromised. After full consideration of all the relevant issues, veterinary surgeons can only advise their clients and act in accordance with their professional judgement. Where, in all conscience, a veterinary surgeon cannot

accede to a client's request for euthanasia he or she should recognise the extreme sensitivity of the situation and make sympathetic efforts to direct the client to alternative sources of advice. Where an animal's welfare is compromised because of an owner's refusal to allow euthanasia, a veterinary surgeon would be justified in informing the client of other action which might be taken.

Euthanasia without the Owner's Consent

(1) The Protection of Animals Act 1911 (Section 1), The Protection of Animals (Scotland) Act 1912 and The Welfare of Animals (Northern Ireland) Act 1972 provide that failure to destroy an animal to prevent further suffering may amount to cruelty. The duty to destroy falls most heavily on the veterinary surgeon who has the skill and training to make the correct assessment. In these circumstances s/he acts as an agent of necessity, and should make a full record of all the circumstances supporting the decision in case of subsequent challenge.

(2) The Acts give statutory powers to a police constable enabling him to order the destruction of a bovine animal, horse, mule, ass, sheep, goat or pig whose condition, in the opinion of a veterinary surgeon, is so severe that it cannot be moved and that it would be cruel to keep it alive. In these circumstances the veterinary surgeon should ask for a written and signed instruction to destroy from the officer in charge, including his identity number and the log number of the incident at a given police station.

(3) Where the veterinary surgeon is asked to destroy an animal injured in a sporting event, the opinion of a professional colleague, if available, should be sought before doing so. Veterinary surgeons officiating at sporting events should consider:

    (a) whether the owner will be present and able to consent to euthanasia if necessary

    (b) whether the owner has delegated authority to another to make that decision in their absence and

    (c) whether if damages were sought for alleged wrongful destruction they would have adequate professional indemnity insurance cover. (Ref: Jockey Club Instruction J17 and FEI Article 1009.15)

Pre-purchase examination

More should be said about clinical examination of an animal prior to purchase as this was once a cornerstone of veterinary practice, especially insofar as horses were concerned, and training in such was provided to all veterinary students. Small wonder that the word 'vetting' continues to be used in other contexts to imply a *thorough* assessment.

In recent years, however, concern over litigation has prompted many veterinarians to decline carrying out such an examination or to be very cautious about doing so. This is a shame as such work is an excellent use of a veterinary surgeon's skills, provides clients with useful information and may contribute to animal welfare (Stashak, 1987). Numerous publications have appeared on the subject over the years, some in languages other than English (see, for example, Adolphsen, 2002; Hladik and Mosing, 2002; Oexmann, 2002; Plewa, 2002 a–c and Krenger and Straub, 2002).

Pre-purchase examination of any animal must be carried out with caution and careful planning. A protocol is essential. Important steps are as follows:

- Discussion with the purchaser.
- The examination.
- Report and communication following the examination.

Discussion with the purchaser of the animal, whether the latter is a horse or a hamster, is essential. It is important to obtain background information about the proposed purchase and what the expectations of the purchaser are. 'Expectations' means 'Why is the client interested in having this animal?' There is a lot of difference between purchasing a child's pony and investing in a good-quality hunter for eventing. It is mandatory to explain to the prospective purchaser what the examination entails and in the UK it is best to follow the system outlined in the RCVS/BVA pre-purchase examination certificate. Less stringent examinations are possible but many veterinarians then insist (in the case of horses) that the client signs a declaration of limited liability examination which states that they understand the limitations.

Examinations for insurance purposes present particular problems – and not only pre-purchase. It is most important to ascertain from the insurance company itself what is required. This may also relate to the value of the animal; specialised techniques may then be required such as endoscopy. In the case of some aspects, for example ophthalmological examination, it has been proposed in Europe that there should be a standard protocol (Gerhards, 2002). In many European countries the majority of horses are insured for veterinary care and useful information is available from insurance databases which can be used as a guide as to the prevalence or importance of certain conditions (Penell *et al.*, 2005).

As full a history as possible is needed before any animal is examined prior to sale. The animal's breed, sex, age and appearance must be recorded. Any registration or other documents need to be checked, as should ear tags, tattoos or other possible indicators of identity. Important information will also include the animal's previous history and whether it has recently been treated with such agents as analgesics or corticosteroids.

The examination itself should be carried out under optimal conditions. This is very different from clinical examinations in forensic cases where there has already been an alleged breach of the law and the work may have to be done *in situ*, using a field kit (see Appendix E). Whether examining a large animal such as a horse or small animals such as fish, the work should be carefully planned and correct equipment made available.

Standard pre-purchase examination of a horse is usually based on:

- Examination at rest – conformation.
- Examination at walk and stopped.
- Examination following a period of strenuous exercise.
- Examination following a period of rest.
- Examination following a second trot and foot examination.

These categories will not be discussed in detail here; reference should be made to standard texts, for example Stashak (1987). However, they provide useful guidelines that can be applicable to other species, especially working animals.

If lameness is detected during the course of examination, it is important that it is graded (scored) using, for example, the grades advocated by the American Association of Equine Practitioners.

Samples for laboratory testing may be taken during examination, some of which will be processed immediately, while others may be retained for possible reference later. In the case of working animals such as horses and greyhounds, the latter are likely to include blood and urine samples which, quite apart from any diagnostic tests, may need to be assayed for the presence of drugs, such as anti-inflammatory agents or tranquillisers.

Endoscopic, radiographic and other investigations can also form part of a pre-purchase examination (Hertsch, 2004) and may themselves prompt legal questions (Bemmann, 2004).

SPECIFIC METHODS OF CLINICAL EXAMINATION

In the same way as there is a standard method of assessing 'soundness' in a horse, there are tried and tested methods of carrying out a basic clinical examination of most other domesticated species. These can be of great help to the veterinarian who is not a specialist and has relatively little experience of legal cases but has been asked to carry out an initial examination. It is important to know something about the background of the patient, especially if it is a working animal, such as a racing greyhound (Molyneux, 2005).

Pre-purchase examination of non-domesticated animals can be particularly challenging. This is largely because of the lack of information about values and significance of lesions or ill-health in many species. The veterinarian asked to carry out such work must be sure that s/he is confident to do so; if in doubt, a knowledgeable colleague, preferably one specialised in the species involved, should take the case. Protocols do not exist for most exotic species and therefore will have to be formulated by the veterinarian – after checking with colleagues and literature.

Let us use as an example the clinical examination of a domesticated rabbit, perhaps a pet animal that is alleged to have been mistreated or neglected. A standard clinical check-sheet for a rabbit might read as follows:

Clinical checklist

(1) History and management.
(2) Clinical examination, with particular attention to:
    (a) Nares
    (b) Ears
    (c) Teeth
    (d) Skin and coat
    (e) Anogenital region
    (f) Body temperature
    (g) Palpate
    (h) Auscultate.
(3) Laboratory tests
    (a) Faeces
    (b) Smears/swabs
    (c) (Blood).

Note that certain key organs or structures are included – the teeth (dental problems are common in lagomorphs), the ears (ear canker is prevalent), skin (parasitic disease is common) and auscultation of respiratory tract ('snuffles', the pasteurellosis complex, is widespread in rabbits). However basic an initial examination may be, it should always include the key organs or structures that are appropriate to that species.

Invertebrates present particular challenges but are increasingly likely to be the basis of a legal or insurance action (some species are worth considerable sums of money) but texts are available on the clinical examination of these species (see, for example, Cooper, 1999a) and in the UK there is even a small, but flourishing, Veterinary Invertebrate Society.

EXAMINATION OF THE REPRODUCTIVE SYSTEM

This can be important both as part of pre-purchase examination and because claims may be made that an animal is not capable of mating and/or reproducing. It usually requires the input of an experienced theriogenologist, but any practising veterinary surgeon should be able to perform a basic, initial examination – sufficient, at least, to ascertain whether or not a dog has two descended testes or that the genitalia of a heifer are morphologically normal.

Detailed clinical examination will focus on the vulva, vagina, cervix, uterus, oviducts, ovaries and mammary glands of a female and the penis, accessory sex glands, testes and epididymides of the male. Additional tests on the male may include observation of libido, mating ability and semen examination (see Chapter 8).

Standard documents may be available for such work – for example, the 'Certificate of veterinary examination of a ram intended for breeding' produced by the British Veterinary Association (see Appendix B).

More specialised investigations in both sexes may involve a whole spectrum of tests, ranging from ultrasonography to karyotyping. A pathologist may be involved, if, for example, developmental abnormalities of the reproductive tract are present, if samples are taken, e.g. uterine biopsies or if animals are culled for investigation – in the study of freemartins, for example (Smith *et al.*, 2003).

Reproductive activity is also discussed in Chapter 7.

THE ORAL CAVITY

The oral cavity constitutes a key part of clinical examination of any animal. It is important in forensic work for many reasons:

- Bite wounds are often a cause of injury, infection or death in humans and other species. The effect of a bite is influenced by both the morphology of the oral cavity and the microorganisms that it harbours.

- Teeth can be used, under certain circumstances, to determine age (Morse *et al.*, 1994).
- The oral cavity can provide other information – for example, about an animal's diet or health status.
- Orofacial trauma is sometimes a feature of abuse of animals, as it is of children (Becker *et al.*, 1978; Sperber, 1989). Bite marks are often a feature of abuse by humans on others (Whittaker, 1989, 1990) but not necessarily so (Warnick *et al.*, 1987).
- Teeth can be examined in order to identify certain *species*, e.g. marine mammals (cetaceans).
- Teeth are used routinely to identify *individuals* in human forensic work, and sometimes so when working with animals.
- Teeth often persist when other tissues have decomposed or been predated (see Chapter 7) and can therefore be a source of valuable forensic evidence.

Space does not permit detailed discussion of each of the above. Bites and wounds that they cause are discussed later in this chapter. In any forensic investigation in which the teeth or the oral cavity are important, reference should be made to relevant medical and dental texts (e.g. Averill, 1991; Barsley, 1993; Prabhu, 2004), including those that cover comparative odontology (Miles and Grigson, 1990) as well as standard publications about veterinary dentistry (Gorrel, 2004; Harvey, 1985; Crossley and Penman, 1995).

Clinical examination of the oral cavity is a routine part of veterinary investigation and, in theory, should present no particular difficulties for a clinician. In forensic work, however, problems can arise because:

- The purpose of examination may be different – often being to link the wounds with a particular species or individual.
- Techniques may have to be used that are not standard in veterinary work – for example, sampling of periodontal pockets for hair, swabbing or casting of damaged teeth.
- Different species may be involved, ranging from sharks to simian primates (see Chapter 2) and their oral anatomy can be very different.

Opening the mouth may in itself be difficult, because of species differences (above) or (*post mortem*) on account of rigor mortis.

The principles of oral examination for forensic purposes are essentially similar to those followed in routine veterinary practice but the following points are especially important:

- Meticulous records of observations must be kept. Use of a dental chart is advisable – a diagram of upper and lower jaws, with teeth, upon which comments can be superimposed. When investigating soft tissue changes (e.g. periodontitis) 'six-point charting', as used by (human) dental surgeons, can be helpful. Photography is important but good, admissible, results need experience (Wander and Gordon, 1987).
- The procedure must be carefully planned beforehand. The animal may need to be sedated or anaesthetised. Appropriate equipment (and assistance) is essential, especially if foreign material has to be collected, swabs taken or casts made.

As with so many aspects of veterinary/comparative forensic medicine, it is wise for the 'expert' to seek specialised advice. Members of the dental profession, ranging from local practitioners to experienced maxillo-facial surgeons, are usually very willing to provide assistance. Indeed, many openly confess to enjoying such contacts with the 'animal world'.

REPORTING AND COMMUNICATION FOLLOWING EXAMINATION

It is most important that all observations made during a clinical examination are noted and that they, together with any verbal comments made during the work, are added to any letter or certificate. Precision is important.

If a potential purchaser is present at the examination, it is possible to discuss the findings with him/her at the time but these comments *must* also be put in writing. Where doubt exists about the significance of the findings, for example, the presence of scar tissue or a raised nodule, this doubt should be recorded and appropriate advice given.

Reports should be professionally sound and scientifically accurate but will need to include lay terminology if intended for the purchaser or owner. Lay terms are best put in inverted commas, in brackets, after the relevant scientific words. It is important to use the correct terminology for a particular species. For example, a report on a horse is likely to describe it in such terms as 'a yearling, chestnut colt' (an uncastrated male animal in its second year of life, red in colour on body, mane and tail). A comparable document about a bird of prey intended for use in falconry might detail the hawk as 'an intermewed tiercel' (a male bird, probably a peregrine or another species of 'long-winged' falcon that has completed its first moult).

Whatever sort of animal is to be examined, the veterinarian should ensure that s/he has professional indemnity insurance (see Chapter 2).

FURTHER OPINIONS

Fields in which expert, second opinions are likely to be needed include dentistry (often relating to specific species such as horses, dogs or wildlife), toxicology, behaviour and neurology. The role of the general practitioner veterinarian should, perhaps, be considered similar to that of the UK medical police surgeon (forensic physician) who will be asked to carry out *screening* of one or more patients (e.g. alleged victims of sexual, physical abuse) in order to ascertain whether or not more specialised examination and investigation by colleagues are needed.

EXAMPLES OF CLINICAL CONDITIONS AND SITUATIONS

There follows discussion of a number of conditions or syndromes that are of particular relevance to forensic work with animals. Conditions which are usually fatal, or where investigation primarily depends upon *post-mortem* examination or detailed laboratory techniques, are covered in the succeeding chapter. There is, however, some overlap and

therefore the reader who does not find what s/he needs here should look in Chapter 7 or refer to the Index.

INFECTIOUS DISEASES

Diseases due to infectious agents (ranging from viruses to metazoan parasites) are very often the cause of litigation, insurance claims, arbitrations, allegations of malpractice, governmental enquiries and a range of other actions.

Space does not permit detailed discussion of infectious diseases. This is not meant to be a veterinary or medical text. However, zoonoses are covered in Chapter 2 because they involve both animals and humans. Another important field is 'import risk analysis': live animals and their products that are moved from one country to another may present a degree of disease risk and this needs to be assessed (OIE, 2004).

Some guidelines for those who have to investigate, collect evidence from or prepare reports about matters concerning infectious diseases are as follows:

- Involve colleagues with appropriate specialist experience and qualifications – microbiologists, immunologists, epidemiologists, statisticians.
- Take all precautions during investigations to minimise the risk of spread of disease to other animals or humans. Be particularly wary of zoonoses and remember that people who are immunocompromised, for whatever reason (see Chapter 2), are likely to be more susceptible to infection.
- Be sensitive to hygiene and whether or not it has been properly implemented in the premises under investigation. Standard sanitary operating procedures (SSOPs) are increasingly being used in veterinary practice (Cherry, 2005). Even if SSOPs are not in place, there should be records of how cleaning, disinfection and waste disposal are being carried out.

NON-INFECTIOUS DISEASES

Situations requiring clinical 'forensic' investigation can be divided into five groups, depending on how

137

they are alleged to have occurred. These groups are insults caused by:

(1) Humans on animals, e.g. beating with a stick, setting of poisons.
(2) Humans on animals *and* other humans, e.g. firing a shotgun irresponsibly.
(3) Animals on humans *and* other animals, e.g. a rabid dog attack.
(4) Animals on animals, e.g. an escaped zoo animal injuring or killing pet rabbits.
(5) Inanimate objects or factors on animals or on humans and other animals, e.g. injury or death from a motor car or a falling tree.

PHYSICAL ASSAULTS

All of the above categories can apply to physical assaults. Some of those that may be inflicted by humans on animals are listed in Chapter 2.

INJURIES

Although there are characteristics of wounds that apply, within limits, to all vertebrate species, specific injuries occur in certain taxa and the investigator should be aware of this. In some cases consultation with an appropriate specialist may be wise.

A few examples of injuries that are taxon-specific or likely to be particularly significant in certain animals are:

- Marine mammals – net-entanglement, injuries caused by boats.
- Birds of prey – trap injuries, abrasions caused by leather jesses or rings (bands) (Figure 5.21).
- Fish – nipped fins and tail, fish-hook damage to mouth.

Even if a particular case requires specialist examination and interpretation, the initial investigator must be prepared to describe (count, measure) the lesions and should ensure that they are photographed, in colour, with a scale and unique reference number.

VIOLENCE, CRUELTY TO CHILDREN AND ANIMAL ABUSE

Over the past twenty years links between violence in the household and abuse of animals have become well established (Arkow, 1992, 1994; Ascione and Arkow, 1999; Felthous and Bernard, 1979; Felthous, 1980, 1981; Olson, 1998). The subject has received particular attention in the UK, elsewhere in Europe, North America and Australia. In the USA, Kellert and Felthous (1985) examined the relationship between childhood cruelty to animals and aggressive behaviour, amongst both criminals and non-criminals, in adulthood. They found that childhood cruelty towards animals was significantly more prevalent amongst aggressive criminals than non-aggressive criminals or those who had not (apparently) committed a crime.

Kellert and Felthous drew up a preliminary classification of motivations for animal cruelty, which ranged from a desire to control an animal to non-specific sadism, with seven other intermediate categories. Interestingly, the study included examples of cruelty to wild species (see later), such as pulling wings off sparrows and 'splitting open the bellies of amphibians' as well as assaults on domesticated mammals. This important paper concludes with the suggestion that:

> *evolution of a more gentle and benign relationship in human society might be enhanced by . . . a more positive and nurturing ethic between children and animals.*

– shades of Alexander Pope, who stated (1713):

> *I cannot but believe a very good use might be made of the fancy which children have for birds and insects.*

Encouraging concern for the well-being of animals is not always easy in poorer, 'developing', countries where there are often pressing human needs. However, the concept can sometimes be promoted with surprising success. In Kenya, for example, the formation by the World Society for the Protection of Animals (WSPA) (see Appendix B) of 'Kindness Clubs' provided a framework for humane education in many parts of Africa.

Recognition of a 'battered-pet syndrome' (Munro, 1996; Munro & Thrusfield, 2001a–d) followed studies on 'battered-child syndrome' that in turn came in the wake of publication of the seminal paper on that subject by Kempe *et al.* (1962). The characteristic of 'battered-pet' syndrome, like its human counterpart, is physical abuse characterised by injuries that are non-accidental – in other words, they have been inflicted intentionally. In their seminal study, Munro and Thrusfield (2001b) recorded 243 cases in dogs and 182 in cats.

Suspicion of 'non-accidental injury' (NAI) in pet animals may be aroused by a number of factors, including unusual distribution or appearance of wounds, untreated lesions, an inconsistent history, suspicious behaviour on the part of the owner(s) and meekness of the animal (McGuinness *et al.*, 2005). In Munro and Thrusfield's studies, lesions encountered included bruises, fractures, burns and scalds, stab wounds, incised wounds and firearm injuries. There was also sexual abuse (see later), asphyxiation and drowning. It was noted that traumatic skeletal injuries in the dogs were more commonly found in the anterior (cranial) part of the skeleton, in contrast to those lesions resulting from traffic accidents. No single injury or group of injuries could be considered pathognomonic but repetitive injuries were highly suggestive of NAI.

The practising veterinarian is in a strong position to recognise animal abuse and should be aware that it may be linked to family violence (Fearon, 2006). S/he can play a part in both detection and prevention (Arkow, 2003, 2004; Arkow and Munro, 2006). Whether or not the findings should be reported, in view of the veterinarian's obligation to maintain client confidentiality, is discussed later. For veterinarians to play their role they need appropriate guidance and this is increasingly the case in certain countries – Australia, Canada, New Zealand, UK and USA for example. Concerns have been expressed however that 'vets could do more' (Anon., 2001; Bonner, 2001) and this is borne out by studies – for example, by Green and Gullone (2005) in Australia – attempting to measure how much veterinarians know about the subject. In the UK students receive training in recognising animal abuse (Anon., 2003a,b) and there is now a pro-

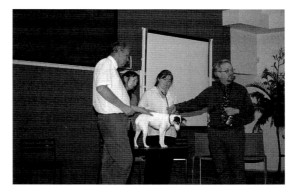

Figure 6.12 A training session in New Zealand. Students are taught how to recognize signs of abuse. This figure also appears in colour in the colour plate section.

gramme for the country's six veterinary schools, in collaboration with the RSPCA (Phil Wilson, pers. comm.). People from other disciplines may also benefit from tuition, especially if in mixed groups, where ideas and experiences can be shared.

Child abuse is sometimes characterised by the administration of drugs by parents and others (Boroda and Gray, 2005). This may have relevance to veterinarians (who are themselves permitted to possess and to prescribe medicines for use in animals) because such substances may also be given to non-human species.

Munchausen syndrome was first described in humans by Asher (1951) and takes its name from the exploits of the 18th century Baron von Munchausen who fabricated stories about himself and then became dependent upon the adulation and attention that he thereby attracted. Asher's original account related to adults who presented themselves with stories of ill-health and, as a result, were subject to numerous, needless, medical investigations. Meadow (1997) stated that the purpose of these claims was to gain sympathy and attention.

Munchausen syndrome by proxy was described in humans by Meadow (1997). It refers to falsification of illness in a child, usually by its mother. Again, the purpose is to attract attention. It can be difficult to detect, sometimes requiring photographic or video evidence (Foreman and Farsides, 1993).

Munro and Thrusfield (2001d) identified nine cases of Munchausen syndrome by proxy ('factitious illness by proxy') in animals as a result of sending a questionnaire to a random sample of 1000 veterinarians, of whom 404 responded. Their cases showed a number of features that are seen in MSBP in humans – attention-seeking behaviour by the owner, deliberate injury, markedly abnormal biochemical profiles, serial incidents, interference with surgical sites, recovery after separation from the owner and 'veterinarian shopping' by the owner. Munro and Thrusfield stressed the need for veterinary practitioners to be aware of this syndrome and urged debate between them and their medical colleagues. Arkow and Munro (2006) encouraged the use of the term 'fabricated or induced illness' (FII), on the grounds that this wording is increasingly being used by paediatricians.

Non-incidental injury is one of the instances where a conflict of interests may occur between client confidentiality and the veterinarian's responsibility to society and the law of the land. The advice in this respect given by the UK's RCVS is:

Animal abuse, child abuse and domestic violence

(1) Veterinary surgeons are one of a number of professionals who may see and hear things during the course of their professional activity which arouse suspicion of animal abuse and/or domestic violence and child abuse. Increasingly domestic violence, child abuse and animal abuse are seen to be linked and efforts are being made to raise awareness within the veterinary profession.

Animal abuse

(2) When a veterinary surgeon is presented with an injured animal whose clinical signs cannot be attributed to the history provided by the client, she/he should include non-accidental injury in their differential diagnosis.

(3) If there is suspicion of animal abuse, as a result of examining an animal, a veterinary surgeon should consider whether the circumstances are sufficiently serious to justify breaching the usual obligations of client confidentiality. In the first instance, in appropriate cases, the veterinary surgeon should attempt to discuss his/her concerns with the client. In cases where this would not be appropriate or where the client's reaction increases rather than allays concerns, the veterinary surgeon should contact the relevant authorities, for example the RSPCA . . . ; SSPCA . . . ; USPCA . . . to report alleged cruelty to an animal.

(4) Such action should only be taken when the veterinary surgeon considers on reasonable grounds that either animals show signs of abuse or are at real and immediate risk of abuse – in effect where the public interest in protecting an animal overrides the professional obligation to maintain client confidentially. A veterinary surgeon may contact the RCVS for advice before any confidential information is divulged.

Child abuse and domestic violence

(5) Given the links between animal and child abuse and domestic violence, a veterinary surgeon reporting suspected animal abuse to the relevant authority should consider whether a child might be at risk. A veterinary surgeon may also consider a child to be at risk in the absence of any animal abuse.

(6) Where a veterinary surgeon is concerned about child abuse or domestic violence, s/he should consider reporting the matter to the relevant authorities. The following authorities can be contacted, the local authority social services department, the NSPCC for England, Wales and Northern Ireland . . . ; CHILDREN FIRST for Scotland . . . or local police Child Protection Unit. A veterinary surgeon may contact the RCVS for advice before any confidential information is divulged.

(7) The NSPCC leaflet *Understanding the Links, child abuse, animal abuse and*

family violence, information for professionals provides further information on domestic violence and telephone numbers for the relevant authorities throughout the UK.

Elsewhere, especially in North America, concerns have been expressed by veterinarians that they, like physicians (Hall, 2006), might expose themselves to criminal or civil action should they make a false accusation, a 'good-faith' report that proves to be unfounded or if they fail to make a report if so required by law. This fear of litigation is discussed in some detail by Arkow and Munro (2006).

It is not only dogs and cats that may be abused (see Table 6.5).

Non-accidental injuries in animals are not necessarily linked with violence to humans. Even the most conscientious and humane person may lose patience with a pet that repeatedly jumps up at visitors or steals food from the kitchen, or a farm animal that stands on an unprotected foot or pins a stockman to the wall.

The motivation for an attack on an animal is not usually the concern of the clinician and should be left to others – the police or the courts – to decide (see Chapter 12).

Arkow and Munro (2006) urge that, when dealing with animals, the terminology used by the medical profession for children should be applied – 'abuse', 'cruelty' and 'maltreatment'. Following this system, there are four types of abuse, any of which may co-exist:

(1) Physical.
(2) Sexual.
(3) Emotional.
(4) Neglect.

These and similar terms are referred to later in this chapter and elsewhere in the book.

Close contact with the medical profession is always advantageous, and much can be learned from experienced paediatricians (David, 2005).

Table 6.5 Examples of abuse of captive and free-living animals.

Species	Type of abuse	Comments
All	Physical assaults, e.g. beating with sticks, gouging of eyes Use of fire, including fireworks Intentional starving, deprivation of water, neglect	Physical assaults are sometimes interpreted as abuse when the real intent was to kill a pest species or to euthanase a casualty Care must be taken in assessing cases
Mammals	Cutting off tail, snipping patagium of wing (bats), pulling-out spines (hedgehogs), etc.	None
Birds	Pulling off wings of young birds	None
Reptiles	Disembowelling, cutting/pulling off tail	Predators, e.g. crows, may also cause disembowelling Some lizards shed tail as a natural defence process (autotomy)
Amphibians	Disembowelling Removal of/damage to limbs by cutting or treading on them Placing toads in a fire to see them 'explode'	As above
Fish	Putting irritant chemicals in water	None
Invertebrates	Various, including dropping worms in a fire, pulling off wings of moths	Sometimes excused by claiming that, e.g. 'insects are not animals . . . cannot feel pain'

SEXUAL ASSAULTS

Arkow and Munro (2006) use the term 'animal sexual abuse' to describe physical assaults on animals that concentrate on the sexual organs, anus or rectum. They include under this heading any use of an animal 'for sexual gratification'.

Interactions of a sexual nature that may be of forensic significance can also be categorised under three headings – human/animal, animal/human and animal/animal.

Human/animal interactions

- Bestiality.
- Sexual stimulation of an animal.
- Sexual damage to an animal.

Sexual assaults on animals have long been recognised but are rarely well documented in the literature, possibly because of embarrassment on the part of authors, even veterinarians (Arkow and Munro, 2006). Often court-hearings provide more detail than do textbooks or journals. Most reports have dealt with larger domesticated livestock, such as donkeys and sheep, and related to bestiality or mutilation of genitalia with sticks or sharp instruments. The latter has sometimes been described, usually anecdotally, in zoo animals.

Sexual abuse of 'small' (companion) animals has been particularly poorly documented until recently. The paper by Munro and Thrusfield (2001c) was an important landmark in the UK in recognising the extent of such activity and linking it with other forms of 'non-accidental injury' (NAI). In their paper the authors described 28 cases of sexual abuse – 6% of the 448 NAIs reported by a random sample of small animal practitioners in the UK. The types of injury reported included vaginal and anorectal penetrative injuries (penile and non-penile), peri-anal damage and trauma to the genital organs. Some injuries, such as castration were severe and a few were fatal. Munro and Thrusfield pointed out that the type and severity of injuries in their survey were similar to those reported in humans.

It is always important to differentiate sexual assaults on animals from human activities that may be part of normal veterinary or husbandry practice (see Chapter 2) – for example, stimulation of male animals for semen collection, rectal or vaginal examination for clinical diagnostic purposes, castration, ovariectomy or vasectomy.

Animal/human interactions

Although well recognised, very little appears to have been published on attempted or successful copulation (usually by male animals on humans of either sex), other than to note that in domesticated animals it is a behavioural aberration (see later). The subject warrants more discussion and far more study.

In some species, where 'imprinting' of young on humans can occur (see early work by Konrad Lorenz, 1952, and others), humans may be solicited or approached as sexual partners. Male animals may attempt to mount – used to advantage in aviculture in order to collect semen for artificial insemination – and females may present themselves for copulation. These activities may appear to be mild and of little consequence but at the very least they may be grounds for complaint, possibly a civil action. Sometimes the offending animal is injured by a person who is attempting to protect him/herself. Where large or powerful species are involved (e.g. eagles, monkeys), serious injuries can result to both human and animal.

Investigation

In the investigation of alleged sexual assaults a range of techniques is used including:

- General clinical examination of the victim (animal or human), including sampling.
- Specific clinical investigation and sampling of reproductive system.
- Laboratory examination – semen, vaginal fluid, hair, blood (see Chapter 8). Collection and examination of semen can follow a combination of techniques used in human forensic medicine (DiMaio and DiMaio, 2001) and in standard veterinary and reproductive biology practice.

MUTILATION OF ANIMALS

Mutilation has been defined by the (UK) Royal College of Veterinary Surgeons (RCVS) as:

... interference with the sensitive tissues or bone structure of the animal, otherwise than for the purpose of its medical treatment.

The term has been used, especially in the UK, to describe non-therapeutic procedures on animals – such as tail-docking of dogs and surgical pinioning of birds – that are, or may be, questionable on ethical grounds. There is guidance for veterinary surgeons as to what may or may not be performed in the RCVS Guide to Professional Conduct (2000). Some 'mutilations' are illegal in one country but permissible in another (see Chapter 3).

Some commentators have suggested that there may be psychological and cultural links between the performance of certain 'mutilations' of animals and surgical (genital) abuse of women.

DEVELOPMENTAL ABNORMALITIES

These are usefully defined as 'defects that result from interference with normal growth and differentiation.' Many are congenital (present at birth) and therefore are associated with abnormal embryonic and fetal metamorphosis but some appear (or may manifest themselves) later in life. The causes of developmental abnormalities in animals are many and various and often multifactorial. They include:

- Genetic factors.
- Infectious agents, e.g. viruses.
- Physical (non-infectious) factors such as irradiation, hyperthermia and (as in freemartins) the fusion of placental structures.

Developmental abnormalities are of forensic importance because they may:

- Provide grounds for legal action against the supplier or breeder of an animal.

- Reduce the actual or insurance value of an animal.
- Be the basis of a charge of cruelty against someone who, for example, as a result of inbreeding produces animals with abnormalities that cause pain or distress (see Chapter 4).
- Be used to support a claim of malpractice against a veterinarian who fails to detect them or to provide appropriate advice.

The field is vast and cannot be discussed in any detail here. It usually involves geneticists and other specialists as well as veterinarians. Recognition, identification and interpretation of developmental abnormalities are often difficult and time-consuming. The challenges are even greater when dealing with non-domesticated species, where often baseline data are lacking, while ectothermic animals (reptiles, amphibians, fish and invertebrates) introduce the added complication of ectothermy. Developmental abnormalities in ectotherms are often associated with adverse or fluctuating temperatures. In some species, even sex determination is temperature-dependent.

In human medicine, 'birth defects' attract much publicity, and litigation or claims of malpractice often ensue. Collation of literature on such defects has proved helpful in legal cases (see, for example, Bergsma, 1982) and similar compilations are needed for both domesticated and commonly-kept wild animals.

Some developmental abnormalities may be induced intentionally. This is particularly the case in laboratory species where a natural or induced animal model (see Chapter 2) may be used to study, for example, spina bifida or polycystic kidneys. In some countries, such as the UK, research is strictly controlled (see Chapters 3 and 4) but the work often raises ethical and legal dilemmas. Less widely recognised, but no less important from a legal point of view, is the breeding of domesticated species, especially dogs and cats, for characteristics ('breed standards') that may enhance their value as show or pet animals but which can be associated with deleterious traits (Robinson, 1990).

RECOGNITION OF PAIN

The diagnosis and measurement of pain in animals are not easy (Hellebrekers, 2000 and Short and Van Poznak, 1992) (see Chapter 4). The assessment is likely to involve an experienced clinician but others, e.g. an ethologist or a pathologist (see Chapter 7), can usefully contribute.

EMERGENCIES

Emergency situations are important from a forensic point of view because:

- They may result from actions which might be questioned or challenged in a court case, by an insurance company or by a professional body – for instance, the administration of an anaesthetic agent or the performance of difficult surgery.
- The response to an emergency, because of the circumstances, may be inadequate, inappropriate or potentially hazardous – all of which may result in questions being asked and possible action taken. Animal welfare (see Chapter 4) and human health and safety (see Chapter 3) may be compromised.

Speed is often essential in an emergency and if the wrong action is to be avoided, it is important that the veterinarian or equivalent (a) is prepared – for example, by having an emergency kit, containing appropriate drugs and equipment and following well-tested protocol (b) keeps up-to-date with current thinking – for instance, cattle may convulse for a variety of reasons (hypomagnesaemia, tetanus, poisoning, nutritional deficiency, meningitis) and each of these is likely to need a different response.

Following any emergency it is important that the circumstances are recorded, either as a report or as data that can be retrieved later if needed.

Emergencies on a larger scale are covered under Disasters (see Chapter 2).

Critical care can produce its own problems and dilemmas, some of which may have legal consequences.

IATROGENIC DISEASE

Disease (infectious or non-infectious) that is caused as a result of human intervention is of great importance from a medicolegal point of view. Animals may develop such iatrogenic diseases following actions that range from the administration of vaccines (see later), through routine medication to minor or major surgery. Alleged cases need careful evaluation, where appropriate in consultation with relevant manufacturers or suppliers of pharmaceutical agents or surgical items.

Sometimes there are well-defined risk factors that should have been taken into account before the procedure was undertaken – and the client advised/warned accordingly and asked to give consent. An example is thrombophlebitis in horses, which can follow jugular cannulation: a recent study (Dolente *et al.*, 2005) showed that the health of the patient was a significant factor in whether or not a horse developed this complication. Other 'non-patient' factors can, however, also play a part – for instance, the make and type of catheter and how it is used (Spurlock and Spurlock, 1990).

Reactions to treatment can be of importance too in food-producing animals. For example, intramuscular injections given to pigs may cause tissue damage that persists until after the 'no-residue withdrawal time' (Klés *et al.*, 2000). This can have legal implications.

ANAESTHETIC AND SURGICAL EMERGENCIES

Emergencies can occur during anaesthesia or surgery – or, indeed, following restraint or treatment (see later and Iatrogenic above). Subsequent ill-health or death may be attributed, in whole or in part, to the procedure performed. This is an area where the threat of litigation or malpractice is very real.

Mortality associated with anaesthesia of humans is usually considered to lie somewhere between 1/10,000 and 1/100,000 (Flaherty and Musk, 2005) but figures vary depending upon the location and facilities available (Ouro-Bang'na Maman *et al.*, 2005). Data for small (domestic) animals dating back to Clarke and Hall (1990) suggested that 1 in 679 healthy dogs and cats and 1 in 31 sick animals died as a result of anaesthesia. A more recent survey (Broadbelt *et al.*, 2005) gave figures of 1 in 1849 (healthy dogs), 1 in 895 (healthy cats), 1 in 75 (sick dogs) and 1 in 71 (sick cats).

Factors that have to be considered when investigating anaesthetic deaths include:

- Whether electronic monitoring equipment was used: in human anaesthesia this aspect is subject to minimal standards. However, physical methods of assessing the depth of anaesthesia and the status of the patient remain a key part of the veterinary anaesthetist's skills and armoury.
- The experience of the anaesthetist ('There are no safe anaesthetic agents, only safe anaesthetists').
- The anaesthetic and premedicant agents used.
- The health status of the patient – and whether or not the animal was adequately assessed beforehand.
- What action was taken when the anaesthetic emergency was detected, including whether or not a properly formulated emergency kit was available and used.

Non-domesticated animals present extra problems, although there have been advances in the anaesthesia of such species, even of invertebrates (Cooper, 2002), in recent years. Ectothermic vertebrates can appear to have died during anaesthesia, only to recover later (see Chapter 4).

Injury and death can also result from medical and surgical procedures. At a meeting of the Royal Society of Medicine in 2005, it was stated that medical mistakes kill or seriously injure more than 15,000 human patients in the UK (www.rsm.ac.uk). Data on animals are difficult to obtain because of (generally) poor documentation. Legal actions and allegations of malpractice against veterinary surgeons are increasing. In a case in Europe in 2005 two veterinary surgeons were ordered to pay £350,000 damages to the owner of a valuable horse that developed laminitis after being injected with corticosteroids and had to be euthanased (Newton, 2005a).

In any allegation, the following points are important:

- Are proper case records available?
- Was the treatment in accordance with current thinking and practice?
- Was the client warned of possible adverse effects – and did s/he sign properly-worded consent forms to that effect?
- Does the veterinary surgeon who was involved admit making any mistakes?
- Are there witnesses, e.g. veterinary nurses, who can confirm or refute any claims?
- Does the practice adhere to clinical care standards (see later) and does it carry out clinical audit?
- Is supporting documentation (paperwork or electronic) available?
- What is the opinion of appropriate 'experts'?

POISONING AND DRUG REACTIONS

Toxicology is the study of poisons and intentional or accidental poisoning is an important part of forensic work (Ferner *et al.*, 1996). The principles of forensic toxicological investigation involving humans were explained by Anderson (2004) who included brief mention of regulatory/animal toxicology. He provided a useful table outlining types of specimen and their value to the toxicologist and much of this is relevant to animal work.

In human forensic work, drugs of addiction are often involved. This is not a major issue in veterinary forensics but animals are sometimes fed drugs (appropriately sealed) in order to smuggle them and a recent survey in the UK (Woodbine, 2005) suggested that 50% of practising veterinary surgeons had seen dogs with ill-effects as a result of eating or being fed cannabis or other agents (see also earlier). Links with botanists may be useful when investigating possible drug cases. Traditional medicines (Figure 5.1) are often exported from Africa and other parts of the world and may contain toxic or hallucinogenic substances.

Cases in which poisoning of an animal is either suspected or confirmed can produce particular problems for the expert witness, particularly if s/he is not experienced in toxicology. In such cases it is wise to have access to a colleague with such experience. Sometimes the case relates to straightforward toxicity, possibly resulting in death (see Chapter 7), sometimes to an allegation that two or more medicines have been administered to an animal and, as a result, had an adverse side effect. The latter is often difficult to investigate. General advice in such case is as follows:

- Contact the manufacturers of the drugs in question (do not rely only on their data sheets), explain the situation and ask for their comments. Ensure that you give the batch number of any suspect agent.
- Check the relevant veterinary practice's treatment records.
- Where a client has administered the treatment, ascertain as far as possible that this has been done in accordance with instructions (compliance).
- Consult standard textbooks.
- Discuss the case with experienced toxicologists, such as (in the UK) those associated with the Veterinary Poisons Information Service.
- Contact the relevant body – in the UK, the Veterinary Medicines Directorate (VMD).

Drug interactions in non-domesticated animals can be even more problematic. The vast majority of agents are not licensed in such species and relatively little information exists about dosages and safety.

Adverse events associated with vaccines are important. They affect what was originally a healthy animal and they can provide grounds for legal action or complaint against both the manufacturer and the veterinary surgeon. So concerned have some authorities been that post-marketing surveillance has been introduced to replace the less reliable system of voluntary reporting (Moore *et al.*, 2005). The increased used by veterinary practices of electronic medical record systems facilitates this and such data, with appropriate safeguards, could be made available in forensic cases.

A word should be said about access to drugs (veterinary pharmaceutical agents). Veterinarians are amongst the privileged few who are permitted to possess and use what have been traditionally termed in Britain 'dangerous drugs' and 'prescription-only medicines'. This brings with it the responsibility to ensure that such pharmaceutical products are stored properly and not used irresponsibly. Veterinary anaesthetics and other agents have been used to commit both suicide and homicide. The liability of veterinarians is increasing exponentially, with health and safety demands playing a large part in dictating how s/he behaves. One example of a relatively new challenge concerns the safe storage and use of cytotoxic drugs that are used in chemotherapy. A recent paper (Hayes, 2005) provides a useful review of the subject and aims to assist veterinary practices in establishing protocols on chemotherapy usage and administration.

In many countries guidelines exist for the 'responsible use' of antimicrobials and other agents – for example, the series issued in the UK by RUMA (the Responsible Use of Medicines in Agriculture Alliance) and these should be followed, in addition to legal controls. Formularies (for small animals, large animals, exotic species) carry less weight but often contain useful guidance for the practitioner and may be quoted in court.

In any forensic case relating to the possible misuse of, or ill-effects from, veterinary medicines, it is useful to consult a suitably-experienced pharmacist.

Veterinarians and others should be aware of changes in national legislation in Europe brought about by the need to comply with EU Directive 2004/28/EC, which came into effect on 30th October 2005. In Britain this is further complicated as a result of the Marsh Report and the findings of the Competition Commission. The new categories of medicines are set out in Table 6.6.

'Batch tracing' is also required. This means that each time a POM-V drug is dispensed, its batch number is recorded. The practice must be aware of which batches are in current use. The requirements for food animals are far more stringent than those for non-food species. These moves have good points but will lead to challenges relating to record-keeping. One advantageous outcome may be more

Table 6.6 Old and new medicine classifications.

Old term	New term
POM	POM-V (Veterinary)
PML	PML-VPS (Veterinary, Pharmacy and Suitably Qualified Person)
P	NFA-VPS (Non-feed animal, Veterinary Pharmacy and Suitably Qualified Person)
GSL	AVM – GSL (Authorised Veterinary Medicine – General Sale List)

computerisation of records in practice which should bring with it benefits in terms of avoiding, or detecting, errors or inconsistencies.

Allegations that contaminated foodstuffs (feed) caused failure to thrive, clinical ill-health or death in livestock are relatively common. Implications of contaminants in the food are not easy to substantiate and are likely to involve:

- Very careful appraisal of the history, when problems first arose, whether or not other animals on the same diet (on different diets but exposed to other, similar, environmental factors such as the same source of water, or identical bedding) have been similarly affected.
- Clinical examination of both normal and 'sick' animals.
- *Post-mortem* examination of both normal and 'sick' animals.
- Standard laboratory tests (blood chemistry, haematology) on animals in the above categories.

Mycotoxins are an important example. These are toxic, sometimes carcinogenic, substances that are produced by fungi and which grow on agricultural commodities. They are ubiquitous and because of the difficulty of ready detection, are an inevitable feature of modern agriculture. A recent book (Diaz, 2005) provides useful information about these toxins, how they form, what they do and how they can be detected and assayed and quotes a recent FAO (Food and Agriculture Organization) report that stated that in at least 99 countries, representing 87% of the world's population, there are mycotoxin guidelines for human and/or animal foodstuffs.

Another important aspect of toxicoses, increasingly relevant to forensic work because of the concerns of consumers, relates to chemical residues that may enter meat or other animal products (milk, eggs, honey) and possibly present a hazard to human health (see, for example, Sharpe and Livesey, 2005).

Poisoning of wildlife can occur accidentally or by intention (PAW, 2005). It can occur on an enormous scale – for instance, the decline of vultures in India, Nepal and Pakistan, primarily on account of ingestion of diclofenac, a drug used in livestock (Oaks *et al.*, 2004). Poisoning of wildlife is reviewed further in Chapter 5. The role of pathological investigations in diagnosis is covered in Chapter 7. Pollutants, including oil, are discussed below.

EXPOSURE TO POLLUTANTS, INCLUDING OIL

An enormous number of pollutants (poisons) can affect the health of humans, animals and plants. They are to be found in the air, in water and in terrestrial environments.

Insidious insults that can cause sub-clinical effects in individual animals or long-term sequelae in populations include:

- Toxic chemicals, including lead from cartridges and anglers' weights (French *et al.*, 1987).
- Chemicals, such as soaps and detergents, that have an adverse effect on, e.g., a bird's plumage (Cooper *et al.*, 1989b) or an insect's ability to walk on the surface of water (Guthrie, 1989), but are not directly toxic.
- Materials such as metal, wire, plastic that can cause physical damage or result in impaction.

Pollution by oil has long been recognised as an environmental problem. Birds, turtles and marine mammals are at the tip of the iceberg. Many other marine animals and plants are affected, sometimes with long-term ecological effects. Increasingly there is pressure to seek compensation from those who spill the oil, whether or not this was intentional. Oil contamination is one consideration in the relatively new field of 'environmental forensics' (Morrison, 1999; Murphy and Morrison, 2002) – see Chapters 2 and 5.

EVIDENCE-BASED MEDICINE

It is important to recognise that although clinical acumen remains of importance, evidence-based veterinary medicine (EBVM) is increasingly likely to be an issue in court cases and similar hearings. Those prosecuting a case are likely to demand confirmation that a treatment that was provided (or perhaps denied) to an animal was in keeping with current scientific evidence. Cockcroft and Holmes (2003) and Holmes and Cockcroft (2004) provided useful guidance to EBVM and emphasised that the key skill required for its practice is the ability to appraise evidence from scientific papers. The next step is to ask 'Is it true?' and then 'Is it relevant to my patient?'

UNORTHODOX TREATMENTS

Legal and professional difficulties may arise over 'unorthodox' treatments. For example, a substantial number of people, including veterinarians, use honey or royal jelly to treat wounds. Such practices are well-established and there is scientific evidence that these substances have antibacterial properties (Overgaauw and Kirpensteijn, 2006). However, in a court, insurance or disciplinary case, such treatments may be questioned.

The situation is even more complex in less-industrialised countries where, of necessity or on account of cultural factors, a whole range of remedies – plant, animal or psychological/spiritual – may be used to treat humans and animals. Again, some of these have proven efficacy – for instance, the use of pawpaw (papaya) (*Carica papaya*) in debriding wounds – but for others there may be no scientific data whatsoever available. This has to be taken into consideration in legal cases.

CONSENT FORMS

These are an increasingly important feature of veterinary practice and of other situations where an owner's animals or property are being handled or managed by a third party. Specimen consent forms are produced by some professional bodies – for example, the RCVS – and the veterinary surgeon would be wise to use these whenever possible.

COMPLEMENTARY AND ALTERNATIVE MEDICINE

The expert in a case where treatment is an issue must be prepared for questions about complementary or alternative medicine, ranging from acupuncture to homeopathy and osteopathy.

Terminology is sometimes complicated, often not consistent and can cause problems (see later). Hektoen (2005), in a paper about homeopathy in veterinary practice, provided a useful résumé, introducing the term 'complementary and alternative medicine' (CAM), which encompasses various types of therapy. These differ widely in their theoretical basis, practice and use. Definitions of CAM also vary but include 'disease treatments and health care practices not taught widely in medical schools, not generally used in hospitals and not usually reimbursed by medical insurance companies' (Bloom *et al.*, 2000). CAM is also sometimes termed:

- Integrative medicine.
- Alternative medicine.
- Unconventional therapies.
- Unproven therapies.

Hektoen drew attention to the two key differences between CAM and academic medicine:

(1) the former lack mechanisms of action that can be explained by the natural sciences.
(2) the clinical effects of CAM have not been verified.

However, the point is made that acupuncture is increasingly recognised as being scientifically-explicable while others, including homeopathy, cannot at present be satisfactorily explained.

Even the words used in CAM can be confusing: there are significant differences between 'aromatherapy' (the unproven use of various odours to treat disease) and 'pheromonatherapy' (scientifically controlled utilisation of naturally produced pheromones)!

Faith-healing is another form of CAM and is sufficiently important to warrant the inclusion in the GPC of the RCVS of the following:

> Faith healers are required in terms of the Code of Practice of the Confederation of Healing Organisations, to ensure that animals have been seen by a veterinary surgeon who is content for healing to be given by the laying on of hands.

An expert should be aware of current thinking. He or she may or may not have experience of CAM and might even be sceptical as to its value. The lawyers should be made aware of such opinions – and indeed of any other strongly-held views that might influence a magistrate, jury or judge – for example, concerning fox-hunting or the use of animals in research.

STARVATION

'Starvation' is a lack of essential nutrients, usually over a prolonged period, and is characterised clinically by profound physiological and metabolic disturbances. The term 'inanition' is also sometimes used but has a slightly different meaning. Inanition is a condition resulting from not just lack of food but also water and/or a defect in assimilation of nutrients.

A third term that is relevant to the theme is 'cachexia'. This usually implies general ill-health and malnutrition, marked by body weakness, emaciation and secondary diseases.

Allegations of starvation are a common reason for the institution of police or animal welfare society enquiries and sometimes prosecution.

Animals that are alleged to have been starved may be examined/seen alive, necessitating clinical examination, or presented dead, necessitating *post-*

mortem examination. In view of the importance of the subject, starvation is considered both here, as a clinical matter, and in the succeeding chapter, under *post-mortem* examination.

It is important to bear in mind that starvation and inanition can be due to a variety of causes, not just omitting to provide food. Starvation in captive animals, whether fatal or not, can be the result of one or more of the following:

* Failure of the keeper to provide any food.
* Failure of the keeper to provide sufficient food in terms of quantity and quality (see below).
* Failure of the animal to accept food, in part or in whole, despite its (food) being offered.
* Failure of the animal to masticate and swallow food, even though food has been offered and, perhaps, taken initially.
* Food not remaining within the stomach (on account of regurgitation or vomiting).
* Food not being adequately digested and absorbed in the intestinal tract (because of malabsorption, increased gut transit time, internal parasites, etc.).
* Food that has been ingested, digested and absorbed not being utilised because of metabolic or other disorders.

The veterinarian who is asked to examine an animal clinically, where there is a suspicion of starvation, should first ascertain the history and the questions that s/he is being asked. It may be, for example, that there is sound evidence that inadequate food was being offered by the owner and this *per se* is sufficient for proceedings to commence. On the other hand, the history and other information that is made available may suggest that the animal was being fed but for some reason was either not taking the food or was not making full use of it in nutritional terms. The clinician must, therefore, liaise closely with those who have background to the case.

Insofar as clinical examination of an animal where starvation is concerned, the following points are important:

* The animal must be weighed accurately and appropriate measurements taken (see earlier).

- A proper condition score should be used (see later), rather than vague statements such as 'in poor condition' or 'clearly emaciated'.
- The condition score should be explained to make it comprehensible to a layman and, if appropriate, a reference to its use given.
- In non-domesticated animals, appropriate comment should be made about clinical observations that might be relevant to an allegation of starvation – for example, 'poverty lines' on the sides of the tail of reptiles, 'hunger traces' on the feathers of birds (see Ptilochronology).
- The breed, strain or variety of an animal must be stated and this taken into account in any assessment – a thin greyhound appears very different from a thin bulldog, even though both are *Canis familiaris*.
- It must be made perfectly clear in any report as to whether a full clinical examination of the animal was carried out (the ideal situation) or whether, perhaps, because of limitation of time, only certain points could be addressed. There are specific features that should be considered in any possible case of starvation (see below) and these should be enumerated and explained in the statement.
- Any additional information relevant to the case should be provided making it clear whether that information was obtained directly by the clinician or was as a result of data provided by an animal welfare officer or policeman or similar. Be very wary of hearsay.

Important criteria in any assessment and reporting where starvation of an animal is suspected or has been alleged include the following:

- Bodyweight (mass).
- Morphometrics.
- Condition score.
- Other features that may be relevant to condition and dietary intake (e.g. skin, hair, pressure sores).
- Assessment of subcutaneous fat, either manually or using ultrasound.
- Assessment of internal body fat, as above.

- Muscle mass and evidence of weakness or other locomotor deficiency.
- Behavioural features that may add weight to or refute a diagnosis of starvation, e.g. marked hunger.
- Change in bodyweight over time following provision of an adequate diet.

Serial weight comparisons are useful evidence if animals are seized. It is important that one person performs follow-up measurements, using the same weighing scales. Variability in balances and scales can be significant when dealing with very small animals. Some commercial companies offer calibration certification.

Scientific papers on the speed of weight loss are few because usually such studies necessitate depriving animals of food. However, some work has been reported on the fasting of animals for veterinary or scientific purposes, e.g. prior to the administration of an anaesthetic agent or to study metabolic changes. There are rodent 'models' (see Chapter 2) for the study of fasting on, for instance, the immune system. Information on humans is available based largely on data from victims of natural and anthropogenic disasters (see Chapter 2), particularly studies in refugee camps. A good review article is that by Allen and Toll (1995) which reported that normal dogs which were fasted lost 21% of their bodyweight by the nineteenth day. Weight loss followed a hyperbolic pattern (i.e. it slowed over time). An experiment with six obese dogs showed an 8% loss by the end of the first week, 5% more in week two and then 3–4% per week thereafter (the experiment stopped at day 42).

Fasting and starvation have an effect on various organs and systems (gastro-intestinal, endocrine, renal – electrolyte and acid-base – cardiovascular, hepatic and metabolic) (Bartges and Osborne, 1995). Both gross and microscopical lesions may be detectable in affected animals, as well as biochemical, haematological and other changes.

There is much published information on the nutrition of animals (see, for example, Kelly and Wills, 1994, for dogs and cats) and this should be consulted, as should specialists in appropriate fields, whenever malnutrition is alleged.

SCORING OF MALNUTRITION

Scoring systems for screening and assessing malnutrition in humans are well established – for elderly patients, for example (Harris and Haboudi, 2005). Techniques employed include:

- Body mass index (BMI) (weight in kg divided by height in metres $\hat{A}^2$). However, BMI can be unreliable in the presence of, for example, ascites and, in addition, measuring accurately the height of elderly frail patients can be difficult.
- Anthropometry – skinfold thickness (using callipers) and arm circumference. These tests are easy to perform but there is considerable variation related to age, sex and ethnicity.
- Biochemical markers – measurement of, e.g., serum albumen, transferrin, lymphocyte numbers, cholesterol and vitamins/trace elements. None of these is adequate *per se*.
- Malfunction screening tools – various techniques aimed at predicting malnutrition, based on a range of different criteria.

Some such methods have been applied to domesticated species and to laboratory animals. Reports of their efficacy and shortcomings are to be found scattered in the literature. A few exotic species have been the subject of similar study, for example for reptiles, the Jackson's Ratio established for the monitoring of Mediterranean tortoises prior to and following hibernation (Jackson, 1980) and other techniques (Calvert, 2004) and subsequently refined for fieldwork by Hailey (2000).

In addition to the taking of photographs as evidence, video recording has much to commend it. The animal should be filmed in recumbency, if that is how it has been found, or standing/walking, as appropriate.

The comments above apply primarily to domesticated mammals but extrapolation is possible to a wide range of other species. Special care must be taken with non-domesticated animals as these may manifest starvation or food deprivation in different ways. Often clinical signs are very subtle. Sometimes specific tests may need to be carried out to access the animal's condition. Free-living wildlife starve for a variety of reasons, often relating to unavailability of food, and diagnosis may necessitate interdisciplinary studies (Cooper and Laurie, 1987).

Great caution needs to be exercised over such matters as how long it takes for clinical signs of starvation to develop, especially if this is to be linked with allegations of 'cruelty' or 'suffering' (see Chapter 4). The food requirements of animals vary greatly and this must be taken into account in any calculation. As was emphasised in Chapter 2, endothermic animals with a high metabolic rate usually need to eat frequently and to take in a substantial proportion of their bodyweight as food each day in order to maintain energy balance. Thus, a small rodent that has been deprived of food for eight hours may be on the brink of hypoglycaemia and death, while a similar period of food deprivation will have little effect on a guinea pig and probably none at all on a dog or a sheep.

Many non-domesticated species can tolerate long periods of 'starvation' so long as they have had an adequate fluid intake. Snakes may survive weeks without food and spiders months. Some animals may refuse food or markedly restrict their intake during times of, e.g. courtship, egg-laying or when feeding their young. The clinical signs of, and pathological lesions associated with, starvation may be very different in non-domesticated species from those that are well-recognised in dogs, cats, horses and farm animals.

DEHYDRATION

This may be concurrent with starvation or separate. It is discussed in Chapter 7.

SHOCK

This is an inadequate perfusion of the tissues and can be a sequel to many different insults. It is not always easy to differentiate *post mortem* from autolytic changes (Rutty, 2004).

OBESITY

Obesity was defined by Markwell and Edney (1994), in the context of dogs and cats, as when 'the accumulation of adipose tissue reaches a stage where there are pathological changes as a direct result.' Such changes are related to the additional load on body systems and can include:

- Osteoarthritis.
- Cardiovascular compromise.
- Increased anaesthetic and surgical risk.
- Increased risk of hyperthermia.
- Diabetes mellitus.
- Hepatic disease (lipidosis).

These other effects reflect the fact that giving an animal too *much* food, or food of the wrong quality, or under-exercising, can contribute to poor animal welfare, which in turn may result in legal proceedings. In practice, relatively few cases are taken against someone whose animals are obese but the situation may change. Criteria for assessing and scoring obesity are available for dogs and cats and for a few other species (Kelly and Wills, 1994).

Overfeeding of some species can be fatal – fish, for example. This is usually due to other effects, such as hypoxia or toxicity, but can be grounds for legal actions, especially if large numbers of valuable animals are affected, such as koi or farmed fish.

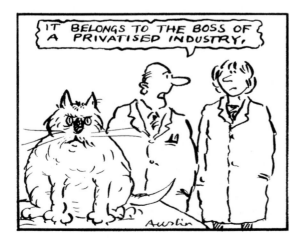

NEGLECT

'Neglect' is defined in the Oxford Dictionary as:

> *. . . a condition when a parent or guardian fails to provide minimal physical and emotional care for a child or other dependent person . . .*

and this can be readily applied to an animal. Arkow and Munro (2006) include neglect in their proposed categorisation of 'cruel' acts perpetrated against animals and define neglect as 'failure to provide the basic physical and/or emotional necessities of life.' They refer to Webster (2005) in stating that animals may have emotions.

The term 'neglect' is sometimes used in legislation but more often is a term that is employed in discussion or description, especially relating to animal welfare. Neglect can be absolute or be restricted to one area of omission only. Examples of where neglect of an animal may be alleged to have occurred include failing:

- To feed.
- To provide water.
- To clean a cage or enclosure.
- To groom the coat.
- To keep at an appropriate temperature.
- To provide environmental enrichment.

The 'Five Freedoms', drawn up originally for farm animals but applicable to most species in captivity, are relevant here (see Chapter 4).

Neglect can be:

(1) intentional.
(2) accidental (by default).

The end result is often the same but the factors leading to it are likely to be different.

Intentional neglect is covered in part elsewhere. It may be linked with abuse or with hoarding of animals (see Chapter 4).

Accidental neglect can occur for many reasons, for example:

- Failure to appreciate the needs of animals (e.g. how much food a dog needs, the dietary needs of a parrot).
- Unavailability of resources, including money.

- Unwillingness to admit that help is needed (e.g. in animal sanctuaries when too many animals are 'rescued' and the staff cannot cope).
- Genuine emergencies, such as illness or bereavement (when humans are likely to be given priority over animals).

SIGNS OF NEGLECT

As 'neglect' is a broad, rather amorphous term, the signs can be equally diverse, to include:

- Loss of weight/condition, leading to starvation.
- Dehydration.
- Soiling/matting of coat.
- Myiasis.
- Unclean environment.

A scoring system, an 'objective scale', can be very helpful when trying to assess neglect or sub-standard care. This is a topic that was covered by Olson (1998): other authors have developed the theme since then. Scoring can be based on existing systems – for example, the condition scores used in clinical veterinary medicine – or may be formulated specifically for the purpose and for the species/breed or individual animal involved. Very simple scoring systems, e.g. for faecal soiling, can be based on a range of 0–3 (Table 6.7).

More comprehensive and precise quantification is possible if, for example, one has a score of 1–5. However, the greater the number of categories, the more chance of inter-observer variation.

A numbering system is recommended as it facilitates electronic storage and analysis of data.

Assessment of faecal soiling is not just a matter of extent. The location of the faeces, their colour, consistency and smell should also be recorded and, wherever feasible, scored.

Myiasis, the presence of dipterous larvae in living tissues, may be used to assess the duration of neglect of animals by determination of the stage of the species involved (Anderson and Huitson, 2004).

Assessment of neglect (or welfare) does not relate to the animal alone. Its home is also significant and the expert must be prepared to assess and comment upon such matters as housing, ventilation (including air changes), temperature, relative humidity, substrate and cleaning practices. Relating the maladies of patients to the environment in which they live is not a new concept. Two thousand years ago Hippocrates, in his teachings on human medicine, wrote:

> *These things one ought to consider most attentively; the mode in which the inhabitants live – whether they are fond of eating and drinking to excess, and given to indolence or fond of exercise and labour, and not given to excess in eating and drinking.*

The great Avicenna, a thousand years later, was a similar exponent of the need to link clinical signs with lifestyle and put this into practice in his work with patients, often resolving problems by careful observation of the patient's behaviour followed by corrective action (Shah-Kazemi, 1998).

Similar detective work is the hallmark of crime scene investigations (see Chapter 9). The most important clues as to why an animal died or how an illegal act was committed may be found in the environment – in the paddock, in the kennel, or in the building where the animal lived.

TRAUMATIC INJURIES

A traumatic injury is produced by a sudden, violent force that results in a compression, stretching, torsion, or penetration of the tissues. The type of injury depends upon the force involved, the amount of energy discharged and the tissues affected.

Humans inflict traumatic injuries on animals, either intentionally or accidentally (see earlier).

Inter-specific and intra-specific interactions can result in traumatic injury to both free-living and

Table 6.7 A simple scale for classifying faecal soiling.

Score	Level of soiling
0	No visible soiling
1	Minimal soiling
2	Moderate soiling
3	Marked soiling

captive animals. Predation, territorial defence, mating-related activities, and fratricide are examples that have long been recognised. Sexual behaviour can be the cause of significant morbidity and mortality.

Collisions between birds and aircraft have resulted in the instigation of bird-control programmes on many large airfields throughout the world (PAW, 2005). Wildlife also may strike buildings, towers, and fences and certain species such as game birds and tortoises are frequently traumatised by mowing machines or agricultural machinery. Injury and/or death of wild animals of all species can be the result of road traffic accidents (Ashley and Robinson, 1996).

There has been much interest in the effect of injuries on the survival and welfare of wildlife, and, in particular, in the incidence and significance of healed fractures and other skeletal pathology. Brandwood *et al.* (1986) compared birds, molluscs, and primates in this respect; bird bones had very low incidences of healed fractures ($\hat{A} \pm 0.003$), mammals higher ($\hat{A} \pm 0.01$), and molluscs much higher ($\hat{A} \pm 1.0$). The structure of animal bones and their tensile strength was studied by Alexander (1984). Several authors have described healed fractures and other pathological changes in archaeological material comprising both captive and free-living animals (Harcourt, 1971).

The importance of self-mutilation or injury by other animals in captivity was emphasised over 70 years ago (Fox, 1923). In recent years, public concern in Europe and North America has prompted research into ways of improving the welfare of animals in zoos and collections, and this has led to the production of management guidelines, some enshrined in law.

Trauma causes damage to essential epithelial, connective, muscular and nervous tissues coupled with secondary effects such as anaemia caused by loss of blood, and sometimes toxaemia. The direct effect of a physical blow will depend on the area of the body involved, the energy discharged at impact and the tissues damaged. Secondary effects may include infection, since the injures serve as portals of entry for pathogens, e.g. infection of fight wounds by *Pasteurella* and *Streptococcus* in carnivores, and multiplication of *Clostridium* in bruised areas of the body of many species.

Clinical signs can range from coma to an almost complete absence of abnormalities. Affected animals usually exhibit pain and/or distress and often external injuries are palpable. There may be evidence of blood loss and shock. Central nervous signs frequently predominate, particularly when the animal has struck its head, and a careful differential diagnosis between physical, infectious and metabolic disease is necessary. The animal may have difficulty in standing and paralysis can occur. In extreme cases, limbs or appendages may be completely lost.

Other signs may be more subtle, e.g. subcutaneous emphysema in a bird, which is suggestive of air-sac damage. Laboratory investigations may assist diagnosis; a drop in PCV (haematocrit) or changes in other blood values may indicate internal haemorrhage. In some cases severe diarrhoea, often blood-stained, is seen, and internal damage to the respiratory tract can result in haemoptysis. In humans an exaggerated immunoinflammatory response may follow injury, sometimes days or weeks later (Smith and Giannoudis, 1998).

LACK OF SUNLIGHT

Lack of exposure to sunlight or its artificial equivalent may be relevant in legal cases relating to (for example) reptiles and marmosets. It may be relevant to the health of 'house rabbits', which often spend their lives indoors. Whilst the prosecution in a case would struggle to obtain a conviction on lack of ultra-violet exposure alone, this could be an important factor in building a case of neglect.

BITES AND BITE WOUNDS

The oral cavity was discussed briefly earlier: here the emphasis is on teeth and their role in causing bite wounds.

Bites from animals are of considerable importance, both from a practical (health/welfare) and a legal point of view. In wild animals biting can be part of normal behaviour, especially during courtship (Duff and Hunt, 1995). Animal bites damage tissues, can introduce infectious agents and can have a profound psychological effect on the victim, whether human or animal (see Chapter 7). Bites are a constant danger in veterinary practices and other places where animals are kept and handled (Drobatz and Smith, 2003).

Bite wounds form an important part of human forensic work where investigation and interpretation of biting incidents and bite wounds constitute a specialised field, involving odontologists and others (Dinkel and Captain, 1976; Prabhu, 2004). From a comparative perspective, bites can be divided into:

- Intra-specific: humans bite humans, dogs bite dogs, badgers bite badgers.
- Cross-specific: dogs bite humans, humans bite dogs (see Chapter 2 – Quotation), vampire bats bite domesticated pigs.

The way in which animals bite – and why they do so – is important. A carnivore bites (and often tears) with its canines; a rodent may nip with its incisors or gnaw with its cheek teeth. A python will bite quickly if defending itself (Cooper, 1967) but hangs on with its teeth if it is trying to retain and constrict a prey item.

Bites are of importance in forensic medicine for the following reasons:

- They can damage tissue and cause injury and/ or death in live animals/humans.
- They can introduce organisms that can cause local or systemic infection in live animals/ humans – ranging from streptococci to lyssa viruses, including rabies.
- They can mutilate carcases *post mortem* (see below).
- They can damage foodstuffs and other materials.

Dog bites are of particular legal significance because of their prevalence (see Chapter 2). Dogs may bite humans and other species *ante mortem* or pre-date bodies *post mortem*. Dogs may act alone or in packs.

The veterinarian or perhaps a zoologist may be asked to examine and give an opinion on alleged bite marks in animals, in humans and in inanimate material, such as food items.

Recognition of the species that caused the bite wound depends upon a combination of the following:

- The shape of the wound.
- The type of wound, e.g. whether canine teeth were involved, producing puncture wounds, or 'cheek' teeth (premolars and molars), causing crushing of tissues.
- The site of the wound, e.g. domesticated cats tend to bite the face or hand of a human.
- Laboratory tests, e.g. on any of the bacteria isolated, or DNA studies on saliva.

Williams *et al.* (1998) recommended photographing bite wounds in black and white as well as in colour. Casts can be taken. As mentioned earlier, skinning a carcase can help to reveal cryptic bite marks and skin punctures that are not easily discerned in haired, feathered or scaled skin (see also Wobeser, 1996). Transillumination often provides useful clues (Dorion, 1987). Reflected light may assist, as can ultraviolet (Barsley *et al.*, 1990).

In human work, bite marks are classified on the basis of whether humans or animals produced the mark and where the mark is exhibited by materials such as foodstuffs or human skin (Cameron and Sims, 1973) (see later).

Bite marks on skin were divided by Holt (1980) into three categories:

(1) Tooth marks themselves.
(2) Arch marks – the pattern presented by upper or lower teeth of the dental arch.
(3) Bite marks – from an aggressive bite.

The appearance and identity of bite marks made by animals can be influenced by many different factors, relating to the characteristics of (a) the bite, and (b) the material or tissue which has been bitten. These will each be discussed briefly.

The bite

Variables include:

- Species of animal (see later).
- Age of animal.
- Health of animal.

- Type of bite – defensive, aggressive (see earlier).
- Other circumstances, e.g. duration of bite.

The material/tissues

Bite marks are more easily distinguished in food-stuffs than in human or animal tissue. The former do not become distorted as do the latter. Forensic odontologists distinguish the types of marks associated with different materials, such as chocolate, fruit and cheese (Prabhu, 2004). In animal work similar differences are seen when, for example, rodents attack food or become trapped and attempt to escape.

Veterinarians who may be involved in legal cases should consider developing their own reference collection of material relating to bites. Teeth and jaws of different species and breeds of animals can be relatively easily prepared and, properly labelled, are easily stored. These can be supplemented with:

- Photographs and radiographs of normal and abnormal mandibular, maxillary and dental structures.
- Casts of normal and abnormal dental structures.

As with bite wounds, every opportunity should be taken to photograph oral lesions. Radiography and casting may need consent from the owner and the former should only be undertaken on live animals if there is a clinical indication for such exposure.

Bites from non-domesticated animals, which in theory can span much of the Animal Kingdom (see Chapter 2), usually require specialist input but the techniques for clinical examination of the bite marks are essentially the same. In a legal case, the first question asked is likely to be 'Which species of animal caused this bite wound?', which may entail comparison of the marks with teeth of known species from museums and elsewhere.

The value of collaboration with the dental profession was mentioned earlier and cannot be overemphasised. Veterinary and dental practitioners who work together find much of common interest. Dental technicians too can provide skilled assistance in collaboration with their counterparts in veterinary practice (Holmstrom *et al.*, 1992; Holmstrom, 2000).

OTHER ANIMAL-INDUCED INJURIES

Investigation of wounds inflicted by animals using their claws/talons, wings or tails requires a comparable, methodical, approach to that of bite wounds.

HYPERTHERMIA

Overheating can easily occur if shelter and housing are inadequate or if animals are overcrowded. Hyperthermia can occur as a result of chase and capture, especially when an animal is pursued or struggles and when the ambient temperature is high. Large, obese animals are more susceptible to hyperthermia than are small, well-proportioned ones. Stress-induced hyperthermia is recognised in some species and gives rise to concern on welfare grounds (Moe and Bakken, 1998).

Exposure to the sun is an important cause of overheating and climate change may be significant in this respect. In the UK the Pet Travel Scheme (PETS) has permitted pet animals to be taken to warm parts of the world where they not only can contract 'exotic', sometimes zoonotic, diseases but also be adversely affected by their exposure to high ambient temperatures.

Ectothermic species are particularly susceptible to hyperthermia if they are unable to lower their body temperature by behavioural means (see Chapter 2). In some reptiles with a low 'critical high' temperature, even modest heat, such as might be experienced when captured and handled (Knight *et al.*, 2004), can prove fatal. Amphibians too can succumb to thermal shock (Green *et al.*, 2003). Certain fish may die or show clinical signs of distress (such as a change in coloration) if they are transferred from water of one temperature to another that is hotter or colder.

Temperature extremes affect tissues in a number of ways, depending upon the severity and duration of the insult and the characteristics of the host, e.g.

coat colour in cattle (Hansen, 1990). Acute heat stress can produce similar effects to burns but may, in addition, cause largely irreversible damage to kidneys, liver, heart and brain, in serum enzymes and electrolytes. Chronic heat stress in domesticated stock (for example, when taken to the tropics) depresses metabolism and production; the underlying mechanisms are not clear. Exposure to high temperatures can affect spermatogenesis and may cause fetal abnormalities. Hyperthermia following exertion or capture appears to produce vascular collapse (shock), necrotic changes in the liver and other organs and hyperkalaemia (Fowler, 1978).

Heat stress can be acute or chronic. Acute effects can include panting or other signs of overheating, and hyperthermia may be detectable. Tachycardia is characteristic. There may be profound metabolic changes (Suliman *et al.*, 1989). In severe cases of sunburn, cutaneous erythema and other skin lesions are present, especially on unpigmented skin. The animal frequently is prostrate, in a stupor or coma, and very dehydrated; it tends to seek cool or sheltered places. Birds show similar panting respiration, and their wings hang loosely.

Chronic heat stress is more subtle in its effects and animals may show only poor growth and high embryonic mortality. Equine anhidrosis, an inability to sweat, occurs in some domesticated horses in the tropics (Morrow and Sewell, 1990), and it may affect other animals.

Humans exposed to high temperatures also suffer both acute and chronic effects. In 'heat stroke' life-threatening clinical signs and/or death can quickly supervene. Data on hyperthermia in humans (e.g. Robbins *et al.*, 1999) can be of assistance in animal cases.

A legal case relating to hyperthermia is likely to be brought on such grounds as:

- Confining an animal, usually a dog, in a motor vehicle where it is exposed to direct sunlight or high temperatures. Data on the temperatures attained in closed vehicles were published in the medical literature some years ago (Zumwalt *et al.*, 1976; Surpure, 1982) and in the veterinary literature more recently (e.g. Gregory and Constantine, 1996). Thermal imaging techniques are proving useful under other circumstances (Warriss *et al.*, 2006).
- Keeping a captive animal (zoo, laboratory, private collection) in a cage or building in which the temperature is excessively high because of extraneous heat, internal heaters or warmth due to overcrowding.
- Tethering of an animal without shade.
- Overexerting an animal.
- Intentional overheating of an animal, either to warm or dry it or perhaps as part of a pattern of abuse (see earlier).

Hyperthermia in animals can be induced intentionally or can result from neglect or ignorance. Even well-intentioned people make mistakes – for example, those involved in marine mammal rescue who may not be aware that a stranded dolphin is becoming overheated on the beach.

The circumstances of overheating can be influenced by such factors as:

- Relative humidity.
- Air movement.
- Dehydration.
- Insulation by hair or feathers.
- Stocking density/proximity to other animals.

It is important to take the factors above into account. All animals have a 'critical high' temperature at which irreversible changes occur, especially in the brain, and death may ensue. It is important in any legal case where overheating is alleged to be aware of such temperatures and, indeed, of the mechanisms and strategies by which different animals thermoregulate.

HYPOTHERMIA

Extreme cold is a danger to both free-living and captive animals, as it is to humans. Many species in very cold or high altitude regions are adapted behaviourally and physiologically to such extremes. Some animals hibernate or go through periods of torpor.

Frostbite is common in captive animals in cold climates. It is a frequent occurrence in birds and has been recorded in free-living opossums and other mammalian species. It can occur when animals are

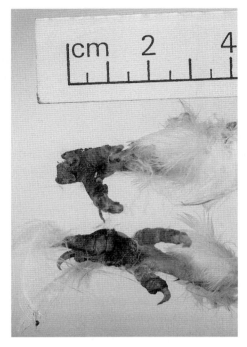

Figure 6.13 The feet of an owl that died following frostbite.

confined without heating in a car or in the hold of an aircraft. Extreme cold is recognised as an important cause of death in game management; ducks and other birds can freeze to the ice by their feet and feathers. Many decades ago, Leopold, the 'father of game management', studied the significance of freezing in animals, and discovered that mortality on a large scale may occur through imprisonment of ground-roosting birds and rabbits by sleet or crusted snow.

Chilling is of ubiquitous significance since even a slight drop in temperature can serve as an important stressor, especially when animals are young. It can prove lethal in both wild animals and free-ranging domesticated stock, e.g. poultry. A sudden drop in temperature in the spring in temperate countries can kill large numbers of birds, both directly and by reducing the quantities of available food if snow or freezing rain accompanies the cold. Storms can have profound effects, especially on wild seabirds, when eggs are destroyed by a combination of cold and parental disturbance.

Hypothermia can be a problem in stray animals that enter water to search for food, causing their body temperature to drop. Hypothermia in water is well-recognised as usually being more rapid and dangerous (to humans and presumably to other mammals) than on land, partly as a result of experiments in Nazi concentration camps and elsewhere (DiMaio and DiMaio, 2001). The situation can be very different in ectotherms, however (see below). Hypothermia can be exacerbated or accelerated if the animals' pelage is damaged – for example, following washing to remove oil (Stoskopf *et al.*, 1997).

In the case of chilling, lowered ambient temperature can result in a drop in the body temperature, especially in young animals where homeothermy often is poorly developed. As a result body metabolism is reduced, and the animal becomes weak and unable to feed; hypoglycaemia may become a feature as carbohydrate reserves are exhausted. More severe exposure to cold can result in frostbite. Pathogenesis is due mainly to dehydration, disruption of cells by ice crystals, thrombosis, and disturbed metabolic activity. As a result there is ischaemia of the superficial tissues that can progress to gangrene and sloughing. A few ectothermic vertebrate species tolerate freezing by producing cryoprotectant chemicals (Lemos-Espinal and Ballinger, 1992; Storey and Storey 1988).

Prolonged exposure to cold may predispose some wild animals to diseases associated with stress. For example, Karstad and Sileo (1971) found gout, amyloidosis, and myocardial infarction most prevalent in waterfowl in cold weather. Cold injury in newborn lambs was investigated by Haughey (1973), who described oedema of the subcutaneous tissues, changes in the adrenal cortex and varying degrees of fat catabolism. Ectothermic vertebrates may or may not show clinical signs or specific lesions as a result of cold. Much depends upon the species, its preferred temperature range and the circumstances of the exposure. However, the metabolism of such species, including immune responses, is usually compromised and infectious diseases may supervene.

There may be only mild, fairly non-specific pathological changes in cases of chilling. The lungs are often congested and an excess of clear fluid may be present in the body cavities; the liver is pale and the stomach is usually empty. In the case of freezing there may be areas of hair or feather loss and specific lesions, such as oedema. Tissues may appear avascular or necrotic, and, in severe cases, have been sloughed or removed by the animal.

In mild chilling the animal may appear cold to the touch, depressed in appearance, and shiver; often no other clinical signs are present. In the case of freezing, the body surface initially feels cold and appears pale; later it may become erythematous and oedematous with the animal exhibiting pain. As with burns, pruritus may accompany healing. In severe cases the affected area becomes ischaemic and sloughs; this has been reported in free-living deer and opossums and in captive mammals and birds (Cooper, 1996a).

Hypothermia in humans is sometimes associated with acute pancreatitis but this relationship has been questioned (Stiff *et al.*, 2003) and a link does not appear to have been postulated in animals.

A legal case relating to hypothermia is likely to be brought on such grounds as:

- Failing to provide adequate heating for housed captive animals.
- Keeping animals outside in cold weather, without proper protection against wind, rain, sleet or snow.
- Intentional abuse, e.g. by putting ice in a domesticated aquarium or turning off electrical heating in a zoo or laboratory animal unit.

BURNING

Burns can be caused by ultraviolet light, heat, chemicals, or friction. Sunburn is due to overexposure of the skin to ultraviolet rays from the sun. It occurs most frequently in captivity in animals that have non-pigmented skin and poor protection. Even fish can be affected.

Bush and grass fires are common causes of death from burning and suffocation in animals. Regular fires are a characteristic feature of certain ecosystems such as tropical savannah. Humans are usually the cause, but lightning and other natural factors can be responsible.

Chemical burns can occur as a result of contact with either man-made or natural areas of acid or alkali. The alkaline lakes of the Rift Valley, East Africa, are the home of alga-feeding flamingos, and it is not uncommon, when the lakes are drying, for groups of birds to be found with soda plastered on their feet. Such birds are generally killed by predators; some die as a result of the skin damage produced by the soda.

Burning by friction sometimes occurs and may be of legal significance. In the wild it can be caused by snares or nets. In captive animals it may occur as a result of a leash or collar that abrades the skin or stereotyped behaviour such as persistent rubbing on a rough surface.

The effects of burning are associated with tissue damage. Cells that are burned become desiccated (dry heat) or their protoplasm coagulates (moist heat). As a result there are local lesions, dehydration, pyrexia due to pyrogens and often secondary infection by resilient organisms such as *Staphylococcus aureus* and *Pseudomonas* spp.

Distinct lesions are usually apparent, and these burns may vary in severity from first- to third-degree burns. First-degree burns involve only the outer layer of the epidermis and cause pain, heat and oedema. Second-degree burns affect the whole epidermis and vesicles are characteristic. In third-degree (full thickness) burns both epidermis and dermis are destroyed. There is severe tissue damage, and because nerve endings are lost, pain is not a major feature. Dehydration, secondary shock and other secondary effects are often present, and if the animal survives over 48 hours after burning, toxic changes may be detectable histopathologically in the liver and kidneys. Inhalation injury affects the respiratory tract, causing mucosal damage, pulmonary oedema and sometimes deposition of particulate material (see Chapter 2).

In burning, distinct first- or second-degree burns – painful to the touch – are usually visible but shaving of hair or plucking of feathers may first be needed. Oedema and distinct vesicles, or in severe cases, sloughing of the skin are present. There is dehydration and the animal is lethargic and depressed as a result of electrolyte imbalance and circulatory shock. Inhalation injury causes coughing, voice changes, expectoration of blood and sometimes carbon particles and dyspnoea.

Any forensic investigation of injuries or death associated with burning should include ascertaining the origin of the fire and whether or not it might have been started intentionally. Daéid (2003) and Ide (2004) discussed fire investigation in some detail.

A legal case relating to burning is likely to be brought on such grounds as:

- Negligently exposing captive animals to household, garden or bush fires.
- Tethering animals so that they sustain friction burns.
- Intentional burning or scalding of an animal, either as part of revenge on a neighbour or as a form of abuse (Figure 4.9).

EXPLOSIONS

Animals and humans can be injured and/or killed in explosions and these may be accidental or illegal. In either case enquiries are likely to follow and expert advice will be needed (Beveridge, 1998). Space does not permit detailed discussion of this specialised and important subject: a useful review was provided by Jones and Marshall (2004).

Amongst investigations that are used to study the effects of blasts is SEM, which may demonstrate characteristic 'clubbing' of nylon fibres: similar changes may be seen on birds' feathers exposed to heat (see Figure 6.9). Anderson (2004) also discussed explosions and emphasised the role of toxicologists in such investigations – for example, examining blood or tissues of victims. Histopathologists also have a part to play by detecting inhaled materials (see Chapter 2).

ELECTROCUTION AND DROWNING

These are often fatal and therefore covered in detail in Chapter 7. When the animal is still alive, clinical signs may assist in diagnosis and these are discussed later.

In electrocution the animal may be comatose, paralysed or show involuntary muscle contractions. There may be apnoea, ventricular fibrillation, dehydration and even fractures. Burns and haemorrhages may be apparent. The clinical history is often very valuable in diagnosis.

The key factors in survival from drowning are the duration of submersion, the water temperature and the speed of resuscitation. Young animals are generally more tolerant of submersion in water than adults, aquatic species more than terrestrial and ectotherms more than endotherms. The diving reflex of mammals occurs in cold water and can permit survival after prolonged submersion: bradycardia occurs and oxygenated blood is shunted to the heart and brain.

The hair or feathers are usually wet and there may be water in the buccal or nasal cavities. If drying has occurred the hair or feathers are matted. If water has been inhaled, respiratory signs predominate and careful examination and manipulation of the animal may result in fluid sounds being heard and excess water being passed out of the trachea or oesophagus.

IONISING RADIATION

Irradiation, either particulate or electromagnetic, can damage tissues. The actual effect of the radiation will depend on the total dose received, dose rate and organs and area affected. As a general rule, whole body doses of 200 rads or more are likely to prove fatal; however, species vary in susceptibility. At doses of over 50 rads many cells die and the multiplication of other cells is inhibited.

As a general rule, the more rapid the rate of mitosis of a cell, the greater the sensitivity to radiation damage. Thus, the haemopoietic tissues usually are affected such that within one to three weeks of exposure the animal shows leucopoenia, thrombocytopoenia, and anaemia. Bacterial infection is a common sequela. The epithelium of the intestine is affected, resulting in diarrhoea and severe loss of fluids and electrolytes. The germinal cells of testes or ovaries may be badly damaged, producing infertility and possibly genetic changes; the severity and duration depend upon the dosage. Fetal tissues similarly can be affected and even low doses, such as 25 rads, may produce developmental effects in the fetus. The nervous system is usually only slightly damaged unless exposed to massive doses (2500 to 12,000 rads).

Lesions depend on the dose of radiation and the area affected. Petechial haemorrhages are common and enteritis may be present. Lymphoid tissues show aplasia and there is destruction of bone marrow. In certain species, or if the dose of radiation is high, central nervous system changes may be apparent, especially cerebral oedema.

Clinical signs vary, depending on the length of exposure and the dosage. In acute exposure (acute radiation syndrome), immediate clinical signs may be slight, but vomiting usually occurs within minutes or hours of exposure. Later, cellular changes begin to take effect and such signs as diarrhoea, severe anaemia, petechiation and alopecia occur. There is increased susceptibility to infection.

More chronic exposure can produce few clinical signs, but reduced fertility, anaemia, leucopoenia, alopecia and neoplasia are well recognised sequelae in humans and such findings may be used to support a claim in respect of exposure of animals. Reference data are available on experimental animals, including monkeys and various rodents. Useful information has also been amassed in the twenty years since the Chernobyl nuclear power plant disaster, including data on animals and plant (WHO/IAEA/UNDP, 2005).

A legal case relating to irradiation is likely to be brought on such grounds as:

- Incorrect or unauthorised use of X-rays – routine radiography or perhaps even as part of enhanced airport security (Gloor *et al.*, 2005).
- Radiation leakage from a power station or laboratory.
- Exposure of animals to 'natural' radiation in the soil.

MAGNETIC FIELDS

Exposure to low-frequency magnetic fields produced by alternating current (a.c.) such as those found in high voltage power lines and electrical appliances have been implicated in ill-health in humans (see, for example, Draper *et al.*, 2005) and birds of prey (see Cooper, 2002).

TRANSPORTATION OF ANIMALS

Much has been published on transportation of animals, the adverse effects that it can have and ways in which its impact can be minimised. Its importance in a welfare context is highlighted in Chapter 4.

A recent report on the transportation of laboratory animals (Swallow *et al.*, 2005) is valuable reading, even for those who are not involved specifically with such species. The authors summarise their two key messages as follows:

(1) Change is stressful to animals, and transport is an especially powerful stressor that should be regarded as a major life event and not undertaken unless absolutely necessary.
(2) Anyone consulted about legal cases concerning transportation should be aware of (a) the diverse adverse effects that transportation can have on the health and welfare of animals, and (b) the multiplicity of factors that can contribute to the equation of whether or not transportation has had such effects.

Brief mention is made of each below.

Effects of transportation

These include:

- Death.
- Clinical ill-health.
- Subclinical effects.

These adverse effects may be categorised as:

- Non-infectious trauma
  ○ Hyperthermia
  ○ Hypothermia
  ○ Dehydration
  ○ Starvation
  ○ Myopathy.

- Infections
  - Skin and other integumentary lesions may become infected
  - Systemic diseases (e.g. shipping fever – pasteurellosis) may be triggered
  - Previously latent or unapparent infections may be activated (e.g. herpesvirus infections).

Clinical signs associated with transportation can include skin lesions, hyperpnoea (e.g. panting), dyspnoea (difficulty in breathing), nasal and other discharges. Subclinical effects compromise haematological and biochemical values, detectable only by laboratory tests but significant in terms of the animal's homeostasis and well-being.

An effect of transportation in some species – dogs, cats, even hawks kept for falconry (Cooper, 2002) – can be 'motion sickness'. This is usually characterised by salivation and regurgitation/ vomiting. It is unlikely to be grounds for legal action *per se* but as its occurrence can be linked with other behavioural traits, such as fear of cars and self-inflicted damage during transportation, it is of possible legal significance.

Horses may react adversely when being transported, sometimes related to whether they are facing the front or the back of the vehicle. This and other factors, including how the animals are loaded, can contribute to nervousness and excitement – with possible damage to the horse, to humans or to the trailer/aircraft in which they are travelling.

Investigation of cases relating to transportation may require detective work on a grand scale. The crime scene (see Chapter 9) may include a farm, a breeding unit, a lorry (truck), aircraft-holding facilities, crates, ramps and so on. Important issues include the fitness to travel of the animal(s), their numbers, environmental conditions, design of premises and the experience and training of staff. Appropriate specialist advice is usually needed (see Chapter 7). Those involved must be aware of legislation and codes that are relevant to transportation (see Chapter 3).

New EU Animal Transport Regulations will come into force in January 2007. They will apply to all live animals carried within the EU and, as Regulations, they will be implemented uniformly across all Member States. The Regulations include

an over-arching condition that no person may cause animals to be transported in a way likely to cause injury or undue suffering. Documentation is an important aspect, as is the use of only authorised transporters and subcontractors.

The International Air Transport Association Regulations (IATA, 2004), published in English, French and Spanish, provide valuable advice on the movement of a whole range of species and the Animal Air Transport Association (see Appendix B) can give guidance.

OTHER STRESSORS

There are numerous other (generally non-infectious) stressors that can have an adverse effect on animals, sometimes prompting concerns and allegations about welfare (see Chapter 4). They include fluctuations in atmospheric pressure, excessive noise, exposure to light/dark or abnormal photoperiods, social deprivation and overcrowding. Brief mention is made below of some of these, with references to further reading.

The effect of pressure changes on humans (for example, as a result of high-altitude illness, decompression or exposure to blast injuries) has been well documented (see, for example, Robbins *et al.*, 1999) and such data can often be applied to animals.

Noise

Noise (excessive sound) has well-recognised adverse effects both physical and psychological on humans and animals. Over the past ten years 'ocean noise pollution' has increasingly been recognised; it is believed to be deleterious to marine mammals and other species (Natural Resources Defense Council, www.nrdc.org/wildlife/marine/sound/contents.asp). Noise may be associated with other stressors, as when animals are frightened by fireworks (see below).

Fireworks

Many species, including wild animals, can be frightened, injure themselves or die as a result of exposure to fireworks. In small pet animals the term 'noise phobia' is often used but fireworks can also harm animals because of the bright lights they emit, the odour that they produce and the fires that are often associated with their use. In the UK, in 2001, an RSPCA survey showed that thousands of animals were treated for firework-related injuries or prescribed sedatives. Sixteen animals were euthanased on account of what were believed to be deliberate attack. In the same year 1362 humans were treated for firework-related injuries (George, 2005). The UK has amended its legislation to make purchase and possession of fireworks more difficult, to control when they are used and to restrict the maximum noise level. Nevertheless, fireworks will continue to be used – and to result in incidents that could lead to legal action or official enquiries. The veterinarian, animal behaviourist and welfare officer who become involved need to be familiar with the subject and may need to make a site visit (see Chapter 10) to see where the incident occurred.

As in all forensics, detective work is often needed. Firework-associated injuries are most likely to occur during relevant festivals, such as Bonfire (Guy Fawkes) Night, 5th November, in Britain, and Divali, New Year, Chinese New Year. Sometimes the firework has an indirect effect: for example, a spent rocket may land on an aviary roof and thus disturb a bird, which then flies into a perch and is killed or injured (a cat walking on the aviary can sometimes have a similar effect).

Light

The effect of light on many animals is poorly understood and may be more complex than hitherto realised. For example, a recent report of myoclonus in starlings exposed to cathode ray tubes and low-frequency light suggests that some birds, like susceptible human beings, may be sensitive to 'flicker' (Smith *et al.*, 2005). The adverse effect of television on certain species of animal has been reported before (Gillett and Blake, 1985).

Both light and dark can serve as stressors, *per se* and because of their secondary effects – for example, by attracting turtles, birds, insects and other species at night and either disorientating them or causing injury and death (Fedun, 1995).

Social interactions

Social behaviour concerns interactions with others, and can be species-specific or inter-specific.

Communication is essential when two individuals come into contact. Some species are mainly solitary, only coming together for mating; while others live in groups. There are two types of grouping behaviour. Groups may be sporadic, transient and involve superficial cooperation and communication, such as in fish schools and migratory groups; or they may be prolonged, intimate and involve detailed cooperation and communication, such as with social insects and wolf packs.

Animals kept in captive environments have no control over group size or composition and natural social behaviour is frequently compromised.

Commercially-produced animals range from being sheltered in high stocking densities to being individually housed. Pigs, poultry, sheep, cattle, goats and horses all have dominance hierarchy systems. Farming systems tend to group animals according to weight, causing intense aggression during the establishment of social relationships because the individuals are similarly matched. Frequent mixing and unstable groups maintain the aggression at severe levels. Overstocking leads to aggression/bullying; competition for food (also, low ranking individuals being unwilling to approach feeding stations); alterations of group membership; loss of contact with familiar conspecifics; exposure

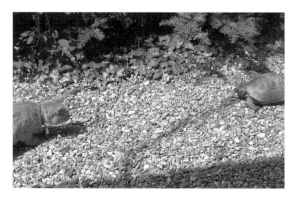

Figure 6.14 Interactions between different species can cause stress or injury and may be grounds for legal action.

to strangers; inability to escape aggressive counterparts by retreating; increased disease transmission; and inability to thermoregulate (overheating). Normal behaviours are restricted by the lack of space and barren environments, preventing such normal patterns as nesting in farrowing pigs and wing-stretching and dust-bathing in poultry. This causes distress, cognitive impairment, damage to health and productivity, and abnormal behaviours including feather pecking, cannibalism and polydipsia (see Chapter 4).

Overcrowding can affect the physical and psychological state of animals and may also facilitate the spread of pathogenic organisms.

Social deprivation can have profound effects on some animals and if the result of human action, may lead to legal action. Animals in quarantine are one example.

The most likely species to be quarantined before entry into a country are dogs, cats and birds. Quarantine regulations often dictate that animals be housed individually to reduce the risk of disease spread, for a period of time specific to the country of importation. Social isolation is stressful to any species that naturally lives in association with conspecifics (see, for example, Elliott and Scott, 1961). Social isolation in quarantine is particularly stressful because the animals have recently been submitted to the demands of long-distance transport, and are now in a strange environment without the comfort of their owners (Rochlitz *et al.*, 1998).

Coping behaviours are often expressed in response, with some animals becoming withdrawn, others hyperactive and others still exhibiting stereotypies and compulsive disorders. The layout of enclosures is important to allow space for retreat, as well as opportunity for interaction with staff. Enrichment of the physical area and more effective management of time may play a part in reducing the likelihood of the formation of behaviour problems.

Theft

The theft of an animal, quite apart from its immediate legal significance, can also have profound effects. The animal may be damaged physically or be exposed to stressors as a result of its being in an unfamiliar location, with different sounds, smells, food and environment. Domesticated animals are usually well catered for in terms of support groups which can sometimes advise on the legal implications. In the UK there is a National Theft Register, now in its tenth year (Hayward, 2004), which records, collates and researches thefts of exotic animals – pets and zoo species.

BEHAVIOURAL PROBLEMS

The field of animal behaviour (ethology) has developed rapidly over the past few years. It is a science that can relate to free-living or captive animals. Of particular relevance to the theme of this book is the research on behavioural disorders of domesticated animals, such as the dog (Heath, 2005) and the horse (Zeitler-Feicht, 2004). Many behavioural aberrations seen in domesticated animals are important to owners and veterinarians – for example, house-soiling, destructiveness, separation anxiety and excessive vocalisation in dogs and crib-biting in horses – but are of limited relevance to forensic work. However, those associated with aggression to humans or other species can be of considerable significance in legal cases (see also Chapter 2 – Bite wounds).

Behavioural problems in pet animals can be a cause of complaint, sometimes prompting civil action against owners. It has been suggested in the UK that owners of unruly pets should be served with anti-social behaviour orders (ASBO). This also could prompt legal challenge and other responses. Both veterinarians and animal behaviourists and perhaps, in some cases, a suitably experienced geneticist, would be likely to be involved as witnesses (Robinson, 1990).

Some behavioural problems are due to, or associated with, infectious or non-infectious disease and this has to be borne in mind in legal cases. The former can range from important parasitic infections, such as acariasis, to the profound neurological changes associated with rabies. Non-infectious diseases which may induce behavioural change include hypothyroidism in dogs, which can manifest itself in a similar way to dominance or fear-related aggression (Fatjó *et al.*, 2002).

Behavioural problems have also been studied extensively in laboratory and zoo animals. In both cases this has led to such measures as the improvement of housing and perceived quality of life by the provision of environmental enrichment and by careful attention to factors such as social grouping (see, for example, Carlstead, 1996).

AVOIDING LITIGATION OR ALLEGATIONS OF MALPRACTICE

How does the veterinary practitioner reduce the risk that s/he is taken to court or reported to a professional body over a clinical case? Concern over this has prompted much discussion and debate, the formulation of guidelines and advice by relevant bodies (e.g. the Veterinary Defence Society in the UK) and relevant lectures and publications by veterinarians and lawyers (Newman, 2004a–c).

It is not easy to predict a legal action or claim of malpractice, as most practising veterinary surgeons will testify. Sometimes the nicest of clients complain bitterly if something goes wrong, or because they meet one of the new generation of lawyers or a 'claims consultant' at a cocktail party and s/he encourages them to sue the veterinarian or to allege professional malpractice. Equally, however, a 'difficult' client sometimes becomes remarkably pragmatic about the outcome of a case.

As a general rule, events can go one of two ways following (for example) the death of an otherwise healthy kitten after what should have been a routine ovariectomy:

(1) The client becomes more distressed and concerned and begins to think and talk in terms of compensation or redress, or
(2) The client, while sad or disappointed, becomes resigned to the outcome.

In any such scenario the rule must be to:

• Assume that legal action or a claim may ensue, and that a complaint will be made to the relevant veterinary professional body.

• Retain records and samples and institute an improved chain of custody on that assumption.
• Think carefully about the appropriate action if a complaint is made by the client
   ○ To the practice, in which case discussion with the aggrieved person may result in conciliation
   ○ To a lawyer or veterinary professional body, in which case it may be better to deal with the latter and the relevant veterinary defence (insurance) company rather than with the client.

Apologising to a client when something has gone wrong would seem to be the proper and professional thing to do. However, it may be interpreted as accepting responsibility and create problems if a civil action or allegation of malpractice ensues. The British medical profession has tackled this problem and in a review of the position, Lilleyman (2006) states:

A prompt apology is a good way to avoid litigation; and even when it fails to do so, both the Medical Protection Society and the Medical Defence Union advise doctors at the earliest stage to provide a full explanation, apologise to the patient and consider what might be done to prevent similar incidents in the future.

Veterinary surgeons likely to find themselves in a similar position should consider having a format for an apology, preferably agreed in advance by their insurance company.

It is also important to think ahead, to anticipate problems and to inform clients/owners of the possible consequences of any action that is to be undertaken. This applies not only to clearly potentially hazardous procedures, such as the anaesthetising of an ill or frail patient, but also what may seem to be a routine, 'safe' task. A good example is the removal of a leg ring (band) from a bird. This can be a stressful procedure and the advice of many – for example, the Association of Avian Veterinarians (AAV) (see Appendix B) – is that the bird should first be examined clinically. Failure to do so might result in a claim or complaint if something goes wrong but, equally, some owners question why such an apparently simple procedure needs extra input by the veterinarian and a correspondingly larger fee. An appropriate consent form, signed as understood by the client, is always necessary (see earlier).

It is important in veterinary practice to maintain the highest standards, in keeping with the advice, recommendations and requirements of professional bodies. The RCVS's GPC provides an indication of how a veterinarian is expected to behave in Britain:

(1) Accessibility, accountability and transparency are expected of every self-regulating profession. All legislation governing the various professions is designed to meet these requirements and to protect the public interest by ensuring a high level of education and training combined with personal and professional integrity. The Veterinary Surgeons Act 1966 which governs the veterinary profession is no exception.

(2) Rights and responsibilities go hand in hand. For this reason on admission to membership of the Royal College of Veterinary Surgeons, and in exchange for the right to practise veterinary surgery in the United Kingdom, every veterinary surgeon makes the following declaration:

'In as much as the privilege of membership of the Royal College of Veterinary Surgeons is about to be conferred upon me I PROMISE AND SOLEMNLY DECLARE that I will abide in all due loyalty to the Royal College of Veterinary Surgeons and will do all in my power to maintain and promote its interests.'

'PROMISE above all that I will pursue the work of my profession with uprightness of conduct and that my constant endeavour will be to ensure the welfare of the animals committed to my care.'

(3) These promises acknowledge the obligation of every veterinary surgeon to observe the provisions of the current RCVS 'Guide to Professional Conduct', and in so doing to make animal welfare their overriding consideration at all times.

The ten guiding principles

Your clients are entitled to expect that you will:

(1) make animal welfare your first consideration in seeking to provide the most appropriate attention for animals committed to your care

(2) ensure that all animals under your care are treated humanely and with respect

(3) maintain and continue to develop your professional knowledge and skills

(4) foster and maintain a good relationship with your clients, earning their trust, respecting their views and protecting client confidentiality

(5) uphold the good reputation of the veterinary profession

(6) ensure the integrity of veterinary certification

(7) foster and endeavour to maintain good relationships with your professional colleagues

(8) understand and comply with your legal obligations in relation to the prescription, safe-keeping and supply of veterinary medicinal products

(9) familiarise yourself with and observe the relevant legislation in relation to veterinary surgeons as individual members of the profession, employers, employees and business owners

(10) respond promptly, fully and courteously to complaints and criticism.

Adherence to those guidelines is an important first step towards reducing the risk of litigation or allegations of malpractice.

The introduction of clinical care standards (CCS) and other quality assurance systems will put extra responsibilities on practitioners. These are already an established feature of medical and dental work in several countries. In the UK the RCVS has introduced its own Practice Standards Scheme which aims to promote and maintain the highest standards of veterinary care as well as giving clients greater choice by making information about practices readily available.

Clinical audit (reviewing performance against a set of criteria and bringing in changes where indicated) can do much to offset allegations of inadequate or inappropriate services (Viner, 2005) and the veterinarian can learn from the experiences in this respect of the medical profession (Viner and Jenner, 2005).

Adherence to legislation is always essential if the practising veterinary surgeon is to avoid trouble – and should include all aspects of practice, such as that relating to health and safety (Irwin, 2005).

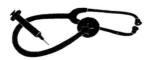

Pathology and Post-Mortem *Examinations*

Hamlet: How long will a man lie i' th' earth ere he rot?
First Clown: . . . A tanner will last you nine year
Hamlet: Why he, more than another?
First Clown: Why sir, his hide is so tann'd with his trade, that he will keep out water a great
*   while. And your water, is a sore decayer of your whoreson dead body . . .*

William Shakespeare

Hic locus est ubi mors gaudet succurrere vitae. (This is the place where death delights to help
the living.)

Traditional – London Mortuary

'Pathology' was defined by Thomson (1978) as 'The science of the study of disease' and thus encompasses the investigation of live patients and samples from them, not just dead animals. In this chapter, however, the emphasis will be on the more 'popular' interpretation of the pathologist's work – *post-mortem* examinations. These can also be called 'necropsies' (singular, 'necropsy') and this term is very often used in animal work.

The word 'autopsy' is generally reserved for the *post-mortem* examination of a human being but in French *'l'autopsie'* can be used for both humans and animals. The origin of the word 'autopsy' is interesting and relevant to forensic medicine. It comes from the Greek *'autopsia'*, meaning 'I see with my eyes' (i.e. 'I observe'), reflecting the fact that the *post-mortem* examination can reveal previously hidden information.

Post-mortem examination of a dead animal or its parts is an important component of veterinary and comparative forensic medicine. A necropsy can provide information on the following:

- Causes of death.
- Causes of ill health.

- Underlying abnormalities/pathology.
- Answers to specific questions, such as the sex of an Amazon parrot or the reproductive status of a red deer.

In terms of comparative forensic studies, a *post-mortem* examination will also yield valuable data on morphometrics, organ weights and organ:body-weight ratios and the gross and histological appearance of tissues. Such data can be of great value when dealing with unusual species. Every effort should be taken to record relevant information and, where circumstances permit, to collect material for study and future reference (see Chapter 5).

SPECIAL EXAMINATIONS

Embryos, eggs, fetuses and neonates need care because of their size and their special features. Neonatal pathology is a well-developed speciality in human medicine (Busuttil and Keeling, 2005): the Report of the Working Party of The Royal College of Obstetricians and Gynaecologists and The Royal College of Pathologists (RCPath) (2001) provides

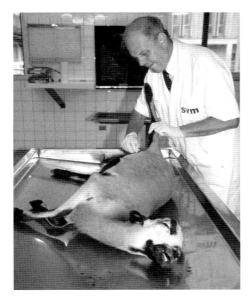

Figure 7.1 A routine *post-mortem* examination in progress. This figure also appears in colour in the colour plate section. (Courtesy of Richard Spence.)

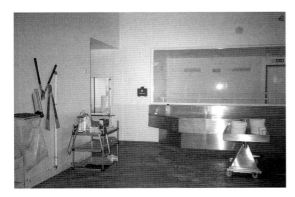

Figure 7.2 Forensic necropsies should, whenever possible, be carried out in a modern *post-mortem* room where safety precautions are in force and contamination of evidence can be minimised.

valuable reading and standards for such work have been established by the RCPath and others. Small specimens – for example, certain amphibians, fish and invertebrates – may require the use of special instruments, such as ophthalmological scissors, and micro techniques – the so-called 'mini-necropsy'. A magnifying loupe or dissection microscope is often essential (see Figure 6.4). Alternatively, or when several specimens are available and can be processed in different ways, small fish, frogs and other species can be embedded and serially sectioned for histological examination – a method pioneered by the late Edward Elkan (Elkan, 1981; Cooper, 1989) (see Figure 2.5) and now used by many comparative pathologists.

From time to time, the remains of a carcase are required for display in a museum or other similar purposes; in this case a 'cosmetic' *post-mortem* examination must be carried out in order to obtain the necessary information and material while inflicting minimum external damage. This necessitates skill and experience. In some cases an endoscope may prove useful. Richard Norman (pers.comm.) recommends 'pre-necropsy negotiation with stakeholders' to ascertain their requirements and the likely compromises before starting *post-mortem* examination.

WILDLIFE

The investigation of wildlife crime (see Chapter 5) often requires the services of a specialist veterinary pathologist (Wobeser, 1996). Some of the responsibilities of a wildlife pathologist and how best to locate a suitable person are discussed in PAW (2005).

BEFORE CARRYING OUT A NECROPSY

Important considerations before embarking on a *post-mortem* examination are as follows:

- Do I have permission to carry out this examination?
- Do I feel confident to perform this necropsy?
- Is a sufficient written history of the case available?
- Is it clear as to what questions I am being asked?
- If the answers to the above are 'no' or there is some uncertainty, should I delay the necropsy until either I or a colleague can do the examination at a later date?

The carrying-out of a necropsy on an animal by a veterinarian is not just a routine matter – and in a forensic case the situation may be even more complex. Most captive animals will have an owner and the professional rules relating to *post-mortem* examination assume this to be the case, putting strong emphasis on the rights of the client – as in the RCVS Guide to Professional Conduct (GPC), where it states:

(1) When a client wishes to have a post-mortem examination carried out – and understands not only the financial implications of that request, but also that the findings may prove inconclusive – the veterinarian concerned should either consent to carry out such examination himself or herself or assist the client by making alternative arrangements with another veterinarian.

(2) In cases in which the owner has retained or repossessed the carcase of an animal which was under treatment by a veterinarian prior to its death and requests another veterinarian to carry out an independent post-mortem examination on the owner's behalf, the normal ethical rules regarding supersession and second opinions do not apply. Nevertheless, the original veterinarian should be advised by his or her colleague that the post-mortem examination is to be carried out and should be invited to provide information regarding previous treatment as an aid to the preparation of an accurate report. The results of the examination must, however, be communicated only to the client and not to the original veterinarian without the client's consent.

(3) Veterinarians wishing to carry out a post-mortem examination upon animals which they have previously treated, in order to satisfy themselves as to the cause of death (rather than at the request of the client), must seek the permission of the client to carry out such an examination.

In a legal case, a request for a necropsy may come from someone other than the client – a police officer, a court or an enforcement agency. Care must be taken in such circumstances. The instruc-

tions should be in writing and signed by an authorised person. If the veterinarian is in any doubt, s/he should seek guidance (if necessary, approval) from the appropriate professional body.

The last of the above questions is often a very important one. In routine diagnostic veterinary work the general rule is that a carcase should be examined as soon as possible after death. It is also usually stressed that freezing, in order to arrest autolysis, should be avoided because of the artefact that it can produce. Both of these points also carry weight in forensic work but there they have to be balanced against the need to ensure that the necropsy is carried out as efficiently and meticulously as possible and that it answers the questions that have been posed. Therefore, although it is still advisable to carry out any necropsy soon after receipt of the carcase, it often proves wiser to delay the examination by, say, 72–96 hours if this means that a more methodical investigation can be performed and better results obtained.

Likewise, although freezing a carcase will have the same deleterious effects (especially in terms of hampering histological studies) as in routine veterinary work, there are occasions when freezing is the only option. This may be the case when there is no possibility of examining the animal for a week or more – for example, because of legal constraints or on account of practical considerations (e.g. necropsy of an elephant or a dolphin is likely to need specialised equipment and a team approach). The logistics of transportation of beach-cast (stranded) marine mammals may require their being sent frozen from a remote location to a suitable laboratory.

STORAGE OF CARCASES PRIOR TO EXAMINATION

The various considerations that may influence how a carcase is stored or treated prior to *post-mortem* examination are given in Table 7.1.

Munro (1998) provided a useful summary of forensic necropsy and emphasised that a forensic *post-mortem* examination must be conducted in a manner that permits all the findings to be used in a court of law.

Table 7.1 Storage and treatment of carcases.

Method of treatment	Advantages	Disadvantages	Comments
Chilled at +4°C	Good preservation for a few days	Autolysis continues to take place, albeit slowly	The autolysis is slow and generally predictable
Frozen	Can be stored indefinitely	Causes artefacts in terms of both gross and histological changes Pathogens generally not killed	Some allowance can be made for gross artefacts (e.g. corneal opacity) but confusion can arise
Fully fixed in formalin or similar fixative	As above Pathogens are usually killed (*not* prions)	Affects appearance of organs – colour changes Permits histopathology but makes DNA studies difficult	Careful interpretation needed, as in embalmed cadavers
Fixed in ethanol or methanol	As above, but DNA extraction is little affected	As above	As above

PERSONNEL

Who should carry out a forensic necropsy is a matter for debate. It is interesting to note that 200 years ago, the 'father of descriptive pathology', Carl van Rokitansky, stressed the importance in human medicine of having a suitably-trained specialist to carry out and interpret necropsies rather than a general medical practitioner. That message is now generally accepted in human work, although from time to time practitioners with little or no specialised training in pathology may have to carry out a human necropsy, especially in an emergency or in countries where pathologists are in short supply.

Similarly, but slowly, the situation is also changing in veterinary work, but the fact remains that the majority of *post-mortem* examinations carried out on animals in order to provide evidence for a court of law are still performed by veterinary practitioners. On top of this, many necropsies of wildlife (see Chapter 5) are performed by biologists from different disciplines only a few of whom have any special training in *post-mortem* techniques. Munro (1998) deplored this situation and urged that appropriately-trained pathologists should be considered the experts when *post-mortem* and supporting laboratory tests are required.

Even if a pathologist performs the necropsy, it is likely that some of the dissection, particularly that requiring special skills, will be carried out by an assistant – perhaps a technician or attendant, sometimes a properly trained 'prosector'. *Post-mortem* record sheets should bear the name and signature of such a person – who should be prepared, if necessary, to give evidence in court.

Post-mortem examination of invertebrates can be carried out by a suitably experienced veterinary pathologist (Cooper and Cunningham, 1991) but sometimes there is merit in a forensic case in having the input of a specialist in, e.g., diseases of insects.

POST-MORTEM METHODS

There are numerous ways of carrying out a *post-mortem* examination and specific methods have been described in the literature for domesticated animals (King *et al.*, 2005). In addition, in recent years recommended approaches for wild species have been published, in some cases promulgated as part of the Action Plan of the appropriate Taxon Advisory Group (TAG) (in Australasia, for example, www.arazpa.org.au).

In comparative forensic work, the wide range of species means that no one technique is likely to be

Table 7.2 Some special features relevant to *post-mortem* examination of non-domesticated species.

Group	Special features
Mammals (Class Mammalia, Phylum Chordata)	Many variations in external and internal anatomy, e.g. presence or absence of tail, structure of gastro-intestinal tract All mammals have hair to a greater or lesser extent
Birds (Class Aves, Phylum Chordata)	Variations in external and internal anatomy, e.g. presence or absence of preen gland, crop, caeca. Certain specialised features, e.g. syrinx in male ducks, subcutaneous air sacs in some storks All birds have feathers All are oviparous
Reptiles (Class Reptilia, Phylum Chordata)	Much anatomical variation between the main Orders e.g.: • Squamata – no functional limbs, elongated organs and only one functional lung in snakes • Chelonia – presence of carapace and plastron and variation in their size and structure • Crocodilia – tough (ectodermal) scales, right aortic arch All reptiles have scaled skin Some are oviparous
Amphibians (Class Amphibia, Phylum Chordata)	Marked distinction in most species between immature (larval – tadpole) stage with gills and other modifications to an aquatic lifestyle and mature (adult) with lungs and a terrestrial lifestyle All amphibians have unscaled mucous skin
Fish (Pisces – three Classes, Phylum Chordata)	Often variation in external and internal anatomy associated with life cycle and habitat (including whether freshwater or marine) Special features of most fish include mesodermal scales, fins, gills and swim bladder
Invertebrates (Invertebrata – at least 30 Phyla)	Much variation, associated with classification, life cycle and habitat Features of relevance shown by some invertebrates include: • Arthropoda – exoskeleton, sometimes thick and strengthened by calcium salts, jointed body and limbs • Mollusca – protective (calcareous) shell often present; body soft; very prone to desiccation • Metazoan invertebrates usually have haemolymph, containing haemocyanin; a few have haemoglobin

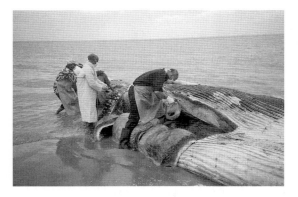

Figure 7.3 Necropsy of a beached whale requires a team effort, adherence to standard protocols and awareness of hazards, such as rising tides. This figure also appears in colour in the colour plate section.

applicable to all species even if they are related. For example, a standard necropsy technique for a trout or salmon, which involves a lateral incision into the animal, is totally inappropriate in a puffer fish where the only ready access to the body cavity is through the ventrum. Special features relating to the necropsy of non-domesticated species are given in Table 7.2 and discussed in more detail later.

CHAIN OF CUSTODY AND FATE OF SAMPLES

The chain of custody (evidence) remains a key part of forensic necropsy. Samples may be taken from a carcase and be sent to diverse laboratories or specialists for analysis (see Chapter 8). Each of these must be traceable to the original carcase from which they came. Chain of custody forms can either be drawn up for specific purposes – for instance marine mammal specimens (Geraci and Lounsbury, 2005) – or be based on standards used by the police and government forensic laboratories (see Chapter 11).

Following *post-mortem* examinations, carcases and tissues may need to be chilled, frozen or (rarely) fixed in formalin. Labelling is important (see also below and Chapter 11). Self-adhesive strips of industrial quality laboratory labelling tape are to be preferred because they are unaffected by freezing. Munro (1998) recommended black letters on a white background or white letters on a blue background in order to make the label easy to read, convenient and permanent.

Labelling of carcases and other specimens is an art in itself and this is discussed in more detail in Chapter 11. It must be remembered that a label on a bag does not necessarily provide an identification of a specimen that is within that bag. Carcases can easily be transposed and therefore it is wise to have a system such as a strip of tape or a tag that can be applied to an extremity of the animal, such as its hock joint. One easy way of marking carcases of dogs, cats and other animals with long tails is to wrap adhesive bandage around the tail. Small pieces of tissue may require alternative methods (see later).

The carcase must be handled and packed carefully following *post-mortem* examination. It may need to be seen again, possibly dissected further, by the original pathologist or by others called by defence or prosecution. Everything on or within the body must be retained, if necessary in separate bags. Trace evidence may be lost if, for example, the animal's head or feet are allowed to hang or are shaken during transportation to the freezer. Medical pathologists put paper bags on the hands to preserve such evidence – paper because plastic bags gather condensation (DiMaio and DiMaio, 2001).

The final disposal of a carcase, when the case is over, will depend upon the circumstances. It is always wise to retain material for a certain period in case it is needed (see Chapter 10). Carcases may need to be returned to their owner, or to a local community (see later), or (usually for legal reasons)

be passed to the appropriate agricultural or wildlife department.

It is not only the carcase and tissues that should be retained in a forensic case. So also should all wrappings, including bags, boxes and padding – the animal equivalent of 'scene markers' (DiMaio and DiMaio, 2001) as they may provide important information about the circumstances of death (see Chapter 11, and Figure 5.8).

The value of retention of material, following legal proceedings, in museum and reference collections is discussed in Chapters 5 and 6.

The keys to success in all forensic work are (1) thoroughness and (2) use of a standard procedure. Necropsy is no exception and adherence to protocols, drawn up in the light of available information (see earlier), is essential.

STAGES OF A POST-MORTEM EXAMINATION

There are several important stages in planning, preparing for and carrying out a forensic necropsy:

- Ascertain the background history and the species to be examined (see Table 7.2).
- Prepare facilities and equipment, including attention to health and safety.
- Obtain adequate assistance.
- Ensure health and safety.
- Plan attendance by other people (e.g. police, RSPCA inspectors) who may need or wish to be present.
- Perform the *post-mortem* examination, including record-keeping.
- Take laboratory samples.
- Retain material and store carcase.
- Clear and clean the facilities, including attention to health and safety.
- Collate records.
- Receive and analyse laboratory findings.
- Produce report.
- Retain all forms, other records (e.g. tapes), specimens and samples (evidence).

Many of the arrangements prior to performing a forensic necropsy are the same as those described for a clinical examination (see Chapter 6). Whether an animal that is the subject of an investigation is alive or dead, the planning and preparation outlined in Chapter 9 (Site Visits, Fieldwork and Collection of Evidence) is relevant.

These will be discussed in more detail, where appropriate, under their own headings.

HISTORY AND CONFIRMING THE IDENTITY/RECORDING THE PROVENANCE OF THE SPECIMEN

These will consist largely of written/computerised notes, together with information provided by the person(s) submitting the specimen.

Access to as full a history as possible is desirable. This may not be available because the animal was found or seized and the owner or keeper who might provide background information is not available. As was stressed in Chapter 6, even if a history is provided, this may not be correct or it may even be fabricated. Often in forensic work the pathologist has to perform an examination on an animal, or carry out tests on samples, not knowing the true background. Sometimes, however, carrying out investigations 'blind' in this way is a good thing. An example is when reading histological sections when preconceived ideas or presumptions may, albeit unwittingly, influence how long is spent on examining certain tissues or how much weight is put on interpretation of equivocal changes in organs.

The general guidance regarding background information about a *post-mortem* case is as follows:

- Always try to obtain a history before embarking on the necropsy – however, brief, inadequate or unreliable this may appear to be.
- Heed the history but do not rely upon it.
- When you have the opportunity to take a history yourself, do so, rather than depending on others who may have a less objective approach to the case.

Important features of a good history include:

- Correct dates and times of incidents or findings: it can make a lot of difference as to whether an animal was found sick or dead early in the morning or later in the day.

- The circumstances regarding the animal(s), how many were involved, the social grouping, accommodation, diet, etc.
- Other aspects, such as the people involved in the *ante-mortem* care of the animal.
- Records, e.g. day books or diaries.
- Photographs or drawings.

PREPARATION OF ROOM

Whenever possible the *post-mortem* room should be prepared in advance. In legal cases extra steps may be needed – for example, to facilitate photography or to ensure appropriate handling of samples that will require special investigations.

PREPARATION OF EQUIPMENT

Equipment also should be carefully prepared and set out before the necropsy. A checklist is useful. Different species may require diverse implements (see Table 7.3).

OBTAINING ADEQUATE ASSISTANCE

When performing a forensic necropsy adequate (and appropriate) assistance is essential both to provide practical help (technicians, attendants) and, if necessary, to offer corroboration of findings. The

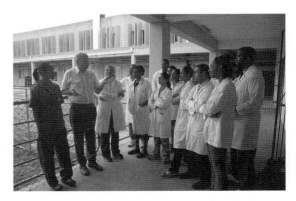

Figure 7.4 In all forensic investigations planning is important. Here a group is briefed before embarking upon the *post-mortem* examination of a bull that was found injured on a public highway.

Table 7.3 Equipment for *post-mortem* examination.

Species	Essential	Useful additions	Special precautions	Comments
All (vertebrate and invertebrate) species	PM table Instruments Protective clothing Incinerator, macerator or other means of disposal Refrigerator, freezer Balance/scales Disinfectants Steriliser or autoclave Bottles and fixatives	Protective hood or flow cabinet X-ray machine	Adequate drainage, disinfection and ventilation	Some requirements are likely to be legal responsibilities under health and safety legislation
Mammals	As above Instruments should include bone forceps and saw for examination of CNS	Vacuum cleaner or similar to remove hair and dander	As above	As above Special care should be taken with certain species, e.g. primates and rodents, especially where infectious disease is suspected
Birds	As above	As above for feathers and feather dust	As above Dowsing carcase in disinfectant may reduce risk of airborne infection but hood or flow cabinet is preferable	As above Special care with psittacines and where infectious disease is suspected
Reptiles	As above Bone forceps and saw facilitate	Container for head of venomous species	As above (All)	As above (All) Care must be taken with venomous species
Amphibians	As above (All) Carcase should be kept damp during examination	As above (All)	As above (All)	As above (All) Care must be taken to avoid contact with parotoid and cutaneous secretions of some species
Fish	Instruments should include long forceps and scissors for dissecting species that have toxic spines	As above (All)	As above (All)	As above (All) Care must be taken with toxic species

(Continued)

175

Table 7.3 *Continued.*

Species	Essential	Useful additions	Special precautions	Comments
Invertebrates	As above (All) Micro instruments (e.g. ophthalmic) are often needed Examination may necessitate use of dissecting microscope or magnifying loop Some aquatic species need to be kept damp or even immersed in saline or water (to prevent desiccation or collapse) during examination	As above (All)	As above (All)	As above (All) Care must be taken with toxic species The small size of many invertebrates can make detailed examination difficult Fixation *in toto* may be advisable, followed by histological examination

amount of assistance needed will depend upon the following:

- Species: a rhinoceros requires more people than does a rattlesnake (but the latter needs skilled personnel – see below).
- Numbers: 20 dead ornamental koi (carp) will take a long time to necropsy and, with the rapid autolysis shown by fish, the first and the twentieth koi will look very different. It is far better to have a team of pathologists and assistants doing the dissections.
- Circumstances: for example, whether in a well-equipped *post-mortem* room or out in the field.

All involved in forensic necropsy must be properly briefed beforehand and reminded that a legal case may result.

ENSURING HEALTH AND SAFETY

See later.

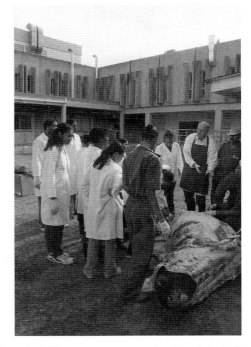

Figure 7.5 The *post-mortem* examination of the bull proceeds. Each assistant has a designated task.

EQUIPMENT

Equipment needed for a forensic *post-mortem* examination will vary depending upon the circumstances. Those involved in animal work may need to be prepared for anything ranging from a tarantula spider or small frog to a stranded whale. Guidelines are given in Table 7.3.

Traditionally, medical forensic pathologists on crime scene visits ensured that they carried a 'murder bag' (not necessarily the right term for those doing veterinary pathology!). This contained useful equipment, including camera, torch (flashlight), notepad and pen and tape-recorder. Veterinarians and others involved in animal work must be more versatile. For example, in wildlife investigations, protective headgear and climbing ropes may even be needed. A full list of equipment is to be found in Appendix E.

If an animal is found dead and has to be moved, it is important to have a photographic record of its original position (see later). This can be usefully supplemented by a chalk or paint outline if, for example, the carcase is on a road, kennel floor or other hard surface.

PLANNING ATTENDANCE OF OTHERS

It is not a good principle to allow others to attend a necropsy as onlookers, for 'interest only'. They can distract from the job in hand, spread micro-organisms, prions or DNA and hamper candid or contentious comments. However, there are instances where attendees are acceptable, possibly even desirable. *Bona fide* persons may include:

- Other pathologists.
- Appropriate colleagues, e.g. clinicians who were involved in the case.
- Support staff, e.g. technicians.
- Police officers.
- Officials from relevant animal welfare or conservation bodies.
- Where appropriate (usually wildlife cases), people from the local community with an inter-

est in, or responsibility for, traditional use or custody of the species.
- Students.

All visitors should be vetted and their names and affiliation appended to the *post-mortem* report. They may need to be shown 'clean and dirty' principles. Extra protective clothing will be needed. Someone unfamiliar with necropsy may need a chair or to be able to retire to a cool place.

CONTACT WITH CLIENTS

In human forensic work the pathologist may be involved in talking to family members or others, including those who may have been bereaved under unpleasant circumstances. This role can be important for legal reasons (obtaining relevant information) but also is part of professionalism – dealing with people (Rutty, 2001).

Such a role exists also in animal forensics. Like his medical counterpart, the animal pathologist can play an important role in contacts with people. Owners want to know why their animal has died, especially if the circumstances were unusual. They may be grieving, anxious or angry. A sensitive pathologist, perhaps joining forces with a clinician, can do much to help.

Notwithstanding the points above, caution must be exercised. Legal cases can be very sensitive and it may be unwise or impossible to divulge certain information. Reference was made to this in the context of clinical examination, where the owner or potential purchaser may be present (see Chapter 6).

PERFORMANCE OF THE NECROPSY

See later.

TAKING AND SUBMISSION OF SAMPLES

See later and Chapter 8.

PREPARATION OF REPORT

See later and Chapter 10.

As emphasised elsewhere in the book, caution must be exercised when it comes to reporting, especially if there is a request for 'preliminary findings' to be divulged. Sometimes such a demand comes from a lawyer, sometimes a police officer, often from the media. The press are always anxious to have some initial information, preferably ahead of their rivals. In one of our cases involving a dog that was found dead under strange circumstances, together with its owner, two national newspapers provided their readers with a diagnosis of the cause of death of the dog – one of them publishing their report before the necropsy had been performed (!) and both accounts totally incorrect.

The moral of this and many other examples is as follows:

- Be very wary of requests for a preliminary *post-mortem* report.
- If you feel obliged to provide *some* information ahead of your final report, do so in the form of a short summary, listing the main findings and stressing that follow-up tests are in progress. Avoid making any verbal statements: they are very likely to be misinterpreted.

It is also wise to check as to who is asking for the report. One should ask enquirers to identify themselves, if necessary by producing an identity card.

RETENTION OF RECORDS

See below and Chapter 10.

RECORD-KEEPING

A whole range of standard *post-mortem* forms is available for animals. Many have been reproduced or published in textbooks and field manuals (see References). They cover not only conventional, domesticated animals but also less familiar species such as reptiles, birds of prey, eggs and embryos and marine mammals (see below).

Although standard diagnostic forms are useful, they are usually broad in scope and have to cater for any eventuality. In many forensic cases, however, specific questions are being asked and therefore (for example) particular attention may need to be paid to the animal's spinal cord or spleen, sometimes at the expense of other organs or tissues. There is often merit in a forensic case in compiling a specific form which can then be used as the basis for a report. Sometimes special forms are available – for example, for marine mammals (Kuiken and Hartman, 1992) – and these may facilitate the correct recording of relevant data. There may even be specified formats for necropsy reports that are of legal significance if, for example, an official (government) necropsy is performed (Korim *et al.*, 1999). In the UK, DEFRA (see Appendix B) has its own *post-mortem* form for carcases where the examination is being undertaken on behalf of the owner because, for example, the bird died during handling for ringing/registration purposes.

A specimen *post-mortem* form is given in Appendix A, together with a model draft report.

Specific aspects of record-keeping are discussed in Chapter 10.

HEALTH AND SAFETY

Health and safety are important in all *post-mortem* examinations and, in the case of those of a forensic nature, also help to ensure that systems are in place that will minimise mixing of materials or contamination. A 'clean and dirty' division is essential and a colour code may be useful to differentiate the two.

It is important, before starting any *post-mortem* examination, to consider any public health considerations (including zoonoses: see Chapter 2) or the possibility that the animal may be harbouring a disease or organisms that may be transmissible to others of the same or different species. By definition, some forensic necropsy cases will be the carcases of animals of unknown or doubtful provenance; this means that they could have been brought in illegally from overseas and be capable of introducing exotic diseases.

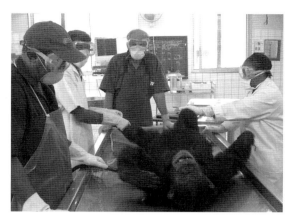

Figure 7.6 Necropsy of certain species requires special precautions to protect against zoonoses. For examination of this chimpanzee, all the pathologists wear goggles. This figure also appears in colour in the colour plate section.

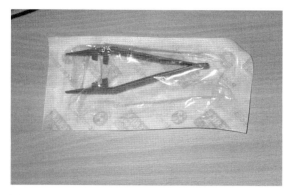

Figure 7.7 Plastic forceps are important in forensic work when bullets have to be removed from live or dead animals.

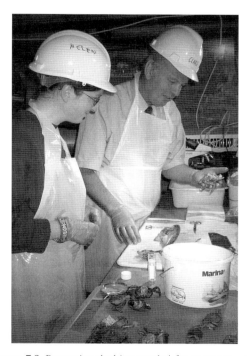

Figure 7.8 Protective clothing needed for necropsy work may include 'hard hats' if there is a danger of collision with equipment or a low roof.

Full precautions should *always* be taken. It is better to protect against risks that do not exist rather than to regret at a later date not having taken adequate precautions. The person carrying out the necropsy should consider consulting the relevant Ministry of Agriculture (DEFRA in the UK) and checking possible risks, using the information provided by the OIE (see Appendix B).

Thought should always be given to using a microbiological safety cabinet for (small) animal necropsies and this may even be a legal requirement when dealing with known cases of zoonotic disease. Fume cupboards are not an adequate substitute, as 'blowbacks' can occur, liberating organisms into the environment. However, in isolated locations or poorer countries, where the correct equipment is not available (nor does legislation demand its use) improvisation may be necessary.

RISK ASSESSMENTS

Risk assessments (referred to by other terms in some countries, e.g. 'hazard management plans', in New Zealand) are an essential process for identifying the hazards and risks in any workplace/activity. They are also a legal requirement in the UK under the Management of Health & Safety at Work Regulations 1999. The notes below give some indication as to how the British system works.

Certain types of work require specific risk assessments, for example workstation assessments for computer work and manual handling assessments for tasks requiring physical effort. *Post-mortem*

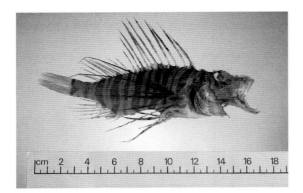

Figure 7.9 Some *post-mortem* specimens can be hazardous to the pathologist. This lion (scorpion) fish bears poisonous spines. This figure also appears in colour in the colour plate section.

examinations and handling of laboratory samples come under the same heading. However, it is necessary to conduct a risk assessment that is suitable and sufficient for any activity where significant hazards have been identified.

Hazards have to be identified and the associated risk evaluated for potential severity and outcome. This then leads to the precautions and controls that must be put in place to ensure that the health and safety of personnel is not put at risk. Arrangements are required to ensure that these precautions are monitored and a record of assessments kept along with a plan to review in the future, especially if any changes occur.

Some special precautions, aimed at protecting both humans and samples taken, will now be discussed in more detail.

DEALING WITH TOXIC SUBSTANCES

When dealing with suspect poisoning cases (see later and Chapter 6), caution must be taken to ensure that samples are handled correctly. This is not just a matter of taking care. It relates also to the method of working and storage of samples. For example, the use of plastic or rubber stoppers on containers may be unwise because the chemicals under investigation may be dissolved (see also Chapters 8 and 11).

Precautions should be taken when examining animals where poisoning is suspected because chemical contamination can occur, giving false results. The precautions to prevent or to minimise such contaminations are similar to those that are used to ensure a clean and dirty system (see earlier, Health and safety). These are listed below:

- The table and environment should be as clean as possible (including freedom from insecticides or disinfectants before the examination starts).
- Each carcase should have a separate laboratory number.
- As a general rule, only one carcase should be on the *post-mortem* table at one time. If more than one table is available or separation can be ensured (for example, carcases in separate trays) a production line system of examination may be considered.
- If not constructed of seamless sheet metal, which is easily cleaned, the table should be covered with plastic or similar sheeting that can be changed between examinations.
- The table should be washed and cleaned between each examination.
- All instruments and protective clothing should be changed between examinations; if necessary several sets of instruments should be available.
- The necropsy technique should be such that minimises contamination, especially spillage of fluids from one organ to another. Tying of loops of intestines or other organs with coloured string will help to reduce this risk and facilitate locating the organs.
- All samples for toxicological assay (blood, urine, tissues) should be placed in separate containers (this is different from histological or electron-microscopical examination where tissues may be placed in the same container of fixative).
- The remains of each animal should be placed in separate storage bags at the end of *post-mortem* examination.
- As in all forensic work, the side (not the lid) of each sample container should be marked with the relevant information: a useful extra precaution, especially when using alcoholic

fixatives, is to place a paper label, with data inscribed in pencil, *inside* the specimen jar – see also Chapter 11.

- Telephones should not be handled by those involved in the necropsy work – if telephone contact is needed, this should be means of a 'non-touch' speaker.

DEALING WITH DNA

Similar precautions to those above apply when samples are to be taken for DNA studies. The origin and purity of any samples are of great importance. Studies in mortuaries have shown how easily surfaces and instruments can become contaminated with 'foreign' DNA. This can be minimised if those involved in the necropsy wear full protective clothing, including face masks, and follow protocols (see earlier).

PERFORMANCE OF THE NECROPSY AND POST-MORTEM TECHNIQUE

Technique is always most important – particularly so in forensic work where a carcase or tissues may need to be re-examined by more than one pathologist. There is value in documenting the necropsy procedure employed for a particular specimen. Useful guidance on some aspects of forensic examination can be obtained from medical texts (see, for example, Burton and Rutty, 2001) but animals present many specific challenges (Cooper, 2003a,b; Echols, 2003; King *et al.*, 2005).

A key message is to observe carefully before handling or even touching. Tissues should always be treated with sensitivity and manipulated with the correct instruments.

It is particularly important in forensic examinations to have (and to use) the appropriate equipment (see also Appendix E). Failure to do so may result in uncertain or equivocal findings and may cast doubt on the experience of the pathologist. Forceps are an example! The choice of instrument is important:

- Rat-toothed forceps – for grasping and restraining tissues that are not likely to be used for histology and similar investigations.
- Non-toothed forceps – for grasping and restraining tissues that are either easily torn or which are destined for histology or electronmicroscopy where forceps damage can cause unacceptable processing artefacts.
- Plastic forceps – for removing lead shot or bullets (where metal forceps may damage the surface, making identification of the weapon less easy) or for taking samples for analysis of certain metals (plastic instruments are also lightweight and disposable, they are therefore useful in fieldwork: see Chapter 9 and Appendix E).
- Small (micro) instruments, such as those used by ophthalmologists, for examination of eggs, embryos and tiny samples (Cooper, 2004a).

Equipment for a forensic necropsy must be more than adequate. It is not a time 'to make do'. Anything that might be needed should be available, for example probes – instruments or tubes, preferably of different colours, that can be placed into hollow structures, such as a blood vessel, or wounds in order to detect their position or the route that a weapon or bullet has taken in the body – not only facilitate investigative work but make it easier to demonstrate significant findings in photographs. If the carcase has to be re-examined at a later date, the probe should be left in place, even if in the interim the tissue has to be frozen or fixed.

Skinning of the carcase is usually an important part of a forensic necropsy, in order to detect injury to the integument and superficial tissues. Most pathologists tend to leave removal of the skin until after the internal examination is completed but Wobeser (1996), in the context of wildlife, advocated skinning the entire animal at the outset. Ultraviolet light may assist at this stage, especially if photographs are to be taken (Barsley *et al.*, 1990).

Incisions must always be performed with care, especially in cases where there is already traumatic injury or, perhaps, a ruptured aneurysm is suspected and therefore dissection may damage important

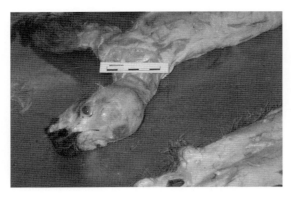

Figure 7.10 Skinning a carcase can reveal important information, as in this puppy where tooth marks were detected in the skull. This figure also appears in colour in the colour plate section.

evidence. Throughout a forensic necropsy one must remember that follow-up examinations may be necessary either by the pathologist him/herself or by someone else called by the prosecution or defence.

As Tables 7.2 and 7.3 and earlier discussion indicate, different types of animal need different approaches. There are many texts available describing *post-mortem* techniques for domesticated species and certain 'exotic' species and a few relate specifically to forensic cases (see, for example, Corradi *et al.*, 2001; Munro, 1998; Wobeser, 1996). Older publications tend only to have photographs in black and white, which can hamper interpretation. More recent texts that include pictures in colour, for example the continuing professional development (CPD) article on necropsy of ruminants (Griffiths, 2005), colour atlases depicting human techniques and cases (Dix, 2000; Gresham, 1975) and relevant material on the Internet, may be of more practical assistance. Clear line drawings (diagrams) are valuable for recording details, especially the positions of lesions.

TIME OF DEATH

Estimation of time of death is always a challenge for the forensic pathologist (Catts, 1992; DiMaio and DiMaio, 2001; Henssge *et al.*, 2002; Shepherd,

Table 7.4 'Spot check' for determining time of death (after Knight, 1996).

Features of body	Likely time of death
Warm and flaccid	Less than 3 hours
Warm and stiff	3–8 hours
Cold and stiff	8–36 hours
Cold and flaccid	More than 36 hours

2003), including those who investigate animal cases (Stroud and Adrian, 1996). In human work the 'spot check' advocated by Knight (1996) is sometimes used (Table 7.4).

These categories of '*post-mortem* interval' (PMI) may be applied very broadly to mammals of the size of an adult human but cannot be considered more than a very rough guide.

There are various specialised methods for attempting to assess the time of death, most of them developed for human work (DiMaio and DiMaio, 2001) and these include temperature measurements, changes in the vitreous humour, muscle studies and evaluation of DNA degradation (Cina, 1994).

The rate of cooling of a cadaver or carcase depends on many different factors (Shepherd, 2003). In the case of animals it is influenced by:

- Size (mass).
- Surface area.
- Insulation – presence/absence of subcutaneous and internal fat.
- Environmental factors such as ambient temperature, wind, rain and whether the body is in water, mud or dry land.

Kienzler *et al.* (1984) provided useful data on temperature changes in dead white-tailed deer.

Munro (1998) described the particular difficulties for the animal pathologist because s/he is likely to be dealing with different species. He referred to some of the limited research that facilitates estimating time of death (see above).

Relatively few methods of assessing time of death are readily available to the veterinary forensic pathologist. S/he must usually depend upon recording and analysis of basic criteria such as:

- Cooling of the carcase.
- *Rigor mortis.*
- Desiccation.
- Discoloration of skin.
- Discoloration of internal organs.
- Maggot activity.
- *Post-mortem* change.
- Scavenging patterns.
- Circumstances of death and storage thereafter.

Oates (1992) produced a software programme for white-tailed deer which utilises such parameters as air temperature, carcase weight and deep thigh temperature. He and others (Oates *et al.*, 1984) also provided information for those working in

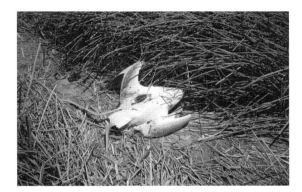

Figure 7.11 A freshly-dead lesser flamingo, probably killed by a predator. Bleeding is apparent. This figure also appears in colour in the colour plate section.

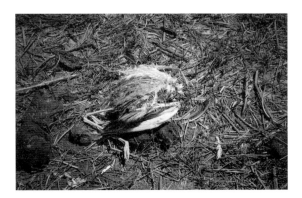

Figure 7.12 A flamingo that died two weeks before the photo was taken. The carcase is dry and little soft tissue remains. This figure also appears in colour in the colour plate section.

the field who are likely to be asked to determine the time of death of other species, including bighorn sheep, antelope, elk, racoons, rabbits and waterfowl.

Zoo-archaeologists sometimes use environmental cues to assess when the death of an animal may have occurred, e.g. tidal lines on marine molluscs (Davis, 1987).

Munro (1998) suggested that, in animals, general estimates are usually all that can be given and advocated use of the following broad categories:

- Recent death – less than 48 hours.
- Several days.
- Weeks.
- Months.
- Years.

Similar periods were suggested in PAW (2005).

Despite these difficulties it is important that the animal pathologist endeavours to provide an estimate or, at the very least, carefully collates relevant data, especially degree of *post-mortem* change (see later), so that they might be analysed.

CAUSE OF DEATH

Ascertaining why an animal died can be of great importance in a legal case. In human forensic pathology in the UK, the pathologist will be asked by the senior investigating officer for a 'cause of death' (Weston, 2004). The death is then classified as an 'accident', 'suicide', 'murder' or 'natural causes'. Such categories are clearly inappropriate to animal work: instead, 'anthropogenic' and 'natural' can be used as a starting point and further designated as necessary and appropriate. It is important to bear in mind that the cause of death is often multifactorial – not always easy to explain in court and often open to rigorous questioning in cross-examination.

CIRCUMSTANCES OF DEATH

Traditionally, medical students were taught that death was brought about by one or more of the following:

- Asphyxia (respiratory failure).
- Syncope (heart failure).
- Coma (brain failure).

The argument was that life depends on the integrity of the three organ systems in brackets above (Ross, 1925). However, the definition of death remains controversial (Shepherd, 2003): there are differing perspectives from clinicians, philosophers, persons with strong religious beliefs and even policy makers (Youngner *et al.*, 1999).

Some physicians still give 'cardiac arrest' as a cause of death but in modern (human) forensic medicine three aspects have to be considered (DiMaio and DiMaio, 2001). These are:

(1) The *cause* of death – for example, a gunshot wound or pneumonia.
(2) The *mechanism* of death – the physiological changes produced by the cause of death that made it fatal; examples could include haemorrhage or a blood-borne infection.
(3) The *manner* of death – how the cause of death came about: 'murder', 'accident', etc. (see above/below).

A similar approach can be applied when an animal has died under strange or unexpected circumstances.

On a broader front, those instructing the pathologist want to know:

- How did this animal die?
- Why did this animal die?
- How long did it take this animal to die?
- When did this animal die?
- Where did this animal die?
- Who was involved, intentionally or inadvertently, in its death?

Not all of these questions will be easy to answer and very often the veterinary pathologist will only be able to offer limited evidence, coupled with opinion.

SUDDEN DEATHS AND UNEXPECTED DEATHS

It is important in any legal case or similar hearing to distinguish these two. They are often confused,

especially by lay people. Sometimes an animal dies suddenly *and* unexpectedly: often only one applies.

An animal that dies suddenly, especially if also unexpectedly, can be the cause of debate, of dispute, and of legal action. Very great care must therefore be taken in dealing with such cases.

There are many possible causes of sudden death. In cattle, for example, such deaths can be due to:

- Acute infections, e.g. anthrax, clostridial diseases.
- Trauma, e.g. damage inflicted by another animal, leading to, e.g., haemorrhage.
- Other physical injuries, such as a road traffic accident (see later).
- Electrocution, including lightning strike (see later).
- Poisons, organic and inorganic chemicals and plants (see later).
- Other non-infectious conditions, e.g. bloat (ruminal tympany) and hypomagnesaemia.
- Anaphylactic shock.

Medical pathologists recognise as rare causes of death, in otherwise healthy individuals, such syndromes as vagal inhibition of the heart, possibly precipitated by a sudden stressor (e.g. as immersion in cold water), and *commotio cordis*, which is essentially ventricular fibrillation following trauma to the chest. Such diagnoses are not recognised routinely in animal work, although vagal inhibition is sometimes the cause of death in animals that are strangled or hanged (see later). The veterinary pathologist's role is often to exclude, as far as is possible, infectious and non-infectious factors and then to state that no obvious cause of death was found (see later).

Investigation of sudden death is an example of where a prompt necropsy can be invaluable (see Appendix D). An adequate history is important. For example, a German Shepherd Dog, previously in excellent health, found dead one morning, might, as the owner suggests, have been poisoned by a neighbour (not an uncommon claim in certain countries). However, an immediate *post-mortem* examination could show that the dog died of acute gastric dilatation. Coupled with a history of a large

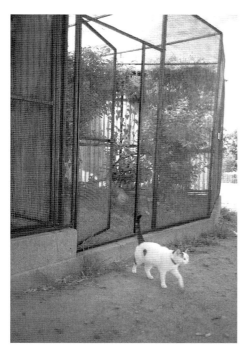

Figure 7.13 The clue to sudden or expected death may be observation. This domestic cat is leaving an aviary where it has been attempting to catch captive birds.

meal late the previous night, this diagnosis would effectively counter any claim of poisoning – and there would be no need for expensive toxicological or other tests.

When sudden death has occurred or is suspected, a site visit is essential (see Chapter 9). The environment may prove as important as the animal. It is best not to investigate the latter until the area has been properly searched and relevant people questioned.

In a court case or insurance claim, the diagnosis or conclusions in cases of sudden death may be challenged, so very detailed records should be kept, including photographs, and as much material as possible retained.

ANAESTHETIC AND SURGICAL DEATHS

These are discussed in Chapter 6.

MAKING A DIAGNOSIS

Not all *post-mortem* examinations provide a diagnosis, even in standard medical or veterinary work. In avian studies, for example, 10–15% of birds examined yielded no specific diagnosis (Cooper, 2002). In forensic work, the cause of death is not necessarily the important finding. As emphasised earlier, all depends on the questions being asked. Sometimes the cause of death is already known (e.g. the cat was euthanased or the badger was killed on the road) in which case the role of the pathologist is to provide information on background pathology or other parameters. Whatever the need, the forensic pathologist must resign him/ herself to the fact that some cases will be inconclusive, even if a whole battery of supporting laboratory tests is carried out. In such cases, the pathologist must be prepared to state this and not be swayed in any way to alter his/her opinion (see earlier, regarding sudden or unexpected death).

Likewise, where there are some significant findings (e.g. culture of bacteria of known pathogenicity to the species), the pathologist must resist the temptation to weave these into a plausible, but poorly-substantiated, explanation of how death may have occurred.

Post-mortem diagnosis of accidents may not always be easy, because in many cases gross lesions are few and histological changes non-specific. There has been little research on this subject in animals and often interpretations must be tentative. This contrasts markedly with human medicine, where forensic science permits accurate and specific diagnosis of many types of trauma (Knight, 1996). In certain cases, a detailed description of the cause of death of an animal may be requested (Cooper and Cooper, 1991; Stroud and Adrian, 1996).

It is particularly important to skin carcases of animals (see earlier). Removal of hair, by clipping, and feathers, by plucking, will help in the detection of superficial lesions. However the body should always be carefully examined externally *before* skinning.

In cases of paralysis, careful dissection of the cranium and spinal cord may be necessary to detect localised damage to the central nervous system (see later).

Radiography and other imaging techniques assist in the diagnosis of certain types of trauma. Laboratory tests, e.g. histopathology, haematology and the examination of urine and faeces for the presence of free blood, may provide valuable supporting information.

GROSS (MACROSCOPICAL) FINDINGS

Descriptive pathology is important (Thomson, 1978) and is usually the basis of a *morphological* diagnosis, such as abscessation of the liver, as opposed to an *aetiological* diagnosis – which often consists of two words, e.g. mycobacterial enteritis.

There are 'typical cases' and 'typical lesions' and these are usually the ones that authors depict in text books, but often what one sees in practice is *not* typical.

Lawyers, jurists and other non-medical personnel often fail to appreciate that not all causes of death manifest themselves as gross *post-mortem* findings. In most such cases, laboratory investigations (histology, bacteriology, toxicology, etc.) will be needed. Examples of diseases in which no specific macroscopical lesions are likely to be visible include rabies, listeriosis, tetanus and various types of poisoning. In some conditions, e.g. lightning strike (see Appendix D), lesions may or may not be detected, depending upon the circumstances. In a few cases (e.g. petroleum poisoning) the diagnosis may even be made as a result of noting a characteristic odour rather than observing gross lesions.

DESCRIPTION OF LESIONS

The basic tenets of descriptive pathology apply to all forensic work, whether one is dealing with a live or a dead animal.

Lesions should be described (Thomson, 1978), using the following main headings:

- Numbers and distribution.
- Location/orientation.
- Raised, flat or depressed.
- On surface only or in deeper tissue.
- Shape.

- Size (cm and mm).
- Colour.
- Consistency.
- Odour.

The shape and size of a lesion can be described in words and measurements or photographed, drawn or traced (see Chapter 6). Such records can be of great value in legal cases, where explanations will have to be given to a magistrate, a judge and, possibly, to a lay jury.

As in clinical work, all senses except taste should be used when examining a carcase – eyes, ears (crepitation, etc.), nose (odours associated with certain infections, parasites and poisons) and touch. The last can be very important: a slight change in the surface morphology of an organ can be best detected by gently running an index finger over it with the eyes closed – as if one is blind. Proper description of the 'feel' of organs or lesions is important. One useful way is to relate this to parts of the human body (cf. zoography – see Chapter 2) so that, for example, 'hard' is likened to the feel of the forehead, 'firm' to the tip of nose, and 'soft' to the lip.

Any changes in appearance following sampling should be noted as should the behaviour of samples when placed in saline or fixative. For instance, do they float or do they sink? Is there a change in colour following immersion (see later)?

The colour of lesions can be important (Hadlow, 1997). Changes in colour have for long been used as an indicator of pathological change and may play a significant part in making a diagnosis. The ability to differentiate colours is important in forensic work and any practitioner who is colour-blind should seek assistance from a colleague. It is wise to standardise descriptions using a colour key – either by compiling a system based on, say, a chart of paint colours (available through most do-it-yourself shops) or one designed for checking photographic colours (see, for example, www.babelcolor.com).

The appearance of lesions can be affected by the presence of pigment, especially melanin but also (e.g. in fish) guanine and xanthine. This primarily concerns the skin but in many ectotherms the liver contains melanin or melanomacrophage foci and in a few species (e.g. certain chameleons), the peritoneum may also be deeply pigmented. The expert who may be challenged in court over this matter – the argument being that it is difficult to discern or interpret some lesions in pigmented tissues – will find it useful to refer to the book *Black and White Skin Diseases* (Archer and Robertson, 1995).

The colour of organs or tissues may change *post mortem*. Some colours are indicative of specific changes, such as bile-staining which results in a green colouring in most tissues but may cause others, e.g. the yolk sac of young turtles, to appear black. Pseudomelanosis can occur – for example, in kidneys – because of contact between the organ(s) and the alimentary tract. The dark coloration that forms and which so easily misleads an inexperienced person is a result of the formation of iron sulphide.

'Patterned' lesions are often a feature of tissues that have been struck with an object such as a hammer. Even bruises may show such patterns (DiMaio and DiMaio, 2001).

Hypostasis (the gravitational pooling of blood in certain areas during or after the animal's demise), also termed *livor mortis* or 'lividity', will produce colour changes and can occasionally be mistaken for bruising. It may be of relevance in ascertaining the circumstances of death. If hypostasis is in an unexpected position (for example, the animal is lying on its left but the right kidney and right lung show hypostatic congestion), this may mean that the carcase has been moved. Differentiation of

hypostatic congestion of the lung and pneumonia is often important in forensic cases. Sometimes both are present. Strafuss (1988) provided a useful table, drawing attention to such features as differences in location, texture and colour.

As in human medicine, a marbling appearance may be associated with the spread of putrefying bacteria in the blood but this is not easy to see through the skin unless the latter is lacking pigmentation (see earlier).

A pink coloration to the tissues is classically associated with carbon monoxide or cyanide poisoning but another important cause is low temperature – either *ante-mortem* hypothermia or *post-mortem* refrigeration (especially at near freezing temperatures). Differentiation can be vital in a forensic case. It is best to *record* such observations but not to interpret them until all the pieces of the 'jigsaw puzzle' are in place. Some significant colours in carcases manifest themselves better a few hours after death or even following immersion of the organ or tissue in saline or formalin.

CONTUSION

Bruises also produce colour changes. They are important clues in any *post-mortem* examination but detection in animals can be difficult because of the presence of hair, feathers, scales or pigmenta-

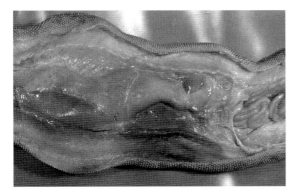

Figure 7.14 Early *post-mortem* change in a reptile is often marked by bile-staining of the ventral skin. This figure also appears in colour in the colour plate section.

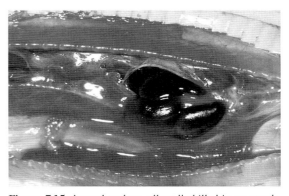

Figure 7.15 A royal python, allegedly killed in an attack by its owner. There is bruising around the heart and, when the animal was first skinned, marks consistent with being gripped in a human hand were faintly visible under the skin. (Courtesy O. F. Jackson.)

tion. Some bruises may be associated with gripping injuries (fingers and thumbs) (Figure 7.15).

A recent (less than 24 hours) bruise is usually purple or red in appearance. Changes in coloration then occur but this is not usually a reliable indicator of time of death. Nor are the changes consistent; in birds, for example, the transition from red to green takes place at varying times in different species. Some bruises may not be readily detected at the *post-mortem* examination but become apparent over the subsequent 24–72 hours. In human pathology such changes are well-recognised, but veterinarians seem less aware of it – a reason for always retaining a carcase, following initial investigation, and then re-examining 2–3 days later when not only bruises but other changes may become more clearly visible.

All injuries should be photographed in colour, with a non-reflecting scale and other relevant information, particularly the case number, date and (where appropriate) 'left' and 'right' markers.

DESCRIPTION OF ANIMALS

As in clinical work (see Chapter 6), accurate identification of animals is essential: failure to do this correctly can prove disastrous in any legal proceedings. Part of identification may be to describe the animal and its markings, plus any significant morphological features, such as overgrown hooves or presence of antlers. Photographs (see above and elsewhere) will help with this but it can also be useful to have on *post-mortem* forms drawings (outlines) of animals – left and right, dorsum and ventrum – on which relevant features, including lesions (see earlier), can be drawn. Medical forensic pathologists take fingerprints from cadavers as part of identification (DiMaio and DiMaio, 2001); comparable records can be taken from some animals – for example, the plastral pattern of tortoises or nose prints of gorillas.

GENDER DETERMINATION (SEXING)

This can be important in forensic work (Dabas and Saxena, 1994; Stroud and Adrian, 1996). Tech-

niques for sexing carcases or their derivatives include recognition of gross characteristics, such as colour of feathers (birds) or features of pelvic anatomy (mammals). Much work has been carried out on sexing and aging of certain taxa, some of which are particularly important from a forensic point of view – birds of prey, for example (Wyllie, 1993). Other methods of sex determination include PCR techniques and hormonal assay (Adrian, 1992).

MORPHOMETRICS

Measurements of animals, their organs and lesions should be *accurate* and *consistent* (see also Chapter 6). It is preferable if the same person does all the measurements and uses the same equipment each time, otherwise individual variation can occur which may give indication of errors. Even sophisticated equipment used for measuring can prove faulty; for example, vernier callipers can be very accurate but that accuracy is easily altered if they are dirty or dusty. Instruments should be cleaned before (and after) use and a useful way of checking that callipers are closing properly is to hold them up to the light.

Although medical pathologists have traditionally 'weighed and measured' (see, for example, Ross, 1925), surprisingly few veterinary texts provide normal (reference) values for the measurements and weights of organs of even the domesticated species. A notable exception is the book by Saxena *et al.* (1998) which includes data on species ranging from hedgehogs to elephants!

A range of instruments can be used to measure animals or lesions or specimens in the *post-mortem* room and each of these has its advantages and disadvantages (see Table 7.5).

If a table is used routinely for *post-mortem* work, especially for 'exotic' species, such as snakes (not easy to measure, dead or alive! – although a plastic or glass tube may assist – see Chapter 6) – centimetre and metre marks can be painted on to the table edge or a rule can be attached to it. This reduces the problem of trying to untangle and straighten an animal and then attempting to measure it. Measuring can be hampered by *rigor mortis.*

Table 7.5 Means of measuring dead animals.

Instrument	Comments
Solid rule	Firm, strong, not always easy to disinfect Not flexible
Transparent rule	Can be held over the body to facilitate location of landmarks and lesions Not flexible
Metal measuring tape	Flexible, compact but may rust
Cloth measuring tape	As above, lettering may fade but will not rust
Vernier callipers	Excellent for precise work Needs sensitive handling and cleaning
Permanent markings on examination table	Very convenient but lettering will fade Animal should be straightened
Centimetre scales on white or black card (laminated)	Can be fashioned out of paper – and subsequently discarded – but may be preferable to have laminated so that they can be washed and used again A (non-permanent) felt pen can be used to add the animal's identity, the date, etc.

Both black on white and white on black rulers/scales should be available if possible, especially when photographs are to be taken, in which case items should be glare-free.

A right-angle rule is often useful. Measuring tapes of different lengths can be supplemented for site visits with a roller system (available commercially for use by architects and others) that measures the ground traversed as the instrument is pushed across the ground.

How the measurement is carried out is important (see Chapter 6): for example, the body length of a tortoise is measured as a straight line (as if the animal is placed between two book-ends) and not as the length of curvature of the carapace. Such a measurement, often referred to as 'standard length', is common in a wide variety of species, including cetaceans and birds. Adhering to conventions established in zoological morphometry will also provide a database in the literature against which one's own measurements can be compared. The measurement of animal bones in a zoo-archaeological context was discussed by Davis (1987) and O'Connor (2000).

Asymmetry is often diagnosed by observation but must be confirmed by measurement, making allowance for observer bias (see Chapter 6 and Gosler, 2004). Fluctuating asymmetry (FA), which reflects small, random deviations from symmetry in otherwise bilaterally symmetrical characters (Stub *et al.*, 2001) can be an indicator of stress (Parsons, 1992) and may, therefore, provide evidence in a welfare case (see Chapter 6).

The assessment of an animal's 'condition', which usually involves measurements and is important in forensic work, is covered in Chapter 6.

DIFFERENTIATION OF HUMAN AND ANIMAL DERIVATIVES

This is an area in which links between the medical and veterinary professions – together with others, such as zoo-archaeologists – are important and where a comparative approach can be of great value. Methods and criteria used include:

- Gross morphology – bones, viscera.
- Light-microscopy – hair, blood (non-mammalian species).
- Electronmicroscopy – muscle (certain species).

- Gel diffusion and electrophoresis – tissues, body fluids.
- DNA analysis – most samples.

Most medical pathologists and forensic osteologists have no difficulty in stating that bones are, or are not, from a human being. However, soft tissues sometimes prove problematic and the input of a veterinary or comparative anatomist can then be crucial. An interesting study, comparing the hand and foot bones of humans and bears, was reported by Sims (1999).

As in all forensic work, duplicate or triplicate samples should be taken so that material can be examined by others involved in the case or sent to specialists elsewhere.

SPECIES DIFFERENTIATION

A whole carcase of a domesticated or familiar species usually presents few problems insofar as identification is concerned, but wildlife can still be problematic (see Chapter 5). Difficulties often arise when parts of an animal are presented. The pathologist will want to know with which species s/he is dealing and this may be a very pertinent question from a legal point of view – if, for example, meat is being sold as one species but trading standard officers suspect that it is from another. Methods for distinguishing carcases (or parts thereof) of horse and ox, cat and rabbit and various other species are well-documented in books covering meat inspection and pathology (see, for example, Saxena *et al.*, 1998). Such texts also provide advice about the 'classification' of carcases for abattoir purposes, including answers to questions relating to whether the animal:

- Had died or been killed.
- Was pregnant or non-pregnant.
- Was mature or immature.
- Was fetal or still-born (see later).
- Was in good, poor or emaciated condition.
- Showed significant *post-mortem* change.

It may be necessary to 'match' portions of carcases – for example, in cases where a number of domesticated or wild animals have been killed, butchered and then had their parts distributed. A useful guide to such work, concentrating on wild mammals, is Stroud and Adrian (1996).

Immunological (mainly gel diffusion) methods, using prepared antisera, have long been the mainstay of differentiating species and continue to be standard in many parts of the world (William and John, 2001).

Various DNA techniques are now being developed to distinguish meats, even those that are canned (see, for example, Rosel, 1999).

MEAT INSPECTION

This is a specific discipline, covered in most countries by legislation, but it can involve the forensic pathologist if there are allegations of fraudulent practice, illegal disposal of condemned carcases and parts, inadequate inspection or failure to recognise and take action over signs of disease in carcases.

Forensic cases relating to meat inspection may relate to either domesticated species or wild animals taken as bushmeat (see Chapter 5). Fish, reptiles and birds may be represented.

AGE DETERMINATION OF ANIMALS AND THEIR DERIVATIVES

Assessing the age at death of animals was discussed in some detail in Chapter 6, where attention was drawn to the skills of zoo-archaeologists in this respect, especially in the context of domesticated animals (Davis, 1987; Chaplin, 1971; Hesse and Wapnish, 1985).

The 'aging' of tissues and remains in terms of how long ago the animal died can be even more difficult. This is often requested, however, and may include the estimation of 'age' of bones found during the demolition of a house or the deep ploughing of a meadow. In human forensic medicine such aging can be particularly important, as bones and other remains over a certain age (50, 70 years depending upon the country and jurisdiction) are unlikely to prompt criminal investigations, on the grounds that anyone culpable is probably now dead.

Table 7.6 Gross changes in tissues.

Specimen	Factor	Likely effects
Bone	Rough handling or damage (e.g. by spade or tractor)	Damage to periosteum, articular surfaces, epiphyses and bone itself
	Exposure to water	Softening, leaching out of minerals
		Microbial and other attack
	Contact with acidic or alkaline soils	As above, plus pitting, reduction in weight
Skins, hides, pelts	Rough handling	Loss of hair, damage to skin
	Damp conditions	Growth of mould (fungi), often with secondary damage by invertebrates and vertebrates
	Excessively dry conditions	Brittleness with fissures or breaks in the skin
	Primary attack by moths, beetles or other invertebrates	Areas of hair and/or skin destruction
	Prolonged exposure to bright lights	Fading of colour

The aging of animal remains can also be necessary, examples being when such remains may provide evidence relevant to a cruelty case (e.g. for how long was a domesticated animal that starved to death locked in a cupboard?) or contravention of conservation legislation (e.g. was a mounted skull prepared before or after the enactment of CITES legislation?).

The aging of animal remains that date back hundreds or thousands of years has traditionally been the preserve of the zoo-archaeologist or palaeontologist and a variety of aging techniques is available, many based on measurement of isotopes.

The expert must always be cautious when initially presented with a bone or a skin of an animal and asked to age it. So many factors can influence the appearance and feel of such specimens. Some examples are given in Table 7.6. It may also be the case that unknown storage conditions or an unusual combination of preservation factors have acted on a carcase, and interpretation can be further confused – as, for example, in the very wide range of ages, diverging between tens and thousands of years, estimated in the literature for seal carcases found far inland in the dry valleys of Antarctica (Richard Norman, pers. comm.).

AGING OF LESIONS

The aging (dating) of skin and soft tissue wounds, contusions and fractures can be of great importance

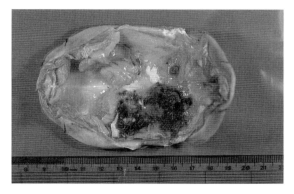

Figure 7.16 Aging of bruises can be complicated. In this case, a tortoise that was the subject of assault, the bruised area has changed colour, largely as a result of refrigeration and brief immersion in formalin. This figure also appears in colour in the colour plate section.

in forensic cases, in both live and dead animals. Two examples of the 'forensic' value of such information are (1) in a live animal, to be able to estimate when a skin wound was inflicted, in a possible cruelty case, and (2) in a dead animal, to be able to age fractures or internal haemorrhage, in an alleged road traffic accident. However, as medical forensic texts testify, the topic is fraught with difficulties.

Relatively few studies have been carried out on the progression and thus the aging of lesions of animals, in contrast to the situation in humans – bruises, for example (DiMaio and DiMaio, 2001;

Langlois and Gresham, 1991; Stephenson and Bialas, 1996). The subject becomes even more complicated once one moves into the realms of comparative forensic medicine because there is then an added dimension relating to body size and whether the species in question is endothermic ('warm-blooded') or ectothermic ('cold-blooded') (see also Chapter 2).

The general rules are:

- The metabolic rate of endotherms (mammals and birds) is inversely related to body mass. Therefore, a skin wound is likely to heal more rapidly in a mouse than in a mountain gorilla.
- Repair and/or regeneration takes place more rapidly at a high than at a low ambient temperature. This partly explains the first point above (small mammals and birds tend to have a higher body temperature than do large animals).
- In the case of ectothermic animals, the ambient temperature is the key factor; snakes with skin wounds will heal more rapidly at 24°C than at 20°C (Smith *et al.*, 1988).

Recognition that certain species heal more rapidly than do others is not new. Over 200 years ago, John Hunter demonstrated the speed of callus formation (and thus of fracture repair) in birds (Turk *et al.*, 2000).

The important questions that anyone who is asked to age lesions in animals should ask are therefore as follows:

- With what species (or taxon/group) of animal am I dealing?
- Is it an endotherm or an ectotherm?
- If an endotherm, what is its likely body temperature? Was it hibernating/aestivating (and thus likely to be at a lower metabolic rate)?
- If an ectotherm, at what temperature was it living/being kept?
- Armed with the information above, plus any extra relevant history and clinical/*post-mortem* observations, can I estimate the age of the wound/contusion/fracture on the basis of:
  - Published or unpublished data on this or related species?
  - My own or colleagues' experience?

  - Extrapolation from human forensic medicine?
- Do I have to make allowance for other factors that may have had an effect, for example the presence of infection or excessive movement, both of which can retard healing?
- Do I have relevant photographs, drawings, radiographs, other images that can be used in a court case and/or sent to experienced colleagues for a second opinion?

Approximate aging of certain traumatic and inflammatory lesions is possible in certain species, mainly humans, domesticated livestock and laboratory mammals, based on published work in comparative pathology journals and medical texts (DiMaio and DiMaio, 2001). The criteria include assessment of:

- Organisation of blood clots.
- Inflammatory infiltrates – acute versus chronic, numbers of pyknotic/karyorrhectic cells, presence or absence of phagocytosed organisms or other material.
- Fibroplasia.
- The healing of abrasions, which takes place in humans in four distinct stages (DiMaio and DiMaio, 2001).
- (In fractures) presence of callus, its degree of ossification, etc.

Even the above can vary significantly depending on such factors as:

- The species, age, sex of the animal – some of this a result of differences in metabolic rate (see Chapter 2).
- Whether a lesion is infected or subjected to movement/trauma, which can delay 'normal' healing.

The difficulties are confounded when one moves to other species. Some data on avian species exist and these confirm that changes take place more rapidly in birds, again attributable to the higher metabolic rate of most of these species. Ectothermic vertebrates present particular difficulties because the processes are temperature-dependent and reptiles, amphibians and fish have different preferred ranges.

TRANSILLUMINATION

In *post-mortem* work, as in clinical investigation, a strong light is of value in detecting lesions. A torch (flashlight), X-ray viewing box or even an endoscope can be used. In the field, especially in the tropics (where many high-profile wildlife crime investigations take place – see Chapter 5), the sun provides an excellent source of illumination through which, e.g., the patagium of the wing of a bird or the abomasum of a gazelle can be viewed.

POST-MORTEM RADIOGRAPHY

Radiography and radiological interpretation play an important part in human autopsy practice (Wilson *et al.*, 2004), and often include computerised radiographic (CR) techniques. Radiography is a valuable tool in veterinary pathology, including forensic examination. Whole-body radiography of small and young animals submitted for necropsy is recommended, especially where the species is unusual (Cooper and West, 1988) or there is a suggestion of abuse (see Chapter 6).

Angiography can sometimes be useful, as it is in humans.

Radiography of carcases and derivatives presents no legal or ethical obstacles because the material being examined is dead. As a result, repeated radiographing is possible and often desirable. However, use of a X-ray machine always carries with

it responsibility for the safety of operators and bystanders.

Other imaging techniques may also be helpful. Neuropathologists in the UK, faced with the dilemma of whether or not consent is likely to be given for traditional autopsy, are beginning to use *post-mortem* magnetic resonance imaging (MRI). These images have the advantage that they include detail that is often lost when the head is opened (Squier, 2005).

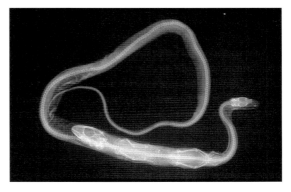

Figure 7.18 An inadvertent contravention of CITES. Radiograph of a rare, endemic snake, imported for pathological investigation, which on arrival was found to have an equally rare species of lizard in its stomach.

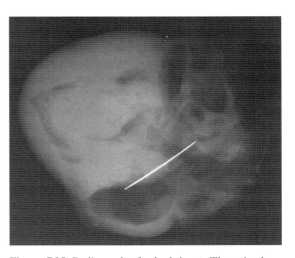

Figure 7.19 Radiograph of a dog's heart. The animal showed clinical signs of cardiovascular failure with no specific diagnosis. *Post-mortem* examination revealed a needle in the dog's heart. (Courtesy of Richard Spence.)

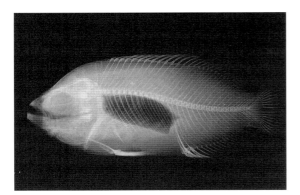

Figure 7.17 A whole-body radiograph of a fish prior to necropsy.

RECOGNITION OF *POST-MORTEM* CHANGE

Accurate differentiation of *ante-mortem* and *post-mortem* changes is important in all necropsies but perhaps never more so than in a forensic case. However, it is not always easy! Often one has to include analysis of the history and circumstances since death (Archer, 2004), coupled with use of laboratory tests, e.g. histology.

Traditional indicators are useful but not always totally reliable and can be challenged in court. For example, it is generally true to state that in a carcase the heart has stopped beating and therefore the animal cannot bleed. However, ectothermic species that are 'dead' may still have a beating heart (Frye, 1999) and even in a mammal blood sometimes comes out of a wound because of the presence of a haematoma or of a well-vascularised lesion, especially if the animal also had a blood-clotting defect. DiMaio and DiMaio (2001) referred to enzyme tests that can be used in humans both to demonstrate that a wound was *ante mortem* as well as to date it.

An example of how *ante-mortem* lesions can be confused with *post-mortem* changes was given by Rutty (2004) who provided an excellent review of shock (in its sense of 'inadequate perfusion of the tissues' – see Chapter 6) and drew attention to how pathological changes, in the lung for example, can be mistaken for autolysis.

An ability to interpret *post-mortem* change is important because it may help to determine the time of death (see earlier).

Progression of *post-mortem* changes can depend upon such factors as:

- Species of animal.
- Health status before death.
- Presence or absence of ingesta in the gastro-intestinal (GI) tract.
- Manner of death.
- Body temperature at time of death.
- Environmental temperature and humidity.
- Location and position of the body.
- Handling and storage following retrieval of the body.

Useful clues to the animal's history, time since death (see earlier) and/or the environmental conditions to which the carcase has been exposed may be provided by:

- Presence or absence of *rigor mortis*, *livor mortis* (hypostasis, pooling of blood, etc.) and *algor mortis* (cooling).
- Appearance of organs and tissues.
- Evidence of predation/scavenging by other animals such as dogs: this may be *ante mortem* or *post mortem*.
- Infestation by maggots, carrion, beetles, etc. (see later).

Organs and tissues undergo *post-mortem* autolysis at different rates. The following is an indication, starting with those organs that rapidly show breakdown and finishing with those that show relatively little decomposition:

- Retina.
- Brain.
- Testis.
- Gastro-intestinal (GI) tract.
- Pancreas.
- Liver.
- Kidney.
- Skin.
- Skeletal and heart muscle.
- Uterus.

There are also species differences. For example, the skin of fish and amphibians tends to autolyse sooner than does that of a mammal or bird.

Although, as a general rule, autolysis is more rapid at a higher temperature, caution must be exercised. As long ago as 1924, Robert Muir, in his *Text-book of Pathology*, pointed out that exposure of pieces of tissue to 55°C for an hour would denature enzymes and, as a result, delay autolysis. A similar situation can occur when a carcase, or part of it, becomes heated.

Studies have been carried out on certain species, especially humans (DiMaio and DiMaio, 2001), but also rats (Seaman, 1987) and poultry (Munger and McGavin, 1972). Remarkably little appears to have been published about *post-mortem* change in ectothermic animals, a notable exception being the study by Frye (1999). Frye's paper was prompted by his being called as an expert in a case involving the death of two captive pythons which necessitated his estimating their likely time of death. Finding nothing helpful (or acceptable in court), he decided to put together his own observations. Frye's article, which deserves to be more widely read, describes changes that can be associated with death in reptiles and amphibians. He emphasised that even when 'clinically dead', these species can exhibit residual cardiac contractions (see earlier). Frye then listed *post-mortem* indicators in reptiles and amphibians; these encompass many of those used in mammals but also include changes associated with the skin, such as bile-staining (see earlier), chromatophore relaxation and expansion and the production of characteristic odour(s).

The parlous shortage of published data on *post-mortem* change in ectothermic animals seriously hampers forensic investigation and needs to be rectified. Scattered information often exists (for example in texts and reports about spoilage of fish and molluscs intended for human consumption) and needs collation.

Seaman's (1984) book on *post-mortem* histological change in the rat reflects a scholarly study. He pointed out in his introduction that most of what is learned about autolysis is by word of mouth from more experienced colleagues: very little had previously been published. Laboratory (Sprague-Dawley) rats were used and six groups of nine individuals were euthanased and sampled at different times over a 16 hour period. Histological sections of a range of tissues were examined microscopically and appearances were described and photographed. Significant differences were noted between, for example, the tongue (where only minor changes were seen over the 16-hour *post-mortem* interval) and the colon (where epithelial loss and saprophytic bacterial invasion occurred early). Changes in some organs, e.g. kidney, showed that *post-mortem* autolysis does not advance uniformly.

The results obtained by Seaman are of considerable value to diagnostic pathologists and to those carrying out toxicological and other studies on rats in the laboratory setting. There is rather less relevance to forensic medicine because the conditions under which animals die and decompose under 'natural' conditions are very different from those in a research institute. The differences include:

- Variation in ambient temperature.
- Carcase(s) often not intact – if, for example, there are *ante-mortem* wounds or *post-mortem* predation.
- Variability in body size and condition.
- Species other than *Rattus norvegicus* are often involved.

There is a clear need for studies similar to Seaman's that, by simulating the forensic situation, take into account the points above (and others) but which, nevertheless, are scientifically sound. This proves far from easy. A project in 2004 at Bogoria, a soda lake in Kenya, East Africa, aimed to study *post-mortem* change in lesser flamingos by using dead chickens (domesticated fowl) as models. The fowls were placed in wire enclosures and pegged to the ground in order to prevent scavenging by baboons, warthogs or birds.

The gross appearance of each carcase was assessed (scored) every 24 hours for sixteen days. Selected tissues were taken each day for histopathological examination and invertebrates were collected for identification and, in the case of larvae, determination of age (instar). The findings are, at the time of writing (October 2005), still being collated but it is clear from initial analysis that many variables influence the gross and histological appearance and the invertebrates present. These include:

- Whether the fowl was exposed in whole or in part to soda water from the lake: this delayed

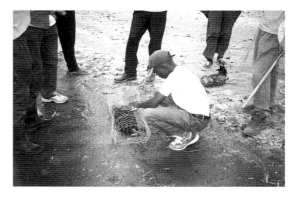

Figure 7.20 Forensic studies in the Rift Valley. A dead chicken in a cage is checked for *post-mortem* change and the presence of invertebrates. This figure also appears in colour in the colour plate section.

post-mortem change and either inhibited or killed carrion-feeding invertebrates.

- The different exposure of parts of the fowl to environmental factors (apart from soda water): the upper surface of the dead bird initially underwent rapid autolysis and invertebrate invasion but this changed if the weather was excessively hot and dry because a layer of desiccated skin formed and appeared thereafter to protect underlying tissues and to deter insects. The lower parts of the fowl were subject to less change and demonstrated a more programmed pattern of autolysis and invertebrate invasion – unless they were exposed to soda water.
- Fluctuating environmental temperatures, sometimes with rain and wind.

These preliminary studies illustrate how complex are the changes that occur under natural conditions, especially in areas of extreme aridity. Without the wire cages there would have been even more variables as carcases would, undoubtedly, have been opened, partly devoured and moved away from the water's edge by predators. The aim was to develop methods of more accurately assessing how long a flamingo had been dead but it is clear that many more experiments will be needed before this is achieved!

Post-mortem change is not only of importance in terms of assessing when an animal might have died and/or how it has been preserved or stored since (see earlier) but is also relevant to the practice of forensic pathology itself. It is not uncommon in standard diagnostic veterinary work for a laboratory to state that the carcase 'was too decomposed for a *post-mortem* examination.' Such a verdict could never apply to a forensic necropsy where no amount of autolysis negates the value of examination. An animal (or human) body may be only a liquefied 'soup' or a skeleton but this is the evidence and it must be properly examined. The words of Sir Arnold Theiler, the eminent South African veterinarian, when teaching osteology to students in the 1930s, are still pertinent: 'Gentlemen . . . you may think it is only an old bone. You have to put your soul into that bone'. Forensic pathology is not for the squeamish. A spirit of enthusiasm and curiosity,

the hallmarks of a detective, rapidly numb the senses to foetid smells, maggot-infested viscera or an uninviting pile of arachnid-ridden crumbling vertebrae.

FORENSIC ENTOMOLOGY

Insects can provide important evidence in the investigation of crime (Brandt, 2001; Erzinclioglu, 2000a,b; Hall and Donovan, 2001; Magana, 2001; Stroud and Adrian, 1996). In particular, the size and age (instar) of larvae or blowflies and certain other species can help in determination of the time, the sequence of events and sometimes the place of death, of both humans and animals (Lothe, 1964; Lundt, 1964). The PMI (*post-mortem* interval) is the time following death that a human corpse or an animal carcase has been exposed to the arthropod community. This discipline of 'forensic entomology' (it will be apparent from the foregoing that it includes invertebrates other than insects – see Chapter 2) is now well-established and many of the techniques are utilised in ecological studies on wildlife (e.g. Ellison, 1990), as well as in legal cases.

Forensic entomologists are not only concerned with death and the PMI. Invertebrates can provide useful clues in other legal cases – for instance, when questions are asked about the origin of imported materials and insect remains are detected. In addition, the finding of dipterous larvae on *live* humans and animals (myiasis) is beginning to be used to assess neglect (Benecke and Lessig, 2001) (see Chapter 6).

In recent years several books and many scientific articles have appeared about the use of invertebrates in legal medicine but the best introduction to the subject remains *A Manual of Forensic Entomology* (Smith, 1986). Smith's scholarly work was dedicated to three pioneers in the field of forensic entomology, Mégnin, Leclercq and Nuorteva, and his references included many by these and others from non-Anglophone countries, especially continental Europe (e.g. Leclercq, 1978; Leclercq and Tinant-Dubois, 1973; Leclercq and Watrin, 1973; Lopatenok *et al.*, 1964; Mégnin, 1894; Nuorteva, 1977). Smith also outlined the history of his subject. He stressed that, while forensic entomology has its roots in Europe, there is evidence that some basic understanding of flies and their role in providing evidence in homicide cases existed centuries before (McKnight, 1981).

The ability of maggots to transform and ultimately to destroy a carcase was recognised in the 18th century, notably by Linnaeus (1788), but the mechanisms and the genesis of the insects were not then understood.

The growth of forensic entomology has been closely linked with better understanding of the biology and natural history of the taxa involved. Leading entomologists in the 19th and 20th centuries threw much-needed light on the life-cycles and identification of the relevant taxa, especially blowflies and other Diptera, and some began to relate this to a possible medicolegal role for these insects (Yovanovitch, 1888).

Smith introduced his text with a lengthy section on the faunal succession on cadavers focusing attention on the significance of geographical location, temperature, humidity, light and shade on the type and speed of succession. These also affect the carcases on which the invertebrates feed. They cannot be covered in detail but are summarised in Table 7.7.

In comparative forensic work, the equation is often complicated by other factors such as the species of animal and the characteristics of their integument (mammal, bird, reptile . . . hair, feathers, scales), the animal's body size and its chemical composition. Entomological studies are increasingly being employed in animal forensic investigations but have not until recently been widely used in wildlife cases (Wobeser, 1996).

PRACTICAL ASPECTS OF FORENSIC ENTOMOLOGY

This is covered in Chapter 9 as it is particularly relevant to site visits and fieldwork.

EXHUMATION

In human forensic work, exhumation of bodies is standard and, depending upon various factors, the pathologist will be presented with anything from a well-preserved, still-clothed cadaver, to an array of bones. As the quotation at the beginning of the chapter points out, how rapidly a body decomposes depends upon many different factors, including how (if) it was encased, depth of burial, ambient temperature, soil type, presence or absence of water and, of course, whether it (the body) was embalmed.

Table 7.7 Factors affecting faunal succession on cadavers.

Factor	*Effect*	*Comments*
Ambient (environmental) temperature	High temperatures tend to hasten metamorphosis	Cyclical alternating temperatures can retard the development of some invertebrate species (Greenberg, 1991)
'Maggot' (intrinsic) temperature	Maggots will themselves generate heat, when feeding *en masse*	See above The temperature drops as maggots emigrate
Presence of toxic substances in or on carcase	May affect maggot development	Some substances kill or retard development of larvae A few, e.g. cocaine, may increase rate of development (Goff *et al.*, 1989)
Soil type, presence or absence of water, burning or chemical treatment of carcase	Various – complex	See literature

In veterinary and comparative forensics, comparable criteria apply. Wildlife cases (see Chapter 5) are often presented as decomposed carcases or parts thereof. Exhumation of an animal's body is occasionally carried out for legal (as opposed to archaeological or research) purposes. With the recent trend in North America and elsewhere to bury pet animals in caskets (some specifically advertised as 'waterproof and leak-proof'), similar factors come into play insofar as decomposition is concerned. The animal pathologist also has his/her equivalent of the embalmed body – the carcase or part thereof, of an animal that has been fixed in formalin, glutaraldehyde or an alcoholic preparation.

Such a carcase presents many of the same challenges as does the embalmed human cadaver. Useful information about embalming and its effects is to be found in Rutty (2001).

Drying and mummifying (see later) are not standard methods of preserving animal carcases but bodies are not infrequently submitted for examination that have been exposed to conditions that lead to desiccation and dry-preservation. Techniques for examination of such carcases are poorly documented but much useful guidance can be obtained from medical texts, gross publications by archaeologists and from the experiences of Egyptologists and

others. Mummified remains often attract an unusual and rather restricted range of invertebrates (Bourel *et al.*, 2000).

IDENTIFICATION OF CARCASES

In human forensic medicine identification of dead bodies is of great importance – perhaps never more so than in the months following the tsunami disaster of late 2004 (described in *The Independent* newspaper of 1 August 2005 as 'the world's biggest forensic operation'). Traditional methods based upon such criteria as clothing, jewellery, tattoos, scars and dentition are supplemented by DNA tests.

In animal work identifying bodies is of less importance although the reliable identification of live animals can be crucial (see Chapter 6). When dead animals or their remains do have to be identified, the methods listed in Table 7.8 can be employed.

Facial reconstruction, from skeletal remains, has become a skilled part of human forensic work but is at present of little relevance to veterinary/comparative forensic medicine other than for taxonomic and palaeontological studies on, for example, the evolution of primates.

Table 7.8 Identification of dead animals or their remains.

Method	Comments
External markings, colour patterns, etc.	Of limited value *per se* as confusion can easily occur Easily masked by *post-mortem* change
External morphological features, e.g. shape of horns, abnormal coloration or wear of hooves	Often of value, especially if linked with other characteristics Horn and hooves (keratin) often persist long after soft tissues have decomposed
Presence of external collars, chains, ear tags, sometimes tattoos and other human-introduced devices	Can be very reliable
Presence of internal devices, e.g. transponders	As above but detection may be difficult without the appropriate instrument or detailed dissection
Surgical evidence, e.g. castration, docked tail	A useful pointer but rarely reliable
Dentition	Will assist in identification of species and in aging (see elsewhere) Usually only of value in identifying individuals when dental work has been performed and good records kept

SKELETAL REMAINS

The particular features of these important samples are discussed later in this chapter.

NON-SKELETAL REMAINS

Sometimes viscera and bones are removed or widely scattered and nothing appears to remain of what was originally an intact dead animal.

In fact, often there are remains that can be found if the area is carefully searched as indicated in Table 7.9.

Detection of the above items requires meticulous sifting of soil and vegetation, where appropriate using equipment to collect trace evidence (see Chapter 10), followed by laboratory investigation. Placing suspect material in warm water will often assist – some components float (e.g. feathers), others sink (e.g. gizzard stones). Radiography (see later) can assist in the detection and recognition of the latter (and of radio-opaque ingesta).

Hair or feathers can provide much valuable information. They may come from the animal itself or something that is has killed or eaten (Stroud and

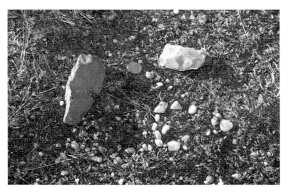

Figure 7.21 A carcase may disappear but evidence remains. A ring of stones from the gizzard of a now extinct moa in New Zealand. This figure also appears in colour in the colour plate section.

Adrian, 1998). Both hair and feathers have been the subject of research which is relevant to their role in forensic science (Ogle and Fox, 1999; Cooper *et al.*, 1989b).

In addition to macroscopical remains there may be other evidence that a carcase has been present at the site:

Table 7.9 Some examples of non-skeletal remains that might provide information in a forensic case.

Remains	*Comments*
Teeth	Often found scattered or buried
Hair, feathers, scales	Commonly present in small amounts (dried or caked with soil), even if the carcase has disappeared
Gizzard stones	Commonly found where certain birds (e.g. galliforms) have died in numbers (Figure 7.21)
Gallstones	Very occasionally found (Agnew *et al.*, 2005)
	Usually readily recognisable, if sectioned, by laminated structure or can be subjected to various analytical investigations, e.g. spectroscopy
Bladder stones	As above
Otoliths	A feature of some fish
	May be present in large numbers where fish have been devoured
Stomach or intestinal contents	May persist, especially if bone, fur, feather, scales or tough vegetation are present
Pellets (castings)	As stomach contents, but usually more compact and drier (Cooper, 2002)
Exoskeletons of invertebrates, including sea urchins	May remain in large numbers if an animal has died with large numbers of invertebrates within its GI tract

- Changes in the soil.
- Changes in the vegetation.
- Changes in the invertebrate fauna.

These investigations usually require expert assistance – forensic geologist, botanist and entomologist respectively.

There is also the question of how best to mark small carcases and pieces of tissue so that they can be used as evidence in court or be readily recognisable when examined in the laboratory. Bags, jars and other containers can be used (see Chapter 8) but once the specimen is removed, it may be lost or transposed. Various methods of identification are available, ranging from the tying (if necessary, suturing) of identity tags or the implantation of microchips, to the cutting in soft tissues (e.g. a piece of fixed spleen) of tiny notches, using a scalpel blade.

TAKING AND SUBMISSION OF LABORATORY SAMPLES AND SUPPORTING INVESTIGATIONS

Forensic *post-mortem* examination may permit a whole range of techniques to be employed that are not usually part of the repertoire of the routine diagnostician.

A small laboratory, adjacent to the clinical or *post-mortem* area, is of great value. It enables certain tests to be carried out immediately and these may yield information while the animal is still being examined: cytological ('touch preparation') samples are an example. The proximity of the laboratory also minimises the risk of sensitive samples drying, e.g. buccal swabs from birds that may be harbouring motile *Trichomonas gallinae* organisms.

A list of basic items to equip such a small laboratory is provided in Appendix E.

SELECTION OF SAMPLES

In forensic work this depends upon the circumstances and the questions that are being asked. Samples that may be taken from live animals, some of them applicable also to *post-mortem* material, are listed in Chapter 6. The choice of sample will be influenced by the purpose for which the test is to be performed. Some may be routine, others more complex. Samples for toxicology often present particular challenges and it may be wise to consult the laboratory before taking material. Species differences may be important: for example, a recent paper (Jeffree *et al.*, 2005) advocated the use of osteoderms (dermal bones) for the measurement of metals in crocodiles!

Samples are not only taken for biomedical investigation. Some, such as explosives, ammunition and weapons will be examined by specialists in forensic and other laboratories.

LABORATORY TESTS

Additions to routine gross (macroscopical) *post-mortem* investigation that may be employed in forensic work are listed in Table 7.10 below. Laboratory tests are discussed in more detail in Chapter 8.

In most cases only a few of these additional investigations will be justified initially. However, it is good practice to retain material (e.g. liver in glutaraldehyde for TEM, brain frozen at 200°C for analysis of pesticides) in case further investigations prove necessary or are requested by a court. Various laboratory techniques are discussed in more detail in Chapter 8.

Correct, secure storage of material taken from a forensic case is vital – as is confidentiality (see Chapter 11). Samples must be handled carefully because of health and safety considerations (see, for example, PAW, 2005) and labelled or marked so that they cannot be misplaced or transposed.

SOME SPECIFIC *POST-MORTEM* FINDINGS

This book is not the place for detailed pathology but some guidelines and comments will be provided on gross findings that are often of relevance in legal, insurance or other cases. Reference should also be made to Chapter 6 for description of some condi-

Table 7.10 Some additional investigations.

Technique	Comment
Direct examination with hand lens, magnifying loupe or dissecting microscope	Recommended initially for any tissue or sample
Radiography (part or whole-body)	Dental or low kV X-ray machines are ideal for small animals or structures
	Digital kits are increasingly being used but check on admissibility in court
Histopathology	Samples (lung, liver, kidney plus abnormalities) should be taken routinely
	Buffered formol saline (BFS) is the standard fixative
Bacteriology	If a bacterial infection is suspected
Mycology	If a fungal infection is suspected
Virology	If a viral infection is suspected, but virology is neither easy nor cheap
Parasitology	A useful routine (ecto- and endoparasites) in all necropsies
	Combine faecal examination with cytology below
	'Ecological tagging' uses helminths to identify the stock from which fish originate
	The presence of parasites may help to pinpoint the origin of other species
Cytology, specific organs, intestinal contents, exudates, etc.	A whole range of simple and rapid tests that can provide useful information in legal cases
Haematology	Small quantities of blood may be obtained from the heart or elsewhere of freshly dead animals
Biochemistry	As above
Toxicology	See text – important in many forensic investigations
DNA studies	Identification, sexing
	Valuable
	Appropriate material should always be stored
Scanning electronmicroscopy (SEM)	Of value in specific cases
	Expensive
Transmission electronmicroscopy (TEM)	As above
Bone preparation, examination and analysis	Bone density and other studies
Digestion studies	Studies on soft tissues
Ashing and mineral analysis, including whole-body studies	Studies on hard tissues (see, for example, Schryver *et al.*, 1974)
Radioisotope studies	See text – aging of remains

tions of forensic importance that can cause clinical signs as well as death.

Starvation

This is discussed in detail later in this chapter.

Dehydration

Dehydration can be a very important finding in legal cases, especially when deprivation of water is alleged (see also Chapter 6).

Dehydration in the live animal is fairly readily assessed using a combination of clinical investigations (e.g. skin 'tenting' and subjective assessment of the viscosity of oral mucus) and laboratory tests (e.g. packed cell volume – PCV). Even so, it is not always easy, especially in ectothermic animals.

Apparent dehydration in a carcase can be misleading and erroneous. In a freshly-dead mammal ('fresh' defined as less than 2–3 hours, but easily affected by temperature, location, etc.), skin tenting and other 'clinical' assessments may still be helpful but PCV estimation, even on apparently still liquid heart blood, is likely to be unreliable because of clotting. Once the animal has been dead for a few hours – and especially if it is in sunshine or exposed to strong winds – any attempt to assess skin tenting is fraught with danger.

Abortions

Abortions are not usually as significant in animal forensic work as they are in human practice but they can still be the subject of a legal case, or an insurance claim or an allegation of professional malpractice, especially when valuable animals such as thoroughbred horses are involved. They may also be a source of zoonotic infections and therefore have implications for human health.

Important features in any investigation include:

- As comprehensive a history as possible, including vaccination records, recent arrivals, age distribution of affected animals, abortion rate and stage of abortion.
- Full clinical examination, including reproductive tract, of the dam.

- *Post-mortem* examination of the aborted fetus and placenta, taking into account the special anatomical features of neonates and checking carefully for developmental, possibly genetic, abnormalities (see Chapter 6) or infectious disease, with supporting laboratory tests on vaginal discharges and blood from the dam where indicated. Knowledge of both normal and abnormal embryological development is important in such work. If anomalies are detected or suspected, reference should be made to texts, some of them based on human studies (e.g. Sadler, 2005) that may help to explain the morphogenesis of such disorders.
- Confirmation as to whether the fetus was indeed aborted (born dead) or, perhaps, lived a short while and then died. This can be important in some legal cases and insurance claims. Whether or not lung floats, coupled with its histological appearance, remains the mainstay of this differentiation but must be interpreted carefully (decomposition with gas production and artificial resuscitation can cause atelectatic lung to float) and be coupled with meticulous examination of the cardiovascular system.

Estimation of age (maturity) of the aborted fetus is important in human forensic medicine (Shepherd, 2003) and such information may be requested in incidents where animals are involved. Data are available for most domesticated species.

In difficult cases, it is wise to involve a specialist theriogenologist.

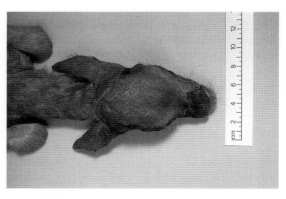

Figure 7.22 Neonates should always be checked for developmental abnormalities. This fawn is brachygnathic.

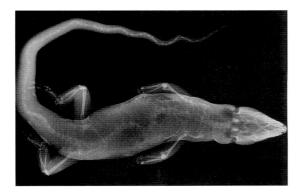

Figure 7.23 Scoliosis in a skink.

Poisoning and chemical burns

Poisons can cause clinical disease (see Chapter 6) and/or death. Toxic substances may either have a directly toxic effect on animals (for example, causing damage in liver or kidney) or they may damage superficial or exposed tissues such as skin, mucous membranes, alimentary system or respiratory tract.

A wide array of substances can prove toxic to animals and may, as a result of intentional or accidental exposure, cause illness or death. Both domesticated stock and wildlife (vertebrate and invertebrate) may be affected, the latter sometimes on a vast scale (PAW, 2005). There is extensive veterinary toxicology literature in many languages and this may need to be consulted in a forensic case. Even more data probably exist in the files of pharmaceutical and agrochemical companies, where results of efficacy and safety tests – many involving laboratory animals – are maintained and may be made available on request. Poisons that can kill animals and which may be ingested, inhaled or absorbed through the skin range from arsenical compounds and herbicides to zinc phosphide and insecticides. Acids and alkalis are still used commonly, by mouth or by topical application, to kill or to injure animals and can sometimes form part of a pattern of animal abuse.

In cases where poisoning is strongly suspected or confirmed and there is a possible question of culpability, many considerations arise. For example, in the case of dogs and cats, factors contributory to poisoning can include:

- Failure to keep human or veterinary medicines in a safe place.
- Use of 'medicines' that were either not intended for the dog or cat or administered incorrectly.
- Access to toxic chemicals because of poor storage of, say, ethylene glycol (antifreeze), herbicides, rodent baits or slug pellets.

In some countries advisory bodies exist that can assist with suspect poisonings – for example, the Veterinary Poisons Information Service in the UK.

The pathologist can play a key role in the diagnosis of poisoning, even if only by excluding other causes of death and then submitting appropriate samples (which may include dead animals and possible sources of poisoning, e.g. baits) to a toxicologist (Shepherd, 2003). Sometimes gross or histological findings may assist in diagnosis of toxicity – in lead poisoning, for example.

Interpretation of findings in believed poisoning cases often benefits from a 'case conference', with input from the pathologist, toxicologist and other specialists. Specialist advice may be needed in cases where ectothermic vertebrates (e.g. fish) or invertebrates (e.g. honey bees) have died. In some cases, the presence of a toxic substance in the body of an animal may be significant even if it does not provide a cause of death *per se* – for example, polychlorinated biphenyls (PCBs) which, because they are immunosuppressive, can predispose some species to infectious disease. In forensic work the possibility that ill-health or death is multifactorial must never be overlooked; this is often a difficult concept to put over to a lawyer or jury.

Poisoning from a clinical point of view is discussed in more detail in Chapter 6.

Trauma

Wounds in humans due to trauma are an important feature of many legal cases (Mason and Purdue, 2000). The aetiology and pathogenesis of trauma in animals were discussed by Cooper (Cooper, J.E., 1996a).

Wounds, whether in live or dead animals, must be carefully described. Healing should also be investigated. Much has been written about wounds in humans (Bucknall and Ellis, 1984). The basic

Table 7.11 Incisions and lacerations – some distinctions.

Feature	Incision	Laceration
Appearance	Sharply outlined Linear, curved or angular Bruising rare Strands of tissue bridging the wound rarely present	Often irregularly outlined Round, oval or stellate Bruising common Tissue bridges often present
Pelage	Little or no loss of hair or feathers around wound	Hair or feathers may be absent
Haemorrhage	Marked	Minimal or apparently absent

approach to investigation in a forensic case is likely to be the same whether one is dealing with a Bactrian camel or a trout. However, there are some important differences, even amongst domesticated animals, and these are reflected in the papers and books dealing with, for example, the particular considerations when managing injuries of horses. Comparative studies on wounds and wound-healing include research on fish and other ectotherms (see, for example, Smith *et al.*, 1988) and these provide a rich database for those who need to understand better the processes that apply in different species.

Both incised and lacerated wounds may be seen in attacks on humans and animals (see earlier). Definitions are important: an incision is a break in the continuity of the skin caused by an object with a sharp edge (Davison, 2004). This is in contrast to a laceration, which is caused by blunt force (see Appendix C). Some distinctions between incisions and lacerations ate shown in Table 7.11. Wounds from weapons are discussed later.

FORENSIC ODONTOLOGY

In human forensic work this is a very well-developed discipline in its own right (Brown *et al.*, 2005; Cameron and Sims, 1973; Cottone and Standish, 1982; Shepherd, 2003; Sopher, 1976; Whittaker and MacDonald, 1989), where it is largely concerned with:

• Identification of cadavers and human remains (Pretty and Addy, 2002).

• Estimation of age of the living and dead (Morse *et al.*, 1994).
• Investigation and interpretation of bite marks and lip prints (see later and Chapter 6).
• Description and investigation of dental and oral lesions, especially those due to trauma, where there are legal implications (Barsley, 1993).

These methods are discussed by a number of authors – see, for example Clark (1994), Nambiar and Nadesan (2004) and Wilson and Brown (1993). Specific forensic techniques are often described in dental journals – radiology and photography being two examples (De Vore, 1977; Havel, 1985).

However, despite the importance of animal bites, both in human and veterinary work, comparative aspects have usually not attracted the same interest. This means that those who are involved in such work must often extrapolate from human odontology and make best use of what has been published in the veterinary, pathological and zoo-archaeological literature.

Some standard veterinary dental texts are available (e.g. Crossley and Penman, 1995; Harvey, 1985). The seminal work by Colyer, revised by Miles and Grigson (1990), is essential reading insofar as comparative aspects of dentition are concerned. References to the odontology of some species are also to be found in specialised journals – for instance, reports of anomalies affecting the teeth in dolphins (Brooks and Anderson, 1998) and a detailed description of dental and mandibular injury in a fur seal (Erb *et al.*, 1996).

Clinical examination of the oral cavity is discussed in Chapter 6. Some similar criteria can be used when investigating *post-mortem* bite wounds. In wildlife cases particular attention may have to be paid to gross *post-mortem* features – in cases, for instance, where it is alleged that dogs have been used illegally for hunting (PAW, 2005). An example of how detailed studies could assist in forensic cases is provided by the paper by Simpson (2006) on patterns and significance of bite wounds in otters.

Lip-print identification (cheiloscopy) is not, apparently, widely used in animal forensics but may have potential. It has parallels with, e.g., the identification of gorillas using their unique nose prints.

Bite-mark analysis is a specialised field (Rothwell, 1995). Its admissibility in court was established some years ago (Hale, 1978). In animal work reference can usefully be made to texts concerning human forensic medicine – the use in some cases of scanning electronmicroscopy (David, 1986), digital imaging (Naru and Dykes, 1996), histology (Millington, 1974), contrast-medium-enhanced radiography (Rawson *et al.*, 1979) and computerised axial tomography (Farrel *et al.*, 1987).

Dental examination is important in *post-mortem* forensic work and is widely used by zoo-archaeologists to identify and age the skeletal remains of animals (Davis, 1987; O'Connor, 2000). Single teeth can assist in the speciation of both domesticated and wild animals – cetaceans are a particularly good example of the latter – and the famous French zoologist Cuvier is reported to have said 'Show me your teeth and I will tell you what you are.'

INTER- AND INTRA-SPECIFIC AGGRESSION

Fighting amongst animals can cause both soft tissue and bony injuries (see later). Studies of fossilised material have revealed evidence of aggression and predation in extinct species, including bite wounds in crocodiles (Mackness and Sutton, 2000).

In wildlife cases it may be important to distinguish lesions caused by dogs – for instance, in hunting or coursing – from those that may be inflicted by another species (PAW, 2005).

ROAD TRAFFIC (VEHICULAR) ACCIDENTS/COLLISIONS

These are a common cause of injury or death in animals and in humans (see Chapter 6). They are sometimes referred to as 'transportation injuries' (see later). Much has been published on vehicular accident investigation and reconstruction because of its importance in human forensics (Van Kirk, 2001).

AIRCRAFT ACCIDENTS

Aircraft crashes are relevant to human medical forensic specialists and may constitute a crime scene if, for example, a terrorist action is suspected (see Chapter 1). A substantial amount has been published about the effects of aircraft accidents (and other incidents such as depressurisation and exposure to low temperatures) on humans but very little appears to be available, certainly in the literature, concerning aircraft and animals.

Animals can also be involved in aircraft incidents:

- If they are being transported legally in the cabin.
- If they are illegally or accidentally transported with the baggage.
- If they (usually wild birds) are the cause of an accident (see later).
- If livestock or other animals on the ground are killed or damaged as a result of a crash, or falling debris.
- If animals on the ground are frightened, possibly panicked, following the flying-over of a noisy (possibly supersonic) or low-flying aircraft (Grubb and Bowerman, 1997).

Any veterinarian or other person involved in investigating such incidents should familiarise him/herself with the extensive literature relating to aircraft and the effects that they can have on humans, animals or property. The various international and national authorities should also be consulted, as should (if appropriate) the military.

TRAPS AND SNARES

These are discussed in Chapter 5, in view of their importance in the context of wildlife crime. They are relevant to both animal welfare and species' protection (PAW, 2005).

Gross and microscopical examination are important in investigating wounds inflicted by items that are used to catch animals – including fish hooks, which can cause severe damage, even death, in both target species and other (protected) animals (Borucinska *et al.*, 2002).

WOUNDS FROM WEAPONS

These will be discussed under two main headings – knife (stab) wounds and gunshot wounds. Various other weapons can be used to inflict damage on animals, ranging from hammers to garden forks. In poorer countries or more rural locations, machetes (cutlasses, pangas), spears and arrows are often the offending items, usually producing a characteristic 'chop wound' (DiMaio and DiMaio, 2001).

Knife (stab) wounds

These are a frequent cause of injury in humans and animals. Their dynamics have been studied using human cadavers (Knight, 1975; O'Callaghan *et al.*, 1999), as have the gross and microscopical features of different types of wound (Humphrey and Hutchinson, 2001; Tucker *et al.*, 2001). Studies on naturally occurring firearm lesions in animals were reported by Corradi *et al.*, (2001), Nozdryn-Potnicki *et al.*, (2005) and Urquhart and McKendrick (2003).

Williams *et al.* (1998) advocated that, when describing stab wounds, the following should be included:

- Position and angle of the wounds.
- Their dimensions.
- The tissues or organs that are affected.

Similar criteria apply to knives and other cutting weapons but here the examination of the wound may rely on the sharpness and structure of the

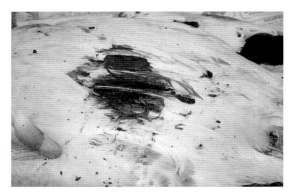

Figure 7.24 A characteristic *ante-mortem* stab wound, in this case in a flamingo, caused by the beak of a marabou stork. This figure also appears in colour in the colour plate section.

weapons, particularly its shape and the number of cutting edges (e.g. serrations) that are present.

As a general rule, a stab wound is deeper than it is long while a slash wound is longer than it is deep. The wounds produced by such weapons may be incisions or lacerations, or sometimes a combination of the two.

Stab wounds can also be a feature of predation or aggression between animals – for example, if a stork stabs and kills another bird (see Figure 7.24). Many of the features are similar to those described above but there are species' differences.

Gunshot wounds

Firearms play an important part in physical assaults against humans, especially in certain countries, and can produce wounds of medical and legal importance (DiMaio, 1999; DiMaio and DiMaio, 2001; Robbins *et al.*, 1999; Warlow, 1996). Guns also contribute to injury and death in animals, both domesticated (Dabas and Saxena, 1994) and wild (PAW, 2005; Stroud and Adrian, 1996; Wobeser, 1996). Scientific interest in gunshot injuries goes back to John Hunter who studied them in the Peninsular War (Hunter, 1794).

Gunshot wounds vary greatly in appearance and this is complicated in animal forensics because of the different morphology of the species that may be involved. Such factors as whether or not feathers or scales are present will influence the appearance of these and other wounds. So also will the type of firearm used: in the UK in recent years there has been an increase in the use for homicide of small calibre weapons, such as modified air-cartridge revolvers and converted blank-firing guns, and this may be reflected in due course in animal injuries. Such weapons present a challenge to the pathologist because they produce 'atypical' gunshot wounds; sometimes, for example, the entry and exit holes are difficult to distinguish.

Airguns are often used to kill or maim domesticated and wild animals and a recent report, *Airgun Agony*, by the Scottish Society for the Prevention of Cruelty to Animals (see Appendix B) showed that 40% of Scottish veterinary surgeons questioned had treated an animal with an airgun wound (Newton, 2005b).

The basic features of gunshot wounds were described by Williams *et al.* (1998), amongst others, and can be summarised as follows:

(1) Contact wounds up to 2 cm diameter: a ragged entrance wound is present; soot or gunpowder may be obvious and carbon monoxide may be detectable in the tissues.

(2) Close range, 2–50 cm: the wound is likely to be circular and concave; soot or gunpowder are unlikely to be detected macroscopically (cf. contact wound) but can be seen microscopically in histological sections; feathers or hairs may be singed by the weapon.

(3) Longer range: the entrance wound is likely again to be circular and concave; there may be grease-soiling on the bullet and soot or gunpowder are not usually visible macroscopically or microscopically.

Shotgun wounds show characteristic features relating to the distance and angle and a tangential shotgun injury may glance off the animal's body producing a wound that resembles a laceration. Usually shotgun wounds present a rounded hole with a narrow rim of soot at close contact. At close range the hole is round or oval and may have a ragged margin of soot deposition and singeing of feathers or hair may be present. At longer range, spread of the shot can result in a central entry hole with multiple peripheral separated holes. The central

hole ultimately disappears leaving a scattering of small holes. Measurements of the scatter pattern can be used to give an approximate range but, as in all ballistic work, it is best if this is correlated with the gun that fired the shot.

There are important differences between the damage caused by a low-velocity weapon, such as a handgun, and those from a high-velocity rifle (Stroud and Adrian, 1996). The latter cause severe injury and shock waves created by the energy of the bullet and can destroy tissues that are not in the pathway.

A very important part of investigation of gunshot wounds is to ascertain the type of weapon that was used (Williams *et al.*, 1998). Electronic databases are available that can help determine the weapon type that was most likely to have discharged a suspect bullet or cartridge case. This is a very specialised field and an expert's advice is usually needed (Wallace and Beavis, 2004). The pathologist must, however, be willing and able to describe the wounds and to investigate them correctly (Table 7.12).

Radiography is important (essential, according to Stroud and Adrian, 1996) in investigation of the wound tract made by a bullet and in recovering fragments from tissues. Wobeser (1996) advocated the use of both radiography and fluoroscopy in wildlife cases.

The microscopical examination of bullets and cartridge cases remains an important part of firearm examination and is increasingly becoming automated. It is crucial that the pathologist removes, handles and stores all ballistic material with care. For example, plastic forceps should be used to

Table 7.12 Differentiation between entry and exit gunshot wounds.

Entry	*Exit*
Well circumscribed, round or oval	Often ragged edges, irregular shape
A 'collar' of abrasion and discharge residue may be visible	Collar and discharge residue rarely present
The same size or smaller than the bullet	Variable size

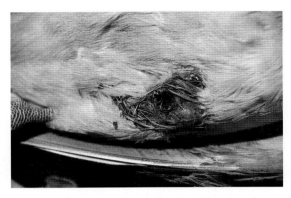

Figure 7.25 An *ante-mortem* shot wound in a parakeet. This figure also appears in colour in the colour plate section.

remove bullets and contact must be avoided with other metallic objects. Bullets and fragments need to be gently rinsed and dried, to avoid oxidation, and then wrapped individually in soft material in a firm container. Other precautions may be wise: ballistics experts can usually advise.

In a court case, questions may be asked as to whether a shot wound was the last tract to have been formed in an animal's carcase – the concept of the 'terminal probability'. This is important in cases regarding the culling of deer, in which the law stipulates minimal legal ballistic requirements and where the sequence of events is relevant to animal welfare (Urquhart and McKendrick, 2006).

It may also be necessary to ascertain whether only one or more than one person was involved in a shooting incident (e.g. during a hunting expedition or a street fight). An animal's carcase may contain bullets, shot or pellets from different guns. Interpretation can be complex and far from straightforward (Mann *et al.*, 1994; Stroud and Adrian, 1996).

PHYSICAL ASSAULT

Physical injuries may be due to assault by animals of the same species, by others of a different species and by human beings. Intra-specific injuries include fight wounds, some inflicted during courtship or competition for mates (Duff and Hunt, 1995). Attacks by other species may involve 'normal'

predation (e.g. a hawk hunts a rabbit – wild or domesticated) or mass killings, as can be a feature when a fox gains access to poultry (Moberly *et al.*, 2004) or finds itself amongst breeding sea-birds (Ennion and Tinbergen, 1967) (see also Chapter 5).

Animals with 'non-accidental' injuries caused by humans (see Chapter 6) may show a number of changes but great care must be exercised in interpretation, especially when large numbers of wild animals are involved (Ralston, 1999). In individual animals kicking or stomping injuries are sometimes a feature of anthropogenic trauma. These are characterised by multiple lesions including bruising and fractured bones. Jumping on the animal's body may cause fractured ribs and damage to internal viscera, including rupture of liver or spleen.

STRANGULATION AND HANGING

Strangulation is a broad term. Compression of the neck can cause death by occluding the trachea (see Table 7.13), by preventing venous return to the heart, by reducing arterial flow to the brain and causing asphyxia (see later) or by exerting specific effects on, e.g., the vagus nerve or carotid sinuses (Shepherd, 2003).

Hanging by the neck can cause death in the same way or by damage to the spinal cord. The vertebral column is often not affected unless the body has dropped a substantial distance (Kumar *et al.*, 2005). Animals may be strangled intentionally by an attack (human or animal) or as a result of self-inflicted damage, e.g. a dog pulling incessantly on a collar or choke-chain.

Both strangulation and hanging can take place in animals and they will need to be differentiated. Medical forensic pathologists use several criteria (DiMaio and DiMaio, 2001; Shepherd, 2003). In animals there are two important differences (Table 7.14).

BLAST INJURIES

Animals may be exposed to blasts accidentally (e.g. because they are trapped in a building that explodes)

Table 7.13 Levels of asphyxia (hypoxia/anoxia).

Level	Example	Comments
External (insufficient oxygen in inhaled air)	Gaseous poisoning Accumulation of carbon dioxide Obstruction of animal's nares, mouth or gills Smothering	Diagnosis may depend upon a combination of history and assessment of the environment
Upper respiratory tract	Foreign bodies or pathological lesions in buccal/nasal cavity, pharynx/larynx or trachea or bronchi Strangulation or hanging	The offending obstruction can usually be located *post mortem* Occasionally it is missing or may have moved (e.g. a migrating ascarid worm)
Lower respiratory tract	Inhaled foreign bodies (see above) or pulmonary pathology	Careful investigation is needed
Cardiovascular system	May impair oxygen exchange	Can be detected macroscopically, e.g. myocarditis, or need detailed investigation, e.g. anaemia
Cellular	Some substances prevent the transportation or diffusion of oxygen across the alveoli or restrict its availability to tissues	Poisons, e.g. cyanide or (fish) nitrites, are often the cause
Thoracic cavity	Crushing or pressure injuries that prevent respiratory movement	See Trauma

Table 7.14 Differentiating strangulation and hanging.

Strangulation	Hanging
Single or multiple marks on skin (including hair loss) and subcutis	A single, usually deep, mark
Animal may attempt to defend itself, by biting or scratching, and thus show other lesions	No defence lesions but animal may attempt to remove the ligature by rubbing or scratching with its forelegs only

or intentionally (e.g. cattle are sometimes used to detect land mines). Dogs trained to detect explosives or to locate cadavers (see Chapter 2) are particularly at risk.

Much has been published on blast injuries in humans (Beveridge, 1998) and much of this can be applied to animals of comparable size. Death is probably more likely in small animals because of their low body mass and their vulnerability to secondary factors, including predation (Table 7.15).

'Shock', characterised by profound psychological as well as physiological effects, is now well-recognised in humans (Guy, 2004). Whether any similar syndrome occurs in animals does not appear to have been explored.

NEONATAL DEATHS

Although neonatal deaths of (human) infants are not, *per se*, unusual – especially in poorer countries – inexplicable mortality is often the subject of debate, sometimes dissent, amongst the medical profession. Legal action may ensue, alleging that the child was killed by a parent. Concerns in the

Table 7.15 Features of blast (explosion) injuries in animals.

Category	Cause	Features
Primary	Direct effects of blast	Pressure wave damages external and internal tissue: often fatal Burns may occur
Secondary	Effects of wood splinters, broken glass, etc.	Flying objects cause external damage
Tertiary	Animal's body is thrown about (especially small/light species, such as birds)	May cause severe external and internal damage and concussion

UK about certain high-profile cases and the stigma that can attach to such terms as 'cot death' or 'unascertained death' have led to public debate and to such incidents being officially reclassified as 'unexplained infant death'. An understanding of research on neonatal deaths in infants and also of the controversy that some of the cases have engendered can be important for those involved in comparative forensic work.

Some neonatal deaths in humans and animals are due to intentional infliction of trauma ('violence'). In the so-called 'shaken baby syndrome' in human infants there is a triad of signs:

(1) Subdural haematoma.
(2) Retinal haemorrhages.
(3) Haemorrhages in the spinal cord.

In child abuse, important features may be:

• Bruising in unusual places.
• Multiple injuries, often of different ages, of both soft tissues and skeleton.
• Derangement of the teeth.
• Bite marks.
• Unusual lesions such as cigarette burns, scalds or linear areas of damage.

Similar findings may be a feature of abuse of animals (see Chapter 6).

Neonatal death in both humans and animals can be due to other non-infectious factors (accidental or intentional) – for example, suffocation, hypothermia, drowning or electrocution, and these are discussed either later in this chapter or in Chapter 6. Infectious disease, of, for example, the respiratory tract, can complicate these and other conditions or cause neonatal disease in its own right. In all *post-mortem* examinations, but especially those of neonates, it is important to look carefully for developmental abnormalities that may have predisposed to death or ill-health (see earlier) (see Figures 7.22 and 7.23).

SPECIFIC INJURIES AND LESIONS

A few specific injuries will be discussed, with references given to appropriate further reading. It is important to remember that all injuries should be photographed in colour, with labels, and measured (see earlier).

Trauma to the brain

Damage to the head, inflicted intentionally or accidentally, can cause brain damage and necessitate particularly careful dissection and interpretation (Graham and Gennarelli, 2000; Murrey, 2000; Whitwell, 2005; Williams *et al.*, 1998). Some of our knowledge of the effects of head injury is based on animal studies (Adams *et al.*, 1983).

Brain damage in animals commonly follows road traffic accidents, fighting and blows to the head or the back of the neck. Clinical investigation of such injuries has advanced greatly in recent years but usually necessitates the use of sophisticated equipment. Correct interpretation of findings requires specialised knowledge (Platt, 2005). Often, however, the injuries prove fatal in which case it is the pathologist who must perform the investigations. Gross *post-mortem* examination must be coupled with histological work. Whenever possible, the latter should include studies on the eyes; brain injuries in both humans and animals can cause haemorrhage in the sclera, choroid and retina.

Trauma to the spinal cord

The spinal cord is also susceptible to injury following trauma. A variety of clinical signs (Webb *et al.*, 2004) and *post-mortem* lesions may be shown. Haemorrhages in the cord are referred to as *haematomyelia* and commonly occur in 'natural' injuries (e.g. when a rabbit damages its back during handling), as well as following an assault or road traffic accident. Radiography and careful dissection may be needed.

Transportation injuries

This term is sometimes used in human forensic medicine to encompass a whole range of injuries associated with accidents involving aircraft, motor vehicles, bicycles and trains (Levinson and Granot, 2002; Williams *et al.*, 1998). In each of these the person may be either a passenger or a pedestrian and a spectrum of pathological lesions, some of them almost pathognomonic, is recognised.

Similar injuries may be caused to animals and a certain amount of extrapolation from human work is both possible and acceptable. There are important differences, however, for example in the position and type of injuries when a dog strikes a windscreen or is hit by the bumper of a slow-moving car.

In animal work 'transportation injuries' has a broader meaning – more allied to the new human discipline of 'travel medicine'. Animals of different species are transported for a variety of reasons and for distances ranging from 100 metres to traversing the globe. Legal action, claims for compensation or other actions may follow complications (alleged or actual) arising from such movement.

The correct and safe despatching and reception of live animals by air, road or water is a specialised subject, requiring both adequate training and practical experience. Any veterinarian asked to give an opinion in cases relating to death or injury to an animal while it was being moved should ensure that s/he has access to appropriate advice, including the relevant legislation, codes of practice and the requirements of the IATA (International Air Transport Association) Regulations (see Appendix B).

Asphyxia

The term refers to a reduction in oxygen (hypoxia) or a total absence of oxygen (anoxia). It is commonly due to an obstruction to air flow and this can occur at various levels (see Table 7.13). Investigation of supposed hypoxic deaths requires careful necropsy (Dabas and Saxena, 1994) and, where appropriate, linking the findings with the environment in which the animal was found.

The ability of animals to resist hypoxia varies greatly. Reptiles, amphibians and fish are particularly resistant (see Chapter 2). In endothermic species such factors as body temperature may be significant: for example, a mammal or bird immersed in ice or snow may survive longer than one at normal body temperature. A few species are even tolerant of whole-body freezing.

Hyperthermia and hypothermia

These are discussed in detail in Chapter 6.

Electrocution

This is discussed in detail in Chapter 6. A useful summary of the effects of an electrical force was by Sornogyi and Tedeschi (1977). Electrocution can be associated with specific entry and exit wounds but usually only if there is a focus of contact with the source of electricity. Shaving of the hair or removal of feathers is an important prerequisite to the examination of a carcase for signs of other changes. Often the skin lesions are very subtle (see later).

The most frequent causes of electrocution in animals are exposure to electrical circuits (Dabas and Saxena, 1994), to lightning (see Appendix D) or to power lines. Power lines are of more importance than lightning to wild birds and can cause physical damage due to collision (see Chapter 7) as well as electrocution. In general, alternating current (a.c.) is more dangerous than direct current (d.c.).

Electrocution damages tissues directly and by producing burns (Sornogyi and Tedeschi, 1977). Respiration can cease completely (apnoea) (see Chapter 6) and ventricular fibrillation is usually the cause of death in fatal cases. Burning or charring of the hair or feathers often is apparent, especially in lightning strike, sometimes with a linear, 'arborizing' (wood-like) patterned appearance (DiMaio and DiMaio, 2001; Robbins *et al.*, 1999). In severe cases, much of the carcase may be burned to the bone, giving a 'fossilised' appearance. Lymph nodes are often haemorrhagic and there can be free blood in the respiratory tract. There may be discoloration and rigor of muscles and the blood may appear black and unclotted. In less severe cases lesions may be few, other than slight burns and petechiae.

The distribution of lesions in electrocution cases depends on the area affected, e.g. the current may have passed only through the legs or from a wing tip to a foot. Other factors also will influence the location and severity, e.g. whether the pelage is wet or dry. Therefore, great care must be taken when carrying out the *post-mortem* examination (Dabas and Saxena, 1994). The pathology of electrocution in domesticated mammals was discussed by Giles and Simmons (1975) and in humans, with a good selection of references, by DiMaio and DiMaio (2001).

A legal case relating to electrocution is likely to be brought on such grounds as:

- Poor maintenance of electrical equipment.
- Allowing a captive animal access to domesticated appliances or power lines.
- Unlawful killing (even in an abattoir, where electric stunning tongs may not be used properly).

Lightning strike

The pathogenesis of this is outlined above. Shepherd (2003) emphasised how varied the lesions associated with lightning can be, often including burns, lacerations and fractures. Occasionally magnetisation, or melting and solidification, of metal objects occur. A case study and a suggested veterinary certificate that might be issued in such cases are given in Appendices D and A respectively.

Burns and death in fires

Fire is a common cause of ill-health and death in both domesticated and wild animals (see Chapter 6; Cooper, 1996a; Dabas and Saxena, 1994). Fires may occur accidentally (in the home, in a zoo, in a laboratory, in the bush) or may be started intentionally, either in order to harm humans or animals or to mask evidence of homicide, killing or other unlawful acts. Much has been published about fires and arson (see, for example, Daéid, 2003).

Factors that influence the *post-mortem* appearance of an animal that has been burned include the duration of exposure, the temperature attained and the size and structure of the body.

It is important to differentiate surface burns, including scalds, from *post-mortem* artefacts associated with incineration.

Diagnosis of burning is assisted by examination of the airways for evidence of heat damage and soot deposition. Toxicological analysis is possible for carbon monoxide or other chemicals and histological examination can provide evidence of inhalation of soot or other products. Hair, feathers and scales may show typical light and electronmicroscopical changes (see Figure 6.8).

Drowning

Drowning is discussed in some detail in Chapter 6 as cases may present while still alive. Drowning usually implies the inhalation of water in sufficient amounts to cause severe injury or death. However, medical pathologists sometimes differentiate between 'dry drowning' (causing vagal cardiac arrest) and 'wet drowning' (inhaled and ingested water). In the case of the latter, vomiting may occur, especially if sea water is swallowed. When water is inhaled, the surface area for gaseous exchange is reduced and bronchioles become blocked, causing anoxia. In addition, an osmotic effect is produced that results in haemolysis in freshwater, or dehydration and pulmonary oedema in hypertonic sea water. Laryngospasm can cause asphyxia. The pathogenesis of drowning in humans is well understood, largely because of experimental work and thus better understanding of the pathological processes involved (Camps and Cameron, 1971). However, there are no pathognomonic findings (DiMaio and DiMaio, 2001).

Post-mortem diagnosis of drowning in animals is based on similar criteria to those for humans above.

Excess frothy fluid is found in the respiratory tract, including the air sacs of birds, and often in the oesophagus and stomach. The lungs are usually distended and slightly congested, and subpleural petechiae may be present. The presence of water in the respiratory tract is usually considered always significant, as can be the finding of inhaled diatoms and other aquatic flora. However, caution must always be exercised. In marine mammals, for instance, the observations above are not at all conclusive (Kuiken *et al.*, 1994) and water and organisms may be inhaled or ingested *post mortem* (Larsen and Holm, 1996). As in humans, prolonged immersion of a carcase in water, whether following drowning or not, can in many species produce swollen, corrugated, skin – so-called 'washerwomen palms' (DiMaio and DiMaio, 2001) – and distended soft tissues.

Exposure to ionising radiation

This can be fatal but in animal legal cases is more likely to be linked with clinical or subclinical signs – lesions, ill-health or reduced performance. It is therefore discussed in Chapter 6.

Inhalation of dust

As was discussed in Chapter 2, pneumoconiosis is important in humans and may be seen in animals, either 'naturally' (as in burrowing or fossorial species, e.g. moles) or accidentally (as in animals kept in urban zoos). Various substances may be inhaled by animals, including different types of soil, sand, diatomite and silicates, and in a court case may provide significant *post-mortem* evidence, particularly relating to provenance.

Impaction of the gastro-intestinal (GI) tract

Ingestion of debris, whether accidental or intentional, causes morbidity or mortality in hundreds of thousands of animals each year. The problem is increasing as more and more non-degradable rubbish builds up on land, in rivers and on the seas. Domesticated animals have long been reported to suffer ill-effects from the ingestion of foreign material. In ruminants, for example, traumatic reticulitis due to metal and plastic objects has long been recognised and may result in peritonitis, pleurisy, myocarditis and death. Traditional causes of the latter, usually on the farm, were nails, screws and pieces of fencing (Neumann, 1979). Tyre wire is now an important factor, certainly in Europe (Harwood, 2004; Monies, 2004; Cramers *et al.*, 2005).

Even marine animals are not spared. The endangered Florida manatee, for example, ingests debris while feeding and, in a survey made between 1978–1986, 63 of 439 animals had rubbish in their GI tract and four had died as a direct result (Beck and Baros, 1991).

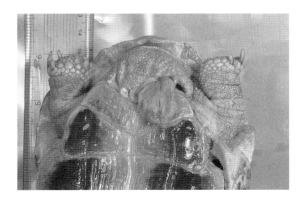

Figure 7.26 Prolonged immersion in water can produce various artefacts, regardless of whether or not the animal drowned. This tortoise, one of two found in a garden pond, has an extruded penis and the soft tissues are waterlogged. This figure also appears in colour in the colour plate section.

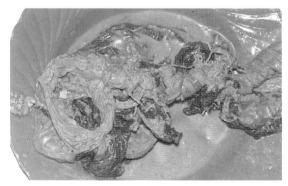

Figure 7.27 The contents of the reticulum of a red brocket deer. An ingested plastic bag has caused an obstruction. This figure also appears in colour in the colour plate section. (Courtesy of Richard Spence.)

Phytobezoars and other concretions found at necropsy may give an indication as to the origin or the feeding habits of an animal.

The presence of material in the GI tract is not necessarily a sign of ill-health. Some items are ingested accidentally, others (e.g. grit in certain birds, stones in crocodiles) may be taken in intentionally. Ostriches will ingest metal and other objects, as will some mammals (including humans), probably as part of a behavioural abnormality but sometimes ('pica') reflecting a need for dietary minerals.

Lesions of skeletons and bones

Although during routine necropsies pathologists detect some fractures, this is usually because either a) the injuries are severe or multiple or in a conspicuous site (e.g. skull) thus not easily missed, or b) the history suggests skeletal damage, in which case a search (sometimes including radiography) (see earlier) is made for lesions. Often, however, fractures (and other skeletal changes) are missed. Even when fractures *are* detected, the pathologist may fail to notice important details.

Skeletal injuries are often overlooked during *post-mortem* examination unless radiography or other imaging techniques are used. There is some merit, when the animal is small or the history suggestive of trauma, in subjecting a *post-mortem* case to whole body or partial radiography (see earlier). The skeleton comes into its own as forensic evidence when a carcase has decomposed and this is discussed later.

In forensic work the situation is very different. In some cases skeletonised remains are all that is available for the pathologist to investigate. This situation has been demonstrated in tragic ways in recent years, by the need to examine the remains of (human) victims of genocide in Rwanda, the former Yugoslavia and elsewhere. In-depth analysis of skeletal change is not, however, a new field of endeavour. Anthropologists, palaeontologists and others have for long been looking at bones of both humans and animals and as a result developed skills in detecting and interpreting even minor lesions (Cox and Mays, 2000). Collaboration with such people can be of great value to those involved in animal forensics (see Chapter 2) and the relationships are depicted below.

The origins and contemporary meaning of the term 'palaeopathology' were discussed by Nunn and Tapp (2000). It was coined by Sir Marc Armand Ruffer a century ago, to describe the science of the diseases that can be determined in ancient human and animal remains (see also Chapter 2). Zoo-

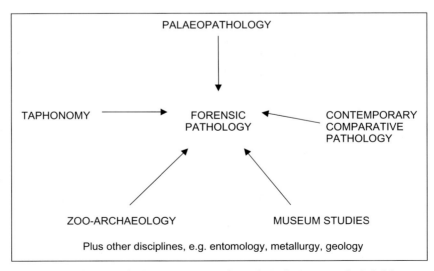

Figure 7.28 Collaboration with those who have experience of osteological science can be helpful.

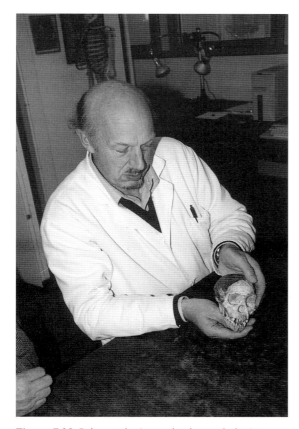

Figure 7.29 Palaeontologists and palaeopathologists have contributed much to our ability to identify and study bones. Here Dr. Ron Clarke examines the famous Taung skull at the University of the Witwatersrand in South Africa.

archaeology (sometimes known as *archaeozoology*) is the study of animal remains from archaeological sites (Davis, 1987; O'Connor, 2000). It tends to cover more recent periods than does palaeopathology, although not necessarily so, and bridges two disciplines – palaeozoology and anthropology/ archaeology. These terms should be familiar to many veterinarians: R.A. Harcourt (1971) and J.R. Baker (Baker and Brothwell, 1980), both British veterinary surgeons, were pioneers in the field insofar as animal remains were concerned. Others have contributed to the subject but the majority of those involved professionally tend to be palaeopathologists and zoo-archaeologists rather than veterinary graduates.

The particular challenges that 'dry bones' present were described graphically by Wood *et al.*, (1992). This and other related publications (see, for example, Duhig, 2003; Miller *et al.*, 1996; Needham *et al.*, 2003; Rothschild and Martin, 1993) are a testimony to the skills of palaeopathologists and zoo-archaeologists, and emphasise the value of establishing links between them and veterinary/ comparative pathologists.

While contact and collaboration with these other disciplines is, indeed, beneficial (and often mutual), caution does have to be exercised. Terminology and categorisation of lesions used by palaeopathologists do not necessarily equate with those employed in diagnostic medicine. A similar situation often applies when contemporary zoologists are referring to animal bones and skeletal pathology. For example, in her excellent study on the pathology of great apes, based on museum research, Lovell (1990) used some terms for lesions that do not concur with current veterinary designations.

O'Connor (2000) discussed the gap that exists between (most) veterinarians and palaeopathologists and provided a useful chapter on sickness and injury in animals, presenting material from both veterinary and zoo-archaeological sources. O'Connor emphasised the need for closer collaboration if animal palaeopathology is to advance.

If called to examine bones, the medical pathologist or forensic anthropologist is likely first to be asked: 'Are these bones human?' If the answer is 'yes', then usually the police are interested and investigations continue; if the bones are not human, then either the case may be dropped or if a crime in which the presence of animal bones is significant is suspected then further questions may follow.

The veterinary/comparative pathologist is likely to have a different orientation and will want to know *which* species is/are present. This should be relatively easy if modern domesticated animals (mammals and birds) are involved (see Chapter 2). A veterinarian should be familiar with such species or be able to seek help from a colleague at a veterinary school; zoo-archaeologists are usually also a valuable source of advice.

Non-domesticated species may present difficulties, especially if they include reptiles, amphibians and fish. Museums may be able to help and there are some good textbooks, including those that deal primarily with prehistoric assemblages, e.g. Lavocat (1966). Davis (1987) stated that, as a general rule, bone fragments of domesticated or hunted species, especially if they are from limb and foot and include an articular surface, can be identifiable to family, often to genus and species. Teeth are usually more distinct.

Skeletons and bones present particular challenges but also special opportunities to the forensic pathologist. Indeed, a special Symposium hosted by the Pathological Society of Great Britain and Ireland in July 2005 was entitled *Forensic Aspects of Bones* and included discussions of such important matters as the interpretation of fractures at autopsy, the identification and ageing of fractures and cleaning and interpreting marks on bones.

Important considerations in the examination of bones include:

- How was the bone prepared? Was this done naturally (e.g. in the soil) or in the laboratory (boiling, chemical treatment, use of *Dermestes* beetles, etc., etc.)? The process can markedly influence appearance.
- How has the bone been handled and stored since collection? Rough manipulation or packing bones together without protection can easily cause *post-mortem* artefact.
- Which species is it? This is discussed above. There are distinct differences in the vulnerability of bones to physical damage. Bones of flying birds, for instance, tend to be light in weight and less easily damaged in transit than are those of a mammal (see also below).
- Which bones are present? Some may be easy to identify, others may only be fragments or splinters. Zoo-archaeologists work on the assumption that 'every scrap of bone should be identified' (Davis, 1987) and this should be the aim in forensic work.
- What was the age at death? This will require careful examination of epiphyses and teeth. Radiography may assist. For many species data are not available.

When the pathologist is presented with a collection of bones, a wise initial approach is to lay them out, on a protective sheet on a table, in an appropriate anatomical position – usually head at one end, tail at the other, vertebral column/sternum down the middle, etc. This systematic approach serves two purposes:

(1) To ascertain how much and which parts of the skeleton are present.
(2) To determine whether more than one animal is represented.

Bones should be handled with gloves in order to reduce spread of organisms and transfer of DNA. Ruminant skeletal material should always be considered potentially hazardous because of the possibility of contamination with prions from brain or spinal cord (see Chapter 2).

Small bones, e.g. sesamoids or carpals, can be easily lost or brushed off the table. It is a wise precaution to put such bones in small, plastic bags. Articulation of skeletal remains can be achieved using strong cord on which vertebrae are strung.

Temporary labelling of bones is best done with soft pencil or by attaching removable labels.

One should never examine more than one set of bones on the table: the protective sheet must be checked and cleared between sessions.

Measurements are a key part of zoo-archaeology (von den Driesch, 1976) and may be necessary in forensic studies. Standard methods should, as always, be used.

The reporting of findings in bones has been well developed and refined by archaeologists and the forensic investigator can gain useful advice from relevant publications (e.g. Jones, 2002).

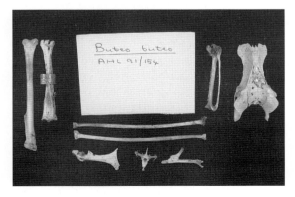

Figure 7.30 The bones of a Eurasian buzzard are carefully sorted, prior to investigation.

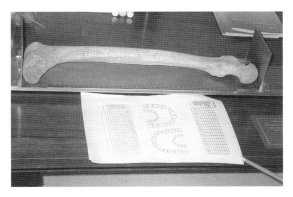

Figure 7.31 Much of relevance to animal forensics can be learned from osteologists who study human bones, for example how to carry out morphometrics.

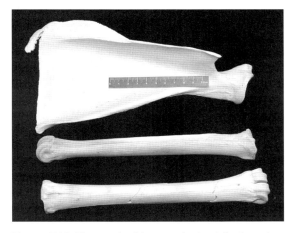

Figure 7.32 Three animal bones submitted for forensic examination. What is the significance of the sharp edge to the scapula (top)? Were the two transverse fractures in the bone (bottom) incurred before death, at the time of death or *post mortem*? (Courtesy of Richard Spence.)

When specifically looking for, or at, fractures, the following points have to be borne in mind:

- Bones are not uniform but have areas of strength and weakness.
- The vulnerability of a bone to the fracture is influenced by many factors including the age of the animal, its sex, its nutritional status and whether it is lactating/producing eggs/ pregnant.
- The type of fracture depends upon other factors, including the force applied and the strength of that particular bone (or part thereof). Some fractures may have a pattern – for example, hammer injury produces a circular lesion.
- Gross and microscopical examination can be usefully supplemented with other investigations including radiography and bone density studies.

Fractures are not the only important injuries to bones.

Animal bones may have been cut or damaged during butchering (for meat) and here the experiences of zoo-archaeologists can be very useful (Davis, 1987; O'Connor, 2000). Recent work on butchered animals using pig material has led to a new method for the qualitative analysis of cut-mark micromorphology (Bello and Soligo, 2005). Stab or machete (panga, cutlass) wounds may cause indentations in the periosteum, either *ante* or *post mortem*. Animal bites may damage bone, leaving tooth marks, again when the victim was alive, or after death, or both. These tooth marks can be used to identify the assailant, whether it be dog, hyaena or crocodile (Williams *et al.*, 1998).

Post-mortem predation (scavenging) of bones is well recognised by zoo-archaeologists: Davis (1987) provided useful information and references and emphasised the destructive effect that domesticated dogs can have on animal remains, by both chewing/ breaking and swallowing bones. Many wild animals attempt to predate bones, possibly in order to obtain dietary calcium (see also earlier): they range from leopard tortoises at antelope kills in Africa (Cooper and Jackson, 1981) to disturbance of Inuit skeletons by polar bears in North America (Haglund and Sorg, 1996).

Natural disease is a common cause of skeletal lesions and can result in new bone growth (e.g. spondylosis, exostoses), loss of bone (e.g. osteoporosis) or a combination of both.

Bones can be easily altered in appearance by chemical and other insults (see also Table 7.6). For example, excess heat (as in a fire) will cause cracking, fragmentation, shrinkage, warping and colour change. Despite loss of key features, burned boned can usually still yield valuable information if examined by an experienced osteologist.

Bones are an oft-overlooked part of forensic work, in both live (clinical) and dead (*post-mortem*) investigations, but they have great potential and can yield much valuable information. Bones from dead animals can be easily stored and re-examined. Repeated sampling for, e.g., histological examination, mineral assay or carbon-dating is possible.

Having said this, special precautions are wise when examining or sampling bones:

- Gloves should be worn to protect both bone and handler.
- When taking samples, whether using a saw, drill or scalpel, goggles and masks should be standard.
- If there is any suspicion that the animal had a spongiform encephalopathy (e.g. bovine spongiform encephalopathy (BSE), scrapie), full precautions are necessary (see also earlier and Chapter 2).

Mummification

The English word 'mummy' derives from the Arabic *mumiya* meaning an embalmed body. Mummification can be either natural or human-induced. The former takes place when environmental conditions permit a body to desiccate (Shepherd, 2003). Artificial mummification, as practised (amongst others) by the ancient Egyptians, involved a number of specialised techniques (Ikram and Dodson, 1998; Nunn and Tapp, 2000). There has long been interest in mummified bodies – their (fairly crude) investigation was a popular pastime in some circles in 18th and early 19th century England and investigators even included John Hunter (Moore, 2005) – but in recent years scientific study has revealed much of medical interest (see, for example, David, 1979). Some of the techniques used to examine mummies are applicable to the desiccated remains of animals, especially the precautions that have to be taken both to conserve the specimen and to protect those involved in the dissection.

Mummies are themselves of forensic interest (Filer, 1995; Nunn and Tapp, 2000) and there is scope for enterprising students of comparative medicine to examine the many thousands of mummified animals in Egypt and in the world's museums. However, care needs to be exercised in order to protect valuable material. Following radiography, minimally invasive endoscopic examination may be a wise first step.

Natural mummification occurs when a carcase is exposed to environmental factors that permit breakdown of tissues but there is no associated microbial multiplication – for example, in a cool, dry, place such as a cupboard in a house or a kennel. Such carcases are dry and may consist of only bones and desiccated tissues (see Figure 7.33).

Forensic examination of mummified carcases is often requested because it has been suggested that the animal died under suspicious circumstances. Investigation of such material can be carried out as follows:

- Careful appraisal of the environment where the animal was found, including measurements of ambient temperature, relative humidity and airflow.
- Equally diligent examination of the exterior of the carcase, to include any newspaper or substrate that is attached to it.
- Collection of skin/hair samples for toxicological and microbiological/parasitological investigations.
- Rehydration in warm normal (physiological) saline, for 72–96 hours, of selected portions of skin and internal soft tissues prior to their being fixed, embedded and sectioned for histological study.
- Microbiological culture of selected tissues, either dehydrated or ground with a sterile pestle and mortar.
- Meticulous inspection of bones.

See also Embalming.

Starvation

A clinical approach to starvation was discussed in some detail in Chapter 6. However, it can result in death; a pathologist as opposed to a clinician may then be asked to examine an animal *post mortem* and to give an opinion as to whether or not the victim starved. Dehydration (see earlier) and starvation may co-exist.

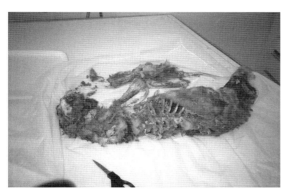

Figure 7.33 A mummified dog, the subject of an animal welfare case, is received for necropsy. This figure also appears in colour in the colour plate section.

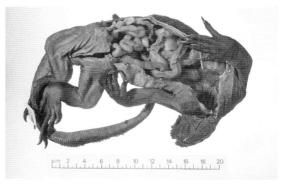

Figure 7.35 Starvation in ectothermic vertebrates can be difficult to diagnose. This marine iguana is one of many that died after an El Niño event. It has no subcutaneous fat and abdominal fat bodies were not located. This figure also appears in colour in the colour plate section.

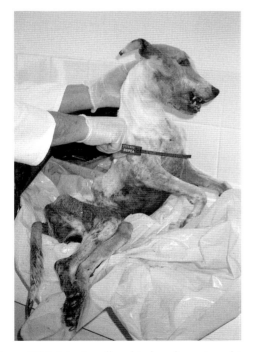

Figure 7.34 A terrier, alleged to have been starved to death. The animal is emaciated. This figure also appears in colour in the colour plate section.

Many of the criteria outlined in the preceding chapter, relating to clinical examination of suspected starvation cases, apply also to necropsy examination and will not be repeated unnecessarily here.

A properly performed gross *post-mortem* examination plays an essential part in cases where, following inadequate food intake or absorption/ utilisation, death has supervened. An emaciated appearance to the carcase, with absence of subcutaneous fat and an empty gastro-intestinal tract, are strongly suggestive of prolonged starvation. In ectothermic vertebrates fat bodies may be absent or depleted. Scoring of all findings is important, as are drawings and/or photographs.

In cases of starvation, organs, particularly the liver, may be appreciably reduced in weight and size. Weighing of the organ and relating it to the animal's total bodyweight (mass) is strongly recommended.

It is not only mammals that show visible changes in appearance of organs and recognition of such is not new. A reduction in size of the liver has long been recognised as a sign of starvation in reptiles by those who kill and eat these animals – in South America, for instance, where over a century ago André (1904) reported that the liver of *Geochelone* tortoises 'shrinks in proportion to the length of time during which its owner has been deprived of nourishment'.

A thorough *post-mortem* examination provides an opportunity to examine internal organs both macroscopically and microscopically. Macroscopical examination will reveal the size and appearance of organs (e.g. if a liver is pale and therefore possibly fatty) and is the time to examine, weigh and evaluate any internal body fat (see above). The gastro-intestinal tract can be examined in detail for presence of ingesta (and its appearance), any lesions or parasites and other possibly relevant abnormalities.

Microscopical (histological) examination enables the pathologist to assess more accurately the appearance of organs – to include whether they contain lipid or show other significant changes and will permit the measuring of hepatocytes or assessment of zymogen granules in pancreatic acini, which can sometimes be used as an indication of impaired nutrient intake.

The pathologist can also play an important part in assessing animals clinically (see Chapter 6). Blood and other samples taken from animals that are alleged to have been starved should be examined by a proficient pathologist. Such changes as anaemia, especially if associated with a low packed cell volume (PCV), may be significant but need to be properly described and investigated.

Nutritional deficiencies and imbalances

Malnutrition may contribute to starvation, or the sequel to it, or be significant in a legal case in its own right as evidence of neglect or cruelty. An important example is metabolic bone disease (MBD) usually caused by a calcium/phosphorus imbalance, which remains common in captive animals, especially primates, birds and reptiles (Fowler, 1978). It can cause severe clinical signs, culminating in death, and its presence is not infrequently considered grounds *de facto* for allegations or charges of cruelty. The details of this and other specific conditions are outside the scope of this book but must be borne in mind by anyone who is asked to give evidence on animals where the quality of nutrition is questioned.

The presence in food of poisonous substances, including mycotoxins, can be of significance in legal or insurance cases (see Chapter 6). Their effects may be detected on gross or histological examina-

tion but confirmation will require toxicological analysis.

Shock

'Shock' (see Chapter 4 and Appendix C) is often difficult to diagnose *post mortem* and yet is often a significant feature of cases that go to court and attract claims of professional negligence. The detection of shock at necropsy is complicated by the fact that it can easily be masked by *post-mortem* change (Rutty, 2004).

Metabolic disorders

Some metabolic diseases are difficult to diagnose accurately in life and present even more problems *post mortem* yet they may be a key point in a legal or insurance hearing, especially if they are congenital. Little appears to have been published on the investigation of metabolic diseases after death in animals but Olpin and Evans (2004) provided useful principles from the human perspective.

Reproductive activity

The breeding status or reproductive potential of an animal is often of importance legally. Clinical assessment of the reproductive system is discussed in Chapter 6.

The pathologist may also be consulted. A question that is often asked in court cases and in insurance claims is whether or not an animal has bred – or, perhaps, whether it would have been capable of breeding (laying eggs, producing young, etc.,) if it had lived longer, been fed better, not been ovariectomised or given veterinary care.

Methods of assessing reproductive activity are given in Table 7.16.

Sexing of skeletal remains is often possible (Davis, 1987).

Other aspects of reproductive biology that may be of legal significance include confirmation of pregnancy, determination of paternity and superfecundity issues as well as causes of abortion or neonatal death (see earlier).

Table 7.16 Methods of assessing previous or existing reproductive activity.

Taxon	Method	Comments
Mammals	*Females*	
	Mammary gland development	Can be deceptive if animal has had a pseudo pregnancy, a hormonal disorder or has been treated with steroids
		Other long-term changes are more reliable indicators than mammary glands alone
	Vaginal cytology	Confirmation of current reproductive activity, sexual receptivity and pregnancy in some species
	Uterine culture and/or biopsy	To confirm presence of infection or other pathology
	Progesterone assays	To detect oestrus, ovulation and pathology
	Males	
	Scrotal circumference (ruminants)	Can be positively correlated with sperm production
	Scrotal width (non-ruminants)	
Birds	Presence of brood patch	Wyllie and Newton (1999) described differences in the appearance of the oviduct of two species of raptor depending upon whether or not they had laid eggs
	Oviduct development	
	Ovarian or testicular changes	
		Ovarian and testicular development have been used in legal cases to provide similar evidence (J.E. Cooper, unpublished)
Reptiles	Oviducal, ovarian or testicular changes	As above

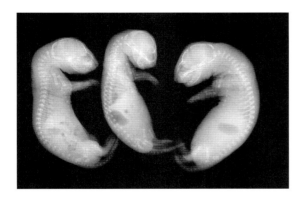

Figure 7.36 Whole-body radiography is advisable when neonatal deaths occur and there is a suggestion of foul play. These are aborted fetuses of ferrets.

GROUP, HERD OR FLOCK EXAMINATIONS

In both *post-mortem* and clinical work it may be impossible to examine all the animals that are presented – when, for example, a pondful of fish shows clinical signs of inco-ordination and gasping or several hundred broilers (chickens) are found dead in a poultry house. Under such circumstances it is usually acceptable to take and examine a *sample* of the animals. It is important, however, to record how the selection was made, in order to counter any criticisms later. Sometimes a random sample is taken, other times a chosen mixture of, e.g., severely affected and apparently normal fish or layer chickens from different pens. The number of animals sampled is also an important consideration. As a general rule, the larger the sample size the better (i.e. the greater the chance of making a diagnosis, or detecting a pathological change) but this has to be balanced against such factors as:

- Time.
- Cost.
- Practicalities, such as the need for the poultry house to be cleaned and disinfected.
- The possibility that another expert may want to examine material.

When dead animals are involved, it is wise to save (chilled, frozen, fixed – see Chapter 10) carcases

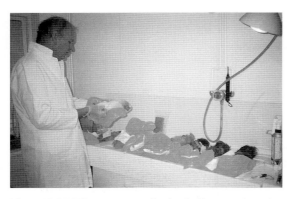

Figure 7.37 When a group of animals dies, care must be taken to avoid transposition of samples or cross-contamination. These guinea pigs have been individually marked for forensic investigation.

that cannot be examined immediately. These can be made available to other experts, if required, or can be examined again by the same pathologist at a later stage, if new questions arise.

When examining large numbers of animals clinically or *post mortem*, there is merit in recording the main findings on a special 'group or flock' form (see Appendix A). This enables findings in different animals to be compared and contrasted rather more readily than if individual forms are used. The data can be hand-written or prepared as a computer spreadsheet.

RETENTION OF TISSUES

Concerns in the UK over the fate of samples of human origin, prompted largely by public inquiries into events at Bristol Royal Infirmary and the Royal Liverpool Children's Hospital (Alder Hey) (Report, 2001), prompted the introduction of guidelines (Department of Health, 2001), legislation (The Human Tissue Act 2004) and the establishment of the Human Tissue Authority (HTA) (see Appendix B).

The HTA advises the public and the government about such issues as storage, use, importation and exportation and disposal of human bodies and tissues. In other countries, controls have generally been less stringent and, indeed, a more healthy approach to organs and other remains applies in some communities, as exemplified by Cyrus (2005) writing from St Vincent in the West Indies (see also Cyrus, 1989). However, all those involved in forensic medicine, especially on an international basis, should be aware of public concern over human remains (see also earlier) and, at the very least, to adopt appropriate codes of practice (see below) and to demonstrate sensitivity in their work.

It is not only recent human remains that have attracted attention. Archaeologists, museum curators and others have had to grapple with the ethical, sometimes legal, implications of working with skeletons and bones of people who died decades or centuries ago. Claims have been made – and increasingly are being honoured – by some groups, for example Australian aborigines, for the return of the skulls and other tissues that came from their ancestors. Much concern has been expressed in recent years over the exhibition of intact, unwrapped mummies, removed from their burial or sacrificial location – for instance, the three 500-year-old Inca children translocated from Llulla-illaco, a mountain in the Andes, and then proposed for display in an Argentine museum (Anon., 2005j). In this and other matters, codes of practice, such as (in the UK) the Department for Culture, Media and Sport publication, *Guidance on the Care of Remains in Museums* (DCMS, 2003) are helpful.

Awareness of the points above and adherence to the legislation and guidelines is, of course, essential for all those who may deal with human remains. This can apply to the veterinary pathologist, especially if s/he is involved in joint studies with medical or dental colleagues and therefore handles tissues.

Animal tissues are not usually as sensitive an issue as those of humans but there are at least two sets of circumstances where particular care should be taken:

(1) When an animal has been a person's close, perhaps sole, companion.
(2) Where wild animal species are of cultural, possibly religious, importance.

The latter can be an intricate relationship. In New Zealand, for example, the kereru, a species of pigeon, is one of a number of species of bird that are sacred to the Maori. How kereru are handled, even during a routine *post-mortem* examination, can unwittingly cause distress or offence (Cooper and Cooper, unpublished data). Further, customary uses of animal remains, such as feathers incorporated in traditional cloaks, may necessitate the return of material after necropsy to local individuals or communities. Appropriate hygiene measures are necessary in such circumstances to reduce risks to human or animal health.

MUSEUMS

Museums always have been a valuable source of information for those involved in forensic work – especially to assist in the identification of bones or other tissues. Their staff are usually helpful and knowledgeable.

Specialised collections are of particular value to those involved in comparative forensics – the Odontological Museum of the Royal College of Surgeons of England, the Colyer collection, being an excellent example (Miles and Grigson, 1990). Medical and veterinary museums sometimes provide a safe haven for material that might otherwise be destroyed in war or civil conflict – as was the situation with mountain gorilla skulls transferred from Uganda to South Africa in the early 1960s (Tobias and Cooper, 2003). Reference collections

of bones, hair and other material are proving invaluable in wildlife forensic work and are therefore discussed in more detail in Chapter 5 (see also PAW, 2005).

The present plight of museums in many parts of the world is a cause of concern for many reasons. The publication *Why Museums Matter: Avian Archives in an Age of Extinction* (Collar *et al.*,

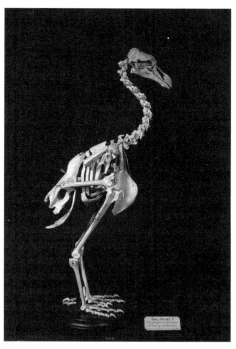

Figure 7.39 Museum specimens yield useful information that can assist in forensic cases.

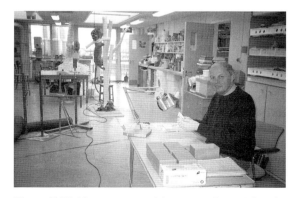

Figure 7.38 Museums are a rich source of material and information relevant to forensic medicine. Here bones are being examined as part of a study on the decline of a rare (Madagascan) species of duck. This figure also appears in colour in the colour plate section.

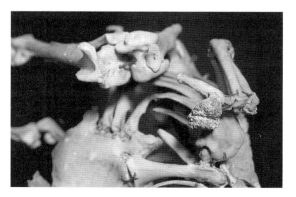

Figure 7.40 A skeletal lesion (right – osteophyte) may help in identifying a particular specimen.

223

2003) provided some very sound arguments for both retaining and extending collections but it is disappointing that such scant mention was made therein of the value of properly-curated animal and human material to diagnostic pathologists (see, for example, Cooper, 1982 and Rothschild and Panza, 2005) and those active in forensic medicine. A useful, 'popular', book explaining the continuing, indeed growing, importance of museums is that by Lincoln and Rainbow (2003); it makes stimulating reading for the comparative pathologist, as a break from routine duties, and it should be on the desks of all policy makers!

DEMONSTRATING PATHOLOGICAL MATERIAL TO LAY PEOPLE

The veterinary surgeon or other expert who has to appear in court or give evidence to a tribunal or committee of enquiry is likely to have to explain aspects of medical work to non-scientific lay people, including magistrates, juries, and judges (see Chapter 12).

Material that can assist on such occasions includes:

- Photographs and electronic images of normal and abnormal appearances.
- Radiographs and other images.
- Specimens in fixative (formalin or alcohol) – whole or treated – in order to demonstrate internal structures, e.g. alizarine red preparations showing embryonic or early post-natal development.
- Properly-prepared feathers and other dry specimens.
- Bones and teeth.

Permission will need to be sought to produce such material in the court room.

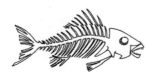

Laboratory Investigations

Adventure on, for from the littlest clue
Has come whatever worth man ever knew;
The next to lighten all men may be you.

John Masefield

Our bones are dried, and our hope is lost; we are cut off for our parts.

Ezekiel 37:11

Laboratory investigations are a key part of forensic science. Some relevant disciplines are almost entirely laboratory-based – for example, toxicology and DNA technology. In routine animal work, however, the investigator is likely to be using (sometimes relying upon) laboratory investigation as an adjunct or back-up to his or her examination of a live or dead animal or its derivatives. However, all those involved in animal cases should be aware of the potential as well as the limitation of laboratory testing and from the outset know where to go and whom to consult for such assistance.

It is impracticable in a book of this size to discuss in detail the many laboratory tests that may be required when investigating an animal forensic case. Whole volumes have been published on these topics, examples of which are given in the References. Instead, this chapter will concentrate on the principles of laboratory investigation, in particular such issues as preparation and dispatch of specimens, chain of custody, health and safety and the production and use of reports.

Any laboratory that is to be used for investigations relating to a forensic case should be:

- Reliable – preferably accredited, with high quality staff (see later).

- Familiar with the legal process and such concepts as a chain of custody.
- Willing to be involved in forensic work, which will include the production of appropriate reports and possible appearance in court.
- Aware of the extra costs, inconvenience and sometimes vulnerability incurred when dealing with material in legal cases.

A more specific list of criteria for wildlife material in the UK was drawn up by PAW (2005) – valid methodology, quality assurance, accreditation, quality control, staff competence and practices complying with good forensic practice. Each of these was discussed and a checklist provided to assist non-scientific staff in making a choice.

Veterinarians and others involved in animal forensics should have a list of laboratories that can assist, including a note of availability, outside hours, at weekends or on public holidays, and endeavour to develop a good working relationship with those laboratories. Sometimes it is easier to deal with one laboratory and for that laboratory to sub-contract work to others that they cannot perform themselves. This can prove satisfactory but it is most important that a proper chain of custody of samples is maintained and that the sub-contracted laboratories fulfil the requirements listed above. If one laboratory is to be utilised, the veterinarian should ideally have visited the premises, met the staff, discussed the sort of work that s/he might be requesting and gone through a mock chain of custody in order to ascertain the standards are adequate. Depending upon the location (country), one should confirm that there is GLP (Good Laboratory Practice) or that the facility follows GLP and has SOPs (Standard Operating Procedures) in place.

Fees should be agreed, as far as possible, beforehand. Often they are far higher than those that apply to routine diagnostic work. In some cases the costs of laboratory tests may be a limiting factor in whether or not to proceed with legal action.

The two key factors in laboratory forensic work are:

(1) Chain of custody.
(2) Quality control.

Chain of custody has been mentioned above and elsewhere in this book. Quality control, which is the hallmark of all forensic work, can be less easy to ensure. In few countries are veterinary laboratories subject to a compulsory accreditation scheme. Where such schemes exist, they tend to be voluntary. However, the lab that can perform a particular much-needed test may not be a part of that voluntary accreditation scheme. These and other factors can conspire to make quality assurance difficult – and if it is, the resulting evidence may be challenged. This is important not only in cases involving domesticated animals but also in wildlife crime investigations (PAW, 2005; Wobeser, 1996).

In cases where a veterinarian is involved, there may be merit in performing some laboratory tests in-house. Modern veterinary practices often include a laboratory in which standard tests are performed on samples from animals. Such laboratories and the staff that run them (see later) are usually experienced and very familiar with the need for confidentiality, record-keeping and proper production of reports. For these reasons, plus the fact that chain of custody can usually be maintained relatively easily, the veterinary practice laboratory may be the best option (see Appendix E). If, however, there is any doubt about these criteria – and, of course, if

special tests are needed – then it is wise to send the material elsewhere (see below). Each case has to be judged on its own merits.

CHOICE OF A LABORATORY

If samples are to be sent to a laboratory, certain safeguards are essential. The three basic criteria (reliability, familiarity and willingness to be involved) were listed on the first page of this chapter but more specific points are as follows:

- Can the laboratory ensure continuity and security of evidence?
- Will the work be carried out to the desired standard?
- Do laboratory staff understand such principles as the unique labelling of exhibits, the correct labelling of photographs and radiographs and the need to retain all wrappings, correspondence, notes and documents?
- Are effective risk-assessment and appropriate safety codes in place?
- Is someone available to be consulted?

It is not wise to use a laboratory without either (a) visiting it, meeting staff and checking systems, or (b) seeking endorsement from someone else who has utilised the laboratory's services.

Three extra tips are:

(1) Agree costs (fees) beforehand, including contingency plans.
(2) Insist that the laboratory creates a file (paper/electronic) from the outset.
(3) Establish a relationship with one person in the laboratory.

The assessment of the reliability and quality of an outside (referral) laboratory was usefully discussed, in a paper for veterinary practitioners, by Wiegers (2004).

PERSONNEL

Staff competence is of the utmost importance in both domesticated animal and wildlife laboratory forensic work (PAW, 2005). The importance of good management of the crime laboratory was emphasised by Tilstone and Lothridge (2003).

SAMPLES

Samples play an important part in forensic work as well as in the routine diagnosis of disease and in the health monitoring of supposedly 'normal' animals. Samples may be taken from live animals, from dead animals or from the crime scene. Any of these may constitute evidence and, as such, need to be properly handled for legal reasons. Chain of custody and packaging are discussed later and in Chapter 11.

What is a 'sample'? It has been defined by Blood and Studdert (1988) as:

> . . . a specimen . . . collected for analysis on the assumption that it represents the composition of the whole.

Correct sampling will yield reliable results and in turn facilitate accurate interpretation followed by appropriate action. In 'forensic' cases such precision is all-important. In addition to ensuring good technique (see below), there may be merit for corroboration in having a witness to the extraction and labelling of samples (Laurence and Newman, 2000).

In a forensic case specimens may need to be taken from live/dead animals, the environment, food samples or elsewhere and mistakes can occur at various stages.

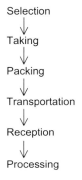

Figure 8.1 Stages in the handling of a sample.

An error or inconsistency introduced at any point in the sequence above can adversely affect subsequent steps and easily prejudice results.

Common causes of error in routine veterinary work (Cooper, J.E., 2002) include, at time of sampling:

- Samples taken at various periods of time after death, when autolytic changes and bacterial multiplication may complicate interpretations.
- Samples taken, packed and transported in diverse ways (e.g. swabs of different type or make, with or without transport medium) and not maintained at appropriate, constant, temperatures.
- Samples taken and/or stored in a totally unacceptable way, e.g. whole blood should never be frozen and hair samples need particularly careful handling to avoid damage and cross-contamination with chemicals or foreign DNA (Robertson, 1999a).

The submission of ALL forensic samples should follow protocols that help to ensure that (a) evidential criteria are met, and (b) health and safety requirements are followed (see Chapter 3). In some countries standard codes of practice for such specimens are available (PAW, 2005).

Common causes of error on arrival at the laboratory include:

- Samples entered incorrectly or inconsistently or not dealt with promptly.
- Variation in methods of storage prior to processing of samples.
- Samples processed in different ways or at varying times after submission.

Techniques for laboratory examination can differ depending upon the species (classification) sampled, its habitat and the purpose of the investigation. Thus, for example, specimens from ectothermic vertebrates, such as reptiles, amphibians and fish, may need to be cultured at 24°C as well as at 37°C if optimal results are to be obtained. Some tests may need to be performed immediately if results are to be reliable – for example, analysis for cyanide and certain pesticides where deterioration may occur at normal freezer temperature (Stroud and Adrian, 1996).

Table 8.1 Samples from live and dead animals.

Sample	Live animal	Dead animal
Faeces	Yes	Yes
Hair, feathers, scales	Yes	Yes
Touch preparations for cytology	Yes	Yes
Swabs, etc. for microbiology of external lesions	Yes	Yes
Swabs, etc. for microbiology of internal lesions	Sometimes, via an endoscope or a surgical incision	Yes
Tissue samples for histology, etc. of external lesions	Yes (biopsy)	Yes
Tissue samples for histology, etc. of internal lesions	Sometimes (biopsy)	Yes
Larger tissue samples for (e.g.) toxicology	Usually not feasible	Yes
Crop and stomach contents for toxicology	Sometimes by lavage or use of emetics	Yes
Blood	Yes	Occasionally (immediately after death)
Ectoparasites	Yes	Sometimes
Eggs and larvae of blowflies and some other insects	Sometimes (myiasis)	Yes

Samples are of different types, depending upon:

- Their source.
- The purpose for which they are taken.
- How they are presented and handled.

Types of sample that may be received by the laboratory from live or dead animals as part of a forensic investigation are listed in Table 8.1.

These examples illustrate that some samples can be taken from either live or dead animals whereas others may only be realistically obtained from one or the other (see Chapters 6 and 7). Samples may be microscopic in size or constitute large portions of tissue, such as bones (Figure 8.2). Environmental samples will include water (Figure 8.3) and soil.

The purpose for which samples are collected is all-important and will influence how they are collected, stored and transported. Examples of the range of investigations that can be carried out are given later, using faeces, blood and biopsies as examples (Table 8.2).

The investigations that are to be carried out often dictate how the sample is taken, presented and handled – for example, blood for haematology may

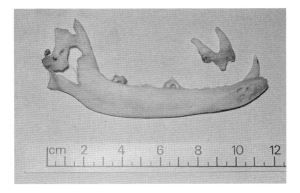

Figure 8.2 The faeces of a free-living rock python, alleged by African villagers to have killed and eaten children and domestic animals, yielded this jaw of a pet dog.

be preserved in one anticoagulant, blood for biochemistry in another. Likewise, techniques in the laboratory will depend upon the request received.

Some samples can serve a multiplicity of purposes, provided that the sample is large enough and/or the technology is sufficiently sensitive and reliable to deal with a small specimen. A feather is an example. It can be used for the following:

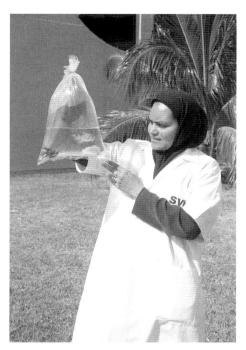

Figure 8.3 Examining fish with the water from which they originated can be an important part of monitoring pollution. This figure also appears in colour in the colour plate section.

Table 8.2 Examples of laboratory investigations that may be carried out on samples.

Sample	Test
Faeces	Microbiology
	Parasitology
	Direct examination for food constituents, sloughed cells, etc.
	DNA studies
	Electronmicroscopy
	Staining for, e.g., fat or glycogen
Blood	Haematology
	Smears for parasitology and differential counts
	Biochemistry
	Serology
	Toxicology
	DNA studies
Biopsies	Histopathology
	Immunohistochemistry
	Electronmicroscopy
	Microbiology
	DNA studies

- Detection of gross abnormalities of shaft, barbs, barbules or follicle.
- Ptilochronology.
- Assessment of moult.
- Collection and identification of ectoparasites.
- Collection and identification of saprophytic organisms (estimation of time).
- Microscopical and SEM examination to investigate lesions.
- Heavy-metal analysis.
- Microscopical, mitochondrial DNA and genomic studies for identification of the species from which the feather came (PAW, 2005).

Feathers and hair and other keratinous structures can provide much information (see Table 8.3) and in the course of such work the forensic investigator must be prepared to consult zoological literature as well as medical and veterinary publications – for example, the studies performed on the effects of digestion, putrefaction and taxidermy on the

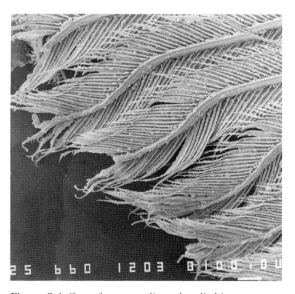

Figure 8.4 One of many starlings that died in a factory explosion (see earlier). Low-power scanning electronmicrogram (SEM) shows mineral deposits on barbs and barbules.

229

Table 8.3 Some laboratory techniques used in forensic work.

Technique	Standard recommended methods
Aerobic bacteriology	Blood agar plates and MacConkey's – incubated at 37°C for 24 hours (72 hours if no growth) Samples from ectothermic animals may also be incubated at 24°C (Cooper, 1999a,b) Other media as appropriate
Anaerobic bacteriology	Same as above, but incubated anaerobically at 37°C for 48 hours (and possibly 24°C)
Mycology	Sabouraud dextrose agar plates – one at 37°C for 7 days, the other at 22°C for up to 21 days Direct microscopy of fresh or prepared material
Mycoplasmology	*Mycoplasma* growth medium
Isolation of *Chlamydia* (now called *Chlamydophila*) tissue samples	PCR, ELISA and fluorescent antibody techniques *Chlamydophila* can be grown in tissue culture, eggs or experimental animals
Virology	Tissue culture Egg inoculation Animal inoculation Fluorescent antibody technique
Serology	Serum neutralisation Gel diffusion precipitation Complement fixation ELISA Fluorescent antibody
Parasitology (see also dipterous larvae, below) • Skin scrapings and/or hair, feathers, scales, faeces, intestinal contents	Direct microscopy plus treatment of sample with 10% KOH prior to examination Wet preparations in physiological saline plus salt or sugar flotation using McMaster counting chamber. Lugol's iodine: identification of cysts $ZnSO_4$ flotation: amoebae, cysts
• Blood	Thin smears fixed in methanol and stained with Giemsa or air-dried and stained with a rapid stain Detection of protozoan and filarial parasites
Histology	Tissues dehydrated in alcohol, embedded in paraffin wax, and sectioned at 6μ or less Stained routinely with haematoxylin and eosin Frozen sections may be rapidly prepared using cryostat.
Immunohistochemistry	Detecting and identifying endogenous and exogenous antigens, including micro-organisms
Cytology – touch preparations, washings, brushings and aspirates	Air-dried for Romanowsky staining Certain rapid stains include a fixative Fixed in methanol for other methods
Haematology • Smears • Blood in EDTA or lithium heparin	Examination of smears for abnormalities, differential counts PCV estimation using standard techniques Haemoglobin may need certain modified methods Total counts using special diluents
See also Parasitology – Blood (above)	Certain Coulter counters can be used for non-mammalian red cell counts Many mammalian species may have cells, Hb and PCV measured with semi-automatic analysers

(Continued)

Table 8.3 *Continued.*

Technique	Standard recommended methods
Clinical chemistry – blood in lithium heparin or EDTA (depends on the species and test required)	Standard procedures for electrolytes and enzymes (colour reaction systems and atomic absorption or flame spectrophotometer methods) Automatic analysers
Electronmicroscopy – tissue samples	Standard TEM and SEM procedures (see also below)
Chemical analysis/toxicology – tissue samples	Standard gas-liquid chromatographic and other procedures Animal studies
DNA studies	Various – depend on samples (see text)
Stable isotope studies on hair	Detecting diet changes and thus migration patterns, for example in elephants (Cerling *et al.*, 2006)
Hair, feather, scale, sloughed skin (reptiles and amphibians) examination	Direct microscopy with or without KOH treatment Culture (bacteriological or mycological) Virology/PCR Hair/feather shafts for mt DNA, follicles for genomic DNA Chemical analysis DNA techniques Histology Electronmicroscopy
Semen examination	Direct microscopy – wet or fixed (stained) preparations Bacteriology Techniques used to examine sperm in connection with artificial insemination can be adapted to forensic needs
Examination of uroliths and other chemical deposits	SEM Optical crystallographic analysis X-ray diffraction Infrared spectroscopy Chemical analysis (Mayer, 2005)
Studies on dipterous larvae and other invertebrates removed from a carcase or found in its vicinity	Smith (1986) provided details Identification: clearing with KOH precedes mounting on a microscope slide; SEM can assist in identification of some species: the specimen must be dehydrated and treated with gold or palladium Live dipterous larvae and other invertebrate species may need to be kept alive – the former may feed on meat and subsequently metamorphose, facilitating identification Unclotted blood can be used as food for ticks, leeches and hippoboscid flies Live invertebrates can be kept alive at 4°C to retard development
Bone examination	Culture, usually following grinding Histology, usually following decalcification DNA techniques
Analysis of food and additives	Various specialised tests for quality and for presence of toxic or unwanted substances
Egg examination	Various (Cooper, J.E., 2002) – for example, speciation using SEM or investigation, using ultraviolet light, to determine whether eggs are from free-range or caged domesticated hens (Gregory *et al.*, 2005)

Key: EDTA = ethylenediaminetetraacetic acid; KOH = potassium hydroxide; PVC = packed cell volume; Hb = haemoglobin; RBC = red blood cell; WBC = white blood cell; SEM = scanning electronmicroscopy; TEM = transmission electronmicroscopy; PCR = polymerase chain reaction

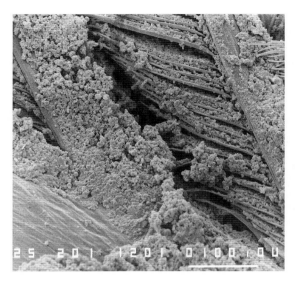

Figure 8.5 Higher power of Figure 8.4.

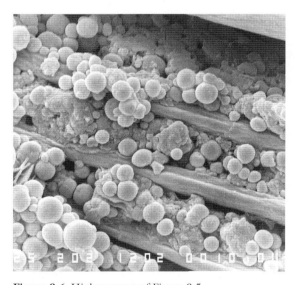

Figure 8.6 Higher power of Figure 8.5.

hair morphology of opossums by Quadros and Monteiro-Filho (1998). Stroud and Adrian (1996) emphasised the value of collecting hair at crime scenes and how it could be used for species identification (Petraco, 1987).

Consistency in sampling methods is vital if results are to be reliable and if different studies are to be comparable. Examples of where method is crucial include:

- Swabs for microbiology – cotton-wool or alginate-coated? The latter are less liable to dry out.
- Large or small? The latter are less likely to pick up extraneous organisms.
- Dry or in transport medium? The latter helps to conserve organisms.
- Faeces for parasitology – whole faecal sample versus only a portion? The latter, taken from the interior, is usually preferred as it reflects better the gut fauna and flora and, in DNA studies, is less likely to contain sloughed gastro-intestinal tract cells.
- Kept at room temperature or chilled? In most forensic work, chilling at domestic refrigerator temperature ($+4°C$) is wise. It slows down bacterial multiplication and decomposition without incurring the damage that ensues from freezing. However, some poisons, such as cyanide, may deteriorate even when the sample is frozen (Stroud and Adrian, 1996).

The time that elapses between taking a sample and processing it is also a fundamental consideration in assessing and interpreting results. Thus, for example, a delay in processing one set of swabs may result in the culture of fewer bacteria, or perhaps an overgrowth of one species (such as *Proteus*), so that the findings cannot then reliably be compared with those from another set of swabs.

The taking and transportation of samples in the field, especially in relatively inaccessible or isolated areas, can present particular problems. This is often the case when working with wildlife (Wobeser, 1996) but at times can be equally applicable to domesticated animals. Special equipment may be required and improvisation is often essential (Cooper and Samour, 1997; Frye *et al.*, 2001). This is discussed in more detail in Chapters 5 and 9. The correct handling and packaging of bones and other animal remains is covered in some zoo-archaeological texts (Davis, 1987). Standard sampling methods should be used where these are available – for example, when testing water (from rivers, fish farms), samples of animal feed or environmental specimens (Cattle *et al.*, 2004).

STANDARDISATION AND QUALITY CONTROL

It is essential to all laboratory procedures to develop and to use protocols, in which the method to be used is clearly defined and followed and will be adhered to in the same way thereafter.

Valid and correctly-applied results are the key to laboratory work. 'Quality control' can be defined as 'tasks that are done during the performance of a test to ensure that best results are valid' while 'quality assurance' is 'pre-planned and scheduled tasks that are performed to ensure that test results are valid' (Wiegers, 2004). An example of the former is the use of positive and negative controls; of the latter, correct calibration of equipment.

Whenever possible, one should check the work and results of technicians and other junior staff. Where this is not feasible, a signed and dated report should be accompanied by retention of relevant material (such as agar plates), available for inspection. In legal proceedings it is dangerous to accept only a verbal assurance from staff: in one of our cases a mastocytoma was misdiagnosed because the pathologist relied on the technician to carry out a toluidine blue stain and she reported 'no sign of mast cells'!

It is important to have control material – in the case of histology, tissues or slides that are positive for, e.g., toluidine blue, Gram, PAS staining.

LEGAL ASPECTS

The collection, transportation and processing of samples are likely to be covered by legislation (see Chapter 3), including Post Office Regulations, health and safety, animal health and possibly (wild animals) CITES (Cooper, M.E., 1987). Even tiny samples may require CITES permits if they originate from species of animals that are listed on Appendices I and II of CITES or (in the EU) on the relevant Annexes of the EU CITES Regulation or (in other countries) are subject to equivalent national CITES legislation and are 'recognisable derivatives' (see Chapter 3).

Packaging is discussed in more detail later and in Chapter 11. Useful advice, directed at wildlife spec-

imens but applicable also to others, is to be found in PAW (2005).

LABORATORY METHODS

Some techniques that may be used in the laboratory on samples from live or dead animals or, in some cases, from their environment, are listed in Table 8.3.

Table 8.3 has a strong veterinary orientation. Some samples that are received may require specialised investigation, even though they originated from live or dead animals – partly digested vegetable matter (Catling and Grayson, 1982), or gunshot residues (Schwoeble and Exline, 2000), for instance.

INTERPRETATION AND REPORTING OF RESULTS

This is a skilled task and, as always, presents particular challenges and pitfalls in forensic work. Some important points are:

- The interpretation must be carried out in the context of what is known of the animal's history and clinical/*post-mortem* findings.

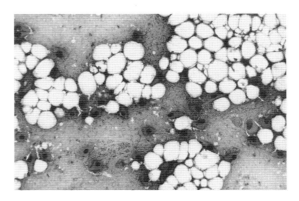

Figure 8.7 Cytological examination provides a rapid means of obtaining information about pathological lesions and is ideally suited to forensic investigations in the field. This liver of a fish shows multiple fat droplets suggestive of lipidosis. This figure also appears in colour in the colour plate section.

233

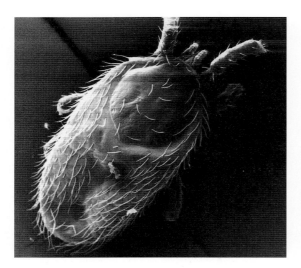

Figure 8.8 Scanning electronmicroscopy has many uses in forensic work, including the identification of invertebrates that are found on or near a carcase.

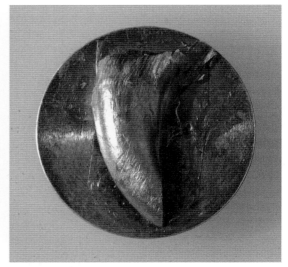

Figure 8.9 Gold spattering, a technique used in scanning electronmicroscopy work, in this case on the beak of a cockerel that was found following an alleged cock-fighting competition. This figure also appears in colour in the colour plate section. (Courtesy of Richard Spence.)

- Discussion with colleagues, including technical staff who performed the test, is invaluable.
- Allowance may have to be made for delays in obtaining the correct samples and for how they were packed and transported. These aspects, even if they reflect badly on those involved, will form part of any report. They should be clearly distinguished from equivocal results as a result of normal processes – for instance, the loss of poisons from stomach contents because of absorption, decomposition, dilution or regurgitation (Stroud and Adrian, 1996).
- If there is any possibility of erroneous or unreliable results, because of a faulty piece of equipment or technician error, this too should be acknowledged and recorded. Where feasible, the tests should be repeated, possibly at another laboratory.
- Where the interpretation is equivocal, or open to challenge, this should be acknowledged. In forensic cases the truth is important and assumptions and decisions that might have to be made in routine diagnostic work, because a patient is at risk, usually have no part to play.
- Caution should be exercised in making claims. 'No parasites seen' is preferable to 'No parasites

present'. Where failure to detect parasites or other features may be attributable to small or unrepresentative sample size, poor laboratory technique or shortage of trained personnel this should be acknowledged and explained (Cooper and Anwar, 2001).
- The person signing the report must be particularly careful in so doing when material has been examined by another person (see also earlier). For example, a veterinary or human pathologist may have experience of domesticated animals or *Homo sapiens* but not be familiar with such particular features of non-mammalian species as the melanomacrophage centres of fish, or the close integration in many reptiles of splenic and pancreatic tissue. A normal structure may therefore erroneously be described as 'pathological' or have incorrect inferences drawn from it. Anyone involved in forensic studies on unfamiliar species should have access to appropriate comparative texts, such as the book by Aughey and Frye (2001).

- When organisms (macro or micro) have to be correctly identified, the name of any colleague (taxonomist) who assisted should be provided. Where doubt exists, an authoritative checklist or catalogue must be consulted. This is particularly important in areas where there is disagreement about speciation – the haemosporidia, for example (Valkiunas, 2004).

The written interpretation should be carefully worded, leaving room for alternative inferences. Haematological, blood chemistry and urinalysis results should be accompanied by normal (reference) ranges, with mention of their provenance.

As a general rule, laboratory reports for forensic use should only be issued when all the results have been obtained and verified. This is rather different from diagnostic work where a preliminary (often verbal) report may be provided in the interests of animal welfare so that treatment can commence, or to reassure the owner. Issuing incomplete, tentative results can be foolhardy in forensic cases because a police officer, even the press, may seize on those findings and thereby possibly influence the legal process.

In reports, one must be wary of abbreviations: the term should be given in full on the first occasion. The acronym 'CBC' is used throughout North America to mean 'complete blood count' but elsewhere in the English-speaking world 'TBC' (total blood count) is often the norm. A rather different example of where confusion can occur if only abbreviations are used concerns the use in text of the letters 'MD' – 'Doctor of Medicine' in the USA but 'Managing Director' in the UK! To someone who is not a native English speaker, acronyms on a report can be even more confusing!

Results should be given in Standard International (SI) Units, to facilitate understanding internationally. Conversion tables can be useful to translate conventional units to SI units. These are given in various texts: the Royal Society of Medicine publication (Baron, 1994) is excellent.

STORAGE OF SAMPLES

The retention of laboratory samples is wise, sometimes essential, because they constitute evidence

(see also Chapter 11). Often this is not feasible because, for example, the whole sample has been used. This should be recorded. Some guidelines regarding retention of samples are as follows:

- If in doubt, assume that the samples will be needed later, even if initially the possibility of a legal case is relatively remote.

- Plan carefully how the samples are to be retained ($+4°C$ refrigeration, standard deep-freeze, ultra-low temperature, fixed). In some cases, e.g. liver that may later require toxicological, virological or TEM examination, it may be wise to divide samples and store them in different ways.

- As a general rule, retain original specimens until initial laboratory results are obtained. For instance, swabs for bacteriological culture should be kept for at least 72 hours (longer if slow-growing or fastidious organisms are being sought), by which time it should be clear as to whether the original sample is still needed.

- Have a proper system (diary, calendar, electronic reminder on a computer) to assist in deciding when a sample can probably safely be destroyed. Ensure that all laboratory staff are aware of the system.

- Appoint a responsible person to 'sign out' specimens when they are destroyed or sent elsewhere (see later).

- Storage of samples can be expensive and take up valuable space. If specimens are definitely needed (the prosecution/defence/court may have requested their retention), ask if the costs of storage (including reagents) can be borne by the relevant authority.

SPECIFIC LABORATORY-BASED STUDIES, WITH PARTICULAR REFERENCE TO HISTOLOGY

There are occasions when one discipline provides an answer to a legal question. A suspect poisoning case is an example: toxicological investigation provides the possibility of detecting significant amounts of a chemical and in some forensic cases this may, *per se*, be sufficient. More often, of course, it is a

Table 8.4 Examples of laboratory-based investigations that may assist in forensic investigations.

Discipline	*Investigation*	*Comments/information that may be obtained*
Parasitology	Identification of ecto- and endoparasites, including blood parasites (haematozoa and microfilariae)	Species present may give clues as to geographical origin of host, time of death or contact with other species, including prey or predator
Haematology	Examination of blood smears	Presence of anucleate red cells will confirm that the blood came from a mammal Other features may pinpoint the species more closely
	Haemoglobin estimations	Elevated values may indicate that an animal has originated from a high altitude
Histology	Standard methods	Many uses, e.g. anthracosis may indicate an industrial origin, a giant cell focus a reaction to a foreign body

combination of results that unravels the situation – in the same way as the cause of clinical disease or a fatality is often multifactorial (see Chapters 6 and 7).

Each case is different and it would be impossible to list all the tests that can be used. Table 8.4 gives some examples.

Histological examination of tissues is a routine part of pathological (*post-mortem*) investigation and often also of material from live animals. The results may give a diagnosis (for example, whether or not a cat that died unexpectedly had pneumonia) or it may provide specific answers to questions which may have legal implications. Examples of where histology can prove useful include:

- Confirmation that a piece of tissue removed during vasectomy was indeed vas deferens.
- Interpretation of tissue reaction around a surgical wound, an implanted transponder or a foreign body.
- Explanation of why a skin wound or fracture failed to heal.
- Age determination of certain species, using studies on sections of bones (see, for example, Broughton *et al.*, 2002).

ARTEFACTS

Artefacts in laboratory preparations, especially histological sections, are well-recognised and can

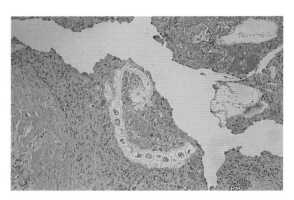

Figure 8.10 Plant material in a histological section. This was introduced when the tissue was collected during a field necropsy. It may provide important information about the location where the animal died. This figure also appears in colour in the colour plate section.

hamper interpretation, especially if they resemble parasites or other structures that may be of diagnostic or forensic importance (Thompson and Luna, 1978). Some apparent artefacts are an integral part of the animal, albeit foreign in nature (e.g. vegetable matter from ingesta that embeds in the wall of the intestine), while others are extraneous (e.g. talc particles introduced during necropsy or surgery) (see below). Many artefacts are due to faulty procedure – during fixation, processing, embedding, cutting, staining or mounting. In a legal case, the finding of artefacts can complicate reporting and may provoke criticism of the techniques used. Equally, however, artefacts can sometimes provide data that assist in analysis of the case, including information about the history or provenance of the animal.

FOREIGN BODIES

A 'foreign body', in its broadest sense, means 'an object that is in the wrong place' and the forensic relevance of such items includes the following:

- Items intentionally introduced or accidentally left in surgical wounds, e.g. transponders ('chips') (Nind, 2005), swabs and instruments (Figure 9.3).
- Reactions in the tissues of animals or humans as a result of ingestion (e.g. metal), contact with dangerous animals (e.g. sea urchins – see Chapter 2) or irritant materials (e.g. talc).
- Unexpected findings in products (e.g. gross contaminants in human foodstuffs or animal feed).

The first two are of clinical importance but will not be discussed in detail here. Histological artefacts are mentioned earlier.

The third category is of considerable significance to forensics because contamination of food, medicines or other products may constitute grounds for criminal action, civil action or both. Various methods are used either to detect such contamination or to identify the contaminant and, depending on circumstances, these can include:

- Chemical analysis.
- Microscopical examination.
- Radiography.

DNA SAMPLES

DNA technology has become a very important part of forensic investigation, both in humans and animals. Indeed, in the minds of many lay people and some scientists, DNA is synonymous with forensics – a far cry from the broadening of the term described in Chapters 1 and 2!

All those who are involved in animal forensic work must be familiar with the potential of DNA technology and at least be able to take and

submit appropriate samples. Useful introductory references are the books by Butler (2001), Rudin and Inman (2002) and Eppler and Lubjuhn (1999). The last of these contains a chapter about DNA-profiling in veterinary medicine (Buitkamp *et al.*, 1999).

DNA-profiling techniques can provide information about a whole range of matters including:

- Parentage and kinship.
- Sex (gender).
- Species.
- Populations.
- Strains.

Analysis of DNA from animals or their derivatives can assist in human forensic investigations. The most famous case, a forerunner, was the murder case in Canada where cat hair implicated and then led to the conviction of a suspect (Menotti-Raymond *et al.*, 1997).

DNA studies have played a particularly important part in the battle against wildlife crime (Fain and LeMay, 1995). They have contributed, for example, to linking a suspect with a crime scene, checking claims of captive-breeding, the identification of species and unequivocal gender determination (PAW, 2005).

General rules for sampling for DNA are as follows:

- Ascertain which available tissue may provide the most informative sample.
- Determine the purpose for which the tissue is required.
- Have a proper protocol and adhere to it.
- Remember that tissue samples from live animals are generally more reliable than from dead.
- Ensure that all instruments and containers are clean (sterile if possible) and free of 'stray' DNA.
- Wear gloves and handle tissues with forceps.
- Place tissues for DNA analysis in sterile plastic containers, paper bags or aluminium foil.
- Label samples correctly and indelibly with a unique number.

The method of transportation and storage of DNA samples is also important. Sarre (2001) recommended the following:

- Transport tissues preserved in ethanol or in bottles, etc., and as cold as possible, preferably at 4°C or −20°C.
- Store frozen tissues at −70°C if possible.
- Keep out of direct sunlight.
- In emergencies – keep cool, keep dry!

Although one of the advantages of PCR-based methods is that tissue samples that contain only limited amounts of DNA (or degraded DNA) can be examined, the value of any DNA study is greatly enhanced by using material of good quality. Quality will be reduced if there is contamination or if there is *post-mortem* change, when the DNA in cells begins to degenerate as a result of exposure to enzymes. The speed at which degradation occurs depends upon the type of tissue and the amount of moisture that is present in the cells – therefore DNA in liver will degrade rapidly compared with muscle on account of the presence of cellular enzymes. Blood shows very slow rates of degradation as long as the temperature is low.

Sampling from carcases and choice of tissue requires particular care. The ears of a dead animal can be particularly valuable as a source of DNA because they generally dry rapidly, thus DNA is preserved. Sarre provided useful guidelines for sample collection. He emphasised the value of blood in comparison with other tissues and the fact that it can be taken from all types of vertebrates. Other sources such as hair shafts degrade slowly and are a useful source of mitochondrial (mt) DNA.

USE OF DNA TECHNOLOGY

At the same time as there has been heated debate, especially in Britain, about the retention of human tissues, a move to establish national databases of DNA, based on a sample (perhaps only a drop of saliva) from everyone in the community, is growing (Sedley, 2005). This subject is not of immediate relevance to those involved in animal forensics but they should be aware of the issues involved, especially the apparently conflicting wishes of society to be able to tackle crime while, adequately at the same time, continuing to respect human rights and privacy. A number of countries have established national DNA databanks, ostensibly as a crime-solving tool – New Zealand, for example (Harbison *et al.*, 2001). The prospects of a global database have been raised but this seems unlikely in the immediate future.

There is no doubt that DNA profiling ('fingerprinting') has revolutionised the judicial process. The discovery by Professor (now Sir) Alec Jeffreys, in 1984, that a distinct, probably unique, DNA profile could be established for each person, led quickly to the use of the technique in legal cases. It is noteworthy that the first use of DNA profiling in a murder investigation resulted in the exoneration of a suspect in addition to identifying the person responsible – a reminder of the role of forensic techniques in protecting the innocent as well as confronting the guilty.

A whole range of DNA analysis techniques is now available – STR DNA profiling, SNP multiplexes, Y-STR and Y-SNP analyses, mitochondrial DNA profiling – but often the samples available in forensic work are so small that a decision has to be made as to which is the most appropriate. PCR has now made it possible to use several types of analysis on single small samples.

Methods of increasing recovery of DNA from material have attracted much interest in recent years. One such technique is laser microdissection (LMD), used in human forensic work in order to improve detection of DNA from spermatozoa.

Watson (2004) discussed the analysis of body fluids (blood, semen, saliva, etc.), with particular reference to DNA techniques.

SENDING SAMPLES ELSEWHERE

Sending forensic material from one country to another is not always easy. A small tube containing dead carrion beetles may pose no health threats, not need a CITES permit and be of 'no commercial value' (NCV) but, almost inevitably, Customs will be interested and delays may result. Having an experienced agent will expedite matters but may entail extra cost.

Samples that may constitute evidence should be placed in separate packages and properly sealed. This implies that its contents cannot be removed, changed or damaged without detection. Evidence seal tape should be used (see Appendix E): the person sending the sample should sign/initial and date the area that is taped. A list of contents should accompany the consignment, with copies available for officials and for the receiving agent.

Perishable evidence will need special attention. It may have to be chilled or frozen *en route*. Various methods can be used and laboratories will advise on this. There are legal and ethical considerations (see earlier). Hazardous material (pathogens, poisons, radioactive or explosive samples, etc.) will be subject in most countries to strict regulation, even if being sent between laboratories (see Chapter 3). Advice must be sought and followed. 'Short-cutting' the system must never be practised as it may compromise both human safety and the judicial process.

Some animal material presents hazards other than those alluded to above (see also Chapter 2). The heads of venomous snakes can still be danger-ous if a fang comes into contact with human skin. The feet of large birds of prey can inflict damage through wrappings, especially if rigid because of freezing. Skunks in the USA and polecats in Europe are amongst species that readily contami-nate material with their pungent and persistent odour, as can formalin used for fixation: the latter is also carcinogenic.

Current fears of terrorism, particularly in the USA, may make it more difficult or less effective to send forensic samples to other countries, or even by air in-country. Gloor *et al.* (2005) suggested, on the basis of a study on feline semen, that new airport security measures at US airports (X-ray scanning of all checked baggage) may cause damage to valuable biological samples when they are trans-ported on passenger aircraft.

TRACKING OF SAMPLES

As in a real chain, there are points of weakness in any chain of custody (evidence). Usually the danger is when a specimen changes hands. The person who receives the material may be a police officer or someone else who is familiar with the legal process. However, sometimes the recipient is not *au fait*

with such matters – a receptionist in a laboratory, for instance, and problems may then arise.

All samples submitted to a laboratory that may constitute evidence should be accompanied by a chain of custody form or docket or have the appro-priate information added to tags on individual samples. A specimen chain of custody form is given in Appendix A.

The laboratory interface is sensitive for other reasons. The person submitting the specimen and the people receiving it may think they comprehend one another but there may be misunderstandings and confusion. Telephoned instructions are never satisfactory. Samples should be accompanied by paperwork that states categorically which tests are required.

Most labs have their own way of working and the veterinarian should be aware of this. Some instructions may need to be spelled out very clearly, preferably in person. For example, a faecal sample submitted to a laboratory may be subjected to a very rigorous examination, but by a parasitologist who concentrates on worms and fails to record, perhaps even notice, that the sample also contains red blood cells, undigested fat and fibres from banana. Not-withstanding the earlier point, a report that says 'No parasites seen' is therefore of limited value. Even less helpful is the bland statement 'Negative' which may mean that nothing was seen down the microscope or, perhaps, that the electricity was not working or the technician was on leave!

Transposition and/or loss of specimens can occur very easily. Correct, unique, labelling and careful storage are important but mistakes often occur when the material is removed from the container for examination or sample-taking. Fixed tissues for histopathological processing are a good example: the small pieces are placed on a surface and can easily be dropped or misplaced.

Some recommended ways of minimising the risk of transposition or loss of specimens, not exclusive of each other, are:

- Set aside time to deal with forensic samples – mistakes are made when one is in a hurry.
- Try to have a colleague or assistant present who can assist and help to ensure that the system is followed.

- Ignore telephone calls (including mobile/cell phones – turn them off!) and discourage visitors and on-lookers: concentrate on the matter in hand.
- Prepare a proper working surface, with a raised lip on the edge to prevent tubes from rolling off, covered with disposable paper which is changed between specimens.
- Where appropriate, count samples in and out.
- *Never* put a piece of tissue back into a container if there is any doubt.

Any errant sample should either be destroyed or stored (separately) elsewhere in case it needs to be retrieved later.

Tracking systems are essential in any forensic operation and imply both the proper marking of specimens and a method of locating where they are at any given time. Electronic (computerised) methods should be supported by means that do not rely on electricity, especially (but not only) in poorer countries. Books for reception and tracing of laboratory specimens that are being processed is one example – as is the careful labelling of refrigerators with details of which specimens go in and which come out. Periodic photocopying of paperwork, so that duplicates can be stored safely elsewhere, as emergency back-up, is wise: original paper copies get lost, and in some countries they may be destroyed by termites.

RETENTION OF LABORATORY SAMPLES

How long material should be retained after reporting is debatable. A legal case may drag on for years. A claim against a pharmaceutical company, a veterinarian, or a diagnostic laboratory, may be made long after relevant samples have been examined. The ability, using modern DNA technology, to perform tests retrospectively makes the saving of material even more important. For example, PCR techniques permit the diagnosis of some diseases and/or the detection of antigens, from formalin-fixed, paraffin wax-embedded tissues, sometimes years after they were processed (Jung *et al.*, 2003). Laboratories that test new pharmaceutical and agricultural products often retain their records and materials for ten years or more, and may even store items in a fireproof basement. In a medical forensic setting, DiMaio and DiMaio (2001) suggested that toxicological samples should be kept for a minimum of two, preferably five years, after analysis.

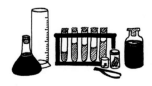

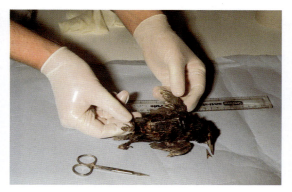

Figure 2.7 One of a number of common starlings killed in an explosion.

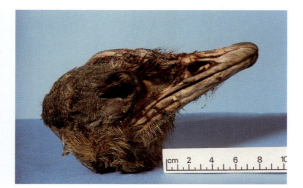

Figure 4.2 The head of a young captive ostrich that was killed by a blow to the head. The question here was 'Did the bird suffer?'

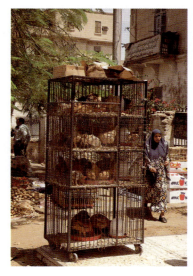

Figure 4.6 In many parts of the world the welfare of livestock is not a priority: a street scene in Egypt.

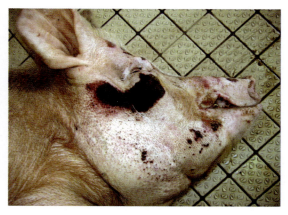

Figure 4.3 The head of a sow that died following a week's recumbency. Skin lesions, that became infected, are apparent. (Courtesy of Richard Spence.)

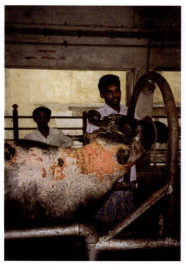

Figure 4.9 A (water) buffalo in India, badly scalded in a revenge attack.

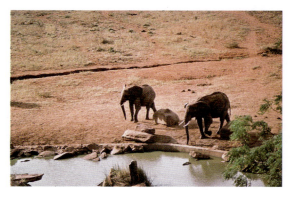

Figure 5.3 Wild animals are particularly susceptible to poaching when under pressure for other reasons – these elephants during a drought in Kenya, for example.

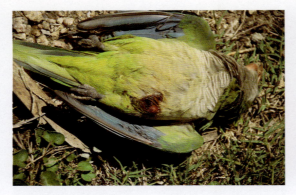

Figure 5.4 A parakeet, one of a number found dead, believed shot, in Uruguay.

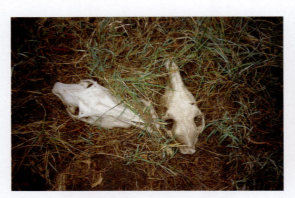

Figure 5.5 Two skulls, from an unidentified equid species, in Kenya. Are they from a zebra or a donkey? Is there a conservation or animal welfare implication?

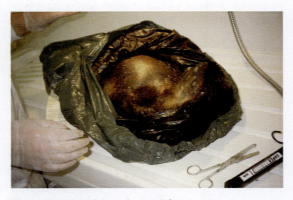

Figure 5.8 A badger, submitted for necropsy to ascertain how it died. There are numerous maggots on the skin and these may assist in determining the *post-mortem* interval (PMI).

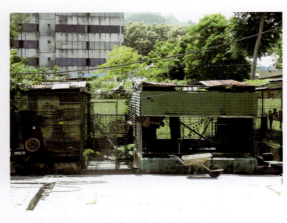

Figure 5.17 Facilities for holding confiscated animals are often sub-standard.

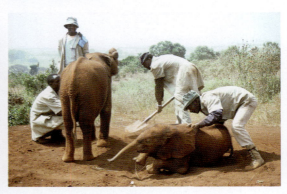

Figure 5.18 Young orphaned animals are tended at an elephant sanctuary in East Africa.

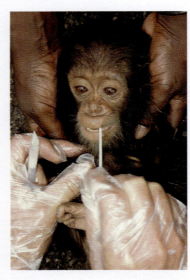

Figure 5.19 A young chimpanzee, orphaned and in need of veterinary attention, because its mother was killed in Central Africa.

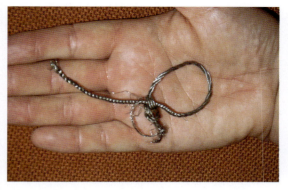

Figure 5.24 Part of a snare, made of braided wire, from Rwanda. This was set to catch small antelope but inadvertently trapped a young mountain gorilla, necessitating amputation of two of its digits.

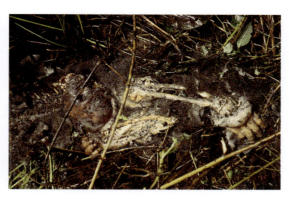

Figure 5.31 All that remained of one of the gorillas – bones, connective tissue and skin.

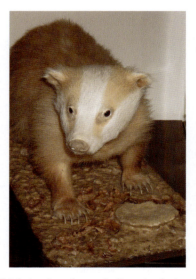

Figure 5.26 A colour form of a Eurasian badger, mounted legally for exhibition by a professional taxidermist.

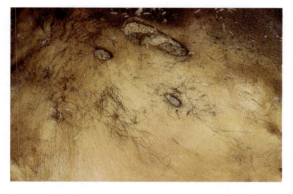

Figure 5.32 Skull wounds in one of the gorillas. The lesions are characteristic of metal arrows, commonly used by local poachers. Live maggots are present.

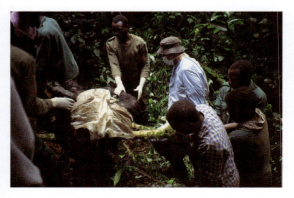

Figure 5.30 One of four mountain gorillas, found dead under mysterious circumstances in Uganda.

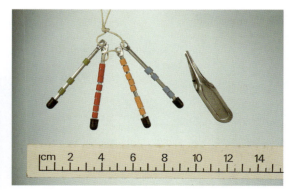

Figure 6.1 Coloured plastic rings, with metal applicator. Such rings are ideal for temporarily marking confiscated birds.

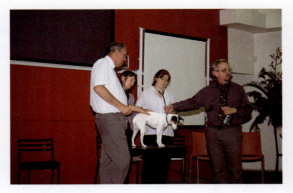

Figure 6.12 A training session in New Zealand. Students are taught how to recognize signs of abuse.

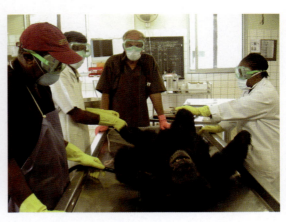

Figure 7.6 Necropsy of certain species requires special precautions to protect against zoonoses. For examination of this chimpanzee, all the pathologists wear goggles.

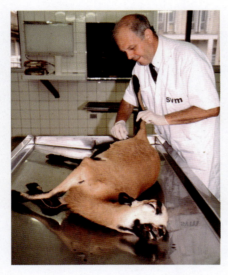

Figure 7.1 A routine *post-mortem* examination in progress. (Courtesy of Richard Spence.)

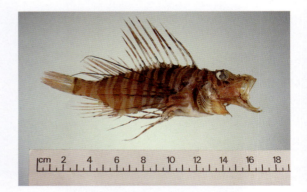

Figure 7.9 Some *post-mortem* specimens can be hazardous to the pathologist. This lion (scorpion) fish bears poisonous spines.

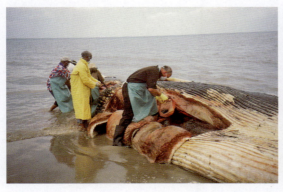

Figure 7.3 Necropsy of a beached whale requires a team effort, adherence to standard protocols and awareness of hazards, such as rising tides.

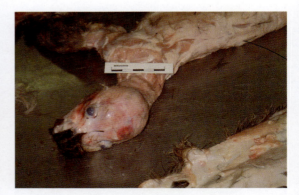

Figure 7.10 Skinning a carcase can reveal important information, as in this puppy where tooth marks were detected in the skull.

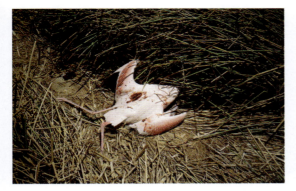

Figure 7.11 A freshly-dead lesser flamingo, probably killed by a predator. Bleeding is apparent.

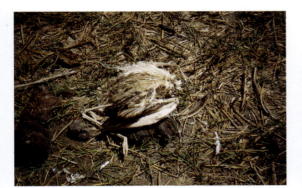

Figure 7.12 A flamingo that died two weeks before the photo was taken. The carcase is dry and little soft tissue remains.

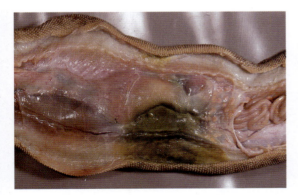

Figure 7.14 Early *post-mortem* change in a reptile is often marked by bile-staining of the ventral skin.

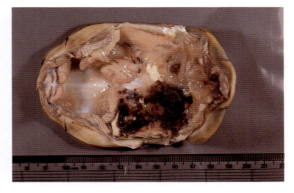

Figure 7.16 Aging of bruises can be complicated. In this case, a tortoise that was the subject of assault, the bruised area has changed colour, largely as a result of refrigeration and brief immersion in formalin.

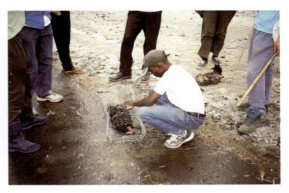

Figure 7.20 Forensic studies in the Rift Valley. A dead chicken in a cage is checked for *post-mortem* change and the presence of invertebrates.

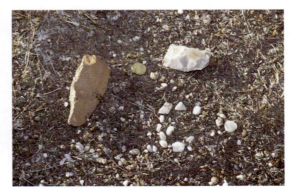

Figure 7.21 A carcase may disappear but evidence remains. A ring of small stones from the gizzard of a now extinct moa in New Zealand.

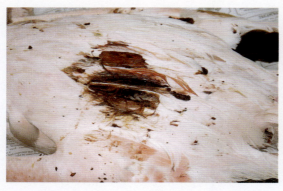

Figure 7.24 A characteristic *ante-mortem* stab wound, in this case in a flamingo, caused by the beak of a marabou stork.

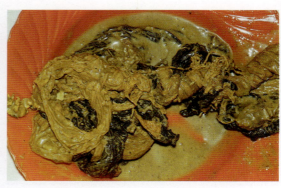

Figure 7.27 The contents of the reticulum of a red brocket deer. An ingested plastic bag has caused an obstruction. (Courtesy of Richard Spence.)

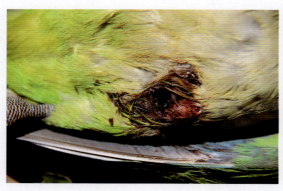

Figure 7.25 An *ante-mortem* shot wound in a parakeet.

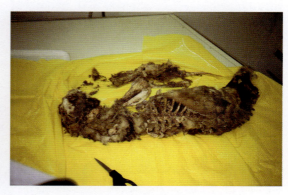

Figure 7.33 A mummified dog, the subject of an animal welfare case, is received for necropsy.

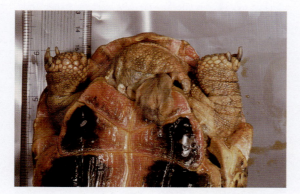

Figure 7.26 Prolonged immersion in water can produce various artefacts, regardless of whether or not the animal drowned. This tortoise, one of two found in a garden pond, has an extruded penis and the soft tissues are waterlogged.

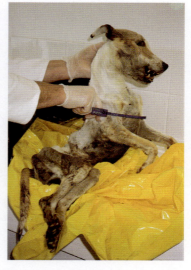

Figure 7.34 A terrier, alleged to have been starved to death. The animal is emaciated.

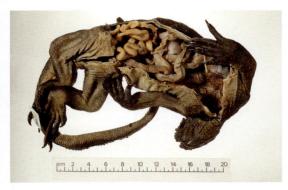

Figure 7.35 Starvation in ectothermic vertebrates can be difficult to diagnose. This marine iguana is one of many that died after an El Niño event. It has no subcutaneous fat and abdominal fat bodies were not located.

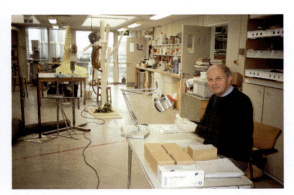

Figure 7.38 Museums are a rich source of material and information relevant to forensic medicine. Here bones are being examined as part of a study on the decline of a rare (Madagascan) species of duck.

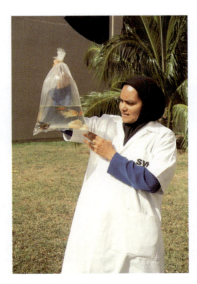

Figure 8.3 Examining fish with the water from which they originated can be an important part of monitoring pollution.

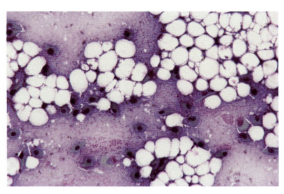

Figure 8.7 Cytological examination provides a rapid means of obtaining information about pathological lesions and is ideally suited to forensic investigations in the field. This liver of a fish shows multiple fat droplets suggestive of lipidosis.

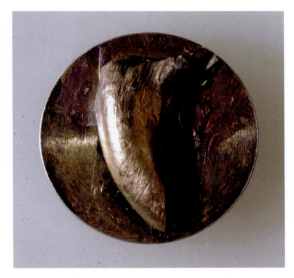

Figure 8.9 Gold spattering, a technique used in scanning electronmicroscopy work, in this case on the beak of a cockerel that was found following an alleged cock-fighting competition. (Courtesy of Richard Spence.)

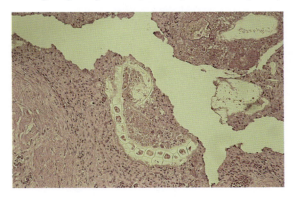

Figure 8.10 Plant material in a histological section. This was introduced when the tissue was collected during a field necropsy. It may provide important information about the location where the animal died.

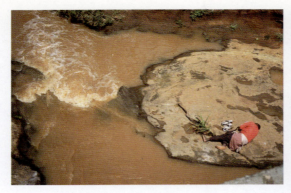

Figure 9.2 In both human and animal forensic work the crime scene can encompass varied natural terrain.

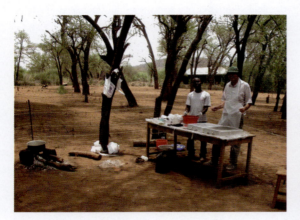

Figure 9.12 Investigations in the field require ingenuity and versatility. In this scene from the Kenyan Rift Valley, a field necropsy site has been established. The 'dirty' area has been demarcated with string and a colour code introduced – red for contaminated material, blue for 'clean'. A fire provides hot water for disinfection.

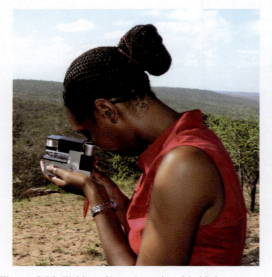

Figure 9.13 Field studies using a hand-held, battery-operated microscope.

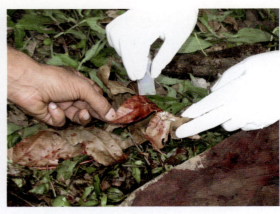

Figure 9.17 Laboratory tests in the field can yield immediate, often significant, results. This is a sequel to visiting the beach depicted earlier. Blood smears are taken from a wooden chopping board: on microscopical examination they prove to be mammalian, all that remains of the stranded dolphin.

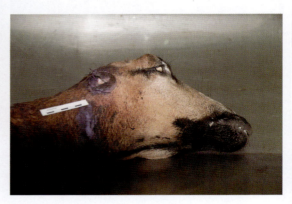

Figure 10.2 Wounds must be properly described and measured. These injuries inflicted by a dog on a Barbados black-bellied sheep were treated subsequently with purple medication.

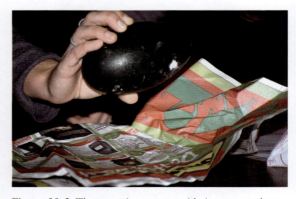

Figure 11.3 The wrapping may provide important clues to the origin of a specimen, as in this case where an egg submitted for examination was wrapped in pages from a local newspaper.

Site Visits, Fieldwork and Collection of Evidence

Detective work combines the use of one's eyes, ears and even one's nose; it means that observations must be accurate; it means having a great deal of patience and, most important of all, avoiding hasty conclusions without being able to prove them.

Maxwell Knight

My bones are not hid from thee: though I be made secretly, and fashioned beneath in the earth.

Psalm 139

Site visits are a key part of human forensic medicine (Pepper, 2005). They are necessary, for example, when a dead body is found or there is a road or rail accident. Those responsible for the protection, preparation and investigation of sites where an offence is alleged to have occurred are specialists in their own field – in the UK termed Crime Scene Investigators (CSIs) or Scenes of Crime Officers (SOCOs) (Townley and Ede, 2004). Veterinarians and others who are involved in animal forensic cases may meet such people during the course of investigations, especially if human death or injury is involved, and can learn much from them.

Site visits are also important in animal forensic work. As a general rule, it is sound practice for anyone involved in legal cases to be prepared to visit the site him/herself and not to depend only upon the descriptions and recollections of others.

Sometimes the issue is an environmental one in which case that location (e.g. where there has been an oil spillage) must be seen. On other occasions a veterinary surgeon may need to visit premises where it is alleged that animals are not being treated humanely or where blood and other samples need to be taken to assess whether captive wildlife are held legally (PAW, 2005). Other examples include:

- Incidents such as assault, involving both humans and animals, when forensic medical personnel are involved and a crime scene has been established.
- Cases relating to captive animals in zoos, aquaria, laboratories or private hands.
- Clinical cases that cannot easily be moved, e.g. a horse in a road accident.
- Wildlife crime relating to free-living animals or derivatives which cannot or should not be captured and need to be examined in their own environment (PAW, 2005).
- *Post-mortem* cases that must be examined *in situ*, e.g. a poached African elephant.

Weston (2004) stated that 'Forensic evidence starts at the scene' and went on to provide a valuable overview of the importance of a crime scene. He emphasised that the investigations can be time-consuming and expensive. The importance of scenes of crime investigations in wildlife cases was stressed in PAW (2005).

The crime scene puts a case into context (Horswell, 2003). An alleged offence can be viewed in a broader way than merely, for example, receiving a specimen and being asked to comment on it. In

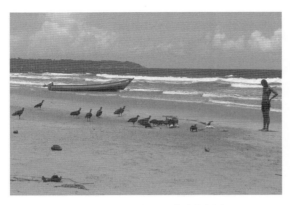

Figure 9.1 A crime scene. A stranded dolphin was unlawfully killed on this beach but only trace evidence remains.

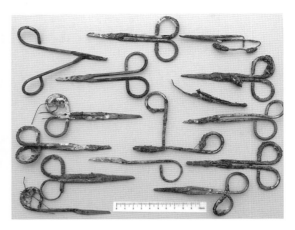

Figure 9.3 Site visits often provide unexpected evidence, such as these surgical instruments found in the ashes of an incinerator at a medical facility. (Courtesy of Richard Spence.)

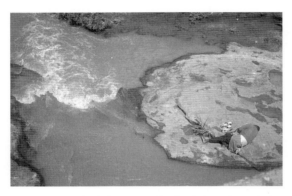

Figure 9.2 In both human and animal forensic work the crime scene can encompass varied natural terrain. This figure also appears in colour in the colour plate section.

PREPARATION FOR A VISIT

Whatever the reason for an expert opinion, certain basic preparation is vital. Some of this is discussed in more detail in Chapter 12. Advice is available to those involved in crime scene investigation from textbooks (see, for example, Townley and Ede, 2004 and White, 2004) and specific guidelines or 'rules of investigation' produced usually by governmental bodies.

Useful basic tips for those likely to be called out are as follows:

- Always have a checklist of essential items that you need to take with you; there are standard items that are always likely to be needed regardless of whether one is seeing a live animal, a dead animal or inspecting a crime scene (see Chapters 6 and 7 and Appendix E).
- Depending upon the information that is being received, supplement the items above with specifics that are needed (for example, examination of the sick or injured animal).
- Dress appropriately – this will depend upon the location (tropical, subtropical, temperate) and on the time of year/season.
- Take spectacles, umbrella, hat, medication and other items that can make life more comfortable.

some cases a visit to the scene is essential – for example, when a large animal is found dead under unusual circumstances. On other occasions a visit may not be vital but is desirable or a wise precaution, as in the case of the brown bear recently killed in France (Penketh, 2005). As a general rule, experts should take every opportunity to be present at the scene for this is the way to understand and to put together better, by evidence-gathering, the jigsaw puzzle that is every legal case.

A drawback to visiting crime scenes is that contamination – the introduction of extraneous, irrelevant material – can, and does, occur (see later).

- Tell someone where you have gone. Legal cases, especially visits to crime scenes, can take a long time and it is important that someone knows where you have gone and for what reasons.

Site visits should be carried out as soon as possible. Exposure to strong sunlight, gusty winds, a sudden shower of rain or a leaking water pipe may destroy, or interfere with, vital evidence (Figure 9.4).

Preparation for fieldwork encompasses the basic rules above but may be more sustained, necessitating extensive planning and carrying or improvisation of equipment (see later).

On any site visit, access to a telephone can be of great importance. However one should not depend on a mobile (cell) phone since these do not always work, particularly in isolated areas as might be the case when investigating a scene of wildlife crime. Therefore the expert should ensure that in addition to a mobile (cell) telephone, s/he has a phone card or money which can be used to gain access to a standard public telephone. This may seem unnecessary to readers from countries where communications are usually reliable but many of those overseas who are involved in forensic work do not have the same luxuries (Olumbe *et al.*, undated).

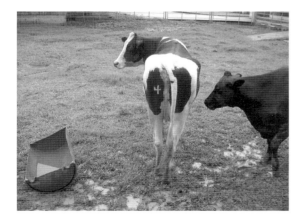

Figure 9.4 Evidence can easily be lost if a site visit is not made immediately. In this scene sudden rain has washed away an important item, relevant to the health of the cattle, which was readily visible thirty minutes earlier.

PLANNING AHEAD

Establishing and maintaining a crime scene in the field can be difficult (see later) especially in animal cases where SOCOs or their equivalent many not be available to investigate and to collect evidence. There are, however, two particular scenarios which sometimes entail a 'forensic' input and where existing planning may ameliorate the situation:

(1) If there is already an established response system, albeit for a different reason – for example, dealing with marine mammal strandings, when trained people who are familiar with protocols operate under a command structure.

(2) When a notifiable or reportable animal disease is suspected (see Chapter 3), as a result of which government animal health officials who have the authority and experience to take control of the situation will be involved.

Working under the circumstances above will greatly ease the work and responsibilities of the forensic investigator(s) – but such situations are likely to be the exception rather than the rule! On most occasions, a veterinarian or other suitably qualified person has to take the lead (see later). For this reason, those regularly involved in animal forensics should regularly practise and perfect crime scene investigation. Advice and assistance will be needed, however, and suitably experienced people, such as those in the two categories referred to above, should be invited to be involved in planning and training (see later).

RECORD-KEEPING AT THE CRIME SCENE

A micro-cassette tape recorder can be used for dictated notes and to record sounds of interest at a crime scene for example. The authors use voice-activated tape recorders. Many moderately priced micro-cassette recorders are available. Inserting the recorder into a bulky stocking or wrapping it in a cloth or a thin polyurethane foam sleeve can reduce excessive wind noise.

Video-recording is a useful way of assembling information at a crime scene and can be supplemented with photography, tape recording and the taking of contemporaneous notes.

Electronic data collection is increasingly important (see Chapter 10) but is not always possible in poorer countries, where wildlife crime is most often prevalent.

There may be different experts at the scene and some liaison between them is inevitable and usually valuable. This may take the form of a 'case conference', usually convened by the lawyer(s) in the case (see later). However, the veterinary expert must always make sure that what s/he records and reports is not influenced by what is heard from others. Ultimately, each expert will be examined and cross-examined separately.

Reconstruction of a crime scene back in the laboratory, office or veterinary practice depended in the past on the use of photographs and drawings. Computer software that can do such tasks is now available for use in human forensic medicine and clearly has potential in animal work. Three-dimensional images are used which can include such features as trees, bushes, furniture, corpses or weapons. The scene can be printed from any perspective and it is often possible to create virtual reality pictures through which the investigator can 'walk' as if in the actual location.

RE-ENACTMENT OF EVENTS

Reconstruction ('re-enactment') of a crime can be very helpful but needs to be carried out in a formal way – properly planned and with attention to detail. Detectives and other crime investigators regularly use such techniques, as do – in a rather different way – archaeologists, palaeontologists and taphonomists who want to test a hypothesis as to (for example) why a pile of bones shows certain unusual fractures.

EQUIPMENT FOR SITE VISITS

Pepper (2005) detailed the many and varied items that might be needed for a crime scene investigation. Many of these are applicable to animal forensic cases but in the same way as the circumstances are different, so also are some of the needs.

A basic checklist for a site visit is given below:

- Background papers, correspondence.
- Forensic submission and chain of custody forms.
- Witness statements.
- Relevant scientific papers/text books.
- Tape recorder and tapes.
- Camera(s).
- Magnifying loupe/hand lens.
- Clipboard and pencils/waterproof pens.
- Chalk.
- Protective clothing.
- Clinical equipment.
- *Post-mortem* equipment.
- Instruments – either several sets or with facilities to clean them between specimens (to prevent cross-contamination).
- Containers for specimens – preferably glassware that has been acid-rinsed, or specially (commercially) cleaned tubes and jars.
- Environmental equipment – as needed (e.g. water-testing kit).
- Entomological equipment (see later).
- Cool boxes, pre-chilled or containing ice.

Some additional useful items are presented in Table 9.1. Detailed and more specific information is found in Appendix E.

All items must be clean before entering the scene – and afterwards thoroughly cleaned, after checking that important evidence has not been removed.

In modern forensic practice, protective coveralls ('boiler suits' in the UK) are often standard. These may or may not incorporate additional features such as protection for the face. There are numerous makes of protective coveralls and they are available in most countries. However, points that they are likely to have in common are:

- Lightweight.
- Liquid-proof.
- Durable.
- Permeable to moisture and gases escaping from the body – less likely to cause overheating.

Table 9.1 Some useful items for crime scene visits.

Item	Comments
Rubber boots	A large size is advisable to facilitate removal
Lightweight shoes	As above May not be suitable if terrain is rough
Plastic overshoes	Always have available for visitors
Other disposables, e.g. rubber gloves	As above
Coveralls	See below and later
Coat	Must be lightweight and appropriate colour (live animals may be disturbed by white clothing)
Umbrella	To protect against rain and sun and to serve as an emergency container Should be lightweight
Vacuum flask	For hand-washing or as a source of clean water, to make tea or coffee
Field equipment (see text)	If detailed investigations have to be carried out at the site

- Anti-static.
- Can be incinerated.

Such coveralls are primarily produced for such purposes as paint-spraying, handling of chemicals, use of agricultural herbicides and waste disposal. However, they are ideal for forensic work, especially when there is uncertainty as to what risks exist at the crime scene.

Increasingly, the expert attending a crime scene must be prepared to don *full* protective clothing including, if circumstances demand, a respirator; terrorist acts, especially where chemical or biological agents are suspected or involved, present a particular hazard.

SPECIALISED EQUIPMENT

Various additional items may be needed at the crime scene. It is possible, depending on the circum-stances and the alleged offence, that the police or other authorities will provide these. Some examples follow.

Light source

Light sources are of great importance, both to search the whole crime scene at night or when overcast and to examine in detail small items, such as animals or their derivatives. A broadband white light is usually ideal, preferably fitted with detach-able colour filters and employing shadow-free beam. Narrow band violet, blue or green illumination can be used to detect hair, bone fragments, fibres, urine, semen, saliva and other body fluids, many of which fluoresce when exposed to it. Such light sources can be assembled, or purchased, often as part of a kit, from commercial companies. The wavelength is important: ordinary ultraviolet, while valuable as a light source for other purposes (e.g. attracting insects), may not have the same effect.

Theft detection products

Theft-detection powders and sprays are available commercially and regularly used in human forensic work in order to incriminate thieves. Most of these products fluoresce under ultraviolet or blue light and as a result a person can be 'tracked' by the powder that s/he disseminates. Although use of theft-detection products is limited in animal work *per se*, veterinarians and others should be aware of the technology as it may be used by the police to detect a criminal act.

Sample collection equipment

A small, hand-held, battery-powered vacuum cleaner is useful for collecting evidence and for such chores as sampling nests for the presence of tiny ectoparasites especially mites. Ideally, the vacuum cleaner should not have an inner dust bag but an impervious, smooth-sided receptacle and a dust filter that can be emptied and washed before being re-used.

Other equipment can also be used to detect or collect samples at the crime scene – for example, brushes. A metal detector can be valuable where metallic objects are sought. An entomologist's aspirator ('pooter') is useful for sucking-up small samples but should not be used by mouth if there is any danger of pathogens or poisons.

PRECAUTIONS AND PROBLEMS AT THE CRIME SCENE

It is most important to remember that a 'crime scene' has a legal significance and should be disturbed as little as possible (Townley and Ede, 2004). At the very least, this means exercising great care when doing a site visit. It must be remembered that in entering any crime scene, one always *leaves* something at the site and one always *takes* something away – a concept based on the work and writings of the great French forensic scientist, Edmond Locard (1877–1966).

An extreme situation where 'contamination' can readily occur is exemplified by human-induced disasters such as acts of terrorism, when the immediate need is to alleviate human (sometimes animal) suffering. But in so doing, forensic evidence is usually lost or disturbed on a large scale. A balance has to be struck.

There are two important points arising from this:

(1) The expert visiting a crime scene must do all possible to minimise the risk of disturbance or removal of evidence or of bringing irrelevant material on to the site (see later). Proper preparation, including the use of appropriately prepared protective clothing, can help here.

(2) The expert who is involved in animal work must be prepared for the fact that, especially

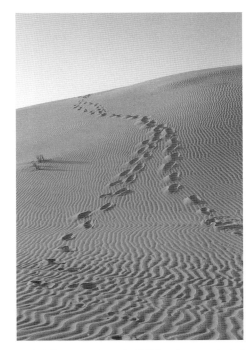

Figure 9.6 Investigation of wildlife crime can be helped by study of footprints – in this case of humans who may have been involved.

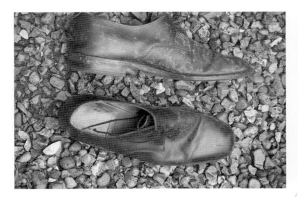

Figure 9.5 Shoes can provide information about a crime but can also contaminate the scene or remove trace evidence.

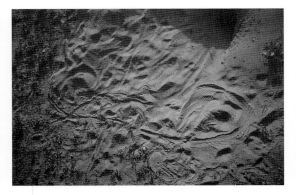

Figure 9.7 Animal tracks may provide useful information. These are marks made by a protected spiny-tailed, 'dhub' lizard in Abu Dhabi.

in a disaster area where humans are at risk or vital evidence is likely to be present, priority will be given to humans rather than animals.

SEARCH WARRANTS

In most countries, these need to be issued before the police or other authorised persons (usually listed by name or position on the warrant) may enter private premises. How a warrant is obtained will depend: in England enforcement authorities need to demonstrate to a magistrate that there are reasonable grounds to believe that an offence has been committed and that evidence of the offence is likely to be found at the premises to be entered.

An expert may be asked to be present when a premise is entered. S/he will be acting under the authority of the relevant body (police, Customs) and must comply with their instructions.

Veterinarians and others may be asked to accompany enforcement agencies and police on unannounced visits to premises where it is believed that an offence concerning animals may have taken place or be in progress. Such actions (sometimes called 'raids') can present dilemmas because they:

- Often have a melodramatic orientation (early morning or late at night, a team approach, participants ready if necessary to respond to threats of, or actual, physical violence). This does not appeal to everyone, however knowledgeable s/he may be about the issue.
- Can introduce an element of partiality because the expert tends to be seen as part of a group that is essentially trying to implicate a person or persons. Teamwork is essential in such circumstances (see later) but must not lead to collusion.

For these reasons it is wise for anyone approached to participate in a 'raid' to ask the following questions:

- Am I happy to be involved in this exercise, bearing in mind the two points above?
- If I am, am I prepared and able to retain, as far as possible, my position as an expert by (for example) not becoming involved in loose talk during the raid, by adopting a professional, unbiased, approach in my dealings with those carrying out the raid *and* the individual(s) under investigation?

Some veterinarians prefer not to be part of the execution of the search warrant but are prepared to be available to examine animals or other evidence immediately afterwards.

SOME RULES WHEN ENTERING A CRIME SCENE

- Plan what you need beforehand in order to avoid entering and leaving the scene unnecessarily. A basic crime scene kit is listed elsewhere but it may need to be supplemented. If in doubt, do not leave it out!
- If a crime scene manager (CSM) or police officer or equivalent is present, follow his/her rules and instructions.
- Minimise all disturbance to the site. Touch nothing unnecessarily, stand still when movement is not required, carry everything you need (and do not put it on the ground). Some examples of actions that can destroy or damage evidence at a crime scene are given in Table 9.2.
- Remember the basic rule that observation is the all-important prelude to action. Stop, stand still and spend at least one minute on surveillance of the site and immediate environment. Use eyes, ears and nose. Remember that some important evidence may be lost if you move too fast – for example, birds at the scene may fly away (Figure 9.8).
- Supplement observation with drawings (sketches), note-taking, photography, video recording and tape recording.

MANAGEMENT OF THE CRIME SCENE

As emphasised earlier, in human forensics, especially when a serious crime (murder, rape, arson) appears to have been committed, the crime scene is secured and managed by trained, competent, persons (Pepper, 2005; Townley and Ede, 2004).

Table 9.2 Some actions to avoid at the crime scene.

Action	*Possible results*
Treading or walking carelessly	Damage to footprints, tyre marks, vegetation
Not wearing gloves	Addition to fingerprints
Wearing gloves but not taking care	Obliteration of fingerprints
Failing to wear adequate protective clothing	Contamination of crime scene with, e.g., foreign DNA Exposure to pathogens, poisons, etc.
Smoking	Contamination of crime scene with ash, etc.
Using domestic facilities at the site such as toilets, wash basin or telephone	Contamination (see above) Addition or obliteration of fingerprints Destruction (by flushing toilet or running water) of evidence
Moving items or turning on/off taps or lights	As above Evidence that, e.g., animals have not been fed, watered or kept warm/cool may be lost or damaged if the facilities are touched or used

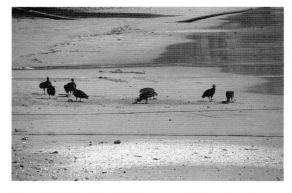

Figure 9.8 New World vultures patrol a beach – often a sign that a dead animal has been washed up.

In animal forensics, things may be different. There are three possible scenarios:

(1) There is an established crime scene because the animal incident is linked with some serious assault on humans or property, e.g. a dog has been shot in the same house as has a family, dead bats are all that remain in a factory that was destroyed in a terrorist attack.

(2) The veterinarian (animal welfare officer, wildlife inspector, etc.) is escorted to the crime scene by a police officer or another official who can organise or assist with the maintenance of a secure crime scene.

(3) The veterinarian is the only official present. For instance, a cat has been reported to have been stoned by youngsters; it is dying in a courtyard. Evidence is present in the location, but as yet no-one else is present to co-ordinate activities.

The last scenario is the most difficult one and may need quick-thinking and decisive action. If the veterinarian has to take charge, even if only initially, s/he must:

- Establish a proper command structure and responsibility by introducing him/herself to others present.
- Ascertain the size and location of the crime scene.
- Demarcate the crime scene by using barrier tape or its equivalent.
- Ensure safety of the scene – for example, by moving bystanders away from buildings that may collapse or animals that may bite.
- Plan collection of evidence and photographic or other records.
- Carry out or arrange special investigations, e.g. blood pattern analysis, invertebrate collection.

- Establish and maintain a proper chain of custody.

Barrier tape or its equivalent will be needed in order to demarcate the crime scene. This can be supplemented with markers, flags, cones and other crime-scene security items (see Appendix E).

If an animal is found dead and has to be moved, it is wise to have a photographic record of its original position (see later). This can be supplemented by a chalk or paint outline if, for example, the carcase is on a road, kennel floor or other hard surface.

RESPONSIBILITY FOR COLLECTION OF EVIDENCE

In many countries collection of evidence in criminal cases will be under the supervision of an appropriately trained person – a Scenes of Crime Officer (SOCO) in Britain. Sometimes, however, especially in poorer countries, evidence has to be collected by those called to the scene (see later). This requires great care to avoid cross-contamination or spoilage of specimens.

HEALTH AND SAFETY

It is important to provide safety for all those in attendance at a crime scene, including those in the field, who are investigating alleged wildlife crime (PAW, 2005). A risk assessment is needed (see Chapter 7) but this can present difficulties as, almost by definition, one does not necessarily know what hazards may be encountered. At a conventional crime scene, for example, risks may include explosives or toxic substances; in the field, however, wild animals, venomous snakes, traps and poachers may be dangers.

Olumbe *et al.* (undated) listed five categories of 'dangers at the crime scene':

(1) Physical, e.g. electricity, fire.
(2) Biological, e.g. pathogenic bacteria.
(3) Chemical, e.g. acids, smoke.
(4) Ergonomic, e.g. strain injuries from lifting bodies.

(5) Psychosocial, e.g. effects on those present of exposure to death and other unpleasant sights.

These can all be applied, with modification and additions, to animal forensic work.

CONTAINING THE CRIME SCENE

Specially-produced barrier tape, usually made of polyethylene, permits the demarcation of a crime scene. Such tape may be labelled, with instruments, not to cross.

PHOTOGRAPHY

Forensic photography is a specialised discipline in its own right (Redsicker and O'Connor, 1997) but in animal work a specialist is not always accessible.

Photographing and examining dead animals and other sensitive material at the crime scene is best carried out without the attention of on-lookers or the press. Privacy screens may be purchased or constructed using canvas or sacking and aluminium poles or strong canes. Sometimes a lightweight tent can be used, especially where there is a need to protect items from rain or snow, but taking care not to damage the crime scene.

Police and other investigators usually photograph the crowds of onlookers that gather at a crime scene. Sometimes the perpetrator of the offence is present, especially in cases of arson where seeing the outcome of one's crime seems to have appeal. This is not specifically relevant to animal work but the concept of photographing onlookers and bystanders may possibly have relevance in (for example) cases where animals have been abused or 'liberated' (see Chapter 4).

Camera accessories, including tripods, facilitate the photographing of material that is illuminated with blue light. The use of reflective ultraviolet photography in forensic work has been described in various publications (see, for example, Kraus, 1985).

Reconstruction of a crime scene, using drawings, photographs or computer software, is discussed elsewhere.

SPECIFIC INVESTIGATIONS AT THE CRIME SCENE

Many of the methods likely to be used are not specific to animal work but relate to the human component (Pepper, 2005) – for example, the taking of fingerprints (Townley and Ede, 2004), the identification of handwriting in notebooks (Huber and Headrick, 1999), the recognition of voices on mobile telephones (Rose, 2002) or the examination of paint and glass (Caddy, 2001).

BLOOD PATTERN ANALYSIS (BPA)

This refers to the examination, identification and interpretation of patterns of blood staining in relation to the actions that caused them (Emes and Price, 2004; James and Eckert, 1998). BPA is extensively used in human forensic medicine (Shepherd, 2003) but has only recently begun to form part of animal work – in the UK, at any rate (Phil Wilson, pers. comm.).

It is generally accepted that there are eight different patterns of blood staining and these range from single drops and impact spatter to contact stains and composite stain patterns. Secondary patterns occur when small drops form and are projected at low velocity on to a surface; for example, a horse with a wound that is dripping blood may also have secondary spatter marks on its lower limbs and hooves. Impact spatter is the most common type of pattern seen in human forensics (Emes and Price, 2004) and can be caused by shooting, kicking and other violent actions.

BPA is a large and complex subject and cannot be discussed in detail here. Those involved in animal forensic work should be aware of the expertise that exists. Useful references include Bevel and Gardner (2002) and MacDonell (1993).

ENTOMOLOGICAL INVESTIGATIONS

The principles and history of forensic entomology were discussed in Chapter 7. A wide range of invertebrates, not all of them insects, can either be part of the faunal succession or contribute in other ways

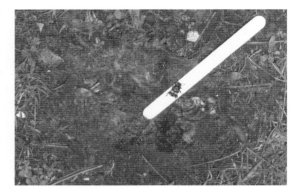

Figure 9.9 A sexton beetle, one of a number of species that can provide information about a carcase.

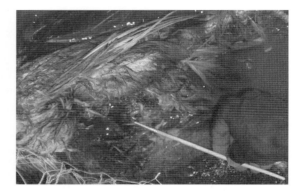

Figure 9.10 Maggots on a carcase.

to forensic studies because (for example) they are transported on an animal's body or are found in its bedding or container.

The main groups of invertebrates of forensic interest are listed in Table 9.3.

Different taxa may predominate in different locations and the expert should be aware of this when working overseas or searching the literature. Thus, the book by Goff (2000) is based mainly on experiences in Hawaii; a useful review of forensic entomology in France and its overseas Départements was provided by Myskowiak *et al.* (1999); Lord and Burger (1984) described arthropods associated with seal carcases on the East coast of the USA while Carvalho *et al.* (2000) published a checklist of arthropods associated with dead pigs and humans in Brazil.

Table 9.3 Some types of invertebrate of possible significance in forensic work.

Classification	Common (English) name	Significance and comments
Phylum: Arthropoda	Arthropods	The group as a whole – the 'jointed-legged' invertebrates
		Some arthropods feed on the carcase itself, others on its inhabitants, yet others use the remains of the animal or human as a 'home'
Class: Insecta	Insects	
Order: Diptera	Flies	
Family:		
Calliphoridae	Blowflies	Most often used in crime scene investigation
Sarcophagidae	Flesh flies	Important in some forensic work
Muscidae	House flies	Important in some forensic work
Phoridae	Coffin flies	The Phoridae may be associated with different stages of decomposition, including the final wave (Leclercq, 1999)
Order: Coleoptera	Beetles	Carrion beetles are part of the faunal succession that responds to the presence of a dead animal
Family:		
Silphidae	Carrion beetles	Some other coleopterous species are associated with dry remains in later stages of decomposition (Pankaj and Satpathy, 2001) or mummified carcases (Bourel *et al.*, 2000)
Staphylinidae	Rove beetles	
Dermestidae	Skin beetles	
Scarabaeidae	Scarab (dung) beetles	Provide information on age, origin and sometimes health status of animal faeces
		Beetles or their larvae may die if faeces contain certain drugs
Order: Lepidoptera	Butterflies and moths	Various larvae may pupate on, or adjacent to, a carcase
Family:		
Tineidae	Clothes moths	Certain tineids may be a feature of mummified bodies (Bourel *et al.*, 2000)
Pyralidae	Grease moths (pyralids)	
Order: Hymenoptera	Bees, wasps and ants	Omnivores that may feed on a carcase and on other animals (mainly invertebrates) that inhabit it
		Ants are often attracted at an early stage by blood and moisture
Order: Dictyoptera	Cockroaches	Omnivores – see above
Orders: Siphonaptera and Phthiraptera	Fleas and lice	May persist on carcase after death but often move away as the temperature drops
		If carcase was poisoned or frozen, dead fleas and lice may be found
Class: Arachnida	Spiders, harvestmen, mites, ticks	Feed on other invertebrates (spiders), on debris (harvestmen)
		Mites and ticks as fleas and lice above
Class: Myriapoda	Centipedes and millipedes	Millipedes often associated with late stages of decomposition, even skeletonisation
Class: Crustacea	Woodlice, crabs, shrimps, *Daphnia*, etc.	Found on or in carcases that are (or have been) in water or damp places
		Some may be inhaled (see Chapter 7)

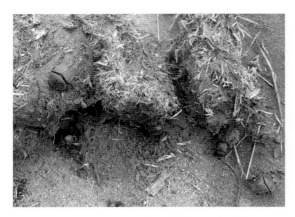

Figure 9.11 The presence of scarab (dung) beetles can assist in determining the age and origin of faeces from wild animals.

It is not just the *presence* of invertebrates on a carcase that is relevant to forensic investigations. Dispersion (movement in order to pupate or to seek additional food) may also be important in assessing the PMI (see, for example, Gomes *et al.*, 2002). The area around the dead body needs to be searched.

Invertebrates are also attracted to animal (and human) faeces, urine and other body products, including exudates and (birds) regurgitated pellets. Insofar as faeces are concerned, scarab beetles are the best known and documented (Figure 9.11).

Bird pellets (castings) can provide useful evidence in forensic cases. As far as invertebrates are concerned, pellets may both *contain* species of interest (the food the bird has eaten, possibly its geographical location) and *attract* beetles, moths etc. – especially when the casting is more than a few days old. Examination of pellets has been discussed in a number of relatively recent texts (see, for example, Cooper, J.E., 2002 and Yalden, 1977), but the best, largely original, information is often to be found in older, less frequently-cited works (e.g. Thompson, 1922; Knight, 1948; Miles, 1952).

COLLECTION OF INVERTEBRATES

It is important that the investigator knows how to collect and how to store insects and other inverte-

brates, even if s/he subsequently submits them to a specialist.

In medical forensic investigations, an entomologist is very likely to be part of the team and this is specifically advocated by some authors (DiMaio and DiMaio, 2001). Also, amongst those present at the crime scene are likely to be personnel who are trained in the correct sampling and collection of invertebrates (Lord and Burger, 1983). In animal forensic work, however, the situation is often very different. Frequently the veterinarian or his equivalent has to make important decisions about how best to collect samples and evidence, including invertebrates. The notes that follow are intended to help those who find themselves in this position. They differ in a number of ways from the more rigorous approach that would probably be adopted by a professional entomologist (see, for example, Smith, 1986; Byrd and Castner, 2000).

Equipment for collection of invertebrates on, or in the location of, a carcase or products such as faeces should include:

- Protective clothing, as appropriate, always including gloves.
- Nets – including sweep net and pond net (for carcases in water).
- Entomologist's beating tray.
- Small (artist's) paint brushes.
- Aspirators ('pooters').
- Forceps, plastic and/or padded to minimise damage to larvae.
- Tubes – glass and plastic.
- A vacuum flask of hot water.
- Ethanol or methanol 70%.
- Thermometer and hygrometer.

Entomological kits may be purchased as such from suppliers of forensic equipment but can also be easily and inexpensively assembled. Any amateur naturalist will know where to purchase nets and other items and if the veterinarian does not him/herself have knowledge in these matters such people should be consulted through a local natural history society or school biology department.

Some general tips regarding the practice of forensic entomology at a believed crime scene are as follows:

- One should approach slowly and attentively: insects of importance may be seen or heard in flight. They can be captured by net.
- Some invertebrates of significance may be present in long grass or overhanging vegetation near the carcase or faeces etc. The beating tray, sweeping net and pooter can be used to search for these.
- The *upper* surface of a carcase should be observed and then examined first.
- Blowfly and other eggs and newly hatched larvae are likely to be at orifices or wounds on a carcase. These sites should be recorded (line-drawings, photos) and specimens collected. Note should be taken of whether larvae are moving or motionless (dead? cold?).
- When the above is completed, the carcase or faeces should be turned over to permit examination of the lower surface and the earth or other substrate on which they lie. Carrion and rove beetles and other non-dipterous species may run out at this stage: they should be collected. Such creatures may also be present under adjacent pieces of stone or corrugated iron.
- When the underside of a carcase or pile of faeces has been thoroughly examined and sampled, soil and associated debris must be searched for larvae that may have migrated in order to pupate or other invertebrates that may have burrowed to escape sun or cold.
- Sampling should proceed as follows:
  - Some larvae and other specimens should be collected alive, in dry containers, so that they can metamorphose. Others are killed to preserve them as they are – best achieved by immersion first in hot water to 'relax' them, then fixing in ethanol. Keeping parasitic invertebrates alive after removal from their host is not always easy (see later).
  - As large a sample as possible should be taken. The larvae collected should be of a range of sizes: they may be of various ages or of different species.

Collection of live parasites is likely to be of more significance when investigating a clinical case or an animal that has recently died/been euthanased – for example, in alleged cruelty cases (see Chapter 6)

– but is mentioned here in a general context. Fleas generally survive if placed in a tube and kept at +4°C. Lice appear to fare better if stored with the hair or feathers from which they come – again preferably at +4°C. Too low a temperature may kill or damage the parasite.

Contact with local weather stations or meteorologists is often important in order to obtain information about temperature and relative humidity over the preceding day or weeks.

The laboratory treatment and examination of invertebrates that are being used in forensic investigations is discussed briefly in Chapter 8.

Basic knowledge of invertebrate taxonomy and biology is an important prerequisite to involvement in forensic studies. Life-cycles vary greatly and an understanding of this is necessary, even for the novice. Thus, blowflies (Diptera) and fleas (Siphonaptera) undergo complete metamorphosis, with ovum, larva, pupa and imago (adult) stages whereas cockroaches (Dictyoptera) and lice (Phthiraptera) have an incomplete metamorphosis: the insect that hatches from the egg resembles the adult.

There remains a need to have invertebrates from carcases properly identified and catalogued (Greenberg, 1991). There are still no keys for identification of many taxa in different parts of the world, as was emphasised in a recent paper on the blowflies of southern Australia (Wallman, 2001).

Maintaining a chain of custody is as important in entomological studies as it is in any other field of forensic work. A useful paper in this respect is that by Adair (1999), all the more so because the article is followed by a note (by Bryan Turner) explaining differences between the system described by Adair in the USA and that followed in the UK.

FIELDWORK – A SPECIALISED VERSION OF THE CRIME SCENE

Forensic work in the field can be either (a) planned, or (b) opportunistic.

Planned fieldwork is essentially similar to a site visit. The investigator or expert knows that s/he is visiting a specific location and, within limits, can plan what equipment to take.

Opportunistic fieldwork is necessary when one is dealing with the unexpected: for example, there may be a report of an injured, sick or dead animal requiring an immediate visit, and one is not fully prepared. In this case, improvisation is necessary, using any equipment that the investigator/expert has with him/her or can purchase or borrow locally. Advanced planning, however, can help to ensure that fieldwork is performed proficiently and is therefore more likely to produce reliable results and stand up to scrutiny in cross-examination.

Each of these situations is discussed in more detail below.

Planned forensic work in the field

Working in the field, using appropriate equipment and techniques, is a well-established technique in both human and veterinarian medicine and much has been published on the subject. It needs careful planning and teamwork (see later). A useful general text is one by Cork and Halliwell (2002) but more specific papers are those by Cooper and Samour (1997), Frye *et al.* (2001), Keymer *et al.* (2001) and Cooper (2004c).

The design and composition of a field kit depend upon the circumstances, in particular:

* The type of case – live animal, dead animal, environmental damage, etc.
* The environmental conditions – low temperatures present very different challenges from working in the heat.
* The location – whether the equipment has to be carried by hand, on a bicycle or motorbike, etc.
* The distance back to appropriate laboratories, clinics or police station, where follow-up investigations can be carried out.

Field kits are discussed later and some suggested contents are catalogued in Appendix E.

Opportunistic forensic work in the field

This requires great versatility and often imagination! Practising veterinary surgeons can usually turn their hands fairly regularly to improvisation because, especially if they are involved in farm or

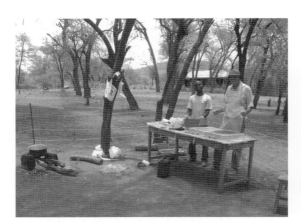

Figure 9.12 Investigations in the field require ingenuity and versatility. In this scene from the Kenyan Rift Valley, a field necropsy site has been established. The 'dirty' area has been demarcated with string and a colour code introduced – red for contaminated material, blue for 'clean'. A fire provides hot water for disinfection. This figure also appears in colour in the colour plate section.

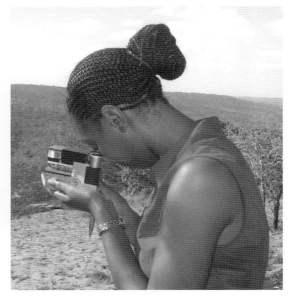

Figure 9.13 Field studies using a hand-held, battery-operated microscope. This figure also appears in colour in the colour plate section.

other visits, they carry certain equipment and chemicals with them and are accustomed to being adaptable. However, even the practising veterinarian, if s/he is regularly involved in forensic work, should consider supplementing standard veterinary equipment with some of the items listed under field kits in Appendix E.

Some examples of improvisation in the field are listed in Table 9.4 below. Where appropriate, more information and/or references are given later.

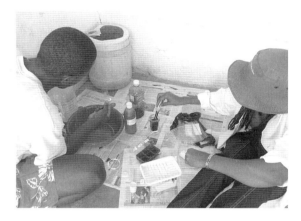

Figure 9.14 A field laboratory, established using locally-purchased materials, permits the staining of blood and tissue specimens.

As a general rule, samples should be maintained at a cool temperature, preferably around +4°C. This may be difficult to achieve in the field, especially in hot climates. Ice will help (see later). Portable refrigerators are available and may be solar-powered but are prohibitively expensive in many poor countries. Refrigerators or freezers may be found in shops or homes in a local town but they may not be appropriate for pathological or toxic material. It is also important to check their reliability: for example, a temperature of around 0°C can prove useful for sensitive forensic evidence but a slight fluctuation (for example, associated with adding or removing specimens) may cause ice crystals to form or samples to warm – either of which can be deleterious.

Numerous ruses may be necessary in order to keep material cold in the field, even for a short period. Secreting samples in a hole in the earth will keep them cool (or prevent their freezing, in a temperate winter environment). Newspaper and vegetation can be employed as insulation. Ice is invaluable – but not always easy to acquire, especially when large amounts are needed – for example, to keep a whole carcase cool. Under such circumstances ingenuity is essential and this may involve soliciting from shopkeepers, from ice-cream vendors (if in the vicinity!) or even from sea fishermen who make use of ice to keep their catch fresh.

Table 9.4 Field techniques – improvisation.

Requirement	Ideal solution	Possible improvisation	Comments
Fixation of tissues	Formalin or commercial alcohol	Alcoholic drinks, including spirits (especially rum), wine and strong beer	See Spratt (1993) and Cyrus (2005)
Handling of contaminated or infected material	Rubber gloves Forceps	Plastic or paper bags Wooden spatulae	See Cooper and Samour (1997)
Sample collection	Laboratory containers	Film pots	See Frye *et al.* (2001) and Cooper (1996b)
Clipboard	Purpose-made of hardboard	A piece of cardboard and a large (bulldog) clip	Lightweight and has the added advantage that the cardboard can, if contaminated, be incinerated after use

SAMPLING

Sometimes it is necessary to take representative or significant samples rather than to transport all the material that is available. The principles of accurate sampling were addressed in Chapter 7. Sampling of live and dead animals when a herd or flock is involved was discussed in Chapters 6 and 7.

It is important that the collection of botanical specimens is in the hands of experienced personnel who know how to select, handle and process samples correctly. Such a person can be an invaluable addition to an animal forensic crime scene investigation.

Care must always be taken when selecting specimens at a crime scene (or its equivalent). For example, if a case revolved around the quality of animal foodstuff, a decision will have to be made as to whether to sample feed bags that are low in the pile or higher up, or a mixture of the two. Representative portions of faeces or other products may need to be chosen (see Chapter 8) rather than all that is available (Figure 9.15).

Samples must be examined and photographed first, before collection (Figure 9.16).

LABORATORY WORK IN THE FIELD

In forensic fieldwork it is necessary to demarcate a specific area for laboratory investigations, preferably in shade/away from rain under a tree or in a sheltered hollow. A disused building, even if not intact, provides flat, easily cleaned, surfaces (Figure 9.14).

Sometimes the boot (trunk) of a vehicle or a trailer is available.

While some forensic laboratory investigations require only a hand lens or operating loupe, others necessitate access to a reliable field microscope. This must have the following characteristics:

- Compact and rugged construction that can withstand vibration.
- High-quality microscopic images (fine resolution and brightness; an edge-to-edge flat field relatively free from aberration).
- Solar or battery-operated light source.

Two field microscopes that have been used successfully are:

(1) The Swift – constructed from durable aluminium and brass.
(2) The McArthur – a conventional aluminium and brass model (see Figure 9.13) and a lightweight plastic version.

Other portable microscopes are currently being produced and will greatly facilitate medical and

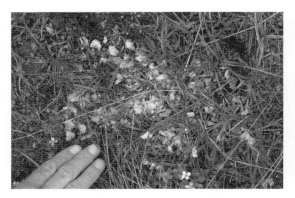

Figure 9.15 Ingesta regurgitated by a jackal. Such material may provide useful information in instances where raiding of livestock is suspected.

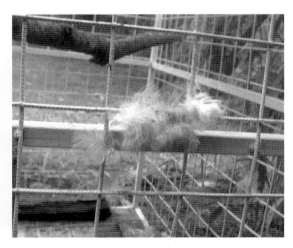

Figure 9.16 A captive owl was pulled out of this cage by dogs. Abundant evidence remains, including these feathers, adherent to the wire.

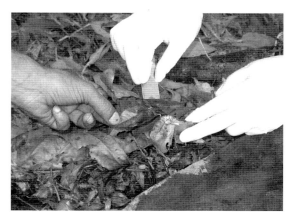

Figure 9.17 Laboratory tests in the field can yield immediate, often significant, results. This is a sequel to visiting the beach depicted earlier. Blood smears are taken from a wooden chopping board: on microscopical examination they prove to be mammalian, all that remains of the stranded dolphin. This figure also appears in colour in the colour plate section.

veterinary fieldwork, both diagnostic and forensic (Roy Rickman, pers. comm).

BATTERY-OPERATED COMPUTER EQUIPMENT

Computers

Data can be recorded and processed on a small battery-powered notebook computer or on a hand-held computer (see also Chapter 10).

The advantages of a hand-held computer are:

- Compact.
- Lightweight.
- Inexpensive.
- Long battery life (typically 3–4 months) using only 2 AA alkaline batteries.
- Substantial digital data storage.
- Ability to transfer stored data back and forth between the computer and a notebook or desktop personal computer and thus provide a back-up facility if the original data are lost.
- Ability to make tapeless digital recording of notes or sounds.

Lightweight flexible solar panels are commercially available. They can be folded or rolled and inserted into protective tubes for storage and transport.

Ultraviolet light source

A battery-powered ultraviolet black light source of illumination is useful for forensic and other investigations, including attracting moths and other insects. Cylindrical tube-type ultraviolet light devices are compact, moderately priced and relatively rugged.

USE OF FIELD EQUIPMENT IN FORENSIC INVESTIGATIONS

Kits for use in the field – for example, wildlife crime investigations – may need to be independent of electricity and water supplies. They should be portable, durable and (especially in poorer locations) relatively inexpensive.

When working in poorer countries, costs can be reduced without necessarily compromising quality. For example, in Rwanda we successfully used local bamboo to make spatulae and utilised plastic film pots as containers for specimens from mountain gorillas, including tissues from poached animals (Cooper, 1996b).

Field kits need to be carefully and securely packed. A rucksack (backpack) can be used but it is preferable to use one of the luggage-type packing cases that are marketed for photographic or endoscopic equipment. Failing that, an all-purpose box of the type designed to carry tools or fishing gear can be employed.

The size and shape of the container are also important. It needs to be readily transported in the field (possibly in a rucksack or on a porter's head) but, at the same time, should be easily stowed in the overhead luggage rack of an aeroplane or local bus.

Field kits must be secured with a padlock. They should also bear warning stickers and the name of the owner. Notices should be in local languages as well as in English and line drawings may help to explain the importance and purpose of the kit to people who may not be able to read, such as baggage handlers or local villagers.

An item that proves invaluable in the field but is rarely mentioned in publications or reports is a lightweight folding umbrella (see Table 9.1)! This is used primarily for protection from sun, snow and other elements but, in addition, can prove ideal for the collection of rainwater, for catching invertebrates and other small animals (an extension of forensic entomology) or searching for and securing trace evidence when 'beating' undergrowth.

Some items on the list, such as the tape recorder and palm-top computer, are not only lightweight but also easily and rapidly hidden. This can be important in war-torn countries or where there is political sensitivity about strangers, especially if they appear to be noting and storing information.

Care must be taken when undertaking international work that the kit does not contain medicines or other items that may not, by law, be transported from one country to another. A list of contents should always be available for inspection (see Appendix E).

The kits described will help to raise standards where forensic work has to be carried out under difficult circumstances. It is not only those who live in poorer countries who stand to benefit from the development of more sophisticated and reliable equipment. Field workers, even those working in less accessible areas of Europe, North America or Australasia, need to have access to reliable *in situ* technology if forensic work is to yield meaningful and reliable results.

PACKAGING AND TRANSPORTATION OF FIELD EQUIPMENT

As mentioned earlier, a lightweight, durable plastic, luggage-type packing case that is designed for holding and protecting photographic and other delicate equipment is ideal for holding and protecting items in the field. A small padlock is useful and discourages unauthorised inspection. One should always pack the equipment oneself: not only does this satisfy airline security requirements, but it also facilitates the location of items, which may be needed quickly.

The outside of the laboratory case must be identified with permanent warning stickers or tags that indicate the fragility of the contents and the owner's name and both home and destination addresses. A similar notice should be plastic-laminated and placed inside the case, in clear view in case it is checked by airport security staff. Upon opening the case, its contents and their purpose should become obvious. Placing an identified sealed pair of sterile surgeon's gloves or a stethoscope in plain view may avoid inspection of each item. (The stethoscope is also clearly seen on radiographic examination and can obviate the need to open the case.) Once the case has been inspected, the hasp that joins the lid with the body can be further secured with a nylon cable tie, which will discourage pilferage if the case must be left unattended.

CARE OF CAMERAS AND FILM

When in the field cameras should be kept in the shade, or at least covered with some shade-affording material. Spare batteries must be packed. Cameras should be protected from excessive moisture, particularly immersion in water. Seawater and alkaline (soda) water are especially harmful to photographic equipment. It is essential that every effort be taken to protect both exposed and unexposed photographic film while working in often hostile environments. A thick-walled padded container offers satisfactory protection for photographic equipment provided that the container is shaded. When in the tropics, an alternative is to wrap the film container in banana or taro leaves, which provide excellent insulation.

FIELDWORK AND SITE VISITS OVERSEAS

Letters of introduction and authorisation can be invaluable in parts of the world where bureaucracy and restrictions are routine. Signatures and appropriate rubber stamps are essential and add weight to such documentation. Apparently simple tasks can often take a long time, especially when they involve more than one country's officials. If one is likely to bring evidence back to a home laboratory, all necessary arrangements should be made before departure. Legislative requirements may involve both animal health officials (Ministry/Department of Agriculture) and those concerned with the conservation of endangered species (Cooper, M.E., 1987). CITES regulations apply not only to live and dead animals but also to recognisable derivatives such as blood smears and small samples for DNA studies – both commonly used as evidence in forensic cases.

TEAMWORK, PLANNING AND TRAINING SESSIONS

Working as a team is often the hallmark of an efficient crime scene investigation. It requires discipline and an understanding of other people's roles and responsibilities without compromising one's own objectivity. Whenever possible, a planning meeting, perhaps as a case conference, is advisable – an opportunity to bring everyone together and to minimise the risk of inadequate communication during the investigation itself. One person has to be in charge and brief the team (see earlier) but everybody must have an opportunity to speak, to comment and to disagree. Cohesion at the scene must be built on mutual respect and understanding, not just the hierarchy.

One surprisingly effective way of concentrating everyone's attention is to use a tape recorder in order to start the proceedings. The date, time and names of the team are recorded on the tape, together with a list of points to be addressed. The very fact that they are being recorded often encourages team members to concentrate on the matter in hand.

Punctuality is important to any meeting or case conference. The person who arrives late misses the introductory remarks and sometimes the planning – not an auspicious start if the aim is to get the team working as one.

There is merit in preparing well for site visits and fieldwork and ensuring that those involved are familiar with the necessary rules and codes of practice. This is particularly important in animal forensics where back-up or direction from the police and other experienced people is often not available.

Training sessions provide an opportunity to plan and, if properly organised, are usually very popular with participants. The choice of a location will depend upon the circumstances but possibilities include:

- A large garden.
- An area of woodland.
- A stretch of disused railway.
- An old airfield.

Excessive numbers of participants should be avoided as they are not conducive to teaching 'good practice' insofar as such matters as not causing unnecessary damage to the scene and disseminating foreign DNA are concerned. A useful ploy is to take small groups, appropriately clad, into the crime scene area and to keep other participants outside the barrier tape where they can observe while awaiting their turn.

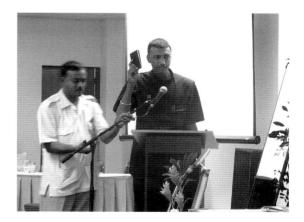

Figure 9.18 Training in court procedure. Two Trinidadian Game Wardens simulate the taking of the oath prior to a mock trial of a man charged with killing a protected monkey.

Teaching techniques also benefit from practice. A 'mock-up' is wise, with different people designated to perform tasks (Figure 9.18).

Reference collections of (for example) feathers, hair or bones can be usefully employed under such circumstances – another reason for establishing and maintaining such collections (see Chapter 7). Human bones are becoming more difficult to obtain in 'developed' countries and sometimes plastic skeletons, which are often of poor quality and relatively expensive, may have to be used as substitutes.

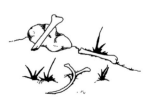

Record-Keeping and Collation and Analysis of Findings

If writing is poor then what is said is not what is meant. If what is said is not what is meant then what ought to be done is not done.

Anonymous – Chinese Proverb

Another error is an impatience of doubting and a blind hurry of asserting without a mature suspension of judgement . . . if we begin with certainties, we shall end in doubts, but if we begin with doubts and are patient in them, we shall end in certainties.

Francis Bacon

However experienced the forensic investigator, the information that s/he obtains from a site visit, clinical examination, *post-mortem* examination or laboratory tests is only likely to prove of value if the findings are properly collated and analysed and if exemplary records are kept. In this chapter this aspect of forensic work involving animals is discussed in some detail. There will be numerous cross-references to other chapters because the salient points will be reiterated in individual sections of the book.

TYPES OF RECORDS

The findings from forensic investigations are likely to be available in various forms. These will include hand-written notes, type-written notes, tape recordings, video recordings, digital images, radiographs, etc. Each of these can be of value in a legal or similar case but has its own limitations. Often it is the combination of data that provides the best evidence. Thus, although a written description of clinical signs shown by an animal that is alleged to have been badly beaten may provide useful evidence, a video recording, audio or photographic record of the animal or incident is often preferable (see later). The whole question of which evidence is acceptable and which is not is changing rapidly. Advances in electronic techniques bring with them better quality methods but also more opportunities for tampering with evidence. This is discussed in more detail later.

Any records, regardless of their type, should be secure and uniquely identifiable by the use of reference numbers, evidence identification tags, scale (metric) and appropriate markings as to what is the left, right, cranial or caudal end of the animal. Once again, much can be gained by following guidelines established for the medical profession. David (2005) set out useful rules for the carrying out of clinical examination of children when physical abuse is suspected. He emphasised the importance of making use of the original radiographs, good quality original photographic prints, etc., etc.

Paper records from elsewhere that are being presented as evidence can be 'questioned', in which case they may need to be checked by a document examiner (Ellen, 1997). This can be a particular challenge in wildlife forensics, where, for example, records of egg collectors, applications for permits and CITES documents may have been falsified or altered (PAW, 2005).

ROUTINE RECORD-KEEPING

Record-keeping is of such importance in judicial proceedings that the veterinarian (or his equivalent), or support staff such as practice telephone receptionists, should begin to start recording the moment that there is the slightest suggestion that a legal case may ensue. This means:

- Making a written note of messages received by telephone or verbally, including date and time.
- Having available additional means of recording evidence, e.g. video camera or tape recorder ('hands-free' if it is to be used in a moving vehicle or while animals are being examined).
- Being extra observant about relevant matters, such as the people who are involved, etc.

SPECIFIC RECORDS

Although there is merit, for various reasons, in having specific clinical, *post-mortem* and laboratory forms for forensic cases, there are occasions when other paperwork has to be completed, perhaps in parallel with the forensic sheets. This particularly applies to wildlife cases (see Chapter 5) where the specimen(s) may be of an endangered or threatened species and therefore, sometimes for legal reasons, needs to be fully documented and the data sent to the appropriate body for cataloguing. Two examples will suffice – birds of prey and marine mammals – where it is important that biological data are recorded, appropriate samples taken for toxicology and material retained for museums or reference collections. All this should be done but it is important not to compromise the forensic investigation, particularly if the case is likely to go to court – for example, by not divulging information on the specimen, or parting with material (even wrappings) that might constitute evidence.

CONTEMPORANEOUS NOTES

In most legal proceedings much emphasis is laid upon 'contemporaneous notes' – made at the time or very shortly after. Such notes should be retained, wrapped in plastic if soiled or contaminated, as they may have to be produced in court (see later). The need to be able to prepare contemporaneous notes, if necessary without warning, reinforces the point that those involved in forensic work should always have paper and pen with them (keeping a diary is good training for this!). Sir William Osler, that giant of 20th century medicine, constantly exhorted his students to take notes. His most appropriate quotation in the context of forensic medicine has to be 'Record that which you have seen; make a note at the time; do not wait.' (Cited in Silverman *et al.*, 2003).

The production of contemporaneous notes is not as simple as might appear. Rules for completion of notes produced by the British police are based on the mnemonic 'elbows' (see Figure 10.1).

Some of this applies also to other methods of record-keeping – tape recordings, for example, where deletion of recorded material is never wise, even if the portion erased is of no apparent relevance to the case because, perhaps, the machine was left to play inadvertently.

CONTAMINATED MATERIAL

From time to time contemporaneous notes or other paperwork becomes contaminated with blood or

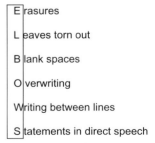

THERE SHOULD BE NO

E rasures
L eaves torn out
B lank spaces
O verwriting
W riting between lines
S tatements in direct speech

Figure 10.1 The British police have produced a mnemonic for the rules pertaining to the keeping of contemporaneous notes.

other tissue fluids. Whereas in other fields of medicine such material would be destroyed, in forensic investigations it is important to retain the original. The soiled papers in their sealed plastic bag should be photocopied and each page marked as such. The photocopies will probably be adequate for most purposes but if there is a request from a court or other authorised body or person for the originals these also can be produced.

ACKNOWLEDGEMENT OF RECEIPT

When a sample is received for laboratory investigation it should be acknowledged with a date and time and the sender provided with the reference number. Such acknowledgement is not only a courtesy but also provides some safeguard against the suggestion subsequently that the material was either not received, or was not dealt with properly. The laboratory should keep a copy of the acknowledgement attached to the paper work.

Such basic courtesies should apply also to the computer. 'Netiquette' governs certain aspects of email and internet usage but not, apparently, the need to acknowledge receipt.

LETTERS OF CERTIFICATION

In veterinary work a signed letter may be produced in order to certify that, for example, a live animal has received a certain vaccine or has been implanted with a transponder (microchip). If not following standard wording (see Chapter 6), such letters must be carefully phrased in order to avoid ambiguity, misunderstanding or legal challenges. An example of a letter used to certify findings in a probable case of lightning strike is given in Appendix A.

PRODUCTION OF A REPORT

Rothwell (2004) outlined the important features of a forensic scientist's report and suggested that it should usually contain the following information:

- Name and address of the expert.
- Outline of circumstances.

- Outline of scientific work carried out.
- List of exhibits examined.
- Description of the work performed.
- Interpretation of the findings.

An example of a report with some of the headings above, plus others, is given in Appendix A.

Rothwell iterated that in Scotland an expert's work must be corroborated (seen and verified) by a colleague and that both scientists put their names on what then becomes a joint report.

Where a standard form exists, or a particular format is recommended, there is merit in adhering to these, although this is not essential. In the UK, for example, the RCVS, The Royal College of Pathologists, and British Veterinary Association are amongst organisations that issue 'standards and guidelines' on various subjects for their members (see Appendix B). Model reports and checklists are available and provide a useful basis for preparation of written expert evidence by the forensic scientist.

Expert reports must also conform to any legal provisions of the appropriate jurisdiction and court. Thus, in England and Wales, the Civil Procedure Rules Part 35 and Practice Direction 35 lay down requirements regarding the content of expert witness reports. These include both a statement of compliance (PD35, 2.2(9)) and a specifically-worded statement of truth (PD35, 2.4). Comparable Criminal Procedure Rules are likely to relate to expert evidence in the future (see Chapter 12).

STATEMENTS

These are generally produced at a later stage, following questioning by a Police Officer or other authorised person. The format is often standard insofar as headings, preamble and style are concerned (see Appendix A).

WRITING, SPELLING AND AMBIGUITY

The importance of both writing and spelling correctly cannot be over-emphasised and is spelt out in the quotation at the beginning of this chapter.

Clear records result in clear reports and these will both impress those who have to use them and reduce the risk of ambiguity or confusion (see later).

Spelling is important. In recent years, standards of spelling have deteriorated in the western world (interestingly, not so in countries in Africa and elsewhere in the 'developing' world) and this means that the expert should be aware as to whether s/he can spell correctly. If in doubt, an electronic spell-checker can be used, but a word of caution here. The computer has many advantages but it cannot always distinguish between similar words with different meanings, e.g. 'discreet' describing the attitude of a witness, and 'discrete' relating to the appearance of a clinical or pathological lesion. Therefore, complete reliance should not be put on the spellchecker. The author of the document must read it him/herself and, if necessary, pass it to someone else for checking (see later).

Spelling presents difficulties to many people, not least those who are dyslexic. Experts who are aware of dyslexia must be particularly careful in the compilation of notes and reports and must be prepared to consult a trusted colleague or friend to assist. As explained above, the computer spellchecker cannot be relied upon to rectify all errors.

The other problem that can arise with a computer spellchecker relates to different dialects of English. One must be aware that some word-processing programmes are switched back to American English without prompting. This can create complications, frustration and embarrassment.

Ambiguity should always be avoided, to the extent of using basic English and repeating words if this clarifies the meaning. A Thesaurus is a key part of an expert's armoury but, in contrast to when writing a scientific document, should be used sparingly in forensic reports. One should explain terms in written reports and verbally to magistrates, judges or juries. 'Battered cod' may mean one thing to a chef or hotelier, something different to an animal welfare inspector or a fish farmer!

As in all fields of forensic work, dates must be unambiguous: 9.11.2001 means the 11th of September 2001 to an American, but the 9th of November, 2001 to most people elsewhere in the world. Confusion over dates, which can even preju-

dice a legal case, is avoided if all those involved in forensic work spell out the date in full, i.e. eleventh (or 11th) September 2001.

The same applies to the time of day. First of all, it is wise in all legal cases to use the 24-hour clock, thus avoiding confusion as to whether 9.00 means nine o'clock in the morning or nine o'clock in the evening: 0900 or 2100 is unambiguous! Having said that, in international cases it is also necessary to say whether the hour relates to, e.g., GMT (Greenwich Mean Time), BST (British Summer Time) or EST (Eastern Standard Time – United States of America).

When abbreviations are used, they should be correct (e.g. 'g', not 'gm', for 'gram') and the full word(s) given on the first occasion. Baron (1994) provided a very useful list of abbreviations of terms that are widely used in medicine and the related biological sciences.

One must be very wary of over-emphasising incidents or findings as this can bring bias to a report or influence those reading it. One way is to use words carefully and to think about their meaning. If in doubt, a dictionary or a Thesaurus should be used. Some examples of words that are now widely used but which are usually too dramatic or exclusive are given in Table 10.1.

Syntax is important in legal documents. The general rule is to use plain English!

As in all aspects of forensic work, precise and unambiguous terminology is essential if confusion is not to arise. The value of employing scientific names, especially when one is involved in international work, is emphasised throughout this book (see also Appendix F). However, correct use of

Table 10.1 Words should be chosen carefully and used with precision.

Popular usage	*Probable meaning*
Impact	Effect
Unique	Unusual
Incredibly	Very
Chaos	Turmoil, confusion
Panic	Fear
Worldwide	In much of the world

standard English terms is also important if written and oral reports are to carry weight. One example is in the equine world, where even the non-specialist should be aware of such terminology as 'cannon bone' or 'gelding'. Inaccurate wording in written reports or responses in court serves both to confuse and, possibly, to discredit the expert. The best example may be the word 'cow' – strictly a female ox, but a term often used loosely and incorrectly when referring to any bovid.

One should particularly avoid unnecessary ambiguity if it is likely to confuse a lay magistrate or jury. For instance, in a court case concerning dog bites, the word 'canine' should be reserved for the offending tooth and not used to mean 'dog'. (The correct noun in zoological parlance is 'canid'.) Biological terminology is very important but, alas, often poorly understood and/or followed by the veterinary profession.

USE OF COMPUTERS

Computers are, of course, an important tool of modern forensic science, including forensic medicine. They are used for report writing, literature searches and sending emails. However, computer security is an increasingly sensitive subject. Access to computers and specific files must be via passwords. Back-up discs of all material should be taken and stored elsewhere under conditions of safety and security. Antivirus and similar programmes should be part of any computer that is used for any forensic work.

Henry (2004) discussed the use of computers to commit crimes and pointed out that such use has redefined where and what a crime scene can be. He emphasised the precautions that must be taken when examining computer-based evidence (in the UK encapsulated within the Association of Chief Police Officers' Good Practice Guide for Computer Based Evidence) and those *preparing* evidence electronically also need to be aware of its limitations and dangers. In particular, no change should be made to data that may subsequently be relied upon in court.

When working in the field, access to computers is not always easy but can be possible using mobile phones, if necessary assisted by a pocket charger powered by solar energy.

COMPUTER ACCESS

If the world population was reduced to a hundred, only one person would own a computer. In 2005, the Anne E. Casey Foundation published a report that stated that, in low-income, central-city neighbourhoods in the USA, 84% of households with children do not own computers. One should not assume, therefore, that all those involved in a case can receive or send emails or search the net, even if they live in 'rich' countries.

TYPING AND THE USE OF ASSISTANTS

Although many people like to type their own reports, others (especially older ones) prefer to make use of a typist. This has many advantages, not least that while the typist prepares the report, the expert can be proceeding with the next case or other important work. Many medical pathologists use a voice-activated tape recorder which is then transcribed by a typist (but see later – Voice recognition). The original tape should be retained safely until the dictated information is no longer required in that form.

There are disadvantages of making use of a typist. Sometimes security is a consideration: anyone who is typing reports of a forensic nature must be well aware that they are of a confidential nature and nothing about them should be divulged nor should unauthorised copies be taken or sent elsewhere. Another danger, however, is that sometimes the typist, particularly perhaps one who has been previously in government service, or has some years of experience, decides to make slight changes to the text – meaning well, but as a result introducing different words or a different meaning to the text. Even changes to spelling or use of language introduced by the typist (or computer!) may not be desirable because the author of the report might be quoting what s/he saw or heard rather than (as it might appear) using incorrect English or spelling.

When a typist is used, the typing which is returned should be checked against the original draft or recording. The omission of a word in a report can have embarrassing consequences – 'not' being the best example. Simple things can also make or mar a report: 'three week old chicks' has two very different possible meanings if hyphens are not included.

Even a minor misspelling of a word can completely alter the meaning of a sentence. This is illustrated graphically by P.G. Wodehouse in his delightful poem 'Printer's Error' where an author is acquitted of murdering a printer who replaced the word 'now' with 'not', thus drastically changing the meaning of the sentence, because the judge shared the accused's horror at such a blunder!

VOICE RECOGNITION

The use of voice-recognition systems has found favour in recent years in certain areas of human medicine – especially radiology and pathology. Lively debate about such usage has appeared in the Bulletin of The Royal College of Pathologists. This was prompted by an introductory article on the subject by Salisbury (2005) who described his own experiences of using a voice-recognition programme, together with a dictionary of pathological terms, over the preceding two years. These developments are inevitably going to influence the production of forensic reports in the future – and veterinarians and others who work with animals need to be aware of, and receptive to, them.

PROOF-READING

It is vital that all statements and reports are properly checked for typographical, spelling and factual errors before being signed and submitted. There are software programmes that can assist with this but ultimately the author should take responsibility (see earlier). If there are co-authors (or corroborators – in Scotland, for instance) these people must not only sign the relevant documents but also read and check them first.

LITERATURE SEARCHES

The expert will need to carry out literature searches and it is important that these are done thoroughly. This can present problems as there are many hundreds of relevant journals, and thousands of possible references. There is also the dilemma of how far back (in years) one goes in searching information that might be relevant and in how many languages. The basic rules are as follows:

- Always do a literature search.
- Make the search as comprehensive as possible and supplement your own library and Internet checks with use of a professional search (e.g. from a medical or veterinary library).
- Remember that older literature (textbooks, government reports) often constitutes primary information; do not neglect it.
- Ensure that the search goes back at least ten, preferably twenty, years and consider looking at a selection of earlier works as a safeguard.
- Remember that pertinent information may be published in languages other than English. To ignore these is negligent; even if you are not able to read many other languages yourself, consider using a database (e.g. those produced by CABI Publishing – Appendix B) that scans languages other than English. Even a summary of a paper in another language, once translated into English, will give an indication as to whether it is worth consulting the whole document. Alternatively, there are Internet 'translation tools' – for example, that produced by Google (www.google.com/language_tools), which provides a rough, but usually adequate, transfer of a piece of text from one language to another.
- Keep a record of all that was done in your literature search. This may be needed or requested when written or oral examination is given; the findings may also be valuable to you or a colleague in a future case.

It is always important to be able to back up statements of 'fact' (as opposed to opinion) with reference to published work. Table 10.2 lists some sources of information, with comments on their reliability – and thus, possibly, their admissibility in

Table 10.2 Sources of information.

Source	Comments
Textbooks	May not have been peer-reviewed before publication
	Information may be out-of-date – books (especially multi-author texts) can take years to appear in print
Scientific and legal journals	May (probably) have been peer-reviewed
	Relatively up-to-date, especially journals that appear weekly or monthly and have a rapid turn-around of submitted manuscripts
Trade and other popular magazines, society newsletters	Unlikely to be peer-reviewed
	Often, however, contain useful practical information, written by hobbyists and enthusiasts, that may be relevant in court
Internet	Very rarely peer-reviewed (although some journals are now published on-line)
	Much interesting, educational and readily available information – but it has to be carefully assessed before being introduced into a report or statement in a legal case

court. The increasing importance of 'evidence-based medicine' is mentioned later and discussed in some detail in Chapter 6.

The World List of Abbreviations was, traditionally, the authoritative source of information on how titles of journals should be cited. Over the years a number of professional journals have produced their own, shorter, guides or recommended alternative systems, such as the annual list of journals produced by *Index Medicus* (Baron, 1994). Recently, however, there has been a tendency for authors or editors to decide for themselves how to list publications. This is unfortunate as it can cause confusion – and the expert should be aware of this.

It may be inferred from Table 10.2 that we do not favour use of the Internet for forensic purposes. This is not the case. The Internet, e.g. Google (www.google.co.uk), provides access to millions of web pages of information. Our message is that the Internet provides plenty of data but not all may be admissible in court.

It is vital, however, that one is critical of scientific papers. The peer-review system is not foolproof and much erroneous or misleading information is published. Many authors do not carry out a proper literature search – and few journals insist upon a description of the search in Materials and Methods (Cooper, 2004b). As a result, relevant publications may be missed, especially if they are in specialist journals or not in English or are not available electronically.

Studies are often based on too small (or biased) samples, or, in veterinary medicine, on a particular breed, variety or subspecies of animal. Projects are also often not subject to good quality control – prompting recent (2005) moves in the UK to insist on conditions before research awards are made from certain government bodies (www.iob.org).

In the past, in both human and veterinary medicine, decisions about treatment were based on personal experience, anecdotes and often invalid comparisons between groups of patients. The introduction of randomised trials has helped to correct those deficiencies but barriers remain. With the current emphasis on 'evidence-based medicine' (see Chapter 6), the need to have access to sound data has never been more important, and forensic reports must reflect this trend. One (important) contribution to improving the quality of scientific data available to the medical and allied professions was the establishment in 1993 of the Cochrane Collaboration which produces, for example, the *Cochrane Database of Systematic Reviews* and the *Cochrane Methodology Register* available on the Internet (http://www.cochrane.org/docs/whycc.htm) and on CD-ROM as part of *The Cochrane Library*.

USE OF TELEPHONES

Mobile (cell) telephones are used on a regular basis and sometimes for the relaying of important information relevant to a case. However, the relative lack of security of a mobile phone has to be borne in mind and caution exercised. A written note of *all* telephone messages that are relevant to a case, whether on a mobile phone or landline, should be retained, together with the date and time of the call. These notes may form part of evidence at a later date. The staff should also be made aware of the importance of recording telephone calls received and telephone calls made, together with date and time – initialling the entry.

Telephone contact between doctor and patient is often standard in human medicine and has many advantages in terms of personal rapport, patient reassurance and cost (Reisman and Stevens, 2002). A similar situation pertains in veterinary work. However, from a legal point of view, 'telephone medicine' has a number of drawbacks – mainly the absence or paucity of a written record of what transpired (see above).

Telephones in clinical and *post-mortem* areas should be 'no touch'.

PHOTOGRAPHS AND DIGITAL IMAGES

Photography has long been a key part of forensic evidence and often provides valuable information. Equally, however, it can be misleading. A useful review of the role of forensic photography was provided by Spring (1996) who emphasised the pitfalls for those involved in such work who are inexperienced or ill-prepared.

Whenever possible, an appropriately-qualified photographer should be involved and this is usually the norm in human forensic medicine. When working with animals, however, the clinician or pathologist may well have to double as the photographer or to ask a colleague to fulfil this role – and therefore careful preparation is required. Munro (1998) provided a useful summary of how best to get results in forensic photography in animal work that would stand up adequately to cross-examination in court. He stressed that there are various precautions that can be taken to minimise the risks of misidentification or transposition of pictures and these include:

- Using film for only one particular case, if necessary discarding the remaining portion of film.
- Including on each role of film a picture depicting the name and address of the film's owner.

The increasing use of digital cameras means a diminution in the utilisation of photographic film (Barrand, 2006). Nevertheless, those involved in forensic work should not assume the day of the camera with film is over (see Chapter 9). Evidence based on digital images is not always acceptable in court (see below) and in some poorer parts of the world, or when working in isolated locations, a digital camera may not be available. The safest approach at present is to use both a film camera and a digital camera and thus be able to produce images of either type in court. However, this advice may be out-of-date soon in many parts of the world as the use of electronic methods becomes more and more routine and admissible.

The question of legal admissibility or evidential weight of information or electronic information has been addressed in many quarters. In the UK, the Lord Chancellor's Department (Department for Constitutional Affairs) has issued a 'Records Management Code of Practice' that is binding on all public bodies. The document seeks to provide good practice guidelines for the electronic creation, storage and retrieval of information with emphasis on the British Standards Institution (BSI) *Code of Practice for Legal Admissibility and Evidential Weight of Information Stored Electronically*, 2nd edn. (www.bsi-global.com). Useful background reading, even for those who live or operate in jurisdictions outside the UK, is to be found in *Science and Technology Fifth Report* ordered by the House of Lords and printed in February 1998 (www.parliament.the-stationery-office.co.uk).

The sending of photographic information to colleagues also requires careful thought and planning. Original film should not be committed to the post (mail) and anything sent should be either registered or dispatched through a courier with full documentation and appropriate copies.

VIDEO RECORDINGS

These are sometimes used as evidence. They can provide useful information that cannot necessarily be gleaned from a series of photos – for example, how long it took an animal to collapse, comments made by those present. However, care must be exercised and it must not be assumed that video evidence will be acceptable in court (see also earlier).

If an expert is asked to view a video and give an opinion on the events that it depicts, caution is essential. Interpretation is never easy, especially if the video was made clandestinely – for instance in a market, hidden under a coat or in poorly-illuminated farm buildings.

TELEMEDICINE

Telemedicine, defined succinctly as 'the practice of medicine at a distance' (Perednia and Allen, 1995), is a relatively new discipline that has advanced greatly in recent years (Wootton, 2002, 2003, 2004). A useful introduction to the subject is by Wootton and Craig (1999).

Telemedicine offers the opportunity to provide medical advice and diagnosis electronically and to link patients, physicians and experts in different parts of the world. It is proving of value to 'developing' countries as well as in the richer nations (Anon., 2002b; Edworthy, 2001). At the University of the West Indies (UWI), in Trinidad and Tobago, for example, there is a Telehealth Programme that links UWI's Faculty of Medical Sciences with the Sick Kids Hospital in Toronto, Canada. West Indian patients are saved travel and waiting time and benefit from access to high-quality tertiary health care that is not available locally. The doctors involved receive professional support and increased access to continuing education, thus reducing professional isolation, which is often a problem in small islands.

Telepathology is increasingly a feature of diagnostic work in human medicine; its use has been analysed and discussed by a number of authors in recent years (see, for example, Jukic *et al.*, 2005 and Dennis *et al.*, 2005). In the UK, The Royal College of Pathologists offers guidance, in the form of a code of practice, for the proper use of telepathology (www.rcpath.org/publications).

Electronic methods are also increasingly being used for on-line training of (human) pathologists – for instance, the Pathnet system introduced by The Royal College of Pathologists (www.pathnet.org.uk).

It is clear that telemedicine is making important contributions to the diagnosis and treatment of human diseases. It is beginning to have an impact in veterinary work too. Veterinary specialists in Europe and North America are starting to use their websites to generate an advisory service to colleagues in such fields as ophthalmology (see, for example, www.davidlwilliams.org.uk). A special issue (Spring, 2005) of the *Journal of Veterinary Medical Education* (see Appendix B) is devoted to e-learning and provides many examples of how electronic transfer of information is affecting veterinary teaching.

In the broader animal health field, telemedicine permits the delivery of information and healthcare to livestock owners in rural communities (Anon., 2003b). New ventures are also springing up that use telemedicine and other electronic methods to send and receive information about the health and diseases of wild animals. These can also be used for forensic purposes – for example, to combat wildlife crime. Perhaps the most enterprising to date is the establishment of a telecentre near Bwindi Impenetrable Forest, Uganda. This collects and disseminates information about the health of the free-living threatened mountain gorillas and the humans who live in local villages. This programme, known as Conservation through Public Health (CTPH), uses solar energy (there is no electricity in the area), high-speed wireless Internet access and voice telephony via satellite communication. It is the first of its kind in Uganda and provides a model for other parts of the world (Nakkazi, 2005).

The sending of electronic images for an opinion is very convenient and inexpensive and in animal work obviates the need to have permits for tissues that may be pathogenic or come from protected species (see Chapter 3). However, it can present problems because of the possibility of distortion or malicious changing of detail and this may weigh against its use in court cases. In addition, there may be legal considerations, as one who is not registered to practise veterinary medicine (which usually includes diagnosis) in one country may, nevertheless, be asked to do so by being sent pictures of a sick or dead animal with lesions.

There have been few, if any, binding judgements concerning the use of telemedicine evidence in court. The consensus at present (Richard Wootton, pers.comm.) is that those involved should keep records, inform their medical (or veterinary?) defence body in advance, register in the relevant country/state and have a proper contract. This issue is discussed in more detail in Wootton (in press). Insofar as teleconsulting in the UK is concerned, reference should be made to the paper by Brahams (1995).

The whole question of telemedicine, its advantages and its drawbacks is well covered in a number of textbooks and in the *Journal of Telemedicine and Telecare* (see Appendix B).

Better visualisation and analysis of electronic images is provided by a number of modern techniques, including digital imaging and texture analysis. They can be used in clinical medicine but are especially valuable in histopathological studies (Isitor and Cooper, 2004). Such methods have great potential in forensic work but need skilled interpretation and standardisation is important (Yagi and Gilbertson, 2005).

Whenever images have been enhanced or altered in any way, the court (or other corresponding body) should be apprised of what has been done, the reasons for so doing and any effects that this might have on the quality of evidence.

DRAWINGS

In this modern, 'electronic', age it is possible to forget the value of pencil or pen and ink drawings in forensic work. They have a number of advantages:

- They need minimal equipment – an old envelope and a pencil may suffice at a crime scene, especially in the field.

- They can be used to illustrate features in three-dimensions (for example, lesions in the tissues of a dead animal that are at different depths below the surface) in a way that is not usually possible in photographs.
- They cannot easily be changed by a third-party without being detected.
- They can be used under circumstances where a camera is either not available or is not permissible. Court scenes in the UK are depicted by reporters in drawings as photography is not allowed; a similar situation may apply to a crime scene in some countries or where there is an issue of national security.

Anthropologists and osteologists make good use of sketches of bones and argue that, properly prepared (e.g. by avoiding too much shaded rendering), these are often preferable to photographs. They can, of course, be readily photocopied or scanned and sent electronically.

Newbery (2006), a veterinary surgeon with particular interests in forensic work, emphasised the usefulness of sketching crime scenes – a farm, a flat (apartment) where an animal had been found dead, for example – and illustrated his article with some of his own drawings. He stressed that one does not need to be an artist to produce reasonable sketches. All drawings and sketches should be signed and dated by the artist.

USE OF THE METRIC SYSTEM

The international nature of forensic science and medicine means that the metric system should be used. Animals should be weighed in grams (or kilograms) and they and their lesions measured in millimetres, centimetres or metres. Standard International (SI) Units are also desirable, if not essential. However, the forensic practitioner should be aware that in the USA and a few other countries, 'conventional' units are still routinely employed and be prepared to request conversion or to do so oneself. A quick and easy way of telling whether or not figures are in SI units is to look at the value for packed cell volume (PCV, haematocrit): if it is a percentage (e.g. 32%), the figures are conventional; in SI units the reading would be 0.32.

QUANTIFICATION OF DATA

As was emphasised in both Chapter 6 and Chapter 7, quantification of findings is important. It is not satisfactory, for example, to describe skin wounds in sheep (Figure 10.2) or 'fret marks' in a bird's feathers (Figure 10.3) without measuring them. Where a feature cannot be measured it should be graded. Thus, congestion of lungs can be described as 'minimal', 'moderate' or 'marked' and designated accordingly 1, 2 or 3. The same simple system can

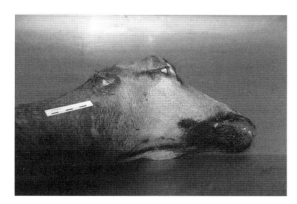

Figure 10.2 Wounds must be properly described and measured. These injuries inflicted by a dog on a Barbados black-bellied sheep were treated subsequently with purple medication. This figure also appears in colour in the colour plate section.

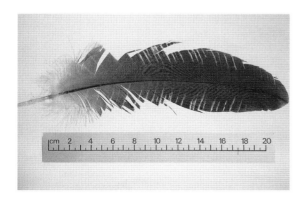

Figure 10.3 Feathers can be a rich source of information about a bird's history. This specimen shows multiple 'fret marks' (fault bars), probably associated with periods of malnutrition.

be used for such parameters as hair loss, nasal discharge, soiling of extremities, hardness/firmness of a swelling or even the colour of a lesion. Scoring systems can be applied to virtually all aspects of forensic work. They are used, for example, to measure pain (see Chapter 4), to assess malnutrition (see Chapter 6) and even, adapted from routine practice, to measure hygiene on dairy farms (Reneau *et al.*, 2005).

Use of scoring systems not only brings more precision into forensic work, it also enables data to be put on a computer and to be used to compare different animals or different circumstances. Even if a basic system, with scores of only 1–3 is used, it reduces inter-observer variation and bias. It avoids confusion over words such as 'quite' ('quite thin') which can have different meanings in different parts of the world.

In cases where epidemiological information is important, standard methods should be used – for example, an 'epidemiological calendar', which standardises time variables and thus permits comparison of events that occurred in a given year or during a specific period with others occurring at a later time or elsewhere (PAHO, 2005). Texts on veterinary epidemiology should be consulted (Thrusfield, 1997).

It is sensible to seek help from a statistician if data are extensive and need to be properly analysed. 'Flawed statistics' prompted the disciplinary action against a leading British paediatrician alluded to in Chapters 2 and 12.

NOMENCLATURE

Scientific names should be used whenever possible, to avoid possible confusion (see Appendix F). They are essential in international cases where the English name, of even a domesticated species, may mean nothing to (for example) a Frenchman. In a legal document, reference to *Cavia porcellus* is preferable to, and less ambiguous than, either 'guinea pig' or 'cochon d'Inde'!

Local names, in different languages or in patois, may be used and knowledge of them can be important especially for those involved in wildlife crime cases. Protected species are sometimes listed by such names in legislation or schedules (see Chapter 3).

DRUG NOMENCLATURE

Directive 92/27/EEC requires use of the Recommended International Non-proprietary Name (RINN) for medicinal substances. In most cases the British Approved Name (BAN) and RINN are identical but where they differ, the BAN has been modified to accord with the RINN. Important examples are the sulphonamides, now spelt with an 'f' so that (for instance) 'sulphathiazole' has become 'sulfathiazole'.

COLLATION AND ANALYSIS OF FINDINGS

The collation and analysis of data can be one of the most daunting parts of forensic work. Often even the (apparently) simplest case requiring an opinion is presented as an enormous bundle of paperwork which the expert has to read and absorb.

There is no one way of coping with this but some tips are:

- To scan the paperwork (and accompanying photographs or other documents) to get an overview of the case.
- To read thoroughly the paperwork from beginning to end, marking important points with a 'highlighter' pen or similar.
- To compile a summary, including flow diagrams or the equivalent to illustrate the sequence and timing of events, the consequences and the people involved.
- In some cases, to consider re-enacting certain of the events in order to clarify the picture insofar as location and personnel are concerned.

Much of the above can be done electronically, on a computer – which can also assist in, e.g., compiling tables or spreadsheets – but many people still use hard copies.

COSTING

One should always record how long it takes to perform each task. Such information may be required in order to claim a fee. Various expert witness organisations provide guidance on charging: some fees are determined by law or agreement, others need to be negotiated.

PRESENTATION OF FINDINGS

As in all forensic work, the veterinarian or his equivalent must be prepared to put reports, or answers to questions in court, in 'lay talk' or 'jury speak' – in other words, in language that ordinary, non-scientific people (such as magistrates and jurors) can understand. Practising veterinary surgeons are usually good at this as they have to adopt different styles in their dealings with clients. This approach not only promotes the concept of clear, fair proceedings but can also enhance the standing of the expert. Part of this can involve putting, say, the weight of a domesticated cat in pounds as well as kilos. The need for this may depend upon the age group of those being addressed: in Britain, for example, the metric system is likely to be understood by all who are under 40 years of age but by only a few born before the mid 1960s.

Reports need to be signed and this should be done in pen (ink or ballpoint). There is some merit in signing in blue (or another colour) rather than black: if the document is photocopied (for whatever purpose), the original version will be obvious. The signature should be legible if possible but not altered just to make it readable. The person's full name can be added in BLOCK CAPITALS.

Rubber stamps or their equivalent should never be used instead of a signature although they do have a place when, for example, government endorsement of a document is needed.

The person signing a document that is likely to form part of a legal case *must* be the one who did the work and who can, if necessary, confirm the facts in court. In some countries, where bureaucracy is still rampant, the system may demand that, say, a government veterinary officer has to sign

Table 10.3 Examples of different meanings.

Word	UK/European English	American English	Comments
Quite (as in 'quite large')	In part/moderate	Very	Avoid!
Bill	Account	Bank note	Avoid!
Billion	Million million	Thousand million	Make clear!
Bomb (colloquial)	Success	Disaster	Avoid!
Gas	Gaseous chemical	Petrol	Make clear! Use another word, e.g. fuel
Dummy	A 'comforter' for a baby	An ignorant, half-witted person	Avoid!

Table 10.4 Some differences between European and American spellings.

UK/European	USA
Oestrus	Estrus
Oesophagus	Esophagus

Table 10.5 Some differences between European and American medical terminology.

UK/European	USA
Liquid paraffin	Mineral oil
Optician	Optometrist
Surgical spirit	Rubbing alcohol
Cattle grid	Texas gate

laboratory reports even though s/he was not involved in the work. This can cause difficulties.

LANGUAGE DIFFERENCES

As long ago as 1493, in Europe, Masters of Grammar were called to interpret Latin in legislation and thus assist the court (cited by Hodgkinson, 1990). Misunderstanding of the written or spoken word not only continues where those involved in a case have different native tongues (for example, an Englishman appearing in a Spanish court) but can also affect comprehension between people who are Anglophones. For example, some everyday words that have different meanings on the two sides of the Atlantic are given in Table 10.3.

Differences in national/regional spelling are not usually a problem in forensic work but there should be standardisation. It does not look good if a word is spelt 'centre' in one paragraph of a report and then 'center' in the next – unless, of course, one is quoting directly.

A few medical words can produce major problems, especially if indexed. These are usually where Europeans have endeavoured to retain the Greek root while Americans have reduced the word to basics. Difficulties occasionally arise when the word starts with the disputed spelling (Table 10.4).

Examples of scientific or medical terms that are significantly different on the two sides of the Atlantic and which may cause confusion are shown in Table 10.5.

European English tends to incorporate more words of French origin and these may not be familiar to Americans and others; for instance, a 'cul-de-sac' is called a 'dead end' in the USA. Some day-to-day words or phrases are familiar to British/European/Commonwealth speakers of English but are largely unknown in the USA. Examples are 'fortnight', meaning 'two weeks', and 'queue', meaning a 'line'. On a British document 'PTO' (please turn over) may appear – usually given as 'Over' in the USA. They and other terms should be avoided in forensic reports – or an explanation/ alternative offered.

The symbol '#' should be avoided in all forensic reports. It can mean 'number' or 'fracture' or, depending upon the context, various other things. It is sometimes called a 'hash sign', sometimes a 'pound sign' (but outside the USA a pound is designated as '£'). It serves only to confuse.

Use of local phraseology or dialect by witnesses can complicate or delay hearings. Popular names of animals and plants may be given (see Chapter 5), and even terms that relate to the judicial process may confuse the visiting expert. A good Caribbean example was given by Errol (1971):

> *So help me God! I goin' down by the courthouse an' take out a summons fer yer. I will make yer prove yer mouth before the doors of court.*

To 'prove your mouth' in Trinidadian dialect means 'to show or prove that what has been said is true (against a charge of slander).' The expert who is appearing overseas – in a wildlife crime case, for example – should be prepared for such differences.

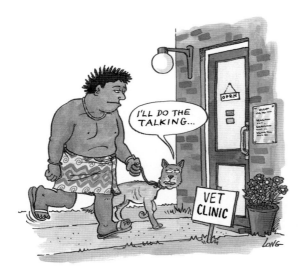

SECURITY

If confidentiality is important, one should be particularly careful about faxes and answerphones. In both cases, information may be readily accessible to other people: an open fax may be read by anyone in the office where it is received and a message via telephone may be picked up by persons other than those for whom the message was intended. When faxing, one should remember that the disparity in size between US paper and international paper (metric) can mean that important information at the bottom of a sheet is lost in transmission.

One should avoid discussing forensic cases when a colleague is on the telephone (even if covering the mouthpiece) or when doors are open and others may hear.

FREEDOM OF INFORMATION

Quite apart from the transparency of court cases, the expert must remember that in many countries – throughout the European Union, for example – freedom of information legislation entitles anyone to ask a public body for recorded information that they hold. This means that, for example, a report on an inspection carried out under the provisions of the relevant legislation (see Chapter 3) of a zoo in the UK, sent to a local authority, can be viewed by anyone, including those who may profess strong views or represent a pressure group.

PHOTOCOPIES

Hard copies of documents are still a key part of most legal cases and other proceedings. This means that often large amounts of photocopying have to be done. It is important to remember that photocopying regulations apply in many countries of the world and that legal proceedings are not exempt from these restrictions. Likewise, permission to use documents for illustrated material should be sought beforehand.

Care must be taken to ensure that photocopies of the reverse of a document (letter, report) or of a separate sheet can be linked to the original. A reference number should be put on all documents before unstapling and copying them. As a general rule, in legal cases, the reverse side should not be used: it can so easily be forgotten.

Sometimes the veracity of a photocopy is questioned in court. Giles (2004) explained the limitations of investigating photocopies, even by an experienced forensic document examiner.

RETENTION OF MATERIAL

It is wise to retain all material that has, or was meant to be, used in court or a similar hearing. For how long it should be kept is arguable (DiMaio and DiMaio, 2001). Five years is probably a good guide but one must bear in mind that it can take longer than this for an appeal to be heard, or a new case brought, or a claim to be made. Computerisation makes storage of records easier but contemporaneous notes and other raw data still need to be preserved.

When using computerised statements and other data, it is wise to retain early drafts, appropriately

dated, in case reference needs to be made to them, especially wording that was subsequently deleted, at a later date. This also enables one to check that changes have not been made to the final document by someone not authorised to do so. However, great care has to be taken to ensure that the version of a document that is used in a statement or in court is the appropriate one. Production of an early, perhaps uncorrected, version of a statement or report can cause embarrassment and may lead to legal wrangling.

Access to data that have not been released but may be needed later must be restricted. Security of both hard copies and electronic information should be stringent (see also Chapter 11).

DISCLAIMER

Technology is moving so fast that advice proffered in this book may well be superseded. However, the information given is considered to be correct at the time of writing.

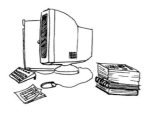

Storage, Labelling and Presentation of Material

These rough notes and our dead bodies must tell the tale.

Robert Falcon Scott (Scott of the Antarctic)

Evidence is a key part of the legal process (Gallop and Stockdale, 2004; Kiely, 2001; Townley and Ede, 2004). In animal work forensic material can range from a hair of an agouti to the frozen carcase of a dead dolphin or data as diverse as a one-page health certificate, vast quantities of paper and electronic farm records.

How evidence should be obtained and documented is often not standard. In Scotland, for example, in contrast to England and Wales, everything has to be verified by a second expert.

'Admissible evidence' is material, such as a dead animal, a photograph or a bullet, the origin of which can be vouched for by a person or persons.

RETENTION OF PROPERTY

This is often a feature of evidence-gathering and in animal forensics may even include the holding of live animals (see Chapter 5). The police and enforcement agencies are usually familiar with the necessary processes.

HANDLING OF EVIDENCE

Some of the principles of handling and dealing with evidence are described in Chapter 8, because laboratory samples are often either evidence themselves or contribute to the significance or admissibility of evidence when it is produced in court.

Important considerations in the handling of evidence are:

- Chain of custody.
- Storage, including security and safety.
- Sealing, labels and labelling.
- Tracking.
- Transfer elsewhere.

Each of these is covered in this chapter and, in some cases (especially chain of custody), also discussed in detail elsewhere in the book.

CHAIN OF CUSTODY

Also known as 'chain of evidence' or 'chain of continuity', this can be defined as the documentation of the transportation and handling of evidence from the time of collection until its presentation in court, including appeals. Each person who is a custodian of the evidence is a link in the chain. If a link is severed or its integrity is compromised, the chain may be broken (Figure 11.1).

Maintenance of the chain demands attention:

On reception of the specimen

- A detailed description of the evidence received, ensuring that it corresponds to what is written in the exhibit book.
- Date and time of receipt.

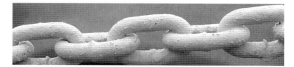

Figure 11.1 A chain of custody (evidence) is only intact if all the links are secure.

- Name and signature of the person releasing the evidence.
- Name and signature of the person receiving the evidence.

While the specimen is in custody, if the recipient (above) is absent

- Date, time and location of where the evidence is stored during that period.
- Name and signature of the person who is temporary custodian of the evidence (this transaction is acceptable in the USA but not usually in the UK and certain other countries – see Adair, 1999).

On release of the specimen

- Date and time of release.
- Name and signature of the person receiving the evidence.
- A detailed description of the evidence being released – also recorded in the exhibit book.

Documentation

In the UK, documentation of movement of evidence ('exhibit') is recorded in an exhibits book or a docket (a continuity document which covers the evidence while it is away from the police). Suitable wording for dockets is given below.

When material is passed to a new custodian (see above), this is recorded in the exhibit book and a docket is opened.

Chain of custody/possession labels (dockets) should include the following data:

> Received from ....
> By ....
> Date (in full) ....

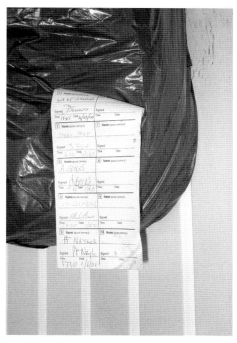

Figure 11.2 A chain of custody label attached to a plastic bag that contains a dead dog. The person handing over the bag has signed the form, as will the recipient.

> Time (international) ....
> Signature...

This information is then repeated down the label (Figure 11.2). A specimen chain of custody form, for receipt of material, is given in Appendix A.

STORAGE

The correct storage of evidence implies:

- Security.
- Safety.
- Ready identification and retrieval.
- Intact chain of custody.

SECURITY

Security implies that material (evidence):

- Cannot be easily removed or tampered with.
- Remains intact, with minimal change or deterioration.

Ideally, it should be stored in a specifically desig- nated and constructed facility but often this is not possible.

Security in the first sense, that of preventing or discouraging unauthorised access, is covered later, under 'Tracking of evidence'. Keys, codes and pass- words are important features of a good, secure system as are physical barriers such as metal bars and reinforced glass windows. Surveillance cameras are increasingly a standard feature. The use of suit- ably trained staff is essential – the person who receives and stores material (often termed an 'evi- dence technician'), for example.

A balance has to be struck between ease of access to facilities and preventing unauthorised entry.

Security in the second sense, of ensuring that the material is intact and of known provenance, is enhanced if the chain of custody is short.

The principles of good storage are discussed below.

SAFETY

The protection of staff and others who may come into contact with evidence is always important and may be subject to legal controls (see Chapter 3). Some examples follow. Safety hoods or cabinets may be mandatory. Correct disposal of 'sharps' may also be obligatory (Sillis, 2003).

When using ultraviolet light, appropriate safety goggles should be worn. Special precautions are necessary when storing items that are dangerous (chemicals, drugs, explosives) or perishable (animal and plant tissues).

Handling procedures are important in terms of both protocol and staff safety – as discussed in the context of soil samples by Saxton and Engel (2005) – and are covered later.

READY IDENTIFICATION AND RETRIEVAL

This is self-explanatory. Both identification and retrieval are facilitated if the evidence is properly marked and sealed. Evidence tape for re-sealing should preferably be unique to the laboratory or facility in question so that it can immediately be distinguished from the tape that originally secured the specimen.

PRINCIPLES OF STORAGE

If evidence is being stored, pending a court case or other hearing, it is vital that it is kept under opti- mal conditions. In a specially-constructed facility this will mean properly controlled facilities with respect to:

- Temperature.
- Relative humidity.
- Protection from strong light, vibration or exces- sive sound (including ultrasound).
- Cleanliness – freedom from gross contamina- tion (dust, soil, splashing, aerosols, odours).

In animal work, purpose-built facilities are often not available and evidence may have to be stored, temporarily at any rate, in a veterinary practice, at a police station or on the premises of an enforce- ment agency. Under these circumstances it is essen- tial that someone is given responsibility for storage. S/he must have the authority both to make deci- sions and to ensure that standard operating proce- dures (SOPs) are put in place and followed.

Refrigerators and freezer units are probably the most frequent source of problems insofar as the presentation of evidence in animal cases is con- cerned. A frozen carcase that thaws or a chilled specimen for necropsy that starts to 'cook' because a freezer has failed is at best an embarrassment, at worst grounds for a case to be dismissed and pos- sibly for an action to be brought against those responsible for maintaining the equipment.

Putting SOPs and less rigid, but pragmatic, pro- tocols and systems in place can do much to prevent such accidents from happening or to ensure prompt remedial action if something goes wrong. In the case of refrigerators and freezers, protocols and systems should include:

- Properly trained staff at all levels, who are aware of the consequences if equipment fails and who will take appropriate action, unprompted, both during normal working hours and at weekends or over public holidays.

- Correctly functioning temperature gauges and thermostats.
- Alarms, to alert staff to significant fluctuations in temperature; these should be both audible, e.g. a bell, and visible, e.g. a red light (preferably one that flashes).
- Back-up facilities – a stand-by generator and/or access to alternative refrigerators or freezers.

Carcases may appear to be an extreme example of why in forensic work equipment must be dependable but damage to laboratory samples can be even more important. A slight change in temperature can affect the survival of micro-organisms or the persistence of a toxic chemical and doubt over the reliability of storage facilities may thereby elicit critical comment and questioning in a courtroom.

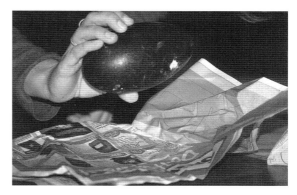

Figure 11.3 The wrapping may provide important clues to the origin of a specimen, as in this case where an egg submitted for examination was wrapped in pages from a local newspaper. This figure also appears in colour in the colour plate section.

HOLDING OF LABORATORY SAMPLES

How specimens are held pending analysis can be very important in forensic work. Use of an unsuitable container or wrapping may cast doubt, especially in cross-examination, about method and the extent to which quality control measures are in place. Table 11.1 gives some examples of different materials, in this case with particular reference to specimens taken for toxicological analysis.

As stressed elsewhere in this book (see Chapters 7 and 8), the *original* wrappings must always be retained, as part of the evidence (Figure 11.3).

INDIVIDUAL CONTAINERS

Once a specimen has been designated as an item of evidence, it will need to be packed separately (see below), in an appropriate container that is properly and permanently labelled and which is as tamper-proof as possible. In criminal cases it is likely that this will be the responsibility of a crime scene manager or his staff.

Bags for evidence need to be in various sizes as they may be used to store material ranging in size from a small feather to a disarticulated skeleton.

Care must be taken when using closed plastic bags to store evidence or to contain laboratory samples (see Table 11.1). They can quickly create a warm humid atmosphere and material may be damaged. Alternative transparent materials that are porous, e.g. cloth bags, are available and some are produced commercially. If necessary, paper bags or paper envelopes can be substituted, the latter preferably with see-through windows so that the contents can be seen.

If plastic bags *are* used, they may need to be heat-sealed in order to make them leak-proof (fluids and odours) and tamper-proof. A heat-sealer is therefore a useful addition to the equipment list (see Appendix E).

Some items of evidence are best stored in metal canisters, some in cardboard boxes, others in clear, transparent, bottles where they can be viewed without needing to be opened. Very delicate material may require wrapping in foam or kept in a 'puff bag' that encases the sample in air. It is most important that containers, regardless of structure, are appropriately leak-proof and crush-proof.

Items of evidence should either be packed separately or if part of the same animal (e.g. airgun pellets or stones from a bird's gizzard) wrapped individually and then placed in a solid container.

Table 11.1 Wrapping and storage of specimens.

Material	Use	Comments
Aluminium foil	Solids (faeces, powders, dried plant material)	Foils should be doubly packaged
Plastic bags	As above	Condensation may form in plastic bags that are exposed to alternating temperatures
Glass containers	Tissue, viscera, swabs, powders, solutions (including volatile liquids)	Best secured with screw-caps A ground glass cap can often be used
Plastic containers	Tissue, viscera, swabs, aqueous solutions, powders	Best secured with screw-caps
Paper bags	Plant material, solids without sharp edges	Use where a poisonous plant is suspected or medicinal products are being analysed If specimen is damp and cannot be air-dried, aluminium foil is preferable
Leaves, e.g. banana, tied with string or fibre	Emergency measure in the field, for faeces and other samples, when no other materials are available	Helps to keep specimens cool in the absence of refrigeration A last resort measure Security is very poor

EVIDENCE CABINETS

Purpose-built cabinets for the storage of evidence are available commercially and have much to commend them. The more sophisticated (and expensive!) designs include secure doors that can be locked, removable shelves and a corrosion-proof interior. Some are designed to store evidence that may emit fumes, e.g. formalin, or particulate material (e.g. pollen or bacteria): these are fitted with HEPA filters.

MARKING EVIDENCE

This is important. Exhibits should be marked in a unique way, preferably in large letters, on different surfaces. The reference number or designation must not then be changed, even if a mistake has been made, such as an error in writing the date of seizure of a gun or an incorrect initial identification of a dead reptile.

Evidence markers can be of different colours and this helps to distinguish separate items (see below). Commercial forensic markers will mark virtually anything – paper, wood, metal, plastic.

SEALING OF EVIDENCE

Tamper-proof ties should be used where appropriate, e.g. for plastic bags that may contain bones, feathers or a small carcase (Figure 11.4).

Where this is not feasible, the adequate sealing of evidence packages with tape is vital. The sealing needs to be strong and it can be rendered more secure by the addition of a signature over the point where the tape finishes. Some commercial tapes are advertised as 'tamper-indicating' because they tear and shred if any attempt is made to remove them.

Coloured labels and tape are useful in order to distinguish different items on different animals. A colour code can be devised and this may assist

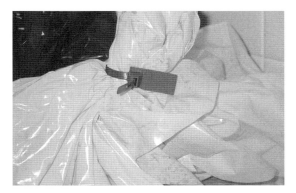

Figure 11.4 A tamper-proof tie that sealed an evidence bag containing a dead rat for *post-mortem* examination. (Courtesy of Richard Spence.)

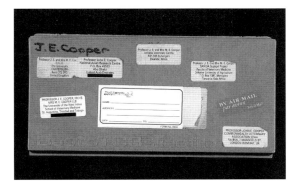

Figure 11.5 Existing marks and labels on evidence must be carefully protected and not overlain by evidence tape. Often it is best to put the item in a sealed bag and to label and seal that. (Courtesy of Richard Spence.)

others, such as laboratory staff, if by any chance details are lost or obscured. Care must be taken to remember that one may need to write on the label or tape: this will influence the colour of the marking pen.

Any containers that bear labels should be carefully managed. In particular, it is vital that any existing labels or identification marks are left intact: no attempt should be made to remove, deface or apply extra labelling to them since they may be an important part of the evidence (Figure 11.5).

As a general rule, advice can be sought from the police or crime scene officers as to how best to handle and store materials and to ensure that any

wrappings are tamper-proof. If, however, the veterinarian or his equivalent is working alone in the field or at a crime scene, with little or no support, the following standard approach is advocated:

- Wrap and place each item of evidence in a strong, transparent, plastic bag.
- Within the plastic bag place a label or copy of relevant paperwork.
- Seal the plastic bag, preferably with a tamper-proof tag or, failing that, tie securely with string or wire.
- Label the outside of the bag, preferably in more than one place, using the same reference or identity number on the paperwork within the bag.

When wire or string has to be used, the type and colour should be standardised so that each bag is closed in a similar fashion. It can also be a useful precaution, in the absence of tamper-proof tags, to use a standard length so that any subsequent interference, such as cutting, bending or tying, can be more readily detected by a change in measurement or appearance.

TAGS

Tags are used where ordinary labels (see below) are inappropriate. Lamination helps to protect them from the excesses of temperature or humidity (see below). A tag usually has a hole punched in it so that it can be attached with strong (preferably nylon) string or wire.

Tags can be attached to animal skins and other soft material using a tagger gun – similar to those used on clothing in department stores. More than one should be applied, in case of damage (see below).

Items marked with a tag should always be handled carefully. Tags tend to become damaged or lost, especially if environmental conditions change.

LABELS AND LABELLING

Labels of various types play a very significant role in forensic medicine. They help to ensure that there is a proper chain of custody (evidence, continuity) and, in the case of exhibits that are to be produced in court, should bear certain important information, such as the signatures of relevant police officers, the name of the case (in the UK, 'R(egina) versus . . .'), a laboratory reference and some description of the contents of the container which they mark (Weston, 2004).

Many types of labels are produced commercially. In animal forensics standard stationery items may need to be adapted for the task.

Self-adhesive labels are usually best for attachment to plastic, glass, wood or metal containers. They should be reliable (i.e. not easily peeled off, even if exposed to extremes of temperature or relative humidity) and tamper-proof while, at the same time, unlikely to damage the underlying surface.

Labelling should be carried out using waterproof, indelible ink. Inks must be avoided that will run if in contact with water (fountain pens) or alcohol (ballpoint pens).

Pencils should, as a general rule, not be used because pencilled information can be so easily erased or changed. However, a pencil can be of value in an emergency when it is necessary to label 'wet specimens', i.e. materials, tissues or parasites that are to be placed in formalin or alcohol fixatives; in this case, the label, written in pencil, is inserted in the fixative together with the specimen (see Chapter 9). Pencil is also ideal for labelling 'frosted' glass slides, especially when taking samples in the field (see Appendix E).

The whole question of labelling is a complex and well-studied one. The person responsible for animal material can glean much useful information from the experiences of those who work in human forensic medicine.

SECURITY AND SAFETY

It is wise to include warning notices on labels, tags and tape both to safeguard the evidence/sample and to protect the person. A warning can read 'Evidence' or, perhaps, 'Pathological Specimen' coupled with – 'Do not touch!' In international work, languages other than English may need to be added. In poorer parts of the world, where many people may be illiterate, an appropriate warning sign, such as a skull or red drops that depict blood, can provide a visual warning. One always has a responsibility for the health and safety of all those who may come into contact with the specimen, as well as the important need in a legal case to protect it from unauthorised handling, damage or contamination.

In the same vein, specific biohazard notices may be needed, bearing the international symbol and additional wording (e.g. 'Handle with gloves' or 'Toxic chemical'), as appropriate.

Material from live or dead animals is often best retained in clinical waste bags. These follow international rules and they are a readily recognisable yellow colour.

SPECIAL CONSIDERATIONS IN FIELDWORK

Storage and labelling can present particular problems if evidence has to remain *in situ* for some time before being transported back to a laboratory or secure holding facility. This may arise in wildlife cases, for instance, where the crime scene may be an extensive area of terrain and material needs to be examined on the spot. Useful guidance on the handling and retention of animal material in the field can be obtained from veterinarians who deal with disease outbreaks, when sick and dead livestock have to be investigated and sampled *in situ*, and also from zoo-archaeologists, many of whom have experience of working in historical sites where great care must be taken in handling, identification and wrapping of specimens (Davis, 1987).

An appropriately constructed trailer can be useful for work in the field. The trailer is towed to the site by motor vehicle and, if appropriate, disconnected at the scene and there used as a temporary forensic laboratory. Ultimately, it is available to transport evidence back to a police station or other secure place.

On a smaller scale, field 'kits' can be used for forensic work (see Chapter 9).

HANDLING OF EVIDENCE

The handling of evidence can be dangerous and unpleasant, whether in the laboratory or the field. Gloves should be worn as a routine and there is often merit in using forceps (lockable variety or artery forceps/haemostats that retain the grip) for small items. For larger pieces of evidence, e.g. the remains of limbs or other blood-stained material, long-handled tongs are useful; those produced commercially for picking up rubbish or for grasping venomous snakes are ideal.

Forceps made of plastic (polypropylene) are advantageous when handling delicate items and can be discarded after use. Disposable plastic forceps can be purchased in bulk from companies that manufacture crime investigation or medical equipment. Small numbers can sometimes be solicited from airlines that use such items to handle hot towels: a useful saving for those on a small budget!

TRACKING OF EVIDENCE

Tracking depends upon:

- An intact chain of custody (see earlier).
- Strict control over access to records.
- A complete audit of movement, recording every change in item or location.

In the past, tracking has depended upon paper records – with all the drawbacks and dangers that this implies. Nowadays the computer is used (see Chapter 10) but it is important to have back-up copies of information in case of an electronic failure. Specific software programmes for tracking are now available and are applied to forensic work by many individuals, police and enforcement bodies. A portable data terminal permits authorised persons to gain access to the tracking system remotely, away from the main terminal – for example, while out at a crime scene.

CHECKLISTS

Checklists are valuable in medical and veterinary forensic work and can form part of the tracking process. They enable the clinician or pathologist to know which samples have been taken and, in due course, to ascertain that those samples have either been sent to one or more laboratories or processed in-house. Checklists can also be adapted for non-medical specimens that are likely to constitute evidence and must not be mislaid or transposed.

It is easy for specimens to be overlooked and, in particular, for laboratory samples to languish in a refrigerator or freezer. This can reduce their scientific value and may elicit embarrassing questions in court. It is wise to attach a copy of any checklist to the refrigerator or freezer and to record on it 'Specimens in . . . , specimens out . . . ' with date and signature. The fridge/freezer should either be dedicated to the one legal hearing or have distinct, well-demarcated compartments or containers therein to ensure that all specimens from the case are kept together. Colour codes can be helpful. Security in the form of locks or seals and restricted access are wise.

VERACITY OF DOCUMENTS

Forgery has been a feature of human society since at least the 3rd century AD (Giles, 2004) and documents produced for a legal case are no exception. Veterinary certificates (see Chapter 6) can be forged or have their wording changed. Fraudulent computer-generated prescriptions, purporting to have come from a veterinary surgeon, have been the subject of recent debate (2005) in the UK, prompting the production of specific forms by the British Veterinary Association (see Appendix B).

If doubt exists about a prescription, letter or report or if a claim is made in court or other proceedings that submitted written evidence is false, it may be necessary to seek the help of an experienced forensic document examiner.

TRANSFER OF EVIDENCE

In the UK and many other countries evidence has to be passed from one person to another by hand. In some other places, including the USA, it can be transferred by post (mail). In the latter case, it is good practice to take the item to the Post Office and obtain some written confirmation that it has been despatched, rather than rely on dropping it in a postbox.

SENDING MATERIAL OVERSEAS/ TO OTHER COUNTRIES

It has been claimed that in today's world, there are no borders, just time zones. This is not entirely true but serves as a pertinent reminder of the need to think laterally when participating in forensic work that may have an international dimension.

Before despatching anything of a forensic nature to another country, one must:

- Ensure that all legal requirements of both exporting and importing countries have been met (Figure 11.6).
- Have spare photocopies and electronic versions of all relevant documents.
- Make allowances for:
  ○ Language/comprehension ('shipping' in the USA means 'despatching', not that the package is going by boat!).
  ○ Time zones (material may arrive in the middle of the night).
  ○ Public holidays (closure of offices and staff shortages may delay processing): this needs prior planning. It is important to consult and to remember that some holidays (e.g. the Muslim celebration of Eid) may be announced at short notice.

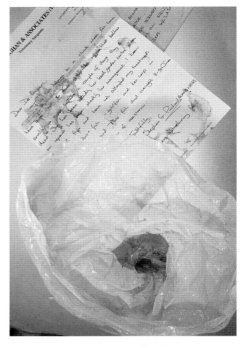

Figure 11.6 How *not* to send a fish for *post-mortem* examination.

PREPARATION OF REPORT

This is described in some detail by Rothwell (2004) and discussed in Chapter 10 of this book. Specific reporting of findings is referred to in Chapter 6 (clinical cases), Chapter 7 (*post-mortem* material) and Chapter 8 (laboratory samples).

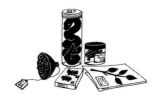

Serving as an Expert and Appearing in Court

Grammatici certant et adhuc sub iudice lis est.
(Grammarians dispute and the case is still before the courts.)

Horace

... the truth, the whole truth and nothing but the truth.

Oaths Act 1978

This statement, used in English courts and, in various forms, in many other jurisdictions, indicates the seriousness of giving evidence in a judicial process. It is the cornerstone of the work of the expert witness.

T. G. Field-Fisher, for many years responsible for the section on animal law in *Halsburys Law's of England* provided, in his succinct, yet highly-readable book *Animals and the Law* (Field-Fisher, 1964) the following advice for veterinary surgeons who act as expert witnesses.

A veterinary surgeon may find himself giving evidence under a variety of circumstances. He may, of course, be merely a witness of fact like any other witness, deposing to matters entirely unconnected with his professional knowledge; or he may still be a witness of fact but deposing to matters which, because of his professional knowledge, he is able to observe better than someone not of his profession, or thirdly, he may be giving evidence of his opinion based either on facts presented to him by others or on facts observed by himself. In the third case only is he giving evidence as an expert, and where his opinion is based on facts observed by himself he is, strictly

speaking, only the expert in regard to his opinion, but clearly it is difficult to separate these functions precisely.

It is as an 'expert' witness that we are considering him here. The term 'expert' may be misleading in that it means only that by reason of training or experience the witness is qualified to express an opinion where an ordinary person is not. It does not imply authority or standing in his own profession. When giving evidence as an expert a veterinary surgeon should realize that his first duty is to assist the court with his honestly-held opinion and the reasons for it, and it is not, strictly speaking, to help one party to the dispute, although clearly it probably will do, since the party concerned would normally know of his opinion before calling him as a witness. He may refer to text-books to refresh his memory while in the witness box, or to correct or confirm his opinion, and if certain passages represent his own opinion he may adopt them and read them.[1]

He may be asked his opinion based either on facts established – whether by him or another witness – or on a hypothesis based upon the evidence. Although he may be asked what would be a proper course of treatment, he should not state whether it is what he would have done himself.[2]

Under cross-examination, an expert witness may not only be queried as to his opinion, but also as to the reasons for his holding it. He may also be challenged as to his competency and his credit may be impeached on the ground that he was not in a fit state to form an opinion, that he is interested, or corrupt, or has expressed a different opinion at other times.[3]

A few golden rules for experts may not come amiss here:

(i)   If you have a firm opinion, be firm about it.
(ii) If there is room for argument, admit it freely.
(iii) Be as concise as possible.
(iv) Use non-technical language if this is possible without sacrificing accuracy of phrase.
(v)   If you have to give ground do so honestly and with a good grace.

Finally, it is of the greatest importance to realize that when an opinion is sought with a view to possible litigation in the future, any written opinion or report given by a veterinary surgeon may well be the whole basis of the case for the party seeking it and therefore no expression of opinion should be given unless the person giving it is prepared to go into the witness box and substantiate it. This is only fair to the person seeking the opinion, for history is littered with stories of unsuccessful litigants whose experts failed to "come up to proof".

This is quoted in full, with permission, because it is the epitome of advice for the veterinary expert witness. While it may be necessary, in the 21st century, to have much more specific rules for the provision of expert evidence, backed up by training,

registration, accreditation and other facilities, the passage demonstrates that the fundamental principles have a long-established pedigree.

INTRODUCTION

The history of the expert witness in England can be traced at least to the 14th century, when special juries of experts were used in the manner of assessors (Hodgkinson and James, 2006). This concept has also evolved in, or been adopted by, numerous countries to the extent that expert evidence is a key element in many judicial systems, even if the rules for the appointment and use of experts may vary greatly.

This chapter deals with the implications of acting as an expert witness in matters relevant to the general scope of this book. It will deal primarily with the law and legal system for England but many of the general principles are relevant elsewhere in the United Kingdom (UK), the Commonwealth (formerly called the British Commonwealth) and in other common law countries.

In the last decade of the 20th century, much dissatisfaction was expressed regarding expert witnesses, the evidence that they proffered and the way that they were used, especially in civil law cases. Eventually, one exasperated court commented that, far from showing impartiality, the expert witnesses were 'on occasion becoming more partisan than the parties'.

A timely reminder to experts of their duties was provided by J. Cresswell in *The Ikarian Reefer* [1993] 2 Lloyd's Rep 68, at 81–82 (conveniently cited in the judgement of Collins J in *Meadow v. General Medical Council* [2006] EWHC 146 (Admin) (http://www.bailii.org/ew/cases/EWHC/Admin/2006/146.html)). These duties were listed and included:

- Independence of evidence.
- Objective and unbiased opinion.
- The presentation of all material facts.
- Disclosure of:
  ○ issues beyond the witness's expertise
  ○ any lack of data or qualification of truth

---

[1]   Concha v. Murieta (1889).
[2]   Ramadge v. Ryan (1832).
[3]   Alcock v. Royal Exchange Co. (1849).

Note: In legal parlance, the masculine includes reference to the feminine, unless otherwise stated.

- any change of opinion
- on exchange of reports with opposing experts, the sharing of material evidence on which the opinion is based.

Collins added that evidence must be given honestly, in good faith and without misleading the court.

Much of the contemporary thinking on practice standards for experts in civil court procedure is derived from the reforms proposed by Lord Woolf in his Report *Access to Justice* (Woolf, 1996). This document led to substantial reforms in the judicial process in England and Wales and at the same time profoundly affected the working practices of expert witnesses. New rules for the criminal justice system are following suit.

Although the fundamental duties involved in providing specialist evidence and opinion remain substantially the same, there have been changes in the manner and standards of its preparation and presentation. There are higher expectations in terms of the quality of experts' reports and presentation of evidence. Written rules have reinstated the once traditional requirement for experts to show independence, integrity and a duty to the court. Control over expert evidence has been transferred from the parties to the court itself.

Where once the skills of the expert were acquired by experience, there is now an emphasis on training, on rules and guidance and on the quality of experts and their evidence. In an article in *Veterinary Times*, Edmondson (2002) described the transition made by one veterinary expert from learning by experience to improving skills through training. However, training will never be the sole route to becoming an expert witness and a blending of the two, together with the appropriate temperament, is the combination most likely to prove successful.

Several approaches to quality control in expert witnesses have been initiated outside the judicial system during and since the 1990s. These include the compilation of registers of experts, some stipulating prior experience, and moves towards accreditation of experts and the consideration of supervision of the forensic science market.

USEFUL DEFINITIONS AND BACKGROUND INFORMATION

There are a number of definitions and distinctions that are useful to anyone who comes into contact with the law, but these may be essential to expert witnesses who intend to become familiar with the legal framework within which they perform their duties.

Legal systems

- There are a number of different legal systems in the world. The predominant ones are the civil law, common law, customary law and Muslim law, although many countries have a mixture of systems. These are explained further and related to individual countries on http://www. droitcivil.uottawa.ca/world-legal-systems/eng-monde.php.
- England and Wales share a legal system, although the National Assembly of Wales (Welsh Assembly) has, since 1999, had power to make secondary legislation within certain areas of policy. In this chapter, for the sake of brevity, references to England and its judicial system include Wales. The same applies to mention of English law, except where Welsh law has diverged (http://www.wales-legislation.org.uk/scripts/) (see below).
- Scotland has a separate legal system that is based partly on common law and partly on civil law. For example, there is distinctive terminology for the courts and legal personnel. It shares legislation with England and Wales on major policy such as defence but, since devolution in 1999, the Scottish Parliament has made separate law on many subjects.
- While England, Wales and Scotland have much shared legislation, Welsh and Scottish laws are gradually diverging. Thus, the Wildlife and Countryside Act 1981 and the Zoo Licensing Act 1981, originally applicable to all three countries, have since been amended separately by each one. It is now necessary to ascertain carefully the country of application of any piece of legislation and subsequent amendments thereto.

- Northern Ireland, the other constituent country of the UK, has a separate but similar legal system although the coverage of law is very similar.
- A useful portal for all UK legislation is http://www.opsi.gov.uk/legislation/about_legislation.htm. For Wales, there is also: http://www.wales-legislation.org.uk/scripts/home.php?lang=E.
- The British Islands (the Channel Islands and the Isle of Man) have their own legal systems as do the 14 British Overseas Territories (such as Montserrat and St Helena), although the UK government may take responsibility for some areas of policy such as foreign affairs or defence or provide a final court of appeal.
- Many Commonwealth nations (http://www.droitcivil.uottawa.ca/world-legal-systems/engcommonwealth.php) and other former British territories (including the USA) originally adopted the English law and judicial system as part of their own. These are often referred to as the 'common law countries'. Such nations have retained some pre-independence English law and this continues to be used, alongside their own statutory, common, religious and customary law together with case law. In addition, reference may be made to the law of other common law countries as an aid to the court in deciding a case. There may be a recognisable similarity in their judicial systems and in certain laws on account of this common origin, for example in animal welfare or in the law on the veterinary profession. Other laws may be similar because they implement international treaty obligations (for example, under the Convention on International Trade in Endangered Species of Wild Fauna and Flora – CITES) or to meet the need for international co-operation, as in animal health controls.
- The constitutions of federal nations usually allow individual states, variously called states (USA, Australia, Nigeria), provinces (Canada), cantons (Switzerland), for example, to legislate on matters such as animals, wildlife and veterinary matters. There may be law at federal, state and local levels in some countries, as, for example, in the conservation provisions for the Florida Everglades in the USA.

Levels of law

There are four main levels at which law is made – international, regional, national and local (see Chapter 3).

Most law is made at national (or, in a federal country, at state) level. National legislation also implements international treaty obligations. In the European Union (EU), the national legislation of Member States includes regulations and implements directives produced by the European Community (EC), the law-making pillar of the EU (Davies, 2001). An extensive body of animal-related legislation emanating from the EU has profoundly influenced the national laws of its Member States.

It is important to make clear the level of law under discussion in expert reports or evidence. For example, when speaking of the 'CITES legislation' it is important to distinguish between the international treaty (the Convention on International Trade in Endangered Species of Wild Fauna and Flora) and the EC CITES Regulations that implement the Convention within the EU. Countries within the EU also have national legislation that provides for the enforcement of CITES. In countries outside the EU, 'CITES legislation' may also refer to their national law on the subject.

Kinds of law

There are many kinds and categories of law and those that are particularly relevant to the expert witness are discussed below.

There are fundamental distinctions between criminal and civil law in most jurisdictions. Different laws, courts and judicial procedures apply to the criminal law and the civil law.

Criminal law

The criminal law deals with relations between persons and the state. Legal persons, as entities recognised in law, may be 'natural persons' (individual human beings) or they may be 'corporations' (companies and other bodies incorporated by statute or charter). Criminal law consists of law that creates duties and obligations, the breach of which is punished by the state (Barker and Padfield, 2002).

Criminal law is, with some exceptions, set out in legislation (see below), for example driving offences, theft or animal mistreatment.

Suspected offences are usually investigated by the police. Other institutions, such as the Customs service, ministerial departments or local government authorities may be invested with law enforcement powers under which they also investigate crimes or they may do so in conjunction with the police.

It is also possible in England and Wales for an individual to bring a 'private prosecution'. Organisations such as animal welfare and wildlife charities sometimes exercise this right to initiate a prosecution when they have a particular interest or when suspected offences are not followed up by the official authorities. On occasions, the charities may collaborate with these authorities in providing information, advice, specialists or by attending the execution of a search warrant.

Offences are prosecuted (brought to the court) by the police (in some countries) or by a prosecuting service, known in England and Wales as the Crown Prosecution Service (http://www.cps.gov.uk/) and in Scotland as the Crown Office and Procurator Fiscal Service. The latter also has prosecutors specially trained in environmental law and wildlife crime (http://www.procuratorfiscal.gov.uk/About/roles/pf-role/specialists).

Successful prosecutions end in punishment by way of fine or imprisonment. There are also other possibilities, such as a conditional or absolute discharge, probation or community service. Some animal and wildlife legislation provides for the confiscation of vehicles and other equipment, such as nets, climbing gear or vehicles that have been used in the crime. There is also, in some cases, the option of disqualification from, for example, keeping or breeding animals, when offences of cruelty or unnecessary suffering have been proved.

Civil law

The civil law normally deals with relations between persons, both natural and incorporated. It includes, *inter alia*, the law of contract and the law of tort (civil wrong). Claims are normally initiated by the persons themselves. Cases are heard in the civil

courts (see below) and the remedy sought is mainly financial compensation, known as 'damages', although there are also other remedies.

In tort, claims are made, for example in trespass, nuisance and negligence or for the consequences of straying animals. Claims under the Animals Act 1971 relate to 'strict liability' for damage, injury and death caused by animals whether or not negligence is involved. Common issues involving animals are injury caused by animals, damage to people or property and for nuisance, caused by excessive noise from dogs or smell from farms (Cooper, 1987; North, 1972; Palmer, 2001; Rogers, 2002) (see Chapter 2). Claims can also arise from death or injury suffered by animals. Usually financial compensation (known as damages) is claimed but, in the case of nuisance, injunctions (for example, to stop or remedy a problem of noise or smell) may also be sought.

The English criminal and civil judicial systems are distinct. Useful descriptions are provided by Bond *et al.* (1999) and Barker and Padfield (2002) and on the internet at: http://www.bbc.co.uk/crime/law/englandcourts.shtml.

Legislation

The national law of any common law country is comprised mainly of 'statute law'. This is:

- Primary legislation, i.e. Acts of Parliament, also called 'statutes'.
- Secondary (delegated or subordinate) legislation called 'statutory instruments'. These are usually described in their titles as Orders, Regulations, Rules or Orders in Council. Statutes confer the power to make secondary legislation on the relevant government ministers and other bodies.

Common law

The remainder of English law comprises the 'common law'. This is the body of law that has evolved over the centuries and is still not enshrined in statute. The common law also includes 'case law', the decisions and judicial reasoning produced in cases brought before the courts. In common law countries, case law is subject to the rule of precedent, which dictates whether a legal decision in a particular case is binding on lower courts in the future. As already mentioned, in some countries, customary and religious law also form part of the body of law.

The courts and the judicial process

Each country has courts in which criminal offences or civil disputes are tried. The court systems of each country have distinctive features. One of the primary differences between the common law countries and others is that the legal systems of the former are *adversarial*, i.e. the parties are opposed and have to persuade the court, by way of evidence, to accept their claim or defence.

By comparison, in the *inquisitorial* system, as in France and Germany, the court and its presiding judge or magistrate direct the management of the case, have a more participatory role, can interrogate the parties and normally appoint the expert witnesses from a list approved by the court. In some such countries, the parties can appoint their own experts in addition to the court expert (EWI, 2004). Needless to say, when examined in detail, the distinction between adversarial and inquisitorial systems tends to become blurred at the edges. For example, the reformed English civil court procedure gives the judge extensive powers to manage a case and in particular to control the use of expert evidence.

Since the position of the expert is different in each jurisdiction, even the experienced expert witness should obtain detailed advice on law, procedure and the role of the expert before appearing in another jurisdiction for the first time.

The presiding authority in the higher courts is usually a judge who, in certain types of case, sits with a jury. At the lowest level of court, magistrates hear cases. There are other fora, such as tribunals or arbitration, in which at least one adjudicator is a lawyer. In the light of this complexity, the term 'presiding authority' will be used to describe the person deciding the case.

In England and Wales, as in many countries, there are separate rules of procedure for criminal and for civil law courts. The etiquette and terminol-

ogy are also different in each system and at different levels of the courts. The expert should take advice on this from the instructing lawyer, court staff, experienced colleagues or from training and literature (such as Bond *et al.*, 1999) before going to court.

The Criminal Procedure Rules 2005 (CrimPR) and the Civil Procedure Rules 1999 (CPR) regulate the conduct of the courts, other than the House of Lords. The CrimPR 2005, for the first time in history, have given the criminal courts a unified set of rules. The CPR made sweeping changes in civil court procedure and drastically changed the management of expert evidence.

While a substantial knowledge of the rules of court procedure is likely to be acquired by only the most experienced experts, all those appearing in the civil courts must be conversant with the section devoted to expert witnesses, namely the CPR Part 35 supplemented by Practice Direction 35. In addition, the expert must comply with the *Protocol for the Instruction of Experts to give Evidence in Civil Claims* (Civil Justice Council, 2005). These are readily available on the website of the Department for Constitutional Affairs (www.dca.gov.uk) and are discussed in the literature on the law of evidence and the duties of expert witnesses. Comparable rules for experts appearing in criminal cases came into force on 6 November 2006 as Rule 33 of the CrimPR.

Other tribunals

Expert witnesses appear primarily in the criminal and civil courts but they are also used in other fora such as town and country planning enquiries (for example, on the impact of a proposed road or building scheme upon endangered species of wildlife or, at an industrial tribunal, for example on the effect of zoonoses or allergens) (see Chapters 2 and 5). There are also parliamentary inquiries and commissions that call for evidence (see Chapter 2). Some experts may also become involved in arbitration or act as assessors.

Veterinary experts may also be called upon to give evidence at disciplinary hearings of, for example, the Royal College of Veterinary Surgeons (RCVS), the governing body of the veterinary profession in the UK, or to assist in insurance claim assessments. In some such hearings the rules of evidence may be less strict and procedure less formal than in the courts but the expert should be aware of the specific rules applied to a particular hearing (Mildred, 1982).

How much law should the expert know?

The instructing lawyer should make the legal aspects of a case sufficiently clear for the expert to understand the relevance of his or her evidence. Experts are likely to build up knowledge of the law relevant to their expertise and may be interested to expand it. There are occasions when the expert may be more aware of the relevant legislation or its application than an instructing lawyer who is new to a field of law. The expert may be able to point out common pitfalls or decisions in past cases.

The expert should also know the relevant parts of the procedural law and official guidance (see above) and should be conversant with any other advice produced for experts.

S/he should also understand the duties owed to the court, the client and the instructing lawyer (see below and Bond *et al.*, 1999). The level of immunity and protection from disclosure accorded to witnesses and their documents should also be understood, although advice on this should be available from the instructing lawyer.

It is important that the expert does not confuse the roles of lawyer and expert. The expert should be concerned with the law, not as a lawyer but to the extent that it enables the expert to comply with relevant requirements and to perform his or her duties effectively.

Evidence

Evidence may be defined as:

- 'One or more reasons for believing that something is or is not true' (*Cambridge Dictionaries Online*: http://dictionary.cambridge.org).
- 'Statements made in a law court to support a case' (*Oxford English Minidictionary*).
- 'Information drawn from personal testimony, a document, or a material object, used to estab-

lish facts in a legal investigation or admissible as testimony in a law court' (*Concise Oxford English Dictionary*).

There are established principles of law as to what is admissible evidence, i.e., that which may be presented to the court and used in its deliberations. The main issue that affects the expert is that of opinion evidence. This is not to be confused with the rules on hearsay evidence. Both are founded in the original common law principle that only oral statements of facts directly observed by a witness are admissible as evidence. This principle has been developed and various exceptions have been established through case law and in statutes (Bond *et al.*, 1999; Cavendish Law Cards, 2002; Tapper, 2003; and other authors on evidence).

Opinion evidence

It is a fundamental rule that a witness should give evidence only of facts. Any inference from facts should be made by the presiding authority of the court, not by witnesses. However, by way of exception, as mentioned above, when technical evidence that is outside the expertise of the presiding authority is presented, an expert witness with special knowledge and experience of the subject is allowed to elucidate and to evaluate the evidence and to express an opinion on it.

Hearsay evidence

Hearsay evidence is defined by the Criminal Evidence Act 1995 as:

> *A statement made otherwise than by a person while giving oral evidence in the proceedings which is tendered as evidence of the matters stated.*

Hearsay evidence is only admissible if it falls within one of the established exceptions laid down in statute or common law. Those that are of importance to expert evidence are:

- S30 Criminal Justice Act 1988: This allows for an expert's report to be produced as evidence in court without the attendance of the expert, subject to leave of the court being given.

- Civil Evidence Act 1995: The Act removes the rule of hearsay in civil proceedings, subject to certain safeguards. Consequently, expert reports may be admitted in evidence without the presence of the expert. In addition, CPR 35 provides that expert evidence should be provided in a report unless the court directs otherwise.

Witness

The term witness may be defined as:

- 'Person who sees or hears something' (*Oxford English Minidictionary*).
- 'Person giving sworn testimony to a court of law' (*Concise Oxford English Dictionary*).

As a basic principle, English law permits a witness to give evidence only of what he or she has personally seen or heard, although as mentioned above, there are exceptions.

There are various kinds of witness.

Witness of fact

Most people who give evidence in court appear as a witness of fact. This may arise from normal daily life, such as witnessing a street fight. Similarly, a veterinarian may provide a description of injuries that s/he has observed while examining an animal involved in a road accident or the condition of an animal that has been presented as a suspected cruelty case. The veterinary witness may speak of the road accident (if s/he actually saw it) and his/her own observations made of the condition of the animal when s/he examined it since these are within his or her direct experience. However, generally, in criminal law, knowledge gathered by the veterinarian from any other source (for example, the owner of the animal in the suspected cruelty case claims to have seen a member of the family beating the animal) is considered to be 'hearsay' and would have to be provided by a person who personally observed the ill-treatment of the animal.

Professional witness

A witness of fact is not generally allowed to express an opinion on the evidence s/he has given. However, a witness of fact who is giving evidence of events that arise as part of his or her employment, such as a police surgeon (now called 'forensic physicians') (see Chapter 1), may be allowed by the court to give an opinion, for example, as to age (Bond *et al.*, 1999). Veterinary surgeons are often asked at the end of their factual evidence in a prosecution for causing an animal unnecessary suffering whether they thought that the animal suffered and whether the suffering was necessary. It may be difficult for professional witnesses to be fully objective (and therefore willing to change their view, if the facts warrant it, in the course of a hearing) when the prosecution was based on their original statement. In such a situation, it may be better for the prosecution to provide a separate expert to give an opinion on unnecessary suffering (see Chapter 4).

Expert witness

An expert witness is so called because of his or her special training, knowledge and expertise in a technical or scientific subject of which the presiding authority does not have sufficient knowledge to assess the facts. An expert witness gives both factual and opinion evidence (see above).

An expert witness is called by a particular party to a case because his or her knowledge and opinion will support that party's arguments. On the other hand, there is a long-standing principle that the expert owes a duty to the court when providing evidence (Field-Fisher, 1964; Porter, 1971). Current commentaries and rules of civil procedure (CPR 35) lay clearly-stated emphasis on the requirements of integrity, independence, objectivity and duty to the court that are expected of the expert witness (Bond *et al.*, 1999 and other authors). This may not always be understood or appreciated by litigants (and some lawyers), not least the party who has called the expert to give evidence and especially so if the expert is obliged, through honesty and objectivity, to agree with the view of the opposite side. It is now clearly stated in the CPR 35 that the expert's duty to assist the court to the extent of his/her expertise overrides that owed to the client.

Some experts tend to appear mainly for one side (e.g. for the prosecution, for the defence, for a particular charity or institution), whereas others give evidence for a mixture of parties.

Single joint expert witness

A new category of expert has arisen in England and Wales from the reforms of the civil law court procedure, namely 'the single joint expert witness', who is appointed by the court as part of the case management process under the Civil Procedure Rules. The single expert is expected to present a report that fairly represents the evidence of both sides, indicating the areas of agreement and disagreement.

The aim, predicated on the Woolf Report, is to reduce the use of expert witnesses in the civil courts as far as reasonable, to use written reports, call a single or a minimum number of experts, and to find as much common ground as possible between either side, thereby reducing the time and cost of a hearing.

LITERATURE

There is no substitute for practical experience and training; nevertheless, an expert witness can gain insight into the legal process and the duties of the expert from the literature available on the subject. Some of the material of a practical nature, e.g. Bond *et al.* (1999), is a valuable resource for all experts, as is the material provided by the expert witness organisations such as the Academy of Experts and the Register of Expert Witnesses. Student texts and revision notes on the law are useful to the non-lawyer in that they provide a good overview of a subject unobscured by detail and learned argument. The professional textbooks may enable the expert to expand his or her knowledge beyond general principles as experience calls for deeper knowledge (see below and References and Further Reading).

All written material becomes out-of-date, including this book. The reader must take the responsibility for ascertaining any more recent material and keeping in touch with changes in the law and court procedures.

There is a considerable body of literature relating to expert evidence. These include:

General legal books useful for the expert witness

- Barker and Padfield (2002) give a good general introduction to English law and the legal system.
- Williams and Smith (2002) explain the legal profession and its resources for a person new to the law.

Literature written for the expert witness

- Bond *et al.* (1999) is a thoroughly practical book dealing with all legal aspects of the work of the expert witness and is based on the authors' training course material. *The Expert Witness in Court. A Practical Guide* deals with the English legal system, both civil and criminal, and the duties of the expert witness in and out of court and also provides model documents, court rules, general guidance and a glossary. It is concise and comprehensible although, surprisingly, it lacks an index and suggestions for further reading.
- Hall (1992) and Mildred (1982) are older books on the expert witness and, while the legislation cited may be out of date, they provide good advice.
- Rothwell (2004) deals with the role of the expert witness and the legal system.
- Leadbeatter (1996) discusses the limitations of expert evidence in a medical context, including issues arising in pathology, dentistry and DNA, and also refers to the training of the medical expert witness.
- Froede (1997) covers the duties of the expert witness in the USA and provides advice on relevant procedures, together with copies of forms and a glossary.
- Townley and Ede (2004) set out in detail the handling of forensic evidence and includes sections on the role of the expert in criminal cases, on veterinary forensic science and with useful forms and checklists.
- Wall and Hamilton (2000) give advice for the expert witness, albeit in relation to the Children Act.
- The professions often produce guidance for their members who act as witnesses: the Royal College of Veterinary Surgeons (2000) has a

section in its *Guide to Professional Conduct* on professional witnesses. The UK-based Institute of Biology includes advice under the heading 'Members as Expert Witnesses' in its code of conduct (Institute of Biology, 2004).

Lawyers' texts on the judicial process and duties of the expert

Many texts written for practising lawyers have sections that may be useful to the experienced expert.

- Tapper (2003) is a text for lawyers on evidence and expert witnesses with some experience will find it helpful, particularly the chapters on opinion and hearsay evidence.
- Keane (2005) has a useful chapter on opinion evidence, especially expert and other admissible evidence; it also has a section on the oath and its variations.
- Murphy (2005) deals with competence and admissibility of evidence.
- Hodgkinson and James (2006) and O'Hare & Browne (2003) are detailed studies of expert evidence and witnesses.
- Murphy (1990) deals with advocacy skills.
- Napley (1991) provides advice to young lawyers on advocacy, including a section on expert witnesses. This provides an insight into the mind and conduct of the lawyers who examine and cross-examine witnesses.

Texts on court procedure

- Atkinson and Moloney (2005) provide a guide to the Criminal Procedure Rules.
- Plant (1999) and Sime (2002) cover the Civil Procedure Rules.
- Rose *et al.* (2005) is a detailed analysis of all aspects of civil procedure.
- Williams (2005) provides a simpler, quicker approach to this subject.

Legislation on court procedure

The Criminal Procedure Rules 2005

- The CrimPR are available on the internet: http://www.dca.gov.uk/criminal/procrules_fin/rulesmenu.htm.

- Rule 24 relates to the disclosure of expert evidence: http://www.dca.gov.uk/criminal/procrules_fin/contents/rules/part_24.htm.
- Criminal Procedure Rule 33, has made new requirements for expert witnesses appearing in criminal proceedings that are similar to CPR 35 in that they relate, *inter alia*, to the expert's duty, report content and the appointment of a single joint expert.

The Civil Procedure Rules 1998

- The Civil Procedure Rules Part 35, 1998. Statutory Instrument 1998 N. 3515 (L.35) (as amended): http://www.dca.gov.uk/civil/procrules_fin/stat_instr.htm Current version: http://www.dca.gov.uk/civil/procrules_fin/current.htm.
- Part 35 Expert witnesses: http://www.opsi.gov.uk/si/si1998/98313215.htm#35.1 http://www.dca.gov.uk/civil/procrules_fin/contents/parts/part35.htm.
- Practice Direction 35. Current version: http://www.dca.gov.uk/civil/procrules_fin/contents/practice_directions/pd_part35.htm.
- Civil Justice Council Protocol for the Instruction of Experts to give Evidence in the Civil Courts: http://www.civiljusticecouncil.gov.uk/914.htm.

These are essential reading for all experts providing evidence for civil law cases. To quote from the last-mentioned document:

> *This protocol applies to any steps taken for the purpose of civil proceedings by experts or those who instruct them on or after 5th September 2005. It applies to all experts who are, or who may be, governed by CPR Part 35 and to those who instruct them. Experts are governed by Part 35 if they are or have been instructed to give or prepare evidence for the purpose of civil proceedings in a court in England and Wales (CPR 35.2).*

Texts written for the veterinary profession

Useful reference papers in the veterinary press for those called as expert witnesses have been written by Forbes (2004), with general advice to veterinary experts, and Laurence and Newman (2000), with very specific guidance to veterinary surgeons acting in animal welfare cases on the examination of an animal, the preparation of a report and giving evidence in court. It is important to distinguish this role from others with a legal orientation in which the veterinarian may be involved.

A useful contribution in this respect was the paper by Davies (1989) in which the role of the veterinary surgeon as a law enforcement officer was examined and discussed. Davies included a section on 'dos and don'ts' and these provide useful advice on how to avoid conflicts of interest and to retain professional independence. This paper is relevant to those who may be called as experts because sometimes the collection of evidence has involved either formal inspections of premises where animals are kept, or the execution of a search warrant in which the veterinary surgeon took part (see Chapters 2 and 9).

Harris (1997, 1998) has provided succinct, valuable advice to USA experts in the veterinary context. Professional conduct in court has been discussed by Ware (2005). What the (UK) Trading Standards Office expects of its witnesses was outlined by Durnford (2005) and the RSPCA provided advice to its experts in Flower (2005). The older literature, such as Porter (1971) and Field-Fisher (1964) (see above), still provides sound advice to the veterinary surgeon on the basic principles of acting as a witness.

EXPERT WITNESSES

Finding an expert

It may not always be easy to find certain kinds of expertise or to verify the qualifications and quality of a given expert. Instructing lawyers may find some experts by personal recommendation. A number of lists and registers are used to find appropriate experts. Such lists usually apply certain criteria for inclusion, set by the compiler, such as qualifications, court experience, and, sometimes, recommendation from an instructing lawyer.

Lists are maintained by organisations such as professional bodies, scientific and other organisa-

tions and expert witness groups. Townley and Ede (2004) provide advice on how to find an expert for criminal proceedings.

Finding the 'hidden' expert

The inclusion of a person's name in such lists does not mean that there are no others who might be approached. Some experts prefer not to publicise themselves or their contact details. Others may have, or think they have, too much work already. Yet others may be specialists in the relevant field but do not consider themselves as 'experts' in the legal sense.

To find the 'hidden expert' the following approach is recommended:

- If the name of the person is known, one can look in the relevant professional list (e.g. Medical Register) or members' handbook, or, alternatively, consult the professional body or organisation.
- If there is no name available but the speciality required is known, the Specialist Lists or their equivalent should be consulted. For example, if one needs a UK expert in small animal dermatology, one should look first at the RCVS Register, available from the RCVS, through any registered member of the profession and at many public libraries. In the Register, one can find lists of those who either hold an RCVS post-graduate qualification in the subject (Certificate in Small Animal Dermatology, Diploma in Veterinary Dermatology) or are RCVS Recognised Specialists in veterinary dermatology. Within the body of the Register, next to the names of members, are given other qualifications that may be relevant, e.g. Dip ECVD (Diplomate of the European College of Veterinary Dermatology) or Dip ACVD (Diplomate of the American College of Veterinary Dermatologists) (see Appendix B).

This is but one example but should help those who are unfamiliar with the world of veterinary specialisation. It can be adapted to other disciplines and other countries with well-developed professional organisations and expert witness systems.

The RCVS Register is also an invaluable source of information about veterinary qualifications within the EU and provides useful addresses of colleges, institutions and companies. Similar guidance concerning veterinarians can be obtained from comparable publications in other countries (e.g. the American Veterinary Medical Association's Membership Directory and Resource Manual).

As mentioned earlier, professional groups (e.g. medical and dental practitioners, pharmacists, nurses, animal technicians and some categories of biologists) may also keep registers or members' lists, which may be available on the Internet.

THE QUALITY OF EXPERT EVIDENCE

Dissatisfaction with the quality of expert witnesses (Woolf, 1996) and, conversely, an emerging interest in the provision of training for expert witnesses, have been evident since the early 1990s and courses have become available. It is also now a recommended item in the requirements for registration with expert witness lists. Some experts mention their training in their *curriculum vitae* (CV) and promotional literature. The (UK) House of Commons Science and Technology Committee's Report *Forensic Science on Trial* (2005) recommended that witnesses should be trained before going into court (www.publications.parliament.uk).

The two key areas in the production of good quality evidence in experts' reports and presentations in court are the quality of the expert and the quality of the science or other information provided. Different institutions have approached these factors, including the courts themselves, expert witness organisations, the professions and government bodies.

Quality of experts

General

There are several elements inherent in the expert witness procedure that are conducive to providing experts of good quality:

- The instructing lawyer should be satisfied that a selected expert is able to provide the required

evidence and has the necessary skills and qualifications.
- The court must satisfy itself similarly and the opposing party is likely to challenge the expert's qualifications, CV and expertise during cross-examination.
- The expert owes a duty to the instructing party to exercise reasonable skill and care and to comply with any relevant professional code of ethics (Civil Justice Council, 2005).

Personal qualities required of the expert are appropriate knowledge and expertise in the speciality professed. In addition, skills and experience in report writing and the presentation of evidence in court are necessary and these have received particular attention in recent years (see Chapters 10 and 11). A suitable temperament may also be considered relevant since court work is particularly demanding and the evidence must be intelligible and convincing to the presiding authority.

The new standards mean that experts, novice or experienced, must ensure that they are well prepared, not only in the area of expertise and specific information relevant to the case but also in the skills appropriate to the preparation of reports and evidence. If training in court skills is not available, a book on the subject, such as Bond *et al.* (1999), together with advice from experienced colleagues, can provide some groundwork.

Training

Training courses are run by expert witness and other organisations, legal offices, universities and professional bodies. Courses are likely to cover the legal and procedural aspects of preparing reports and giving evidence and will often include some role-play practice. Some courses may include aspects of forensic science and crime scene procedures.

Societies (such as the Veterinary Association for Arbitration and Jurisprudence) (see Appendix B) may run short, very focused courses for members within the context of their specialisation. Butler-Sloss and Hall (2002) have mentioned that the judiciary has begun to arrange 'mini-pupillages' and the courts have started to provide 'witness training days' for medical experts to gain experience and to increase the pool of experts. Some Royal Colleges also run courses for prospective medical experts. There has been debate as to whether the government or professional bodies should fund the training of experts in view of the reluctance of their members to give expert evidence. Some universities provide short courses tailored for experts and there is a large variety of degree courses in forensic science (http://www.castleviewuk.com/).

It is necessary to distinguish between general training for expert witness work from what is known as the 'coaching' of witnesses, i.e. preparing a particular witness in how to give his or her evidence in a specific case. The latter is not permitted in England and may lead to exclusion of the evidence from the hearing.

Quality assurance

Another approach to improving expert witness standards is through quality assurance.

In the light of concern about the quality of experts, the British government has established the Council for the Registration of Forensic Practitioners (CRFP) (see Appendix B). The CRFP has set up a registration scheme for experts from certain professions, including veterinary surgeons. Experts must meet certain criteria and abide by a Code of Practice (see Appendix G). An expert in breach of the Code may be struck off. This scheme is not currently compulsory and it does not cover all categories of expertise.

The CRFP's role has not necessarily been welcomed in all quarters (Ware, 2005). Lord Woolf (1996) also expressed reservations about compulsory accreditation, in that it could prevent the use of good experts who chose not to join the scheme or who were only needed occasionally. In view of the fact that some organisations have their own accreditation schemes, the CRFP has produced a list of twelve criteria for accreditation schemes.

The quality of evidence

Assessment of the quality of expert evidence – the courts

Expert evidence must be based on scientific (or other) facts that are presented in each case by expert witnesses. The current legal standard for the quality of scientific evidence in English courts is whether it is generally accepted by the scientific community.

In the USA, a new standard for the admissibility and quality of evidence was laid down by the Supreme Court in *Daubert v. Merrell Dow Pharmaceuticals Inc. (1993)*. This case provided that each set of scientific evidence must be assessed according to the six 'Daubert criteria'. This was subsequently adopted in the Federal Rule of Evidence 702 and by many state courts. The rule replaced a more flexible test established in 1923 in *Frye v. United States (1923)* which held that science or method that is widely accepted as established amongst scientists in the relevant field is admissible as evidence (see Parliamentary Office of Science and Technology (2005) for a summary of the two tests). As a consequence, cases now include a pre-trial hearing to apply the Daubert standards to the evidence as a test (Bohan & Heels, 1995). In England, the Court of Appeal approved of *Frye* in a case in 2001, but failed to mention the Daubert case. There is considerable debate in the UK and USA on the value of the Daubert criteria and it remains to be seen whether the English courts, or those of other common law jurisdictions, will move towards them (Murphy, P. 2005).

Meanwhile, in the Republic of Trinidad and Tobago, as if to emphasise the variation between countries in the development of the use of scientific evidence, the first admission of DNA as evidence in a criminal case was reported in the *Trinidad Guardian* for 5 Jan 2006. Legislation providing for a court to order a person to give specimens for DNA was at that time going through Parliament. Experts who undertake to give evidence outside their normal jurisdiction, although prepared for differences, may be surprised at the extent to which some common law countries' legal systems have not developed or have yet to modernise in line with other parts of the world.

Overseeing scientific evidence

Concerns regarding the quality of science in court prompted a review in the UK by the House of Commons Science and Technology Committee

(House of Commons Science and Technology Committee, 2005). As a result, consideration is being given to the establishment of a Forensic Sciences Advisory Council (FSAC) 'to oversee the regulation of the forensic science market and provide independent and impartial advice on forensic science'. This, too, is the subject of much debate.

A useful summary of the current state of forensic science in England has been produced in a Postnote (Parliamentary Office of Science and Technology, 2005) by the Department of Constitutional Affairs (www.dca.gov.uk).

PREPARING TO ACT AS A VETERINARY EXPERT WITNESS

Some advice and basic ground rules for those taking on a forensic case are offered below. These should be used in conjunction with training, relevant literature and taking advice from experienced experts as mentioned above.

Before taking on a case, the veterinarian should:

- Consider whether s/he wants to act as an expert witness: it calls for a certain temperament, since cross-examination in court can be traumatic and may put professional reputation at risk. A legal case should only be accepted if the person feels competent to deal with it and is willing, if necessary, to appear in court. As a general rule, it is best to decline if a person feels inadequate professionally, is not comfortable being challenged, especially in cross-examination, or does not want to be exposed to the publicity, scrutiny and repercussions that some cases bring in their wake.
- Consider whether the undertaking is feasible. The legal process can be protracted, particularly if there are appeals or re-hearings or if additional evidence becomes available. Travel may be involved, especially if part of the alleged offence took place overseas or relevant evidence is in custody in another part of the country. The veterinary expert has to consider the possible cost in personal terms or in relation to his/her practice with regard to time, lost practice earnings, reputation or any other consequence of

being involved in the judicial process (Forbes, 2004).

- Ascertain what is required, even before providing any preliminary comment. This may be very different from making a diagnosis or recommending treatment. The veterinarian should also determine the ownership of any live or dead animal involved in the case because this may be relevant professionally in terms of accepting instructions, divulging confidential information and possible conflicts of interest. For example, it may transpire that a client of the veterinary expert is involved in the case.
- Ensure that his/her expertise is appropriate and adequate. The instructing lawyer should also satisfy him/herself of the foregoing points.
- Ascertain that s/he has been offered sufficient time to carry out the necessary research or examination and to write the report to a high enough standard. One should enquire whether a preliminary report is required (to enable the lawyers to assess the strength of their client's case) or an in-depth report (that contains all the evidence). If cases are brought to court relatively quickly, experts need to be instructed in good time in order to prepare the best evidence for the court. Further, an early report may also prevent an unnecessary case going forward if it is clear that the evidence is not adequate or does not support an allegation.
- Ensure s/he is available for the hearing and when the dates are known, reserve them and advise his/her employer or practice.
- Be prepared if a lawyer is new to the legislation (e.g. wildlife or cruelty cases), to ensure s/he understands any pitfalls that the prospective expert can foresee from previous experience.
- Ensure that, once s/he has agreed to act as an expert, a letter of instruction is issued by the instructing lawyer, containing key points such as the work required, essential dates and deadlines, fees and expenses. It may be necessary to request the inclusion of any omitted items or other matters of importance. The Criminal Justice Council *Protocol* specifies the essential terms of appointment, and model letters of instruction and advice on the content are available.

- Set out and agree a basis for calculating fees and an estimate of the expenses for work such as examining the evidence, writing a report and attending court. For example, laboratory and other tests are expensive and it should be ascertained beforehand that resources are available to cover such costs.
- Be aware that his/her contract is with the instructing lawyer who is also responsible for payment of the expert's fees and expenses. It is important to obtain a written confirmation of this together with an agreed time for payment (e.g. 2–4 weeks) after the required work is carried out. There may be limits on the level of fees allowed, especially in legal aid cases when the instructing solicitor will want to get approval for the amount before agreeing to it. It may be difficult to know how much to charge at first but experienced colleagues should be able to provide guidance.
- Ensure that his/her professional insurance covers work as an expert witness and that the level of cover is adequate (see Chapter 2 and McKeating, 2005)

Preparation by the expert witness

While carrying out veterinary, welfare or conservation forensic work in the course of examining the evidence or carrying out research, the expert should consider the following:

- When taking possession of live or dead animals or their derivatives (such as samples) that comprise evidence, the expert should ensure that they are held legally. In certain countries, it may be against the law to possess a wild animal, whether alive or dead, that has been illegally captured, killed or imported – even if it is evidence in the hands of a veterinarian. It is important to clarify whether this is so and, if appropriate, to apply to the relevant authority for a licence or written approval to retain the live animal or carcase (see Chapters 3 and 5). After examination is completed, it may be advisable to return the evidence to the authority that provided it in order to reduce the risk of loss or deterioration in the hands of the expert. On

change of possession, the evidence should be sealed and signed for according to established chain of custody procedures (see Chapter 9).
- Accurate information about the circumstances of the alleged offence (a 'history') should be obtained, preferably in writing. This should include details of the relevant legislation.
- Prior discussion should be held with those involved in initiating the investigation or in bringing charges.
- The veterinarian must be prepared to consult colleagues, especially those with specialised knowledge of forensic matters, warning them beforehand that the enquiry relates to litigation and giving consideration to confidentiality.
- Correct identification of the species involved (see Chapter 6). The scientific name should be provided and any recent taxonomic change included. There may be special names for different sexes or ages of an animal. Any other common or vernacular names, particularly of wildlife, used should be noted since witnesses from different social, national or ethnic backgrounds may use a variety of names for the same species (see Chapter 10). These can be recorded in the glossary of the expert's report.
- A site visit may be necessary to the location where the offence is alleged to have occurred or the premises where (for example) the live animals can be viewed or the dead animals can be examined (see Chapter 9).
- Obtaining access to the evidence and any further authorisation, in addition to permits mentioned above.
- Proper collection, transport, storage and submission of evidence (see Chapter 9).
- Collection and evaluation of trace evidence (see Chapter 9).
- Careful documentation and record keeping, including appropriate photographic records, leading to production of a report (see Chapters 9 and 10).
- The maintenance throughout of meticulous records. Whenever possible, these should be contemporaneous. Tape recorders, cameras, handwritten, typed and computerised notes and the raw data all play their part. Even if

observations or records seem to be irrelevant at the time, they should be stored until the case is over (see Chapters 9 and 10).

- Clinical and *post-mortem* material should, whenever possible, be carefully retained and not discarded (see Chapter 6 and Chapter 7). The best rule is: if in doubt, keep everything. Carcases, tissues and plasma can be frozen and tissues can be fixed in formalin for subsequent examination or re-examination. Samples such as hair and feathers can usually be stored without preservative but must be properly packed and labelled (see Chapter 11).
- Clinical examination of live animals should be carried out thoroughly and meticulously (this aspect is covered in more detail in Chapter 6).
- Dead animals, likewise, require a painstaking approach, and the practitioner must remember that the investigation and standards will be different from those used when carrying out a routine diagnostic *post-mortem* examination (see Chapter 7).
- Laboratory investigations must be performed promptly and diligently with high standards of quality control, also ensuring that the 'chain of custody' is properly maintained and recorded (see Chapter 9).
- It is important to remain up-to-date on relevant subjects, to carry out relevant literature searches and to consult colleagues (subject to restrictions of confidentiality). Continuing professional development (CPD) is a useful method of both maintaining the high level of knowledge expected of an expert as well as reducing the risk of professional negligence (malpractice) (see below).

Legal aspects

The expert should:

- Read the legal documents, such as the charge or claim provided by the instructing lawyer. The expert should also be supplied with, or look up, the relevant legislation and be familiar with any changes (Irwin, 2005).
- Understand the expert witness's duties and legal liabilities (see below).

- In civil law cases, be conversant with the Civil Procedure Rule 35, the associated Practice Direction and the CJC *Protocol* (see above).
- Have some knowledge of the legal system and the courts that will hear the case (see below).
- Be guarded in expressing any opinion to the press or other outsiders, including the police and other authorities.

Duties and liabilities of the expert

- The expert acts under contract with, and is paid by, the instructing lawyer.
- The expert owes a duty to the instructing lawyer and the client to perform to the standard expected of an expert of his or her standing.
- An expert who falls short of this standard could be sued for negligence or breach of contract. Bond *et al.* (1999) have discussed the most common forms of failure. Serious cases of negligence may be referred to the expert's professional body for consideration of disciplinary action. However, in February 2006, in the course of the decision on Sir Roy Meadow's successful appeal against being struck off the Medical Register (see Chapter 2), it was held that expert evidence given in court is normally subject to immunity from civil suit and disciplinary action. Further, only a court could make a complaint of serious professional misconduct in respect of an expert's evidence (*Meadow v. General Medical Council* [2006] EWHC 146 (Admin) (see above)). In October 2006 it was subsequently held on further appeal in *General Medical Council v. Meadow* [2006] EWCA Civ 1390 that there is no immunity for expert witnesses from professional disciplinary proceedings: http://www.bailii.org/ew/cases/EWCA/Civ/2006/1390.html.
- The CPR 35.3 expressly states that the expert owes a duty to the court and that this overrides the duty to the client.
- The expert has a duty of confidentiality: the expert's report and communications with the instructing lawyer are confidential until the client authorises disclosure (unless there is a joint report).

- Legal professional privilege (confidentiality) extends beyond communications between a lawyer and client to anything written or oral produced by the expert in contemplation of that client's litigation. However, by way of exception, the CPR requires the disclosure of the instructions given to the expert.
- The expert should avoid defamatory statements in reports.
- The veterinary expert should be insured against liability and legal costs, remain in compliance with the RCVS *Guide to Professional Conduct*, maintain registration as a veterinary surgeon (and any other authorisation to practise or to be termed a 'specialist'), as well as accreditation as an expert and membership of medicolegal associations, networks and expert witness organisations.

The expert's report

- The expert has to prepare a report for the instructing lawyers. It will contain the evidence that will be presented to the court.
- A preliminary report may be required – this serves as a basis for a decision whether to proceed with the case.
- There are now specific requirements for some aspects of an expert's report in civil law cases (see CPR 35 and associated documents). It is likely that similar provisions will apply to criminal court experts in the future. It is wise to follow one of the standard formats that are available (Bond *et al.*, 1999) in order to ensure compliance with the requirements. The report will include, *inter alia*, credentials, the basis of the case, relevant issues, the investigation carried out, the findings and the expert's opinion. The report comprises the evidence that the expert will present to the court, if required.

Court

- There are two aspects to giving evidence; the content (the material that is in the report) and the presentation (the manner in which the expert gives evidence to the court). The latter

can affect the impact of the evidence on the person(s) deciding the case.
- It is important to prepare for the event by undertaking training, reading a training manual or getting advice from experienced colleagues, as well as refreshing the memory from the report.
- It is advantageous to visit the court in advance to see the courtroom and facilities and, if possible, to observe a case. Local traffic flow and parking, public or religious holidays or other major events should be ascertained as these can easily disrupt well-laid plans (Figure 12.1). This will be particularly helpful when the court or judicial system is new to the expert (Figure 12.2).

On the day of the hearing

- It is important to have all necessary information, papers, a copy of the report and any other materials that may be used in giving evidence.
- Punctuality and appropriate, sober dress are essential.
- Once at the court the expert should find the instructing lawyer, re-read the report, relax and

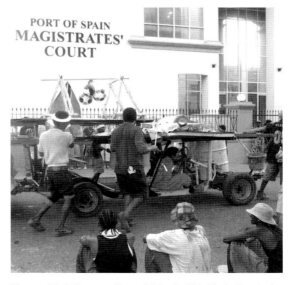

Figure 12.1 Jouvert (Dawn) Mas in Trinidad. Carnival is not a public holiday but will override the working plans of any unsuspecting visiting expert witness.

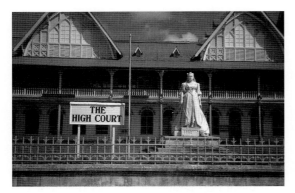

Figure 12.2 Reconnaissance of an unfamiliar court is recommended.

have some alternative work or reading in case of delays.

Giving evidence

The procedure as it affects the veterinary professional witness is provided on the RCVS website. The procedure for the expert witness is as follows:

- The expert takes the oath to tell the truth: there are forms of oath to suit various religions and an option to 'affirm' if a witness does not wish to take an oath.
- The examination-in-chief follows. The lawyer for the side for which the expert is appearing puts questions that enable the expert to present to the court first, his/her credentials and then the evidence. The expert should speak directly to the judge (and, if present, the jury) or magistrate(s) and throughout bear in mind that the expert's duty is to the court (CPR 35).
- Cross-examination by the lawyer for the other side. This will relate to all aspects of the evidence provided by the expert. The approach is likely to be tough and, despite the respect due to an expert, various techniques will be used to challenge, even destroy, the expert's evidence, reputation and expertise. The scrutiny will include findings and opinions, science, method, handling of the evidence, chain of custody, any delegated work such as laboratory tests and record-keeping. It is often easier to find fatal weaknesses in techniques rather than in expert

opinion. In the face of cross-examination it is important that the expert maintains the duty owed to the court, as well as objectivity, honesty, integrity and poise. It may help to view criticism as part of necessary judicial theatre and take it objectively rather than personally.
- Re-examination: the first lawyer may use this to enable the expert to clarify points raised earlier.
- After giving evidence, the expert may be permitted to leave the court or can be requested to stay in case further advice is needed.

Other considerations

The veterinarian who is likely to do forensic work regularly should consider enhancing resources by:

- Building up a reference collection that includes pathological specimens, radiographs, literature, books and reprints – this is discussed further in Chapters 6 and 7.
- Participating in continuing professional development (CPD) (see below).

CPD can be defined as the continuous progression of capability and competence, but need not necessarily lead to a qualification. Some professions make CPD compulsory for those in practice. This may involve attending courses or meetings, reading, publishing relevant literature and any other method of keeping up-to-date (see Chapter 13). CPD serves many functions:

- Satisfies professional obligations.
- Maintains and improves competence.
- Increases job satisfaction.
- Improves career prospects.
- May be helpful in litigious circumstances.
- Develops managerial and organisational skills.
- Helps to keep up-to-date with ongoing changes and developments in knowledge, skills and operating environments.

The expert witness is first and foremost an expert in his or her own field. Appearing as a witness or producing a report is but one facet of that; it should not dominate a person's outlook but be carried out within the context of the expert's professional life and work.

Acting as an expert witness with the required level of integrity and objectivity has never been easy. A medical case, over 200 years ago, illustrates how applying these qualities in court can have a tragic outcome. John Hunter was ridiculed by Mr. Justice Buller in the Donellan case of 1781 (see Chapter 1) because he, rightly, refused to speculate beyond the evidence he could tender. When questioned about this Hunter responded, 'I can give nothing decisive'. The jury was directed to believe the less experienced but more dogmatic doctors called by the prosecution and, as a result, the defendant was executed. Nevertheless, Hunter was described by Moore (2005) as 'a model of medico-legal professionalism' since he had been honest about the limitations of the evidence available.

CONCLUSIONS

A succinct summary and assessment of the present state of forensic science and expert evidence in the UK since the early 1990s, together with a view on future developments, is provided in the 'Postnote' by the Parliamentary Office of Science and Technology on *Science in Court* (Parliamentary Office of Science and Technology, 2005). This indicates that much has already been done on the civil law side, soon to be followed in criminal procedure, to improve the expert witness system. The extensive changes have aimed to raise the standards of expert witnesses and their evidence. In addition, many organisations have helped to improve training and standards and the government has established a body to oversee expert witnesses and may do likewise for forensic science. The expert now has access to much more support and advice but, conversely, is also subject to closer scrutiny and control than in the past. These are all steps towards the fulfilment of Lord Woolf's vision of a better, swifter and less costly judicial process. If these measures prove successful, they may also provide a useful model for other countries that seek to improve their citizens' access to justice.

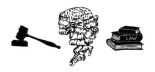

CHAPTER 13

The Future

Venienti occurite morbo. (Go and meet the approaching malady.)

Persius

The next few years are likely to see an ever increasing escalation in lawsuits concerning animals, their products and the environment. This is due to a number of factors, among them an increasing tendency for owners to resort to litigation, the escalating financial value of many animals, the global trade (some of it illegal) in wild species and greater public concern over conservation, biodiversity and ecosystems (Cooper and Cooper, 1998).

In parallel with an increase in legal proceedings, there will probably be additional contested insurance claims and a greater tendency to threaten or to bring disciplinary proceedings against those who are perceived to provide inadequate or unprofessional services. These developments all mean that the veterinarian, and others involved with animals, will need to be better prepared and more knowledgeable on legal matters.

As 'wildlife crime' (see Chapter 5) becomes more widespread, increasingly lucrative and further linked with other criminal activities, so also will governmental and non-governmental organisations need to become better prepared to tackle it. Such efforts will necessitate closer collaboration between different bodies and with the public, as illustrated in the UK, where the government-supported Partnership for Action against Wildlife Crime and non-governmental groups like the Royal Society for the Protection of Birds work closely to combat those who contravene wild animal legislation (see Appendix B).

In the richer countries, and increasingly elsewhere, public concern over conservation and environmental problems encompasses unease about damage to ecosystems by, for example, deforestation, urban and rural chemical pollutants, radioactivity and pathogens. There is often a demand that the parties responsible for such acts, whether malicious or not, should be brought to task. This in turn means investigations, enquiries and criminal or civil legal action. Because animals are often affected, as individuals or populations, there is usually a need for veterinary and other specialist input.

Global environmental effects, mostly precipitated by human activities, such as production of greenhouse gases, land degradation and the involution of farming systems, may be more difficult to attribute to an individual or an organisation but are increasingly important to human, animal and ecosystem health (Rapport *et al.*, 1998). Human-induced climate change is controversial and likely to attract debate and litigation for years to come. There is increasing evidence that higher environmental temperatures are having profound effects on habitats and also the animals and plants that live there – for example, by serving as a 'driver' to emerging infectious diseases (Anderson *et al.*, 2004). Migration patterns of some birds and insects are changing, provoking fears that warmer seas could affect birth rates of whales and sex ratios of sea turtles.

Concern over animal welfare will undoubtedly play a big part in the anticipated rise in legal cases concerning animals. Some of this might be linked to environmental matters: animals can suffer pain, discomfort, or distress when a wildlife crime is committed or following the spillage of oil or other chemicals into the environmental. Assessment of welfare and how best to define such words as 'cruelty' and 'suffering' are likely to continue to tax scientists and lawyers alike (see Chapter 4).

As iterated in Chapter 3, many countries have welfare legislation, and prosecution of those who are believed to have harmed animals is routine in the richer parts of the world. However, as pointed out in Chapter 6, it has proved very difficult to decide when an animal's welfare has been compromised and guidelines for assessment are often far from reliable. In such cases, whether involving live or dead animals, veterinarians and their colleagues are increasingly likely to need to be able to carry out appropriate behavioural and laboratory investigations, the results of which will play a part in developing the necessary standards.

It has been shown that owners of animals in North America, Western Europe and other industrialised regions are becoming more litigious, and that this trait is not confined to those who keep dogs, cats, horses or farm animals. Exotic birds, mammals, reptiles and fish, even invertebrates, can be worth large sums of money and the loss of an individual or a whole collection can often prompt the threat of legal action against the supplier, the neighbours or the veterinarian. For the same reason, there is likely to be an increase in insurance claims, the challenging of professional opinions and certification, and in reporting of actions and attitudes to veterinary and other disciplinary bodies.

One consequence of greater involvement in legal work that will continue to test the veterinary profession and others is that of how far expert witnesses should or should not align themselves with one side of a dispute. Traditionally, they have been impartial, with the function of assisting the court (see Chapter 12). However, in recent years, veterinarians and other specialists have increasingly been called upon to advise in the preparation of cases (for the prosecution or the defence) and to collect and present evidence. A step further on is the involvement of veterinarians in law enforcement, including crime-scene investigation and the execution of search warrants (sometimes termed 'raids') on premises where animals or their derivatives are kept. In such instances, the expert becomes part of a team and there is the risk of divided loyalties – between that of an impartial but conscientious professional and that of assisting the team to win its case. Forbes (1998) discussed this dilemma in some detail and drew attention to the need for the veterinarian to adhere strictly to the law and to retain professional integrity.

Of course, veterinary involvement in law enforcement is not a new development, but has to be seen in a different light from providing unbiased, expert, opinion: some of the implications discussed by Davies (1989) were referred to earlier in the book. In many countries veterinary surgeons already serve as inspectors of boarding kennels, breeding establishments, zoos and laboratories, and tighter legislation on the conservation and welfare of animals is likely to lead to an expansion of this role in future.

All of this means that the veterinarian of the 21st century (Figure 13.1) cannot afford to be complacent. Whether interested in legal cases or not, s/he is likely to become involved – and certainly must be prepared for that eventuality. This requires some familiarity with the demands of forensic work and the detailed investigations and meticulous record-keeping that are its essential concomitants.

Some forensic work involving animals is carried out at a local level. This is usually the case when dealing with domestic species. Things can be very different when wildlife and species conservation are at stake, however. As a result, there is already substantial cooperation between countries, including some of the poorer nations of Africa, Asia and South America, as well as the richer 'developed' parts of the world. Such collaboration is proving fruitful, especially in respect of species and products covered by the Convention on International Trade in Endangered Species of Wild Fauna and Flora (CITES), for example rhino horn and ivory (Europe, Africa and Asia) and threatened psittacine birds (United States, Mexico and South America).

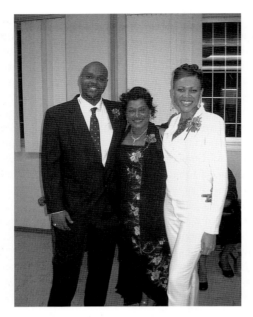

Figure 13.1 Three students at the University of the West Indies celebrate their admission to the veterinary profession. Future generations are the key to the development of comparative forensic medicine.

FUTURE NEEDS

What, then, are the needs for the future? A number can be identified, of which the most important are:

- Raising the awareness of veterinarians and others to the potential and challenge of forensic work.
- Teaching and specialised training in appropriate topics.
- Greater access to reliable information.
- Establishment, use and standardisation of systems and protocols.
- Research and development of relevant techniques.
- Increasing collaboration.

Each of these will be discussed in turn.

Increasing awareness

Surprisingly few veterinarians are cognisant of the need to be prepared for legal cases. Some are remarkably unaware of their own vulnerability,

especially when dealing with valuable animals or demanding owners. There are particular pitfalls in working with non-domesticated species and yet these are becoming increasingly popular as pets and therefore further potential subjects of litigation. It has been estimated that in the UK, in addition to nine million cats and six million dogs, there are seventy million fish, five million reptiles and over two million captive birds. The lack of awareness by some veterinarians of this and other trends in pet-keeping needs to change.

Veterinary teaching and specialised training

'Teaching' in the context of this chapter is considered to be part of the standard education of any qualified veterinarian (Doctor of Veterinary Medicine, Member of the Royal College of Veterinary Surgeons, etc.) while 'specialised training' refers to post-graduate study. Although most veterinary students are taught jurisprudence, including a little on the very important subject of appearing in court as a witness, scant attention is usually paid to the role of the expert. There is a need to rectify this situation by incorporating into the veterinary course relevant lectures and practical demonstrations, either as a specific part of the curriculum or as an adjunct to other subjects such as pathology, toxicology and clinical medicine.

At present, specialised post-graduate training in veterinary forensic medicine as such is not readily available. This means that veterinarians generally have to rely largely on experience, external tuition or advice from others, rather than receiving specific training as part of a veterinary course that might lead to recognition as specialists. Wobeser (1996), in discussing wildlife, stated that necropsies should be performed by 'pathologists with formal training and experience', and the same may reasonably be said of other veterinary and animal-orientated disciplines that contribute to the legal process, but opportunities to obtain such training and experience are remarkably few.

In the UK there are as yet very few short courses for veterinary practitioners in routine diagnostic *post-mortem* work, let alone the special features of forensic pathology, and yet most animal necropsies are still carried out by such people, not by specialists. As public expectations of forensic investigation grow, so too will pressure mount for higher standards of veterinary pathology. The owners of animals, and the courts, will expect *post-mortem* examinations to be carried out in a way that leaves less latitude for doubt or dispute. This may mean use of specialist pathologists or specific training of practitioners in necropsy work.

Some training programmes for veterinarians in appearing as an expert witness are increasingly being offered – for example, in the UK by the Veterinary Association for Arbitration and Jurisprudence (see Appendix B) – but these are of short duration, relate to court procedure rather than forensic method and confer no specific certification or qualification.

Enrolment in post-graduate degrees, diplomas and certificates that are primarily targeted at the medical profession or forensic scientists is something of which veterinarians or other professionals concerned with animals may be able to take advantage, if this is appropriate. Examples are the short courses on forensics organised by the Armed Forces Institute of Pathology in the USA (see Appendix B).

In view of the small numbers involved, there may be merit in considering the development of training courses for veterinarians that are run in collaboration with the medical profession. In the UK, for example, The Royal College of Pathologists has a Specialist Committee on Forensic Pathology that is charged with advising on training and standards in forensic pathology. The College already includes veterinarians among its Members and Fellows, and joint training sessions could be a means of providing veterinary and comparative forensic instruction. It might also be possible to develop a programme for veterinary practitioners on the lines of, and perhaps in collaboration with, the Diploma in Medical Jurisprudence that already caters for forensic odontologists, pathologists and physicians.

Quite apart from specialist qualifications, membership of appropriate societies is to be encouraged. Not only does such an association help keep experts in touch but they may be interrogated in cross-examination as to their suitability as expert witnesses, including whether or not they are affiliated to certain bodies. Thus, one would probably expect a British veterinarian who claims specialist knowledge of skin diseases to be a member of the European Society of Veterinary Dermatology, or a clinician with a reputation in the field of exotic species to belong to, say, the British Veterinary Zoological Society (see Appendix B).

Continued membership of and involvement in relevant societies, including reading and using their literature, may be especially important when a witness is 'retired', i.e. is no longer practising full-time his/her original profession. Under such circumstances questions may be asked in court as to whether that person is, indeed, still up-to-date.

Accreditation of those involved in forensic work is likely to become a feature in future in the few countries where such systems are in place. In the UK the Council for the Registration of Forensic Practitioners (CRFP) (see Appendix B) has adopted this role and although doubts have been expressed in some quarters about the need for such a body, veterinarians in certain specialities are amongst those beginning to be listed on the CRFP Register.

The training of non-veterinarians

The discussion in this section has been predominantly related to the veterinary profession but there is also a need for training of others who are likely to be involved from a legal point of view with animals or the environment. University degree courses in forensic science are proliferating in Britain, on the continent of Europe and in North America but few of these include specific tuition on animal matters. The Forensic Science Society (see Appendix B) offers Diplomas in some subjects, such as Crime Scene Investigation, Document Examination, Fire Investigation, Firearms Examination and Forensic Imaging and there would seem to be a niche for such topics as animal and environmental forensics.

All of the foregoing is likely to become increasingly important as society demands higher standards of expert witnesses and questions whether the expert has had any appropriate training. The UK House of Commons Science and Technology Committee's Enquiry *Forensic Science on Trial* (www.publications.parliament.uk) expressed concern over the relative lack of training and recommended that this should be made available from public funds. The British government's response was brief but pointed – 'Such training is the responsibility of the professions to which expert witnesses belong'. The Committee also expressed concern that in some recent cases expert witnesses were penalised far more publicly than were the judge or the lawyers. As Wallace (2005) pointed out, focusing criticism in this manner on the expert could have very detrimental effects.

Not everyone believes that training witnesses will improve the system. For example, Cross (2005), a consulting forensic ecologist, argued that 'experts are made by experience, not training' and that accreditation might lead to over-confidence and a tendency to protect one's reputation – to the detriment of the judicial system.

Ultimately it is the court that has to satisfy itself that an expert witness is suitable for the case in hand. This is probably best left to the discretion of the court rather than being set in rigid standards.

Greater access to information

Acquisition of knowledge and knowing where to obtain it is complementary to formal programmes of education. However, even before improved teaching and specialised training are widely available, veterinarians and others can arm themselves with relevant information. Articles relating to forensic work with domestic animals and wildlife are appearing in increasing numbers. Books and papers directed primarily at forensic work involving humans can also be very valuable even if the reader is generally concerned with animals other than *Homo sapiens*. Publications about the duties of expert witnesses are useful (see Chapter 12 and Appendix B). Many medicolegal texts and journals are available. Websites abound but must be used with caution; few are peer-reviewed although some provide sound information.

Veterinarians will find it useful to join some of the numerous forensic societies and organisations (see Appendix B), membership of which often comprises lawyers as well as medical and biomedical scientists. Many of these bodies hold meetings that provide professional or technical contacts and offer access to publications and guidelines, some of which are valuable in non-human work.

There are numerous organisations and societies available to the expert. Some of these have a professional status, with a code of practice and perhaps even a disciplinary system. Others are essentially clubs that one can join on payment of a subscription, supported, in some instances, by references. The expert can gain much from participating in the activities of societies where there is the opportunity to exchange views with others, including those from different disciplines, and to attend meetings where topics as varied as preparation of reports, claiming fees and current legislation are likely to be discussed.

Establishment, use and standardisation of systems and protocols

One of the main factors retarding the development of veterinary and comparative forensic medicine is the dearth of standard systems and protocols. The need to be systematic and to dutifully follow protocols when dealing with live or dead animals or their derivatives has been stressed elsewhere. However, there are as yet few proven guidelines as to, for example, which samples should be taken from animal material destined for legal cases or even how they should be labelled, transported and stored. Those who are not working regularly in the forensic field are usually unaware of the importance of maintaining a chain of custody and may not know of the existence of tamper-evident boxes, which might be of use when transporting evidence. This can put them at a disadvantage, particularly if working on wildlife crime, where legal cases have a regional and often international dimension and impact.

This paucity of defined and tested systems and protocols needs to be addressed as a matter of urgency. It is hoped that the data presented in this book will play a part in encouraging the establishment of sound protocols that, in turn, will serve the veterinarian and others when dealing with forensic cases. The expert's system, not his or her opinion, is often the Achilles heel in a court case: in other words, it is easier to find fault with technical work (e.g. procedures, delegated duties or record-keeping) than it is to challenge an expert's opinion. Veterinary and comparative forensic medicine are, however, evolving disciplines and it is important that those who use or develop protocols disseminate the information widely and request feedback so that appropriate amendments and improvements can be made.

Coupled with the lack of systems identified above, is a pressing need to establish databases, as emphasised in Chapter 10. These should include written and electronic literature (records, reports, books and journals) and also material such as pathological specimens, blood smears, parasites, hides and skins and electronmicrographs of relevant tissues, paraffin blocks and histological sections. Put together, these comprise a valuable resource – a 'forensic reference collection'.

When threatened or endangered species are involved, the nucleus of such collections is sometimes already available, having been established previously to provide information and specimens for conservation, diagnostic or health monitoring purposes (see Chapter 5). When no collections exist, and this is usually the case for species that are not threatened with extinction or are not yet considered important for other reasons, it may be necessary to establish specific animal forensic archives. These might be housed at veterinary schools or research institutes, with the material made available both for research and evidential purposes.

Research and development of relevant techniques

There has been remarkably little basic or applied research in the field of animal forensics. Extrapolation from human work is useful but not always ideal. This is where comparative forensic medicine should come in to its own, allowing lessons to be learned and applied from a wide range of species and disciplines. *Post-mortem* changes and their interpretation, especially when ascertaining time of death, are one example of where proper study and evaluation are required. Another fertile area for research is the effect of weapons such as crossbows and shotguns on animals, especially wildlife shot from a distance. Examples of where questions need to be answered are legion and while some may

necessitate expensive equipment, others require little more than weighing, measuring, recording and publishing basic biological data.

Increasing collaboration

As the pages of this book demonstrate, animal forensics is not a specialised subject. It overlaps with many other fields because animals are kept and utilised by humans, are important components of biodiversity, serve as sentinels and models in the wild and in captivity and respond to many insults in a similar way to *Homo sapiens*. Animal forensic medicine may require the input of the medical and dental professions as well as veterinarians – in the investigation of abuse or the study of bite wounds, for example. Cases relating to environmental pollution necessitate close links with ecologists and others from a biological background. Forensic laboratory investigations involve chemists, microbiologists, immunologists, DNA technologists and other specialists.

Advances in veterinary and comparative forensic medicine will be greatly enhanced if studies are carried out in collaboration with scientists from other disciplines, including those referred to above. The medical and dental professions are particularly important links because many of the techniques used in humans can be applied to animal work or because humans and other creatures suffer similar insults.

Cooperation with non-medical groups can be equally rewarding, however, and prove beneficial in terms of the quality of evidence available in court. In the field of wildlife ecology, for example, many research workers are as interested as are veterinarians in why animals died or sustained injuries and the circumstances of those incidents, albeit often for different reasons. Examples of studies by biologists that are of direct relevance to animal forensics include the aging of game carcases, the effects of aircraft on behaviour and breeding success of wild birds and the use of hair morphology to differentiate species of free-living mammals.

The demand for interdisciplinary collaboration is likely to grow for other reasons as well. Developments in science will bring in their wake ethical dilemmas that will necessitate legislation, or codes of practice, or both. Areas of contention will include:

- Genetic engineering, including gene exchange and the production of genetically modified organisms.
- The welfare of transgenic animals.
- The establishment and use of gene banks and gene libraries.
- Cloning technology.
- Stem cell research.
- Organ and tissue transplantation from animals to humans (xenotransplantation and xenotransfusion).

Current concern about emerging diseases, terrorism and other potential 'disasters' mean that risk-analysis is increasingly necessary – for example, on the likelihood of introduction and spread of exotic organisms if animals and their products, including genetic material, are moved from one country to another. This and other fields relating to biosecurity will have legal implications and thus become part of the rapidly broadening spectrum of animal forensics.

NETWORKING

Throughout this book there has been strong emphasis on the increasingly international nature of forensic medicine. Veterinary and comparative forensics are no exception and some fields, such as conservation and wildlife crime, are, by definition, truly global.

The term 'networking' is very much in vogue at present. It implies communication with others who have similar interests and where an exchange of information may be advantageous. This is often perceived as meaning Internet and email contacts, which are certainly of enormous value in permitting people from widespread locations to correspond inexpensively and rapidly in a way that would have been impossible twenty years ago.

However networking is more than this. It includes corresponding by letter or fax, exchanging of literature and, when possible, meeting in person. Not all people can attend the major conferences, such as those of the International Association of Forensic

Sciences (see Appendix B), but there may be opportunities for forensic scientists from poorer countries to obtain grants or other assistance. Regional and national meetings are also useful for networking, the former especially in areas such as the European Union, where legislation is becoming harmonised and therefore forensic matters are more of a shared concern.

Mention was made earlier of 'exchange of literature'. This refers not only to published and unpublished work but also to data that are unlikely ever to appear in print but could be made available to others for reference. This is a further reason why the habit of just photocopying or down-loading printed papers is of limited value. It is probably only the tip of an iceberg. It may be more productive to contact the author, requesting a reprint or electronic copy and asking if other literature on similar subjects is available. As a result:

- Direct contact is made with a colleague, which can lead to further fruitful exchange of ideas.
- Extra information may be obtained.
- An original reprint or electronic version with good quality photographs might be obtained.

CONCLUSIONS

Forensic veterinary medicine is a rapidly evolving subject that will increasingly influence society. It has in the past been predominantly concerned with domesticated animals but is likely to expand, as part of the broader field of comparative forensic medicine, because of concern over global pollution and declining biodiversity and the growing public insistence that action should be taken to challenge illegal and irresponsible damage to the planet (Figure 13.2).

Although the whole field of forensic medicine offers exciting challenges, it is, as yet, not a true *bona fide* discipline within the veterinary curriculum nor is it widely recognised in other areas of animal-based endeavours. This lack of status, coupled with the paucity and scatter of literature and data, often hampers the ability of veterinarians and their colleagues to contribute skills and knowledge to the necessary standard.

In the past, reticence by veterinarians in particular to become involved in forensic work encouraged

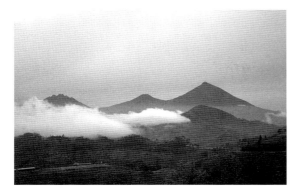

Figure 13.2 The Virungas in Central Africa. Such areas, which have a high biodiversity and provide a home for endangered species, are often themselves under threat. Environmental forensics is likely to play an important part in their protection.

less-experienced and less-qualified people to offer their services, even in legal cases that clearly required a background in animal health and welfare. Thus the *quality* of expert witnesses began to be questioned (see Chapter 12). Concern is regularly expressed in many parts of the world that the field of forensic science and the lure of fees from court appearances may be attracting people from a variety of backgrounds who have inadequate expertise.

It was nearly a decade ago that claims were first made, both in the scientific literature and popular press, that incompetent and dishonest forensic scientists were undermining the criminal justice system in Great Britain and that 'quacks' were infesting the courts because of the unregulated way services were marketed (Erzincliogu, 1998). Many eminent lawyers, notably Lord Woolf, advocated that the system should be overhauled, if fair access to justice was to be achieved. Amongst proposals were that a fully staffed statutory body of forensic science should be set up and proper accreditation of experts introduced.

The debate culminated in the report *Access to Justice* (Woolf, 1996). In the succeeding years, there have indeed been innovations and improvements in procedure and the need for a forensic accreditation body appears to have been met by the establishment of the Council for the Registration of Forensic Practitioners (see earlier).

It is clear, therefore, that the forensic scene is changing in the United Kingdom. Similar developments are under way in some other countries. Nevertheless, it remains true that in many parts of the world, in both rich and poor regions, 'expert' opinion on various subjects, including animals and the environment, can still be provided by individuals who may not be entirely objective, who have little or no training and who lack access to relevant, accurate information. It is our hope that this book will go some way towards redressing this situation.

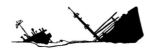

Appendices, References and Further Reading

Submission and Report Forms

These are suggested formats that can be changed, as necessary, to suit the requirements. Much of the initial, background information on the form below can, for example, be used not only when submitting or receiving a carcase for necropsy but also for live (clinical) cases and laboratory samples (but see also Form 2).

1 – Submission for Post-Mortem Examination

Submitting Client/Agency .... Reference No......................................

Lab Ref... Date (in full) ....

Address ....

.... Post (Zip) Code ....

Tel........................... Fax............................... Email ....

Veterinary Surgeon (where applicable) ....

Address and contact details ....

Other relevant persons, e.g. police officer, wildlife inspector ....

Species of animal (English and scientific name) ....

Local name .... Breed/variety ....

Colour/markings ....

Age .... Sex..................... Pet name (if appropriate)..................................

Ownership of animal or sample(s) ....

Number/Ring (Band)/Tattoo/Microchip/Other methods of identification

....

Background to the case/history...

....

....

....

Sample submitted..

Sent by hand/courier/post/other ....

Method and description of packing...

Tag No........................ . Prior storage condition..

Signature of courier ....Date ....

Signature:...   *Sheet Number 1/3*

Date: ....

Time: ....

316

Carcase ....

Organs (state) ....

Other tissues ....

Parasites ....

Blood (and details of how presented) ....

Swabs ....

Other ....

Comment on chain of custody (attach relevant paperwork) ....

....

Questions being asked (expand as necessary)

- Why did this animal die? ....
- When did this animal die? ....
- How did this animal die? ....
- Did this animal suffer pain or distress? ....
- What species is this? ....
- What is its provenance/parentage, etc.? ....
- What is this material? Species? Sex? ....
- Other questions ....

Investigations required ....

Post-mortem examination ....

Laboratory tests:

      Toxicology ....

      Bacteriology..

      Histology..

      Other...

Other tests as necessary to answer the questions above ....

....

....

Signature:...   *Sheet Number 2/3*

Date: ....

Time: ....

Results to be sent to ....

....

Special instructions regarding the storage/transfer/disposal of samples/wrappings/carcase

....

....

....

....

Other comments, e.g. cruelty case, civil action, insurance claim, professional malpractice hearing, etc.

....

....

....

....

....

Signed by recipient at (location)...

Date .... Time ....

Signature:..   *Sheet Number 3/3*
Date: ....
Time: ....

2 – Submission Form (and Report): Laboratory Examination

(Include background history from Form 1, as appropriate)

Species.. Reference No ....

Sample.. Collected by ....

Location..Date................................Time..........................

Relevant History ....

Lab ID .... Stored in...

Sample submitted by ....Date........................Time..........................

Sample received by ....Date........................Time..........................

Laboratory Investigation Report

Gross Examination..

....

Microscopical Examination ....

....

Further Test(s)

Test	Submitted (date)	Results (Received date)	Comments
Microscopy			
Bacteriology			
Cytology			
Parasitology			
Haematology			
Biochemistry			
Other (specify)			

Summary of findings...

Results/Comments/Interpretation ....

Reported by ....Date........................Time ....

Signature:...   Countersignature ....

Date: ....   (if appropriate)

Time: ....

3 – Submission of Exhibits: Chain of Custody Record

Laboratory Case No:..

Submitter's Reference No:..

Exhibits submitted:

Item No.	Lab Exhibit No.	Brief Description

Chain of Custody: Received in Sealed Condition

Item No.	Received From	Received By	Date

Laboratory Stamp Received   Laboratory Stamp Delivered

4 – Group or Flock Examination

(Include background history from Form 1, as appropriate)

Species.................................... Source.................................... Reference....................................

Purpose(s) of Examination .... Date of Examination ....

No.	Sex, Age, Size	External Findings	Internal Findings	Other Observations	Comments

Summary_____

Further work needed.................................... Signature.................................... Date.................................... Time....................................

Countersignature (if appropriate)....................................

321

5 – Initial Recording of Histopathological Findings

Slide No.	Comments on preparation, including stain	Tissues on slide	Observations	Scoring of changes (where appropriate)	Comments	Interpretation

Some suggested abbreviations: AICI = acute inflammatory cell infiltration; CICI = chronic inflammatory cell infiltration; wnl = within normal limits. Scoring system: 1 = minimal; 2 = moderate; 3 = marked

Summary

Further work needed............................ Signature........................... Date.................... Time...................

Countersignature (if appropriate) ....

6 – A Suitable Certificate for a Case of Lightning Strike

Attend early – there is less chance of *post-mortem* changes or of your word not being accepted

Supercare Veterinary
Hospital
Front Street
Old Town
Rockshire

Your full address and date

Tel: 01 234 678 890

29th February 2003

'Certify'; it is a certificate

This is to certify that at 8.00 this morning, at the request of Mr. Winston White of Hill Farm, Uppington, Rockshire, I attended field no. 223, also known as top 20 acres, Hill Farm, where I examined a Friesian cow ear tag No. R3056/807 belonging to Mr White, which was lying dead.

Identify the owner/ the person who called you

Identify the animal

The cow was freshly dead and positioned under a lone Elm tree in the middle of the field.

Say exactly where you examined the animal

There was strip of bark torn off the trunk of the tree – typically the result of lightning strike. An electrical storm had affected the locality late yesterday evening (28th February 2003).

Indicate the evidence: there was a thunderstorm and the tree had been struck by lightning

On the right side of the cow from the head to the front foot there was a line of scorched hairs and subcutaneously, below this scorching, there were haemorrhages.

No evidence of any other disease condition was visible externally on this cow's body.

Record the evidence of your findings and the lack of any other reasons for the animal's death

It is my considered opinion that this cow died as a result of a lightning strike.

Signed

NEVER say that the cow certainly was killed by the lightning. Despite all the evidence you did not do a full *post-mortem* examination and there is still a miniscule chance of some other cause of death

A. N. Other, MRCVS
(Partner in Supercare Veterinary Hospital)

Identify yourself and KEEP A COPY

(Courtesy of J.D. Watkins, MRCVS)

7 – Example of a Witness Statement (UK)

It is important to ensure that statements comply with any legal requirements and other guidance on form and content that is appropriate to the jurisdiction and court concerned.

Statement of Witness

(C.J. Act 1967, Sec.9: M.C. Act 1980, ss 5A (3) (A) and 5 (B), M.C. Rules 1981, Rule 70.)

Statement of

Age   Over 18

Occupation   Veterinary Surgeon, specialising in small animal dermatology

This statement consisting of page(s) each signed by me is true to the best of my knowledge and belief and I make it knowing that, if it is tendered in evidence, I shall be liable to prosecution if I have willfully stated in it anything which I know to be false or do not believe to be true.

Dated the   day of   200 . . .

States:

WITNESS REPORT   Page 1/n

Date: Signature: Continued yes/no

8 – EXPERT WITNESS REPORT

This is a suggested format for detailed reports or opinions by an expert witness. The information cited is fictitious but is intended to give some indication of the type and scope required in a legal case.

It is important to ensure that reports comply with any legal requirements and other guidance on form and content that is appropriate to the jurisdiction and court concerned. The use of well-established models may help to ensure that reports are correctly prepared and presented.

ANTHONY JOHN HASLAM, DVM, FRCVS

Prepared 6th June, 2005

Address of witness, including telephone and fax numbers
(international code) and e-mail/website details.

WITNESS REPORT   Page 1/n

Date: Signature: Continued yes/no

Contents of Report

Statement of witness
   Introduction
   Background
   Request

Material available prior to visit

Discussions held

Technical investigation

Findings

Records

Statements

The facts on which the opinion is based

Appendices

Appendix 1 – Experience

Appendix 2 – Findings and Interpretation

Appendix 3 – Photographic Evidence

References or Relevant Supporting Literature

WITNESS REPORT   Page 2/n

Date: Signature: Continued yes/no

Report

1.0 INTRODUCTION

1.1 Formal details

1.2 I am a Veterinary Surgeon practising from the above address. I hold a BVSc (Bachelor of Veterinary Science) degree from .... University and a DVM (Doctor of Veterinary Medicine) from .... University. I was elected MRCVS in .... gained an MSc (Master of Science) in Tropical Veterinary Medicine from .... University. I became an RCVS Recognised Specialist in .... in ....and a European/American Diplomate in Veterinary Pathology in ....

1.3 I have provided Expert Witness services for both prosecution and defence for twenty years. I have acted for and advised various bodies including the European Union, Customs and Excise and numerous Police Forces. I am listed as an Expert Witness within my field on various registers. I am accredited/have applied for accreditation by the CRFP (Council for the Registration of Forensic Practitioners) *(or other bodies, if appropriate)*.

1.4 I was asked a) to study relevant document b) to meet .... c) to visit the premises of..

1.5 Synopsis

1.6 Instructions

1.7 I was provided with a statement by............................ and was to give my opinion in writing.

1.8 Following study of this statement I was of the opinion that... ....

1.9 The visit and sources of information

1.10 At the time of the visit, I was in the company of ....
My statement is a compilation from the following sources:
   a. My contemporaneous notes and drawings, photographs and digital images (see attached)
   b. Video of ....
   c. Statement of ....
   d. Bundle of documents reference .....
   e. Statement of ....
   f. Statement of ....
   g. Photographic album exhibit reference (see Appendix 3)...............

2.0 THE BACKGROUND

2.1 The relevant parties

2.2 Listed below are the persons and their alleged role in the relevant events

2.3 PC (Police Constable).....................

2.4 The RSPCA, represented by ....

2.5 The Expert Witness ....myself

2.6 Supported by a colleague.................

2.7 Others ....

3.0 TECHNICAL INVESTIGATION

3.1 Background Information
The relevant legislation

3.2 Section................. of the ....provides that

4. Material available to the Expert Witness prior to the visit

5. Interview Records of

THE FACTS ON WHICH THE OPINION IS BASED

6. **CONCLUSIONS**
   The facts on which my opinion is based are detailed above.

7. My Opinion

8. Apportionment of Responsibility
    8.1
    8.2

9. I confirm in so far as the facts stated in my report are within my knowledge I have made clear which they are and I believe them to be true and that the opinions I have expressed represent my true and complete professional opinions

10. Note that any compliance statement should conform to the current, legal requirement appropriate to the particular court such as (for England and Wales) the Civil Procedure Rules Part 35 and Practice Direction 35. These demand both a statement of compliance (PD35, 2.2(9)) and a specified statement of truth (PD35, 2.4).

I confirm that this statement has been compiled in accordance with the Code of Practice of the Council for the Registration of Forensic Practitioners (CRFP) *(or other relevant guidelines)*.

DATE:

TIME:

NAME AND SIGNATURE:

WITNESS REPORT   Page 5/n

Date: Signature: Continued yes/no

Appendix 1

Experience
(Details of Expert)

Appendix 2

Findings and Interpretation
(Table of Findings)

Appendix 3

Photographic Evidence
(List of illustrations)

Reference	Location	Description

References or Relevant Supporting Literature

Journals, Societies, Organisations, Useful Addresses and Sources of Information

For textbooks, theses/dissertations and specific articles (scientific and popular) see References and Further Reading.

JOURNALS AND OTHER PUBLICATIONS (PERIODICALS)

(While every effort has been taken to verify the addresses given, it is possible that some may be incorrect, especially where an international publishing house, with numerous offices, is concerned. If in doubt, websites should be checked.)

American Journal of Forensic Medicine and Pathology, Lippincott-Raven Publishers, 227 E. Washington Square, Philadelphia, PA, 19106, USA.

Animal Welfare, Universities Federation for Animal Welfare, The Old School, Brewhouse Hill, Wheathampstead, Herts AL4 8AN, UK.

Australian Journal of Forensic Sciences, Australian Academy of Forensic Sciences, c/o McGraw-Hill Book Company Australia, 4 Barcoo St. Roseville, New South Wales 2069, Australia.

AVMLA Newsletter, American Veterinary Medical Law Association (see later – Websites).

Beitraege Zur Gerichtlichen Medizin, Franz Deuticke Verlag GmbH, Rockhgasse 6, A-1010 Vienna, Austria.

Bulletin of Medical Ethics, Royal Society of Medicine Press Limited, PO Box 9002, London W1A 0ZA, UK.

CAB Abstracts, CABI (see later – Websites).

Citation, American Medical Association, Health Law Division, 515 N. State St, Chicago, IL 60610, USA.

Clinical Ethics, The Royal Society of Medicine Press, c/o Portland Customer Services, Commerce Way, Colchester CO2 8HP, UK.

Clinical Risk, The Royal Society of Medicine Press, PO Box 9002, London W1A 0ZA, UK.

Crime Laboratory Digest, Federal Bureau of Investigation Laboratory, FSRTC, FBI Academy, Quantico, VA 22135, USA.

Fayixue Zazhi/Journal of Forensic Sciences, Ministry of Justice, Institute of Evidence Technology, 1347 Guanghu Zilu, Shanghai 200063, China.

Forensic Science International, Elsevier Science Ireland, PO Box 85, Limerick, Ireland.

Hoigaku No Jissai To Kenkyu/Research and Practice in Forensic Medicine, Tohoku University, School of Medicine, Department of Forensic Medicine, Sendai shi, Miyagi-ken 980, Japan.

Horse Law, Equine & Animal Lawyers Association (see later – Websites).

Index Veterinarius, CABI (see later – Websites).

Indian Journal of Forensic Sciences, Forensic Science Society of India, Forensic House, Karnarajar Salai, Madras 600 004, India.

Inform Quarterly Newsletter, International Reference Organization in Forensic Medicine & Sciences, c/o Dr William G. Eckert, Editor, Box 8282, Wichita, KS 67208, USA.

Interfaces, Forensic Science Society (see later – Websites and Information about Specific Organisations).

International Academy of Legal Medicine and of Social Medicine, Elizabeth Francson, Treasurer, Avenue Nicolai, 49A-8, B-4802 Verviers, Belgium.

Japanese Journal of Legal Medicine/Nippon Hoigaku Zasshi, Medico-Legal Society of Japan – Nohon Hoi Galdcai, Faculty of Medicine, University of Tokyo, 7-3-1 Hongo, Bunkyo-ku, Tokyo 13, Japan.

Journal de Médecine Légale Droit Médical, Editions Alexandra Lacassagne, 69003 Lyon, France.

Journal of Clinical Forensic Medicine, Official Journal of the Association of Forensic Physicians, the Australia and New Zealand Forensic Medicine Society and the British Association of Forensic Medicine, Elsevier, Oxford, UK.

Journal of Comparative Pathology, Elsevier, 6277 Sea Harbour Drive, Orlando, Florida 32887-4900, USA.

Journal of Forensic Sciences, 1916 Race St, Philadelphia, PA 19103, USA.

Journal of International Wildlife Law & Policy, 1210 Floribunda Avenue, 7 Burlingame, CA 94010, USA.

Journal of Telemedicine and Telecare, Royal Society of Medicine Press, PO Box 9002, London W1A 0ZA, UK.

Journal of Veterinary Medical Education, The Association of American Veterinary Medical Colleges, 1101 Vermont Ave, NW Suite 301, Washington DC 20005, USA.

Legal Medicine, Official Journal of the Japan Society of Legal Medicine, Elsevier, Oxford, UK.

Medicine, Science and the Law, Chiltern Publishing, 34 Aylesbury End, Beaconsfield, Bucks HP9 1LW, UK.

Medico-Legal Journal, Dramrite Printers Ltd, 175 Bermondsey St, Southwark, London SE1 3UW, UK.

Medico-Legal Society of Sri Lanka, Proceedings, Medico-Legal Society of Sri Lanka, 111 Francis Rd, Colombo 10, Sri Lanka.

Medizinrecht, Springer-Verlag, Heidelberger Platz 3, 14197 Berlin, Germany.

PAW Bulletin, Partnership for Action against Wildlife Crime (PAW) (see later – Websites and Information about Specific Organisations).

Proceedings of the Veterinary Association for Arbitration & Jurisprudence (see later – Websites).

Revista Española de Medicina Legal, Asociación Nacional de Médicos Forenses, Goya 99, Madrid 9, Spain.

Revista Italiana de Medicina Legale, Casa Editrice Dolt, A Giuffre, Via Busto Arsizio 40, 20151 Milan, Italy.

Royal Society of Medicine, PO Box 9002, London, W1A 0ZA, UK.

RSPB Legal Eagle, Royal Society for the Protection of Birds, The Lodge, Sandy, Bedfordshire, SG19 20L, UK.

Science & Justice, Forensic Science Society, 18-A Mount Parade, Harrogate, N. Yorkshire HG1 1BX, UK (see later – Websites and Information about Specific Organisations).

Seminars in Avian and Exotic Pet Medicine, Elsevier, P.O. Box 6283239, Orlando, Florida, 32862-8239, USA.

Societa Lombarda di Medicina Legale e delle Assicurazioni Archivio, Universita degli Studi di Milano, Istituto di Medicina Legale, Via Mangiagalle, 37 Milan, Italy.

Sudebnomeditsinskaya Ekspertiza/Medico-Legal Expert Testimony, Izdatel'stvo Meditsina, Petroverigskï pertulok 6-8, 101838 Moscow, Russia.

The CITES Bulletin, Wildlife Licensing and Registration Service, DEFRA (see later – Websites).

The Expert and the Law, National Forensic Center, 17 Temple Terrace, Lawrenceville, New Jersey, 08648, USA.

Vet CD (a CD-ROM database of citations and abstracts, updated quarterly), CABI (see later – Websites).

Veterinary Bulletin, CABI (see later – Websites).

Veterinary Clinics: Equine Practice, 1600 John F. Kennedy Blvd, Suite 1800, Philadelphia, PA, USA.

Veterinary Clinics: Exotic Animal Practice, 1600 John F. Kennedy Blvd, Suite 1800, Philadelphia, PA, USA.

Veterinary Clinics: Food Animal Practice, 1600 John F. Kennedy Blvd, Suite 1800, Philadelphia, PA, USA.

Veterinary Clinics: Small Animal Practice, 1600 John F. Kennedy Blvd, Suite 1800, Philadelphia, PA, USA.

Veterinary Record, British Veterinary Association, 7 Mansfield Street, London, W1G 9NQ, UK.

Wound Ballistics Review, International Wound Ballistics Association, Box 634, Pinole, CA 94564, USA.

Your Witness, UK Register of Expert Witnesses, JS Publications, PO Box 505, Newmarket, Suffolk, CB8 7TF, UK.

Zacchia, Societa Editrice Universo, Via GB Morgani 1, 00161, Rome, Italy.

SOCIETIES, ORGANISATIONS, USEFUL ADDRESSES AND SOURCES OF INFORMATION

Some professional and academic organisations that are of relevance to forensic work are described in more detail at the end of this Appendix. Royal Colleges and certain other bodies are prefixed with the definite article, 'The'. A small selection of veterinary associations is listed, in most cases those of countries to which a specific reference is made in the text.

Agriculture Department of the Welsh Office, Park Avenue, Aberystwyth SY23 1NG, UK.

American Academy of Forensic Sciences, PO Box 669, Colorado Springs, CO 80901, USA.

American Board of Medical Specialists, One Rotary Center, Ste 805, Evanston, IL 60201, USA.

American Humane Association, 63 Inverness Drive East, Englewood, CO 80112, USA.

American Medical Association, Health Law Division, 515 N. State St, Chicago, IL 60610, USA.

American Society for Testing and Materials, 1916 Race St, Philadelphia, PA 19103, USA.

American Veterinary Medical Association, Headquarters 1931 North Meacham Road – Suite 100, Schaumburg, IL 60173, USA.

Animal Welfare Institute, P.O. Box 3650, Washington, DC 20007, USA.

Armed Forces Institute of Pathology (AFIP), Room 1077, 14th Street & Alaska Avenue, NW, Washington, DC 20306-6000, USA.

Association of Personal Injury Lawyers (APIL), 11 Castle Quay, Nottingham NG7 1FW, UK.

Australian Veterinary Association, Unit 40, 2A Herbert Street, St. Leonards, NSW 2065, Australia.

Berne Convention Secretariat, Council of Europe, BP431R6, F-67006, Strasbourg Cédex, France.

British Association for Shooting and Conservation, Marford Mill, Rossett, Wrexham, Clwyd LL12 OHL, UK.

British Association in Forensic Medicine, Department of Forensic Pathology, The Medico-Legal Centre, Watery St, Sheffield S3 7ES, UK.

British Museum of Natural History, Veterinary & Forensic Services, Cromwell Road, London SW7 5BD, UK.

British Veterinary Association, 7 Mansfield Street, London, WIG 9NQ, UK.

CABI Publishing, Nosworthy Way, Wallingford, Oxfordshire OX10 8DE, UK.

Canadian Council on Animal Care, 1510–130 Albert, Ottawa, Ontario K1P 5G4, Canada.

Canadian Society of Forensic Science, 2660 Southvale Crescent, Ste 215, Ottawa, Ontario, K1B 4W5, Canada.

Canadian Veterinary Medical Association, 339 Booth Street, Ottawa, Ontario K1R 7K, Canada.

Canadian Wildlife Service, 9942 108 Street, Edmonton, Alberta, Canada.

Centre for Online Health, Level 3, Foundation Building, Royal Children's Hospital, Herston 4029, Australia.

CITES Secretariat, International Environment House, Chemin des Anémones, CH 1219 Chatelaine, Geneva, Switzerland.

Commission on Environmental Policy, Law and Administration, Adenauerallee 214, D5300 Bonn, Federal Republic of Germany.

Council of Europe, BP 431 R6, 67006 Strasbourg Cédex, France.

DEFRA, Animal Health Division, Government Buildings, Hook Rise South, Tolworth, Surbiton, Surrey KT6 7NF, UK.

Department of Agriculture and Fisheries for Scotland, Chesser House West, 500 Gorgie Road, Edinburgh EH11 3AW, UK.

Direction des Journaux Officiels, 26 rue Desaix, 75727 Paris Cédex 15, France.

Environmental Law Centre, Adenauerallee 214, D5300 Bonn, Federal Republic of Germany.

Eurogroup for Animal Welfare, 38 rue Georges Moreau, 1070 Brussels, Belgium.

Farm Animal Welfare Council (FAWC), Government Buildings, Hook Rise South, Tolworth, Surbiton, Surrey KT6 7NF, UK.

Fauna & Flora International, Great Eastern House, Tenison Road, Cambridge, CB1 2TT, UK.

Federation of Veterinarians in Europe (FVE), 1 rue Defacqz, B-1000 Brussels, Belgium.

Forensic Access, Building F4, Culham Science Centre, Abingdon, Oxfordshire OX14 3ED, UK.

Forensic Alliance, Building F5, Culham Science Centre, Abingdon, Oxfordshire OX14 3ED, UK.

Forensic Science Service, Metropolitan Laboratory Library, 109 Lambeth Rd, London SE1 7LP, UK.

Health and Safety Executive (HSE) Secretariat, General Enquiry Point, Regina House, Old Marylebone Road, London NW1 5RA, UK.

Home Office, Queen Anne's Gate, London SW1H 9AT, UK.

Humane Society of the United States (HSUS), 2001 L St. NW, Washington DC 20057, USA.

Indian Veterinary Association, 123 7th Main Road, IV Block (West), Jayanagar, Bangalore 56011, India.

Institut Juridique International pour la Protection des Animaux, 86 rue du Pas Saint Georges, 33000 Bordeaux, France.

Institute of Animal Technology (IAT), 5 South Parade, Summertown, Oxford OX2 7JL, UK.

Institute of Biology, 20 Queensberry Place, London SW7 2DZ, UK.

International Air Transport Association (IATA), 26 Chemin de Joinville, P.O. Box 160, 1216 Cointrin, Geneva, Switzerland; 2000 Peel Street, Montreal, Quebec, Canada H3A 2R4.

International Union for Conservation of Nature and Natural Resources (IUCN), 1196 Gland, Switzerland.

Latham Foundation, 1826 Clement Avenue, Alameda, CA 95401, USA.

National Animal Ethics Advisory Committee, c/o Ministry of Agriculture and Forestry, P.O. Box 2526, Wellington, New Zealand.

National Fish & Wildlife Forensics Laboratory, USFWS, 1490 East Main Street, Ashland, Oregon 97520, USA.

Partnership for Action against Wildlife Crime (PAW), DEFRA, Global Wildlife Division, Temple Quay House, 2 The Square, Temple Quay, Bristol BS1 6EB, UK.

Pathological Society of Great Britain and Ireland, 2 Carlton House Terrace, London SW1Y 5AF, UK

Ramsar Secretariat, International Union for Conservation of Nature and Natural Resources, 1196 Gland, Switzerland.

Royal Society for the Prevention of Cruelty to Animals (RSPCA), Wilberforce Way, Southwater, Horsham RH13 9RS, Sussex, UK.

Royal Society for the Protection of Birds (RSPB), The Lodge, Sandy, Bedfordshire, SG19 2DL, UK.

Scientists' Center for Animal Welfare, P.O. Box 9581, Washington, DC 20016, USA.

Scottish Home and Health Department, New St. Andrew's House, Edinburgh EH1 3YF, UK.

Secretariat of the World Heritage Committee, UNESCO, 7 Place de Fonenoy, F-75700 Paris, France.

South African Veterinary Association, P.O. Box 40510, Arcadia 0007, South Africa.

South African Veterinary Council, P.O. Box 25033, Monument Park, Pretoria 0105, South Africa.

Superintendent of Documents, US Government Printing Office (Supplier of Federal legislation), Washington DC 20402, USA.

Tanzania Veterinary Association, Sokoine University of Agriculture, P.O. Box 3174, Morogoro, Tanzania.

Tanzania Veterinary Board, Ministry of Agriculture, P.O. Box 2077 or 9152, Dar-es-Salaam, Tanzania.

The Academy of Experts, 2 South Square, Gray's Inn, London WC1R 5HT, UK.

The British Academy of Forensic Sciences, Anaesthetic Unit, The Royal London Hospital Medical College, Turner Street, London E1 2AO, UK.

The Commonwealth Veterinary Association (CVA), 93 Mt. Edward Road, Charlottetown, Prince Edward Island, C1A 5T1, Canada.

The Council for the Registration of Forensic Practitioners (CRFP), Tavistock House, Tavistock Square, London WC1H 9HX, UK.

The Expert Witness Institute, Africa House, 64–78 Kingsway, London WC2B 6BD, UK.

The Forensic Science Service, Trident Court, 2920 Solihull Parkway, Birmingham Business Park, Birmingham B37 7YN, UK.

The Forensic Science Society, Clarke House, 18A Mount Parade, Harrogate, N. Yorkshire HG1 1BX, UK.

The Kenya Veterinary Association, P.O. Box 29089, Kabete, Nairobi, Kenya.

The Linnean Society of London, Burlington House, Piccadilly, London WIJ OBF, UK.

The Royal College of Pathologists, 2 Carlton House Terrace, London SW1Y 5AF, UK.

The Royal College of Surgeons of England, 35–43 Lincoln's Inn Fields, London WC2A 3PN, UK.

The Royal College of Veterinary Surgeons (RCVS), Belgravia House, 62–64 Horseferry Road, London SW1P 2AF, UK.

The Royal Entomological Society, 41 Queen's Gate, London SW7 5HR, UK.

The Worshipful Society of Apothecaries of London, Faculty of Conflict and Catastrophe Medicine, Black Friars Lane, London EC4V 6E5, UK.

Trinidad and Tobago Veterinary Association, c/o Trinidad & Tobago Group of Professional Associations, The Professional Centre, 11–13 Fitz Blackman Drive, Wrightson Road, Port of Spain, Trinidad.

Uganda VeterinaryAssociation, c/o Faculty of Veterinary Medicine, Makere University, PO Box 7062, Kampala, Uganda.

Uganda Veterinary Board, Department of Veterinary Services and Animal Industry, P.O. Box 102, Entebbe, Uganda.

UNEP/CMS Secretariat: Bonn Convention, Ahrstrasse 45, D-5300 Bonn 2, Federal Republic of Germany.

United States Department of Agriculture (USDA), Washington DC 20250, USA.

United States Fish and Wildlife Service (USFWS), US Department of the Interior, 18th and C Streets NW, Washington DC 20240, USA.

Universities Federation for Animal Welfare, The Old School, Brewhouse Hill, Wheathampstead AL4 8AN, Herts, UK.

Veterinary Council of New Zealand, P.O. Box 10563, Wellington, New Zealand.

Veterinary Council of India, 116/15 W.E.A., Arya Samaj Road, Karol Bagh, New Delhi – 110 005, India.

Veterinary Defence Society (VDS), 4 Haig Court, Parkgate Estate, Knutsford WA16 8XZ, Cheshire, UK.

Wildlife Licensing Section, Global Wildlife Division, DEFRA, 1/17 Temple Quay House, 2 The Square, Temple Quay, Bristol BS1 6EB, UK.

Wildlife Trade Monitoring Unit, IUCN Conservation Monitoring Centre, 219c Huntingdon Road, Cambridge CB3 ODL, UK.

World Association of Wildlife Veterinarians (WAWV), c/o Dr Francis Scullion, 16 Cranlone Road, Ballygawley, Dungannon, County Tyrone, BT70 2HS, Northern Ireland.

World Society for the Protection of Animals (WSPA), 89 Albert Embarkment, London SE1 7TP, UK.

World Veterinary Association, Endraque 28A, DK-2100 Copenhagen O, Denmark.

Worldwide Fund for Nature (WWF), 1196 Gland, Switzerland.

WEBSITES

American Academy of Forensic Sciences – www.aafs.org

American College of Veterinary Pathology – www.acvp.org

American Humane Association – www.americanhumane.org

American Veterinary Medical Law Association (AVMLA) – www.avmla.org

American Zoo and Aquarium Association – www.aza.org

Amnesty International – www.amnesty.org.uk

Animal Transportation Association (AATA) – www.aata-animaltransport.org

Armed Forces Institute of Pathology (AFIP) – www.afip.org

Blue Cross – www.bluecross.org.uk

British Association for Biological Anthropology and Osteoarchaeology (BABAO) – www.babao.org.uk

British Association of Forensic Physicians – www.afpweb.org.uk

British Association for Forensic Odontology – www.bafo.org.uk

British Bird Council – www.britishbirdcouncil.com

British and Irish Association of Zoos and Aquariums (BIAZA) – www.biaza.org.uk

British Veterinary Zoological Society (BVZS) – www.bvzs.org

CABI Publishing – www.cabi-publishing.org

California Association of Criminalists – www.cacnews.org

Canadian Council on Animal Care (CCAC) – www.ccac.ca

Canadian Wildlife Service – www.cws-scf.ec.gc.ca

Centre for Online Health – www.eq.edu.au/coh

Church of England – www.cofe.anglican.org

Compassion in World Farming (CIWF) – www.ciwf.org

Conservation Breeding Specialist Group of the IUCN/SSC (CBSG) – www.cbsg.org

Convention on Biological Diversity (1992) (CBD) – www.biodiv.org

Convention on International Trade in Endangered Species of Wild Fauna and Flora (1973) (CITES) – www.cites.org

Convention on Migratory Species (1979) (CMS) – www.cms.int

Department for Culture, Media and Sports (DCMS) – www.culture.gov.uk

Department for Environment, Food and Rural Affairs (DEFRA) – www.defra.gov.uk/wildlife-countryside/gwd/zoo.htm

Durrell Wildlife Conservation Trust (Jersey Zoo) – www.durrellwildlife.org

Elsevier – www.elsevierhealth.com

English Heritage – www.english-heritage.org.uk

Equine & Animal Lawyers Association – www.animallawyers.co.uk

European Association of Zoos and Aquaria – www.eaza.net

European College of Veterinary Pathologists (ECVP) – www.ecvpath.org

European Network of Forensic Science Institutes (ENFSI) – www.enfsi.org

Fauna & Flora International (FFI) – www.fauna-flora.org

Federation of Veterinarians in Europe (FVE) – www.fve.org

Food and Agriculture Organization of the United Nations – www.fao.org

Forensic Access – www.forensic-access.co.uk

Forensic Alliance – www.aeat.com/forensic-alliance/contact

Forensic Archaeology.Com – www.forensicarchaeology.com

Forensic Medicine for Medical Students – www.forensicmed.co.uk

Forensic Science Service – www.forensic.gov.uk

Humane Slaughter Association – www.hsa.org.uk

Humane Society of the United States – www.hsus.org

International Air Transport Association (IATA) – www.iata.org

International Association for the Study of Pain (IASP) – www.iasp-pain.org

International Association of Forensic Sciences – www.iafs2005.com/eng/index.php

International Fund for Animal Welfare – www.ifaw.org

International Organization for Standardization (IOS) – www.iso.org

International Species Information System – www.isis.org

International Whaling Commission – www.iwcoffice.org

IUCN (The World Conservation Union) – www.iucn.org

Latham Foundation – www.latham.org

National Greyhound Racing Club (NGRC) – www.ngrc.org.uk

Netherlands Forensic Institute – www.forensischinstituut.nl

Oiled Wildlife Care Network – www.owcn.org

Organisation International des Epizooties (OIE) – www.oie.int

Partnership for Action against Wildlife Crime (PAW) – www.defra.gov.uk/paw

Ramsar Convention on Wetlands (1971) – www.ramsar.org

Re-introductions Specialist Group of the IUCN/SSC – www.iucnsscrsg.org/pages/l/index.htm

Scottish Society for the Prevention of Cruelty to Animals (SSPCA) – www.scottishspca.org

Species Survival Commission of the IUCN/SSC – www.iucn.org/themes/ssc

The Academy of Experts – www.academy-experts.org

The American Academy of Forensic Sciences – www.aafs.org

The Association of Forensic Physicians – www.afpweb.org.uk

The Association of Public Analysts – www.the-apa.co.uk

The Commonwealth Veterinary Association – www.commonwealthvetassoc.org

The Council for the Registration of Forensic Practitioners (CRFP) – www.crfp.org.uk

The Directory of Expert Witnesses – www.lawsociety.org.uk

The Expert Witness Institute – www.ewi.org.uk

The Forensic Science Service – www.forensic.gov.uk

The Forensic Science Society – www.forensicscience-society.org.uk

The Human Tissue Authority (UK) – www.hta.gov.uk

The Hunterian Museum at The Royal College of Surgeons – http://www.rcseng.ac.uk/museums

The Law Society – www.lawsociety.org.uk

The International Association of Forensic Toxicologists – www.tiaft.org

The Linnean Society of London – www.linnean.org

The Royal Botanic Gardens – www.kew.org

The Royal College of Pathologists – www.rcpath.org

The Royal College of Surgeons of England (Hunterian and other museums) – www.rcseng.ac.uk/services/museums/collections_html

The Royal College of Veterinary Surgeons (RCVS) – www.rcvs.org.uk

The Royal Society of Chemistry – www.rsc.org

The Royal Society of Medicine, Section of Clinical Forensic & Legal Medicine – www.rsm.ac.uk/forensic

The World Organisation for Animal Health (OIE) – www.oie.int

The Worshipful Society of Apothecaries of London – www.apothecaries.org

UNEP – World Conservation Monitoring Centre – www.unep-wcmc.org

United Nations (UN) – www.un.org

United Nations Development Programme (UNDP) – www.undp.org

United Nations Educational, Scientific and Cultural Organization (UNESCO) – www.unesco.org

United Nations Environment Programme (UNEP) – www.unep.org

United States Fish and Wildlife Forensics Laboratory – www.lab.fws.gov

Universities Federation for Animal Welfare – www.ufaw.org.uk

Veterinary Association of Arbitration and Jurisprudence (VAAJ) – www.vaaj.co.uk/index.htm

Veterinary Council of New Zealand – www.vetcouncil.org.nz

Veterinary Defence Society (VDS) – www.veterinarydefencesociety.co.uk

Wildlife Conservation Society (WCS) – www.wcs.org

Wildlife Incident Unit – www.cls.gov.uk

Wildlife Licensing and Registration Service, DEFRA – www.ukcites.gov.uk

Wildlife Licensing Section, Global Wildlife Division (DEFRA) – wildlife.licensing@defra.gsi.gov.uk

World Association of Zoos and Aquariums – www.waza.org

World Heritage Convention (1972) – www.unesco.org/whc

World Society for the Protection of Animals (WSPA) – www.wspa-international.org

World Veterinary Association – www.worldvet.org

WWF – The Global Conservation Organization – www.wwf.org www.defra.gov.uk

INFORMATION ABOUT SPECIFIC ORGANISATIONS

The work and roles of some bodies that are of relevance to forensic work are described below. The information is based on returns from organisations who were invited to contribute. Those that were contacted but failed to respond are listed earlier in the Appendix, without details.

The Council for the Registration of Forensic Practitioners (CRFP)

The Council for the Registration of Forensic Practitioners (CRFP) is an independent regulatory body, set up with UK Government support with the objective of promoting public confidence in UK forensic practice. CRFP's essential functions are to:

- Publish a register of competent practitioners in all the mainstream forensic specialties.
- Ensure, through periodic revalidation, that forensic practitioners keep up-to-date and maintain competence.
- Deal with registered practitioners who fail to meet the necessary standards.

The Register of Forensic Practitioners can be consulted through their website, www.crfp.org.uk, which also contains full information about the organisation and what it is trying to do.

Address: Tavistock House, Tavistock Square, London WC1H 9HX, UK
Telephone: +44 (0)20 7874 1922
Fax: +44 (0)20 7383 0888
E-mail: info@crfp.org

The Forensic Science Society

The Forensic Science Society was founded in October 1959, with the objectives: 'to advance the study and application of Forensic Science and to facilitate co-operation among persons interested in forensic science'.

The Society became a Professional body in November 2004. The criteria for admission as Student, Affiliate, Member and Fellow are available on application.

The society publishes a peer-reviewed journal and *Interfaces* (a newsletter) as well as offering diplomas, an accreditation scheme and holding a minimum of three conferences per year.

Address: The Forensic Science Society, Clarke House, 18a Mount Parade, Harrogate, North Yorkshire, HG1 1BX, England
Telephone: 44 (0)1423 506068
E-mail: membership@forensic-science-society. org.uk

Partnership for Action against Wildlife Crime (PAW)

The Partnership for Action against Wildlife Crime (PAW) comprises representatives of all the statutory and voluntary organisations involved in wildlife law enforcement in the UK. The functions of PAW include:

- Providing opportunities for member organisations to work together to combat wildlife crime.
- Promoting the enforcement of wildlife conservation legislation, particularly through supporting the networks of police Wildlife Crime Officers and Customs Officers.

PAW's Forensics Working Group:

- Keeps abreast of developments and works to provide tools to assist enforcers in their investigations.
- Advises on how forensic techniques used in other situations might be applied to wildlife investigations.

Address: Partnership for Action against Wildlife Crime (PAW), DEFRA, Global Wildlife Division, Temple Quay, Bristol BS1 6EB, UK
E-mail: paw.secretariat@defra.gov.uk

Centre for Online Health

The Centre for Online Health is an academic research centre of the University of Queensland.

The Centre's main areas of activity are:

- Research in the areas of telehealth and homecare.
- Teaching about online health.
- The delivery of online health services.

The Centre's overall goal is to research and develop best practice models in online health care that are applicable to Australia and other countries. Although primarily aimed at human health care, much of the work is directly relevant to veterinary work, especially the diagnosis of animal disease, particularly but not exclusively in poorer parts of the world.

The Centre's expertise also has relevance to forensic work, particularly the electronic transfer of evidence, without the need for health and CITES permits, and the submission of important clinical and pathological images to appropriate experts for an opinion.

Address: Centre for Online Health, Level 3, Foundation Building, Royal Children's Hospital, Herston 4029, Australia
Telephone: +61 (0) 7 3346 4754
Fax: +61 (0) 7 3346 4705

European Network of Forensic Science Institutes (ENFSI)

ENFSI was formally founded in 1994. The number of members has increased steadily over the years from 11 in 1994 to over 50 in 2005. The aim of ENFSI is to ensure that the quality of development and delivery of forensic science throughout Europe is at the forefront of the world. ENFSI is governed by a Board elected by the member institutes. The 16 Expert Working Groups are the backbone of ENFSI in terms of scientific knowledge and interests.

Address: P.O. Box 24044, NL-2490 AA, The Hague, the Netherlands
E-mail: secretariat@enfsi.org

Wildlife Health Services (including Comparative Pathology and Comparative Forensic Services)

Wildlife Health Services (WHS) is a UK-based organisation with a strong international orienta-tion. As its name suggests, it is essentially an advisory body, with particular interests in the health, welfare and conservation of wildlife.

WHS operates in three main areas:

(1) Consultancy, including forensic investigation of alleged wildlife crime.
(2) Diagnostic and investigative pathology, of all animal taxa, especially involving forensic cases, insurance claims and allegations of malpractice.
(3) Teaching and lecturing, mainly of ecosystem health, wildlife disease, animal law and ethics.

Address: Wildlife Health Services, P.O. Box 153, Wellingborough, Northamptonshire, NN8 2ZA, UK
E-mail: NGAGI@vetaid.net

The Association of Forensic Physicians (AFP)

The Association of Police Surgeons of Great Britain was formed in 1951, becoming the Association of Forensic Physicians in 2003.

Their stated objectives are:

- To promote the discipline and knowledge of clinical forensic medicine.
- Look after the best interests of all police surgeons.
- Encourage advancement in medicolegal knowledge in all its aspects as applied to their work.

AFP has its own peer-reviewed publication – the *Journal of Clinical Forensic Medicine* (see earlier) – has general information regarding the AFP and a message board. Importantly, there have been a number of comprehensive guidelines produced that members might refer to.

Address: 1 Tennant Avenue, College Milton South, East Kilbride, Glasgow G74 5NA, UK
Telephone: +44 (0)1355 244101
Fax: +44 (0)1355 249959
Email: admin@afpweb
Web site: www.afpweb.org.uk

The Hunterian Museum at The Royal College of Surgeons

The Hunterian Museum at The Royal College of Surgeons is one of the earliest and most important medical collections in the world. It is based on the collection of the surgeon and naturalist John Hunter (1728–1793), and includes many wet and dry pathological specimens from domestic animals and both captive and wild exotic species. The museum collections also contain many more specimens of comparative anatomy and pathology added in the 19th and 20th centuries. The Museum is open to the public without charge from 10.00–17.00 Tuesdays–Saturdays.

Access for teaching and research is encouraged. Details – including an online catalogue – are available at: http://www.rcseng.ac.uk/museums.

Address: The Royal College of Surgeons of England, 35–43 Lincoln's Inn Fields, London WC2A 3PN, UK

The Wildlife Incident Unit, Central Science Laboratory

The Wildlife Incident Unit investigates, using modern analytical methods, the presence and significance of pesticide residues in wildlife, including companion animals, honeybees and suspected baits. Work is carried out as part of the Wildlife Incident Investigation Scheme (WIIS) and other studies. The results of the work have been used to help in the registration process of agrochemicals and enforce legislation.

Other work includes the investigation of residues of pesticides and drugs implicated in the deaths of wildlife from around the world.

Address: Central Science Laboratory, Sand Hutton, York YO41 1LZ, UK
Telephone: +44 (0)1904 462457
Wildlife Incident Unit Mobile:
           +44 (0)7776 497305
Fax: +44 (0)1904 462251
Web: http://www.csl.gov.uk

The American Academy of Forensic Sciences

The American Academy of Forensic Sciences, a non-profit professional society organised in 1948, is devoted to the improvement, the administration, and the achievement of justice through the application of science to the processes of law.

For nearly 60 years, the AAFS has served a distinguished and diverse membership. Its 6000 members are divided into ten sections spanning the forensic enterprise. Included among the AAFS's members are physicians, attorneys, dentists, toxicologists, physical anthropologists, document examiners, psychiatrists, engineers, physicists, chemists, criminalists, educators and others. Representing all 50 United States, Canada and 56 other countries worldwide, AAFS members actively practise forensic science and, in many cases, teach and conduct research in the field as well. Each section provides opportunities for professional development, personal contacts, awards and recognition. Many sections publish periodic newsletters and mailings which keep their members abreast of activities and developments in their fields.

As a professional society dedicated to the application of science to the law, the AAFS is committed to the promotion of education and the elevation of accuracy, precision and specificity in the forensic sciences. It does so via the *Journal of Forensic Sciences* (its internationally recognised scientific journal), newsletters, its annual scientific meeting, the conduct of seminars and meetings and the initiation of actions and reactions to various issues of concern. For its members, AAFS provides placement services as well as scientific reference studies. Founded in 1948, the AAFS is headquartered in Colorado Springs, Colorado, USA.

Address: James P. 'Jim' Hurley, Director of Accreditation & Development, American Academy of Forensic Sciences, 410 North 21st Street, Colorado Springs, Colorado 80904-2798, USA
Telephone: +1 (719) 636-1100
E-mail: jhurley@aafs.org
Website: www.aafs.org

Glossary of Terms

The following list is not comprehensive but may serve to assist readers who are unfamiliar with medical and biological terms. Some are adapted, with permission, from the Glossary drawn up by Dr. Richard Shepherd of St. George's Hospital, London. Further definitions are to be found in the text, by using the Index or chapter headings.

Abrasion – an injury to the skin involving the outer surface (epidermis) only. In common parlance termed a 'scratch' or a 'graze'. Abrasions are caused by contact with or against a blunt object and are one of the triad of injuries caused by blunt force (see also Bruise and Laceration). In pathology parlance, an erosion is a shallow abrasion (of any tissue); an ulcer, a deeper abrasion that penetrates the surface layer.

Abrasion collar – the rim of abrasion around an entry gunshot wound.

Acute – describes diseases or clinical signs that start abruptly, are usually characterised by marked intensity and then subside after a relatively short time. From Latin *acutus* – sharp.

Aetiology – the study of the cause of a disease.

Allergic alveolitis – a hypersensitivity reaction, usually in humans, to, e.g., feathers or dust from birds; often given such names as 'pigeon-fancier's lung'.

Anaphylaxis – an acute allergic reaction, sometimes resulting in severe clinical signs or even death.

Aneurysm – an abnormal dilatation of a blood vessel, which may rupture.

Anorexia – absence of appetite (also Inappetant).

Anterior – the front of the body, limb, organ, etc. (see also Cranial).

Apnoea – cessation of breathing.

Aquarist – one who keeps fish.

Asphyxia – lack of oxygen to the cells of the body caused by reduced oxygen in the inspired air. Often caused by obstruction of the external or internal airways (as in strangulation); inability of the blood to carry oxygen or of the cells and tissues to utilise oxygen.

Atrophy – decrease in size of a tissue or organ.

Autolysis – *post-mortem* breakdown of tissues, usually as a result of cell death, may involve the whole or part of the body. Can complicate *post-mortem* examination but may assist in determination of time of death.

Autopsy – *post-mortem* examination, usually of a human (see also Necropsy).

Aviculturist – one who keeps birds.

Bacteraemia – the presence of bacteria in the blood.

Barotrauma – injury to internal organs caused by sudden and rapid changes in environmental pressure, e.g. by explosions.

Battered baby – deliberately injured child (see also Child abuse). A 'battered-pet' syndrome is also recognised.

Bestiality – sexual activity between a human being and an animal. Exact definitions differ between countries and have varied over the centuries. Sometimes called 'zoophilia'.

Biodiversity – biological diversity; the variety of living things.

Biosecurity – the management of deliberate or accidental unwanted animal and plant pests and diseases.

Bite – injury caused by the mouth and/or teeth of an assailant (human or animal). Often has a characteristic appearance and may contain indentations or bruises caused by the teeth which can be used to compare with the dental chart or dentition of the suspect.

Blackening – The deposition of soot as a result of a discharge of a firearm. Its presence is used to determine the range of fire of a gunshot wound.

Blast – a short episode of high pressure, usually caused by an explosion, commonly followed by a shorter period of lowered pressure. Can cause Barotrauma.

Bleeding – leakage of blood caused by damage to blood vessels (see also Contusion, Haemorrhage).

Blisters (vesicles) – collection of fluid derived from blood below the outermost layer of the skin (epidermis). Caused by some infectious diseases and by many types of trauma, particularly heat and electricity. Also associated with hypothermia and barbiturate poisoning.

Blowflies – bluebottles, greenbottles and other sarcophagous flies in the order Diptera, class Insecta. Their larvae (maggots) and pupae can be used to assist in the determination of the time of death in cases of advanced decomposition.

Blunt injuries – term used to describe the group of three types of injury caused by blunt objects: abrasions (grazes), contusions (bruises) and lacerations. Many objects may act as blunt weapons, ranging from the ground (a fall) to a human fist or a horse's hoof.

Brain death – complete absence of any functional activity in the brain. Diagnosed after a specified series of neurological tests have been performed at least twice and the effects of drugs, alcohol, hypothermia, etc. have been excluded.

Bruise – see Contusion.

Buggery – carnal intercourse by a male person with another person or an animal, consisting of penetration *per anum* (also Sodomy).

Bullets – projectiles fired singly from rifled weapons.

Burns – injury caused by either wet or dry heat. There are degrees of severity: first – outer surface of skin only; second – full thickness of skin; third – deeper tissues. Chemical and friction burns also occur.

Bushmeat – non-domesticated animals (wildlife) used as food.

Cadaveric spasm – extremely rare form of *rigor mortis*, recognised mainly in humans, which is of instantaneous onset, said to be associated with traumatic death following exertion.

Captive (animal) – animal kept under some form of restraint (by humans), varying from permanent caging to general supervision.

Caudal – relating to the cauda or tail. Also used for Posterior (see later).

Chain of custody – an (official) record of the movements/handovers of specimens/items of evidence.

Child abuse – infliction of injury, usually over a period of time, on a child or infant. May be physical, sexual or psychological. Similar abuse can be inflicted on animals.

Choking – accidental or deliberate obstruction of the upper airways leading to asphyxiation.

Chronic – describes diseases or clinical signs that may arise slowly and persist for a relatively long time. From Greek *chronos* – time.

Clinical signs – the features of a disease that can be observed, for instance, lameness, diarrhoea, etc. (see also Symptoms).

Comparative forensic medicine – that branch of forensic science relating to different species of animals, including humans, and its application to the judicial and other processes.

Concussion – lay term for the effects of a head injury. No generally agreed medical definition exists. However, in humans a group of symptoms including amnesia, confusion and altered consciousness are referred to as Post Concussional Syndrome.

Congenital – defect present at birth. The effects may be immediately apparent or may not become manifest until later in life.

Congestion – accumulation of blood in a tissue or organ. This is not bleeding as the blood is still in the blood vessels.

Contrecoup – injury to the brain on the opposite side to the site of an injury to the head. Some believe that contrecoup injuries indicate that the head was free to move when struck, others dispute this.

Contusion – leakage of blood from a damaged blood vessel, most commonly the smallest vessels, capillaries.

Cot death – Sudden Infant Death Syndrome (SIDS), also called Crib Death in the USA.

Cranial – relating to the cranium or skull. Also used for Anterior (see earlier).

Cut – in popular parlance, a break in the surface of the skin. Correct forensic terminology depends on the cause of the skin injury; blunt trauma causes lacerations, sharp trauma causes incisions.

Cyanosis – blueness of the skin caused by reduced oxygen in the blood.

Death – the cessation of life. Usually ascertained by the absence of heartbeat and respiration.

Decomposition – decay of body after death (see also Autolysis). Very variable and exact type and speed of decomposition will depend on body type, environmental temperature, availability of water, etc.

Defence wounds – injuries received by victims while defending themselves. Most commonly seen with attacks involving a sharp weapon but any object can be the cause of defence wounds. In humans defence wounds are typically on the palm of the hand and/or outer border of the forearm: in animals they can be on the side of the neck or the rear end (depends on species).

Dehydration – lack of water in the body. Can occur in starvation, neglect, hyperthermia, etc.

Demographics – study of factors that affect a population, such as birth and death rates.

Diarrhoea – loose faeces.

Disease – disordered state of an organism or organ. Anything that causes impairment of normal function. Diseases can be caused by infectious agents (e.g. viruses) or non-infectious factors (e.g. burns).

Disseminated intravascular coagulation (DIC) – a complex disease process in which there is uncontrolled clotting of the blood inside blood vessels. It can be caused by many factors including septicaemia, trauma, etc.

Domestic (animals) – in this book used to describe animals that live in or around human habitation, not necessarily 'domesticated' (see below).

Domesticated (animals) – species that have long lived in association with human beings for purposes such as food production or companionship. In biological parlance, domesticated means captive-bred for many generations with corresponding changes in appearance, morphology, behaviour, etc. from the wild progenitors (see Chapter 5).

Drowning – death caused by immersion in a fluid, usually water. Pathological features may be absent if death was rapid and they differ for fresh and salt water drowning.

Dysentery – blood in faeces, may be fresh (red) or partly digested (dark and tarry).

Dysphagia – difficulty in swallowing.

Dyspnoea – difficult breathing.

Ecology – the study of the interrelationships of organisms and their environment.

Ecosystem – a dynamic complex of plant, animal and micro-organism communities and their non-living environment that serve as a functional unit.

Electrocution – death or injury caused by the passage of an electrical charge. Effects depend on the voltage, amps and the time for which the current flows. High voltages can result in great tissue damage while low voltages may leave only minimal marks.

Embolism – blockage of a blood vessel, usually an artery, by an extraneous object or material. In humans the commonest form is the blockage of the arteries of the lungs by fragments of blood clot which have become detached from areas of deep venous thrombosis (DVT) in the legs.

Enclosed animals – usually used in respect of deer or similar species kept in a park: they are primarily fenced in but in some cases may have some freedom to come and go.

Entomologist – one who studies insects.

Entomology – study of insects. Can be useful in forensic studies for the estimation of the time of death from blowflies, beetles, etc. present on the body and their stage of development (see also Blowflies).

Ethology – the study of animal behaviour.

Exhumation – recovery of a body from a grave or burial place.

Exit wound – site where a weapon, most commonly a bullet, leaves the body.

Exotic – strictly non-indigenous animals, often excluding those already established in the wild in a particular country. The term 'exotic' is also used, especially by the veterinary profession, to describe unusual or non-domesticated species.

Farm animals – a generalisation not used in legislation (cf. livestock) for animals commonly used in commercial agriculture, being an alternative to listing separate species when convenience is more important than precision.

Farmed or ranched animals – applied to deer, mink, foxes, etc. kept for animal husbandry.

Fat embolism – blockage of blood vessels, particularly of the lungs and kidneys, by portions of fat, e.g. bone marrow. Seen following trauma, particularly fractures.

Feral animals – animals (usually domesticated) living in a wild state after leaving captivity. Escaped wild animals are usually described as having 'reverted to the wild' or as being in 'a free-living state'.

Firearms – weapons that fire projectiles such as bullets and pellets.

Flotation test – the placing of tissues in water to see if they float or sink. Sometimes used to determine if a baby or young animal was born alive – inflated lung floats – but this is not a totally reliable test. Pneumonic lung sometimes sinks, sometimes floats, depending upon the changes present. Liver that floats may be fatty or contain air/gas.

Foci (singular 'focus') – a small, usually distinct, lesion such as a micro-abscess in the liver.

Forensic veterinarians – registered veterinary practitioners who have a particular knowledge and experience of a field of veterinary science, the recovery of forensic samples and the provision of opinion, preparation of evidence for court or the giving of oral or written evidence based on that opinion.

Forensic veterinary medicine – covers all situations in which veterinarians collect information or samples, give opinion on, prepare expert witness statements on, or give evidence in court on any aspect of their professional fields of expertise.

Free-living (animals) – animals not living in captivity. This would normally relate to Wild or Exotic species (q.v.) but it may also be applied to domestic animals, although the adjective Feral (q.v.) is often used. Thus a feral cat is a domestic cat (*Felis catus*) living independently of human control whereas the (Scottish) wild cat is a separate species *(Felis sylvestris)* and usually occurs as a free-living creature, although it is also occasionally kept in zoological collections.

Haematoma – used to describe a significant collection of blood outside blood vessels and in the tissues of the body.

Haematemesis – vomiting of blood.

Haemoglobin – pigment in red cells responsible for carrying oxygen.

Haemoptysis – coughing-up of blood.

Haemorrhage – bleeding.

Hanging – form of ligature strangulation where the pressure on the neck is produced by the weight of the body.

Health – a state of physical and mental well-being (NB: not merely the absence of disease).

Health and Safety (H&S) – important considerations, especially in the workplace. Legal implications.

Health monitoring (Screening) – ongoing evaluation of health status; may involve clinical examination, haematology, parasitology, etc.

Herpetologist – one who keeps or studies reptiles and amphibians.

Hide and Die Syndrome – sometimes a feature of death from hypothermia where the individual (human or animal) hides away in a small space, e.g. cupboard, etc., either in an attempt to keep warm or through confusion induced by low body temperature.

Histology – microscopic study of the composition of tissues and organs.

Homeostasis – constancy in the internal environment (the *milieu interieur* of the French physiologist, Claude Bernard) of the body, naturally maintained by adaptive responses that promote healthy survival.

Hyperaemia – increase in blood supply to an organ or tissue.

Hyperpnoea – increase in respiratory rate.

Hyperthermia – an increase in body temperature.

Hypertrophy – increase in size of a tissue or organ.

Hypoglycaemia – low blood sugar.

Hypostasis (adjective: *hypostatic*) – the red staining of the skin of a carcase caused by the settling of blood under the influence of gravity. Areas of the body that are in contact with surfaces will be unaffected and will remain white (if the skin is not heavily pigmented).

Hypothermia – decreased body temperature.

Hypoxia – low levels of oxygen in the blood and tissues.

Iatrogenic – an adverse reaction that results from treatment, induced by human intervention.

Ichthyologist – one who studies fish.

Incidence – the number of new cases of a particular disease during a stated period of time.

Incision – break in the continuity of the skin caused by an object with a sharp edge.

Incubation period – the time between acquisition of infection and onset of clinical signs, *or* the period between a fertile egg (of a bird, reptile, etc.) being laid and hatching.

Indigenous (animals) – a term, not used in legislation, referring to animals that have always existed in a given geographical area.

Infarct – an area of tissue that has been deprived of a blood supply.

Infection – the entry of an organism into a susceptible host (human or animal) in which it may persist. Detectable clinical or pathological effects may or may not be apparent.

Infectious disease – a disease caused by the actions of a living organism (virus, bacterium, etc.), as opposed to (for example) physical injuries, endocrinological disorders or genetic abnormalities.

Inflammation – the normal response of the body to damage, whether biological, chemical or physical.

Injury – tissue damage (see also Wound).

Introduced (animals) – non-indigenous species that are established in the wild in areas where they have not always existed.

Invertebrate – an animal without a vertebral column. The majority (89%) of living creatures, encompassing such groups as the insects, arachnids, crustaceans, molluscs and worms.

ISO 14001 – international standards on environmental management.

Kinetic energy – potential energy of a moving object.

Laceration – break in the continuity of the skin or organ caused by application of blunt force. One of the triad of injuries associated with this type of force. Lacerations are usually characterised by jagged edges. They are not caused by sharp objects, which produce incisions.

Latent infection – an unapparent infection in which the pathogen persists within a host, but may be activated to produce clinical disease by such factors as stressors or impaired host resistance.

Lesion – an abnormality caused by disease of a tissue. Usually it is characterised by changes in appearance of that tissue, e.g. a raised nodule on the skin.

Ligature – a cord or other material that is tightly tied or applied to part of the body, e.g. the neck, a limb or (in surgery) a bleeding blood vessel.

Ligature mark – a form of friction abrasion due to the effect of a ligature.

Lumen – cavity of a hollow organ, e.g. lumen of the stomach or uterus.

Maceration – destruction of tissues or a body caused by a combination of trauma and decomposition.

Maggot – developing (larval) stage of some insects (see also Entomology and Blowflies).

Morbidity rate – the proportion of clinical cases during a given time.

Mortality rate – the proportion of deaths during a given time.

Mummification – a form of decomposition that is associated with warm dry conditions whereby the body dehydrates. Often results in remarkably good preservation. Usually involves the whole body but may involve only part, most commonly the extremities.

Munchausen Syndrome – a complex psychiatric syndrome associated with a desire to obtain medical treatment (often invasive) by complaining of fictitious illnesses. May also involve the children or animals of the individual when it is called Munchausen Syndrome by Proxy.

Necropsy – autopsy, *post-mortem* examination (of an animal).

Necrosis – death of a cell/tissue/organ.

Oedema (American: Edema) – abnormal accumulation of fluid under the skin or elsewhere (e.g. pulmonary oedema).

Ornithologist – one who studies birds.

Parasitaemia – the presence of parasites in the blood.

Parasites – organisms that live in or on another and benefit from it. Nowadays, especially by biologists, divided into *macroparasites*, such as worms and ticks, and *microparasites*, such as bacteria and protozoa.

Pathogen – an organism capable of producing disease. Can range from a microscopical organism, such as a bacterium, to a worm or a flea.

Pathogenesis – the mechanisms by which disease develops.

Pathology – strictly (from its Greek roots), the science of the study of disease. In common parlance tends to be related to *post-mortem* examination and related laboratory studies.

Penetrating injuries – injuries which pass through the skin.

Petechiae (singular: petechia) – pinpoint haemorrhages, due to rupture of small venules.

Poison – a substance which can harm the body if taken in sufficient quantity.

Posterior – the back of the body, limb, organ, etc. (see also Caudal).

Prevalence – the total number of cases of a particular disease at a given moment of time.

Prognosis – forecast of the probable course and outcome of a disease.

Propellant – the chemical substance used to provide energy to fire a projectile from a firearm, e.g. gunpowder.

Protected (animals) – animals that have the protection of some form of law, usually conservation legislation. A specific term in the UK in the Animals (Scientific Procedures) Act 1986.

Pruritus – itching.

Putrefaction – decomposition.

Rifled firearms – firearms that have grooves in the barrel that cause the bullet to twist as it leaves the barrel.

Rigor mortis – stiffening of the muscles after death. Very variable process which is affected by many factors and generally cannot be used to give an accurate time of death but may give some clue as to *ante-mortem* history.

Scald – a type of burn due to hot liquid, usually water.

Septicaemia – multiplication of organisms in the blood, usually with pathological effects on organs.

Shock – a physiological response to trauma, haemorrhage, infection, toxaemia and stressors, characterised by inadequate blood flow to the body's tissues (largely a deterioration of capillary perfusion) and sometimes life-threatening cellular dysfunction.

Smooth bore firearms – firearms that do not have rifling or groves in their barrels, e.g. shotguns.

Smothering – blockage of the external air passages (nose and mouth).

Sodomy – see Buggery.

Stab – a penetrating injury caused by a sharp object that is deeper than it is wide.

Starvation – lack of food.

Stillbirth – birth of a dead human baby after 24 weeks gestation or of an animal (mammal) late in gestation.

Strangulation – application of pressure to the neck resulting in obstruction of the airways with or without obstruction of the blood vessels.

Studbook – detailed records of births, deaths and genetic relationships and other biological data.

Sudden death – no specific definition. Usually death without premonitory signs. Some medical authorities state that the time period should be less than a few minutes. Must not be confused with 'unexpected death' where the human or animal may have been unwell for some time.

Sudden Infant Death Syndrome (SIDS) – sudden unexpected death of a child of less than two years (in some definitions, one year) which is unexplained despite extensive investigation and tests (see text).

Suffocation – asphyxiation caused by obstruction of the external airways or lack of oxygen in the inspired air.

Superior – the upper part of the body, limb, organ, etc.

Symptoms – the features of a disease that are experienced and can be recounted by a human patient, for instance, giddiness, abdominal pain. Not used for animals.

Systematics – the processes that describe species, which encompass three disciplines: description of species (identification), taxonomy, and description of relationships among and between taxa (phylogenetics).

Systemic disease – affecting the whole body (cf. local disease).

Tachypnoea – rapid breathing.

Taphonomy – from Greek *taphos* (grave): the *post-mortem* fate of biological remains. Forensic taphonomy is the application of such studies to assist legal investigations.

Taxon – a group of organisms such as species, genus or family.

Taxonomy – the science of classifying and naming organisms.

Thrombosis – blockage of a blood vessel by a blood clot in a live animal (distinguish from *post-mortem* blood-clotting).

Throttling – see Strangulation.

Toxaemia – the presence of a toxin in the blood.

Translocation – deliberate movement of wild animals from one part of their range to another.

Trauma – injury.

Traumatic asphyxia – asphyxiation caused by restriction of the movements of the chest wall, e.g. crushing.

Vagal inhibition – slowing or stoppage of the heart caused by stimulation of the vagus nerve; can be caused by pressure on the neck. Sometimes sudden death, in the absence of specific signs, is attributed to vagal inhibition.

Vertebrate – an animal with a vertebral column (mammals, birds, reptiles, amphibians and fish).

Veterinarian – one trained and qualified in veterinary medicine. In Britain and some other, mainly Commonwealth, countries veterinarians are usually, for historical reasons, called 'veterinary surgeons'.

Veterinary forensic medicine – that branch of forensic science relating to domesticated animals.

Viraemia – the presence of a virus in the blood.

Wad – felt, cardboard or plastic material that is used to separate shotgun pellets from the propellant.

Whiplash – type of injury to the neck usually caused by sudden backwards and forwards movement(s).

Wild animals – defined by the common law and also given specific meaning (as to wild birds and protected wild animals) in (for example) the (UK) Wildlife and Countryside Act 1981. Although normally occurring as free-living animals, they may be found in captivity.

Wound – a breach of the integrity of the skin or other surrounding structure (see also Injury).

Zoonosis (adjective: zoonotic) – an infection or disease that is naturally transmitted between vertebrate animals and humans.

Zoophilia – sexual activity between a human being and an animal (see also Bestiality).

Some Case Studies, Demonstrating Approach and Techniques

The following are examples of cases, provided by colleagues. They have deliberately been solicited from different parts of the world in order to demonstrate the international importance of veterinary and comparative forensic medicine. Some relate to circumstances in which legal action or complaint of malpractice ensued. The majority, however, are examples in which meticulous investigation, using the detective work alluded to so frequently in the text, provided answers to questions and either resolved the matter or suggested a non-litigious way forward.

The names and locations (and, where requested, the designation) of the veterinary colleagues who provided each case study are given. The authors are grateful to all of them for their contributions. Every effort has been exercised to retain each person's style of writing and expression. The only slight changes that have been made are to format and typography in order to bring a degree of consistency to this Appendix.

LIST OF CASES

CASE 1 – UNEXPECTED DEATH OF A PUPPY

Background

The carcase of a four-month-old puppy (domestic dog) of mixed breed was received for *post-mortem* examination. The puppy was one of two that had been vaccinated 36 hours previously. The two puppies had been confined since vaccination to a large garage and small, adjacent yard. Both seemed well until this puppy was found dead.

The owners claimed that the puppy had died as a result of the vaccination and demanded compensation from the veterinary surgeon.

The veterinary surgeon (VS) managed to persuade the owners to have the dog necropsied, at his (the VS's) expense.

Instructions received

(1) To carry out as full a necropsy as possible, in order to ascertain the cause of death and any factors that might have contributed to it.

(2) To produce a written report, to include specific mention of the culpability or otherwise of the VS.

(3) To retain the puppy's body in case a second examination was requested.

Action taken

A full *post-mortem* examination was carried out within a few hours of the puppy's death. As requested by the pathologist, the animal's body had been carefully wrapped and sealed, exactly as it was found, within two plastic sacks.

Gross findings showed no evidence of a local (subcutaneous or intra-muscular) reaction in the site where the vaccination was said to have been given.

External findings included marked congestion/hyperaemia of conjunctivae, buccal cavity and thinly haired parts of the body (e.g. axillae). The head and neck were 'wet' – an excess of clear, mucous, material.

Internal findings were of marked congestion and haemorrhage of all internal organs and tissues. There was no gross evidence of infectious, traumatic or neoplastic disease.

A toxicosis was suspected and, in view of the gross findings, kidneys were submitted for paraquat analysis. This proved negative.

Routine samples (lung, liver, kidney and others) had been taken for histological examination, pending further instructions from the VS/owner.

A tentative diagnosis of 'toad' (bufotoxin) poisoning was made, based on the gross *post-mortem* findings that have been reported in affected dogs (Bedford, 1974; Simmons and Sohan, 2001).

Outcome

Following the *post-mortem* examination, the owners accepted that the puppy's death was in no way associated with the vaccination. When told that, in the absence of detectable paraquat, the presumed diagnosis was bufotoxicosis, they immediately volunteered information that the puppy had been seen to play with toads in the yard, even prior to vaccination.

The owners stated that they were satisfied with the results and did not wish to pursue the matter. Further, they announced that they had purchased a replacement puppy and would like the VS to vaccinate it as soon as possible!

Comments

A happy outcome, largely because of the willingness of the owners to accept the report of the pathologist and the speed with which a necropsy was performed.

References

Bedford, P.G.C. (1974) Toad venom toxicity and its clinical occurrence in small animals in the United Kingdom. *Veterinary Record*, **94**, 613–14.

Simmons, V.C.G. & Sohan, L. (2001) A retrospective study of the treatment of toad poisoning in dogs in Trinidad. *Journal of the Caribbean Veterinary Medical Association*, **1** (1), 23–8.

Case provided by John E. Cooper, FRCVS, Trinidad and Tobago.

CASE 2 – CATTLE ON A RAILWAY LINE

Background

The neighbouring single-handed elderly practitioner called our veterinary practice for help early one summer morning and asked if we could attend a level-crossing on the main railway line from the West Country to London (England). A gate had been left open and a herd of forty-odd cattle had strayed on to the line and been hit by the overnight express which would have been travelling at over 100 miles (170 km) per hour.

Findings

The farmer said that eleven cows were missing and a glance down the line showed some of them, dead, in various states and at distances stretching away eastwards. One carcase was without any mark at all, just lying on the side of the track; three others were variously damaged but dead as 'whole' bodies, three cows were badly injured but alive and two of these were standing. A shotgun was available and they were dispatched immediately, on humane grounds. Seven 'down' and four to go. While walking along the track it became apparent some of the casualties had gone directly under the express train and been bowled over and minced along a great distance. Body parts extended over at least two miles and it was possible to identify two animals by almost whole heads and another by a part of the cranium; however the eleventh victim was only located by finding an ear and then counting back along the track and totalling only 21.

Fortunately the express train was not damaged nor were any passengers injured. In fact, the driver saw the cattle but could not pull up in time and reported just a heavy 'bump'. When the train stopped some miles further on, a pressure hose had to be used to wash the remaining bits and pieces of minced cattle from the underneath of the engine and carriages.

Outcome

A veterinary report was written and the railway company was exonerated as it was the farmer's responsibility to make sure the gate was closed. However, his insurance company paid for the eleven cows, despite the fact that an ear was the only evidence for one of them.

Case provided by John D. Watkins, MRCVS, UK

CASE 3 – WELFARE OF A RAM

Background

Autumn sheep fairs are a long-time traditional part of the British agricultural scene and the one in South Wiltshire is large and famous, trading in thousands of sheep.

A client in Somerset put together a small group of surplus stock and at the last minute included an old ram which was coming to the end of his breeding life but which might be useful to someone with a small flock.

At the fair a Veterinary Inspector checked the sheep. He decided that the old ram was lame, in distress, should not have been brought such a distance or to the fair, ordered its slaughter on humane grounds and served the farmer with a summons under the Protection of Animals Act 1911 for causing unnecessary suffering. The farmer pleaded 'not guilty' and chose to face the magistrates in South Wiltshire.

Outcome

The charges were that the ram was lying down in the pen, would not get up when prodded, his feet were overgrown and his knees stained with grass and faeces, indicating a long-standing chronic lameness.

The Defence did not deny that the ram had overgrown hooves and may also have had a respiratory condition possibly caused by the journey of some 40-odd miles (60 km) to the fair. But the ram was a Texel, a breed originally from northern France or Holland and used to produce very chunky, meaty offspring. Photographs were produced showing numerous animals of the breed and especially lambs, which had stained knees because it is almost a habit in these sheep to kneel down to eat or suck. However, the charges were dismissed and the farmer acquitted when the magistrates quizzed the Veterinary Inspector and learned that he had ordered the ram to be slaughtered not nearby, but be taken to an abattoir in another county, Dorset, a distance almost as great as the original journey from the farm to the fair!

Case provided by John D. Watkins, MRCVS, UK

CASE 4 – LIGHTNING STRIKE

Background

It was a period of hot humid 'muggy' weather, often encountered in England in the summertime, and although there was no rain, rumblings of thunder had occurred overnight round and about the North Wiltshire area.

Nearly all farm insurances cover death of animals by lightning strike and it was no surprise to arrive at the practice and to find that one farmer wanted a certificate so he could make a claim. Sometimes the claimant would ask for a certificate without expecting a visit to verify that the animal had actually died or indeed checking that lightning was the cause of the death, but this morning the farmer expected a visit and indicated where we should meet him as the dead animal was some distance from the farmhouse.

Findings

We went together across several fields and up on to the top of one of the rolling Downs, so typical of the beautiful countryside of that area.

The Top Field was indeed on the top of the Down and there was the body of the cow lying dead, immediately underneath the solitary tree in the middle of the field. Certainly we had much which suggested the cause of death, and on getting closer, no blood was seen to be leaving the nose or anus (possible anthrax), nor was there a swollen crepitating leg (indicative of the clostridial disease 'blackleg'). No other indications of disease could be found but the cow had a streak of singed, hair-smelling, coat extending from the head down the right shoulder and extending to the right forelimb. Incising the skin under the 'singe' revealed a strip of bruising and on looking up at the tree, a line of stripped bark could clearly be seen running down the trunk. The cow's number was on the metal ear tag (in the right ear, so did it form the attraction for the electricity?) and no difficulty was envisaged as a veterinary certificate was written, allowing the claim to be made.

Case provided by John D. Watkins, MRCVS, UK

For further reading concerning electrocution and lightning strike, see Chapters 6 and 7.

CASE 5 – BANK HOLIDAYS ARE A JOY BUT OCCASIONALLY THEY ARE ACCOMPANIED BY PROBLEMS

Background

One Easter Thursday (the day before Good Friday), a farmer noticed that one of his beef animals was lame but decided to wait to see what happened. On the Saturday he phoned his veterinary practice for a Certificate as the animal was still lame and the farmer considered that it was best slaughtered before it lost any weight. The veterinary practice, very correctly, would not issue a certificate unless they saw the animal and the farmer did not want to pay for this so one was not obtained. Easter Sunday came

and went, as did Easter Tuesday; then, on the Wednesday, phone calls were made to get the animal killed. An abattoir, often used by the farmer, agreed to do the job, more or less as a favour to the farmer. The animal was transported on the Thursday and was killed as soon as it arrived at the abattoir. On the Friday morning the Meat Inspector checking the carcase contacted the Royal Society for the Prevention of Cruelty to Animals (RSPCA) who called in an experienced veterinary surgeon for an opinion and as a possible expert witness.

The RSPCA brought an action against the farmer both for allowing an animal with a broken leg to go without veterinary attention or humane slaughter for eight days and for transporting the animal alive some 120 miles (190 km) to the abattoir – at the same time passing six other abattoirs which could have carried out the slaughter and thus saved the pain of the long journey.

Outcome

The farmer pleaded 'Not Guilty', but was found so. He was fined a large sum and court costs were awarded against him – a verdict arrived at because of the distance travelled by the suffering animal. The amount of healing which had taken place around the broken humerus in the eight days between the injury and the slaughter helped to prove the duration of neglect.

Case provided by John D. Watkins, MRCVS, UK

CASE 6 – SKELETAL REMAINS CREATE HAVOC

Background

A group of contract workers, while on a reforestation programme, encountered several cloth bags at their worksite. Upon investigation, they found the skeletal remains of animals in and around these bags. Immediately they reported it to the local government agency that contracted them. As word spread, the local media became involved, went to the site and took photographs and interviewed the workers who discovered the bones.

Being a small island community, rumour quickly spread and the entire town close-by concluded that the bones were of canine origin – 'dog bones'. In this country, previous to this discovery, there had been a rumour that certain restaurants, especially those owned by people of Asian origin and who sold Chinese food, prepared dogs for public consumption. This was said to have occurred without people's knowledge, the meat being passed off as beef or 'wild meat' (meat derived from hunting of wild, native species).

In the nearby town there was one restaurant in particular which had a reputation in some quarters for selling prepared dog meat. Naturally, upon residents hearing about the discovery of bones, these restaurants suffered great financial losses over the following weekend.

The evening newspapers presented photographs and interviews with all involved and concluded that the find was indeed that of dog bones. The newspaper headlines and reports on the following day came to the same conclusion.

The Local Government Authority contacted Health Officials in the area for assistance but they did not have the expertise to handle the case and only after two weeks of searching did they consult the Veterinary Public Health Division of the Ministry of Health. The Veterinary Public Health Coordinator requested the help of the local Veterinary Pathologists at the Ministry of Agriculture. The Local Government Authority then requested that the bones be identified as to the type of animal to which they belonged.

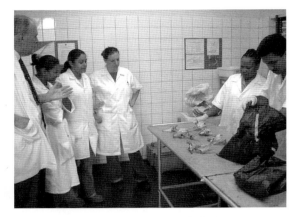

Figure D.1 A team of veterinary pathologists starts to examine the sample of bones that has been submitted for identification. (Courtesy R. Suepaul.)

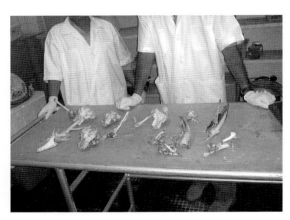

Figure D.2 The bones in D.1 are clearly of avian origin. (Courtesy Rod Suepaul.)

Findings

The following are the findings of the report of the Veterinary Pathologist.

> *The material presented was in two black, sealed and labelled plastic bags. It included: sacrum x 4, keel x 3, humerus, skull x 2, and skull with vertebral column attached [Figures D.1 and D.2].*
>
> *The skeletal remains are all of AVIAN origin and the following findings support this statement:*

(1) *All four (4) sacra were of the synsacrum type, a characteristic of avian species and a small number of reptiles.*

(2) *All bones seemed light in weight. Avian species have pneumatic long bones and other parts of their skeleton have a higher percentage of cancellous bone to dense bone than other species. As a result, it has more air spaces and is lighter, to assist in flight.*

(3) *Three sternal bones with pronounced vertical keels were found, another characteristic of avian species.*

(4) *Attached to one keel bone, described in (3), was a complete avian wing skeleton, consisting of a clavicle, a humerus, radius and ulna, metacarpals and phalanges.*

(5) *Attached to the phalanges were four light-coloured, almost white, primary wing feathers.*

(6) *All three skulls, including the one attached to the vertebral column, were small in size (less than 5 cm from rostral to caudal extremities and 3.5 cm at greatest width) and had the general characteristics of avian species*

These primary findings were presented to the Local Government Authority. Photographs were taken.

Outcome

The Local Government Authority presented the veterinary report on national television and speculated that the bones originated from New World vultures attracted to a nearby waste disposal site, although this was not mentioned in the veterinary pathologist's report. There was much public scepticism over the veterinary report and few believed it. This could have been partially due to the manner in which the photographs were presented by the television and print media. They passed off the sacra as skulls with the acetabular fossae resembling orbital fossae on skulls. Also, the photographs made the bones look larger than they actually were. Another factor was that local zoological experts vigorously challenged the veterinary statement that the skeletal remains were of avian origin and insisted that they were canine in origin. This speculation was based primarily on the photographs released by the media, not on examination of the bones themselves.

The Ministry of Agriculture communication specialists decided to leave the matter alone and there was little further debate. It should be noted that further comparisons indicated that the skeletal remains were of large galliform birds, probably domestic turkeys; these are commonly reared in the area.

Comments

This is an example of the problems that can arise if the media focus on an incident, especially in a small community. Such interest and speculation by news-

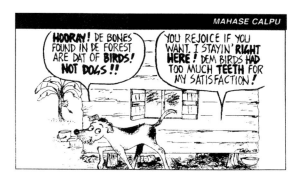

papers, radio and television can, if a legal case ensues, seriously undermine the judicial process. In this instance no criminal charges were brought, nor did the restaurant owners seek civil redress from the media. The veterinary pathologist wisely made no statement or comment that might further have inflamed the situation.

The case is a reminder that the expert (the veterinary pathologist in this case) must confine him/herself to the questions being asked and the material presented. In this instance the specimens in the two bags were unequivocally bones of birds. What else might have been shown on television was not relevant.

Case provided by Rod Suepaul, DVM, Trinidad & Tobago

CASE 7 – A COW ELEPHANT THAT WAS KILLED BY GUNSHOT

Background

On January 3rd 2002 the Forest Department officials approached me to conduct a *post-mortem* examination on a cow elephant carcase that was found dead in a coffee field. Based on the request, I conducted a necropsy on the spot where the carcase was found.

Findings and report

Date and time of receiving information: January 3rd 2002 at 7.00 a.m. (07.00)

Date and time of necropsy being conducted: January 3rd 2002 between 12.30 p.m. and 4.30 p.m. (12.30–16.30)

Location: The animal was found dead in a coffee and pepper field within the Odakkolly forest block, near the Mudumalai Wildlife Sanctuary, which is part of the UN-designated Nilgiri Biosphere Reserve, a vital habitat for the Asian elephant and other endangered species.

Date and time of death: Probably before 48 hours, that is on January 1st in the early hours.

Description of the animal: Asian elephant, black, cow elephant; around 18–20 years of age, left fore-limb circumference 101 cm, hind, 215 cm. Five nails on the forelimbs and four nails on the hind limbs. A nursing cow; her udder was full.

External examination

(1) The carcase was found lying on the left side. Marks of struggle and kicks by the ill-fated animal were noticed on the ground where the carcase was found. A few coffee plants and small trees were found broken from her struggles. The animal had dragged her hind-quarters for around 10 metres on the ground.

(2) No injury or wounds were seen on the right side and the visible areas during my thorough examination.

(3) We turned over the carcase on to the right side with the help of ropes and assistants.

(4) While examining the left side of the body, we noticed lacerated wounds on the foot, body and on the head.

No abnormality was detected on external examination except a wound around 3 cm diameter that was found to be deep (more than 30 cm) on probing with a lancet.

Internal examination

The carcase was partially decomposed; the death had probably occurred 48 hours before. Flies had laid eggs and some had become tiny maggots.

(1) Examination of head and neck revealed no clue to the cause of death.

(2) I instructed the assistants to open the area nearer the wound found on the left side and follow its course.

(3) During the examination we followed the blood-tainted course of the wound and found that the 10th rib was fractured around 50 cm below the lateral spine of the corresponding vertebrae. The rib had a complete fracture, with fragments.

(4) We further followed the course of the wound and that was leading to the peritoneum, stomach, passed through the left kidney, causing a lot of haemorrhage, and to the vertebral column between the 10th and 11th vertebrae. The length of the wound was around 110 cm.

(5) We separated the part of the vertebral column carefully including the 9th and 12th vertebrae and placed this on a sheet and carefully opened the course of the wound and recovered a lead bullet of 1.2 cm diameter ×1.5 cm length that had penetrated the spinal cord and struck at the site firmly between the 11th and 12th vertebral articulation.

(6) On examination of the other vital organs, the heart and lungs were highly congested. No abnormalities were found in the liver, uterus and bladder. The intestines contained a lot of roundworms of *Toxocara* spp. The brain showed no abnormality on gross examination.

(7) A pair of tusher (rudimentary tusks) was removed from the upper jaw.

Diagnosis and cause of death of the animal

The cause of death of the animal was shock, due to fatal injuries to the vital organs caused by the bullet.

Organs and materials handed over to the Forest Officials

(1) The lead bullet recovered from the body.

(2) The injured organs, namely the fractured vertebra (10th left) with the affected portion of spinal cord, left kidney.

(3) A pair of tusher (rudimentary tusks) recovered from the animal.

I gave my report to the Forest Officials on the very next day. The owners of the plantation, and also the neighbour, were arrested, based on this report. On interrogation, the landowner agreed that he had shot the animal with a country-made gun because the animal was with a herd of elephants that was damaging his crops.

The gun was seized and the culprit was imprisoned for three years and had to pay Rupees 100,000 as his penalty.

Special notes

(1) In the case of most of the wild animal deaths in and around the Mudumalai Wildlife preserve – a protected area – forest officials experience a lot of difficulties in receiving information on poaching, illegal killings and in finding the carcases.

(2) Decomposed carcases are often found because of the pervasive odour of putrefaction, by which time the cause of death can be difficult to determine on autopsy.

(3) Identifying and recovering the bullet from a huge decomposed carcase is an up-hill task.

(4) Without proper evidence, the culprits would not have been apprehended.

Hence, our work is of great help to the Forest Department Officials and the wildlife, whose continuing demise, especially of endangered species like the Asian elephant and tiger, of which there are still viable populations in the Nilgiris, calls for greater international support and collaboration to help the Forest Department to meet its conservation mandate. Without the continuing support of caring individuals like Mr. Gary Fink, Ms. Deanna Krantz and Dr. Michael W. Fox in the US, the wildlife in this bioregion would have no future.

Outcomes of the case

(1) The Government ordered a through search for illegal weapons in and around the wildlife area and confiscated them.

(2) The sentence against the culprit in this case became a lesson to others and such type of killing of wild animals has since been reduced to zero over the last three years.

Case provided by Dr. M. Sugumaran, BVSc, Senior Veterinarian, Gudalur, Tamil Nadu, S. India, who works collaboratively in-field and with support from Deanna Krantz and her husband, Dr. Michael W. Fox, to help improve the health and welfare of domestic animals belonging to the poor, and wildlife conservation efforts in the UN-designated Nilgiri Biosphere Reserve.

CASE 8 – A COW INJURED BY A COUNTRY BOMB

Background

On August 28th 2004 I was called to a farmer's cattle shed at the request of the local police. I was shocked to see a cow that was suffering from fatal injury on the right side of her mouth.

History of the case

The owner of the cow, Mr. P.M. Ponnu, told me that his cow went for grazing on the adjacent field in the morning around 9.00 (09.00). In the afternoon around 2.00 (14.00), the cow returned home with the injury. Someone who was grazing her own cow saw the ill-fated cow grazing in the neighbour's field before the cow was injured. She also told that they heard a loud cracking noise around noon. The owner of the cow lodged a complaint at the police station about the blast occurring in the neighbour's field that had injured his cow. He also demanded compensation. The police officials filed a case against the landowner, Mr. Joseph, on whose property the blast had occurred. The charges were (a) possessing and placing deadly blast illegally (b) an offence under the Prevention of Cruelty to Animals Act 1960.

Veterinary opinion

I carefully examined the cow and the following were my findings:

Description of the animal

A cow aged around 5 years, black in colour, 167 cm height, Holstein Friesian cross-breed, full-term pregnant, udder fully grown.

Description of the wound

(1) A huge wound with haemorrhage on the right side of the mouth. The shape of the wound was complicated. Length of the wound was 34 cm and the width was 28 cm (Figure D.3).
(2) A complete fracture of mandible on the affected side (left).
(3) Two molars and all the premolars were shed out.
(4) Upper and lower lips were severely injured.
(5) Muscles and salivary glands were injured.
(6) Base of the tongue was affected and the tongue was protruding.
(7) Marks of burns were seen on the edge of the wound.

Prognosis of the case

As the organ of prehension and the adjacent muscle and bony structures were severely damaged, the cow would be unable to eat fodder and drink water. She would suffer from severe pain, starvation, dehydration, secondary infection, including screw-worm infestation, if she did not quickly succumb to shock and die. Hence, I advised the owner and the police to dispose of the cow after I had delivered the calf through a caesarean section, and then euthanised the mother. I conducted the caesarean operation and delivered a live female calf. (The calf was reared by hand-feeding and she is doing well to date.) I

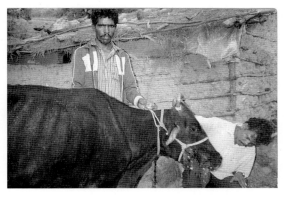

Figure D.3 The injured cow, showing the extent of the damage to its jaw. (Courtesy Dr M. Sugumaran, BVSc.)

performed euthanasia in the presence of the owner and the police and buried the ill-fated animal.

Outcome of the court case

The landowner who had placed the fatal country bomb denied the charges. A case was filed and he was remanded for 15 days under judicial custody. During interrogation he eventually admitted that he had placed the country bomb to kill the wild pigs that were damaging his paddy field.

The culprit was put in jail for 3 months and compensated the owner of the cow with a sum of Rupees 12,000. I appeared in the court as a professional expert witness to clarify my certificate produced by the police. The news was published in the local newspaper and I hope awareness was created about the seriousness and danger of using such bombs as an injurious wildlife deterrent.

Special note

Many people were using such blast materials made up of gunpowder, silica stones, old nails packed tightly in a tin capsule that was used to pack snuff. The tightly packed capsule is wrapped in a piece of animal intestine and smeared with animal fat. This ready-to-use bomb is placed on the route of the wild pigs. If picked up into the mouth, the animal's mouth and face will be blasted open and the animal will die of the injury. I have conducted *post-mortem* examinations on many Asian elephant carcasses in the Nilgiri Biosphere Reserve and have reported some that were fatally injured by this type of bomb and died slowly and in agony, from starvation.

Case provided by Dr. M. Sugumaran, BVSc, Senior Veterinarian, Gudalur, Tamil Nadu, S. India (for details see Case 7)

CASE 9 – CATTLE WITH IMPACTION

Background to case

Over a long period of time numerous cattle were rescued by an animal welfare charity as a result of information received from the public. The public complaint was usually that a street cow, or bull, was recumbent on the street and apparently could not rise. No further history was usually available. Once rescued the clinical examination of these cases revealed similar findings. The cattle were usually recumbent, of poor body condition with starey coats and a distended abdomen. They were afebrile or hypothermic, dehydrated, often had diarrhoea, most would eat, some had foul-smelling breath, cudding was absent or very much reduced. Rumen sounds were slow or non existent, rectal palpation revealed a large firmly distended rumen; most females were not pregnant. Where it was possible to perform a 'grunt' test for traumatic reticulo-pericarditis, this was done with negative results. Many animals would attempt to stand but be unable to do so. Various treatments were attempted including intra-venous rehydration, antibiotics, steroid therapy for shock, calcium, magnesium and other salt replacement. Some were stomach-tubed and given fluids by mouth, some were physically lifted and given physiotherapy. Others received magnesium sulphate by mouth. None of these treatments was successful and the patients died between a few hours to a week after admission.

Instructions received

After a number of such cases and a variety of treatments, a typical case was selected for *post-mortem* examination with the aim of determining the cause of the problem in these animals. Only gross *post-mortem* examination was possible. The animal chosen was a female of local mixed breed cow of middle age (full mouth of well worn teeth). External findings were of emaciation with decubital ulcers on elbows, stifles and hips. Slight, recent abrasions were present on the rib cage. The coat was starey. There was faecal soiling around the tail and hindquarters. Udder was non-lactating. The eyes were sunken.

Internal findings

The carcase lacked any subcutaneous body fat. Skin tented easily. There was some haemorrhage around the jugular veins. Lungs were slightly blackened; mediastinal lymph nodes were blackened on inci-

sion. Heart was normal with normal amounts of normal pericardial fluid. Liver was unremarkable. Gastro-intestinal (GI) tract consisted of a rumen and reticulum grossly distended and impacted, omasum was normal, abomasum was empty. Intestines were normal but lacked faecal balls. Incision into the GI tract revealed a mass of tangled, foreign, non-food, material in the rumen. This was removed and estimated to weigh 25–30 kg. The mass consisted mainly of plastic bags with some pieces of cloth, leather and sacking. There were almost no normal ruminal contents present. The reticulum contained some normal ingesta and a considerable quantity of foreign objects and gravel. These objects were removed and analysed. They consisted of:

106 nails, 22 screws, 4 drawing pins, 1 earring, 2 zips, 1 metal watch strap, 6 nuts, 6 ball point pen nibs, 1 cog, 2 hearing aid batteries, 6 paperclips, 1 curtain ring, 5 crown bottle tops, 7 pieces of Emery paper, 1 mango stone, 5 pieces of coaxial/electric cable, 1 medal, 1 silver chain, 4 coins (total value 2 Rupees), a pen clip and a number of ball bearings. Kidneys were unremarkable. Uterus was non-gravid but showed signs of previous pregnancy. Bladder was partially full. There were no signs of infection.

Conclusions

The skin lesions were due to prolonged recumbency on hard surfaces. The fresh wounds on the ribs were due to loading trauma at the time of rescue exacerbated by dehydration reducing the flexibility of the skin. Lung pathology was ascribed to prolonged exposure to traffic pollution, particularly particulate matter from diesel engines (anthracosis). The probable cause of death was thought to be rumen stasis and atony leading to starvation. The rumen stasis was attributed to the filling and distension of the rumen with foreign material in particular plastic bags which became entangled by rumen movements thus preventing passage along the GI tract and eventual removal by defaecation.

Outcome

Following the *post-mortem* examination, the charity and others mounted a public awareness campaign of the hazards posed by carelessly discarded plastic bags, particularly those containing edible material. This campaign involved school children, women's groups and others. In places shopping bags made of jute were distributed. The eventual outcome of this campaign was a ban by the State Government on some plastic bags, particularly those made of plastic of less than 20 microns thick. Any positive effects of this partial ban have yet to be seen due to the high levels of plastic waste already in the environment, and the shift by retailers from thinner bags to ones of thicker plastic. The Government has subsequently announced a further restriction on the use of plastic.

Case provided by Dr. Sunil Chawla, BVSc&AH, Chief Veterinary Surgeon, Help in Suffering, Jaipur, India and J.F. Reece, BSc, BVSc, MRCVS, India/ UK

CASE 10 – THE SHOOTING OF A SEA LION

History

Post-mortem examination report

Path. Register No.: W294-93
Date of this report: 14-04-93

Cadaver of animal found at Seal Bay, Kangaroo Island on the morning of 26th January, 1993. Cadaver transported to NPWS ranger station at Murray's Lagoon. Examination begun on the afternoon of 26th January, 1993 by Dr Richard Norman, with Dr Elizabeth Norman and Mr Anthony Maguire in attendance.

Species: Australian sea lion (*Neophoca cinerea*)
Age: approximately 3 years
Sex: male
Date of examination: 26-01-93

Gross findings

General description

The cadaver was that of a subadult male recently in good health. Male secondary sexual characteristics were not developed to any noticeable degree. The cadaver was in partial rigor, with the dorsal epaxial

muscles and the pectoral muscles still strongly contracted. The weight was estimated to be approximately 40–60 kg. The standard body length from the tip of the snout to the base of the tail was approximately 1 m.

There was an area of haemorrhage over the right side of the face surrounding the orbit and extending almost to the right commissure of the mouth. The tissues of the orbit were inflamed. There was a large and deep skin defect on the left shoulder, and a small firm nodule encrusted with clotted blood on the right shoulder. The cadaver was generally, but lightly, covered with sand. The fur was dry except for an area on the left flank and shoulder surrounding the skin defect.

Integument and musculoskeletal system

The pelage was in good condition, without areas of wear or alopecia. The skin defect on the left shoulder was roughly oval shaped, elongated in the ventrodorsal direction. The diameter was 3.5 cm in the craniocaudal direction, and 4.5 cm in the ventrodorsal direction. Necrotic and devitalised muscle was visible in the depth of this wound, along with a substantial quantity of sand. Exploration of this wound revealed a generous subcutaneous adipose layer coursed with fine capillaries and oozing serous fluid. Deep to this layer was a zone of devitalised superficial muscle 10 cm in diameter with a central wound tract. This wide zone of devitalisation proved to not extend deeper than the superficial muscle layer, and instead the deeper part of the wound tract was surrounded by a narrow zone of necrotic muscle. The caudal angle of the left scapula impinged on the wound tract, and an avulsed fragment of the angle remained partially adherent by periosteum and muscle. An abscess containing thick pink-tinged pus dissected across the medial surface of the left scapula. There were no sea-lice (marine isopods) present in the wound. On the right shoulder overlying the dorsal part of the scapula, a small mat of crusted dried blood and fur obscured a puncture wound through the full thickness of the skin. Dissection revealed a strait and narrowed bloody tract approximately 3 mm in diameter which continued through the subcutaneous fat. The right scapula had a neat circular hole

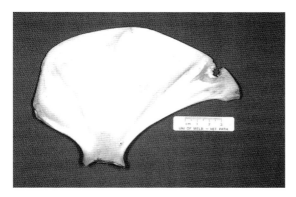

Figure D.4 Scapula of the sea lion, showing a circular hole consistent with its being perforated by a bullet. (Courtesy Richard Norman.)

approximately 6 mm in diameter in the line of the wound tract close to the dorsal border of the infraspinous fossa. Preparation of the right scapula as a bone specimen demonstrated subperiosteal new bone growth extending 10–20 mm away from the hole on both the lateral and medial aspects of the bone (Figure D.4).

A sliver of the dorsal border of the scapula was lost during its preparation. There was no evidence of cavitation or secondary missile tracts. No cestode plerocercoid cysts were found in the subcutaneous tissues despite extensive dissection and incision of the adipose layer.

Eyes

There was no abnormality of the left eye or adnexa. The right peri-orbital tissues were severely inflamed, with diffuse swelling extending in a zone some 10–15 cm in diameter. The right conjunctivae were haemorrhagic and there was a mild hyphaema. There was a small ragged break in the dorsal palpebral conjunctiva which suggested a penetrating injury. Dissection, radiographic examination of the skull, and preparation of the skull as a bone specimen demonstrated no projectile, or bony injury to support this view.

Respiratory

Upper respiratory tract mites, *Orthohalarachne attenuate,* embedded in nasopharyngeal mucosa,

provoking severe local inflammatory reaction. Lower respiratory tract mites, *Orthohalarachne diminuata,* in trachea and extending down through primary bronchi and bronchial tree. The lungs were heavily congested with pneumonic areas spread throughout. The cut surface oozed blood or serous fluid. Pieces of lung floated when placed in fixative. The thoracic cavity had not been traversed by any projectile.

Cardiovascular

The heart was flaccid and dilated and contained clotted blood.

Alimentary

The oral cavity, pharynx and oesophagus were normal. The stomach contained three large smooth-surfaced pebbles and squid beaks. The stomach was generously dilated with clear pink-tinged fluid. There was no trace of food. Intestine also without food. Parts distended with gas and with attenuated translucent wall. Generally prominent capillaries, petechiae and ecchymoses over serosal aspect of intestine wall. Ecchymoses scattered over entire length of intestinal mucosa. Moderate numbers of *Corynosoma* sp. acanthocephalans attached to intestinal mucosa. Knot of three well-developed *Diphyllobothrium* sp. cestodes in distal small intestine. Liver generally deep brown but with areas of pallor and generalised lobular pattern. Normal incisures over diaphragmatic surface present. Thin-walled fluid-filled cyst approximately 20 mm in diameter adjacent to neck of gall bladder.

Endocrine

Adrenal glands congested.

Lymphoreticular

No abnormality detected.

Urogenital

Testes located in inguinal canal and scrotum not discernible. Immature os penis. Kidneys a little softened and congested.

Neurological

Brain not examined to preserve skull intact for radiography. No projectile present in radiograph. Radiograph has an air space artefact in left temporo-occipital region. Preparation of the skull demonstrated it to be intact and without evidence of projectile injury to it.

Histopathology

Multiple foci of bacterial growth present in a wide range of tissues including lung, liver, kidney and lymph nodes. The lesions tended to be more mature in the lungs, with each consisting of a central focus of short chains of cocci or coccobacilli with satellite bacterial foci all bathed in a narrow band of eosinophilic material, and surrounded by a zone of necrosis with a moderate inflammatory response. Lesions in other tissues, particularly kidney and liver, appeared as bacterial emboli, generally without any associated inflammatory response. Lungs were heavily congested and atelectatic in zones. A section of an *Orthohalarachne diminuata* was seen in a bronchiole bathed in a mixed exudate. Intestine showed loss of villi, extravasation of blood and a thick adherent layer of mucus and cellular debris with proliferating bacteria. Stomach was unremarkable. Lymph nodes were hyperplastic and hyperaemic.

Diagnosis

A firearm projectile passed through the right shoulder of the sea lion and exited through the left shoulder. In penetrating the skin of the right shoulder, the skin stretched with the result that after passage of the projectile a hole of a diameter smaller than the diameter of the projectile remained.

The injury to the right scapula, the simple wound tract, and the absence of secondary missile tracts suggest a low to medium velocity bullet in stable flight was responsible. A .22 long rifle cartridge fired from a rifle could cause an injury comparable to that observed here. Further, the diameter of the hole in the right scapula supports the suggestion that a .22 calibre was involved.

The exit wound suggests that the bullet had become unstable during its passage through the animal, possibly only after striking the angle of the left scapula. It is unclear whether the fragment of bone from the angle of the left scapula was the result of the bullet striking the bone, or whether it would have been avulsed by sudden muscular contraction. There was no evidence of cavitation as occurs with high velocity bullet wounds.

The subperiosteal new bone growth (Figure D.5) indicates the periosteum was lifted from the bone at the site of perforation between 10 and 14 days before the animal died. The gross finding of the extensive dissecting abscess on the medial aspect of the left scapula supports this time course. Therefore, the animal was shot between Tuesday, 12th January 1993 and Saturday, 16th January 1993. The severe trauma to the right eye may have occurred at the same time as the gunshot wound; however, the association is not conclusive. The swelling, bruising and hyperaemia were of at least three days duration. Blunt trauma such as with a heavy collision would cause a similar injury.

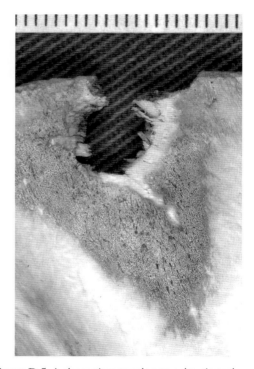

Figure D.5 A closer view reveals new subperiosteal bone, confirming that the injury was at least ten days old. (Courtesy Richard Norman.)

The extensive microvascular injury, particularly evidenced in the petechiation and ecchymoses of the intestinal serosa and mucosa, suggested septicaemia as a terminal sequel to the gunshot wound. Histological sections confirm this finding with massive bacterial embolism of many tissues during the 24 hours before the death of the animal, and with a range of more mature lesions, particularly in the lungs, demonstrating the earlier progress of the infection.

The overall necropsy picture is therefore that of a healthy young male Australian sea lion shot with a .22 rifle, which died up to two weeks later of a septicaemia resulting from the gunshot wound.

Disposition of specimens

The following specimens have been retained at the University of Melbourne, Veterinary Clinical Centre. The specimens were collected and are retained under the provisions of National Parks and Wildlife Service Permit to undertake research in a reserve W23259-01:

- Fixed (10% formalin): Lung, heart, kidney, spleen, liver, pancreas, intestinal wall, mesenteric lymph nodes, axillary lymph nodes, prescapular lymph nodes, testis, right eye.
- Fixed (70% alcohol): Bile duct cyst.
- Paraffin blocks: Lung, heart, kidney, adrenal gland, spleen, liver, pancreas, intestinal wall, axillary lymph node ×3, prescapular, mesenteric, testis.
- Frozen: Liver.
- Skeletal specimens in preparation: Scapulae, skull, partial pectoral limb, partial pelvic limb.
- Parasitology (specimens in 70% alcohol and frozen at −85°C): *Orthohalarachne attenuate, Orthohalarachne diminuata, Corynosoma* sp., *Diphyllobothrium* sp.

References

French, R.W.B. & Callender, G.R. (1962) Ballistic characteristics of wounding agents. In: *Wound Ballistics* (eds J.B. Coates and J.C. Beyer). Office of the Surgeon General, Department of the Army, Washington, D.C., USA.

Harvey, E.N., McMillen, J.H., Butler, E.G. & Puckett, W.O. (1962) Mechanism of wounding. In: *Wound Ballistics* (eds J.B. Coates and J.C. Beyer). Office of the Surgeon General, Department of the Army, Washington, DC, USA.

Owen-Smith, M.S. (1981) *High Velocity Missile Wounds.* Edward Arnold, London.

Pavletic, M.M. (1986) Gunshot wounds in veterinary medicine: Projectile ballistics – Part I. *The Compendium on Continuing Education,* **8** (1), 47–60.

Pavletic, M.M. (1986) Gunshot wounds in veterinary medicine: Projectile ballistics – Part II. *The Compendium on Continuing Education,* **8** (2), 125–34.

Case provided by Richard Norman, PhD, MACVSc MRCVS, New Zealand.

CASE 11 – HUNTING OUT OF SEASON?

Background

There was no indication initially that this incident might have legal implications. The author was running a veterinary diagnostic laboratory in the UK at the time and, amongst other things, offered a faecal parasitological service for owners of birds of prey.

In early August a faecal ('mute') sample was received by post for laboratory investigation from a 'hawk' – a peregrine *(Falco peregrinus)* – trained for hunting and owned by an experienced falconer in Scotland.

Instructions (request) received

To carry out a parasitological examination on the faecal sample 'to look for worms, before the hunting season begins.'

Laboratory findings

Gross examination (including use of a hand lens) was carried out following standard techniques (Cooper, 2002). This revealed normal droppings (a mixture of dark brown faeces and pure white urates), with no evidence of a foetid smell or unusual consistency. Two wet preparations were made, in normal saline, for direct examination, and a weighed portion of the faecal material ground was coarsely filtered and suspended in super-saturated NaCl solution for examination by flotation.

The flotation method revealed small numbers of eggs of two genera of nematodes – an *Ascaridia* sp. and a *Capillaria (Eucoleus)* sp.

The wet preparations confirmed the presence of eggs of the above worms plus assorted plant material, down feather barbs characteristic of day-old (cockerel) chicks, other adult galliform barbs and barbules and several biting lice of the family Philopteridae. The latter were of a genus, *Goniodes,* which is found on grouse (*Lagopus* spp.) (Price *et al.,* 2003). The faecal material appeared within normal limits with no evidence of, e.g., free blood or undigested fat.

Follow-up

A report was sent to the person who submitted the sample, describing the findings, explaining the possible significance of *Ascaridia* and *Capillaria* in a trained, working hawk. A postscript was added by hand: 'Why were you flying your hawk at grouse before the season starts on 12th August?!'

Outcome

Within a few minutes of receiving his report the falconer was on the telephone asking, 'How did you know that my hawk caught and partly ate a grouse last week? I didn't tell you that in my letter!'

The laboratory findings were explained: the presence of the biting lice, together with feather material from a heavily pigmented galliform bird, was, 'beyond reasonable doubt', indicative that the hawk had devoured a grouse, probably the Scottish red grouse, shortly before the mute sample had been taken and submitted for examination.

The falconer audibly gulped and admitted that his hawk had, indeed caught and killed a grouse before the open season had started. He explained that he had 'slipped' (released) his hawk for it to chase a pigeon but, instead, it had pursued a young red grouse – which, because of the latter's inexperience, it had easily caught. By the time the falconer arrived, found and was able to 'take up' (retrieve) his hawk, it had devoured some of the grouse. The latter was lacking breast and leg muscle and the hawk had visible and palpable food in its crop. The falconer said that he was embarrassed by the whole incident.

No further action was taken but the falconer said that he would take extra care in the future not to fly his hawks near young grouse before 12th August – and would view veterinary pathologists in a new light in future!

Comments

This was a case that did not get to court and probably, in view of the circumstances, would never have done so. Professional ethics dictated that the laboratory findings were confidential to the client and could not be divulged to an outsider. However, a decision had been made to draw the matter to the attention of the falconer as a footnote to the report.

The killing of the grouse before 12th August was, strictly, unlawful. However, the falconer might, if taken to court, have been able to plead in defence that the hawk flew and caught the grouse but that this was done without any intention on his part.

References

Cooper, J.E. (2002) *Birds of Prey: Health & Disease.* Blackwell, Oxford.

Price, R.D., Hellenthal, R.A., Palma, R.L., Johnson, K.P. & Clayton, D.H. (2003) *The Chewing Lice. World Checklist and Biological Overview.* Illinois Natural History Survey. Special Publication 2:501.

Case provided by John E. Cooper, FRCVS, UK.

Facilities and Equipment Lists

FACILITIES

Facilities needed for forensic work involving animals range from a fully-equipped laboratory with a national or regional role, governmental or non-governmental (private), to a small, specially-designated, area of a veterinary practice, animal welfare centre or wildlife unit. In some circumstances the facilities may consist of portable equipment in a vehicle, a trailer or a portable field kit (see Chapter 9). However, the basic principles of design and system are the same and these relate to:

- Security.
- Safety.
- Chain of custody.
- Accuracy of reports and reporting.

The needs and features of a large facility, including site building and laboratory design, a mechanical plumbing and electricity systems checklist and extensive guidance on construction and occupation were amply described by the U.S. Department of Justice (1998). Within this publication is information that is relevant also to smaller or improvised units, such as those needed in the field.

A small, specially designated, animal forensic unit is likely to comprise a building or room that contains the following:

Basic

- Reception area.
- Refrigerator and deep freeze.
- Computer.

- Storage facilities for fixed or dry material, paperwork and back-up computer discs.

As necessary

- Stainless steel examination table(s), with hydraulic lift system (when space is limited, folding tables, attached to a wall, are particularly valuable for forensic work).
- Appropriate lighting, including ultraviolet, both portable and ceiling-mounted.
- Laboratory bench and sink with appropriate facilities for disinfection, disposal of clinical waste and ventilation (see also below).
- Scavenging equipment (for anaesthetic gases, fumes, etc.).
- Clinical facilities, including X-ray machine and viewer, heavy-gauge steel dangerous drugs cabinet, endoscope(s), surgical instruments, etc., etc. These may be part of an adjacent veterinary practice, in which case they need not be incorporated into the forensic unit as such.

Appropriate arrangements, in accordance with relevant laws and codes of practice (see Chapter 3), must be made for provision of water and gas and for drainage. In temperate countries central-heating may be required; in the tropics or subtropics, air-conditioning. If these facilities cannot be provided, full use should be made of natural ventilation, insulation or shade, as appropriate. Much has been published on the design of laboratories in isolated areas, especially in tropical regions, and advantage can be taken of this when planning forensic facilities.

OBTAINING EQUIPMENT

If one has the chance to set up a forensic unit *de novo* then no expense should be spared to ensure that the correct and best equipment is available. Items for clinical and other work with animals can be purchased from veterinary suppliers but for pathological investigations it is wise also to consult catalogues from companies that supply tables and other equipment for mortuaries and for human forensic work. The range that is offered by such companies is usually extensive and often better tailored to the needs of a forensic investigation than are standard veterinary items.

The four principles listed above apply to all facilities, large or small. Specifically, security is of great importance. The forensic unit must be lockable, with limited access, as should the reception and storage facilities it contains. There should be only one key for sensitive locations and surveillance cameras are a wise precaution.

Safety, chain of custody and accuracy of reports and reporting are discussed in some detail in relevant chapters.

EQUIPMENT – GENERAL ITEMS FOR FORENSIC WORK AT THE CRIME SCENE

Recommended equipment for work at the crime scene is listed below. More specific items for working the field – for instance, when investigating wildlife crime – are catalogued later. Reference should also be made to different chapters in the book, some of which are mentioned below, where needs for certain types of investigation are outlined.

- Protective clothing, including boiler suits (coveralls), gloves (surgical, thick kitchen, long rubber, etc.), masks, goggles, boots and overshoes.
- Barrier tape, flags, markers, cones and other crime-scene security items.
- Protective gloves and clothing, barrier tape, and tools, such as tongs and hooks for handling hazardous materials.
- Disinfectant and deodoriser to neutralise smells from carcases, etc. (both used with caution at crime scenes as they may destroy trace evidence).
- Collection kits (pre-packed) for taking samples for laboratory investigation, including toxicology, DNA, haematology, etc.
- Appropriate labels, tamper-proof tags, evidence seals, etc.
- Marking pens.
- Scales/balances, callipers and micrometer for weighing animals, tissues and samples (see Chapter 6).
- Rules, tapes, centimetre scales, etc. for measuring (see Chapter 7).
- Equipment for taking casts of dentition, imprints in bones, animal tracks, etc., including plaster of Paris, other powders and silicone-based materials, waxes plus retention frames or stiff cardboard.
- Trace-evidence collection equipment (see Chapter 9).
- Evidence packing, e.g. bags, boxes, tubes, envelopes and other supplies for packaging and storing evidence.
- Photographic kit, including (as appropriate) digital/still cameras, video cameras, magnifier, night vision equipment, aerial camera system, camcorder.
- Binoculars/field glasses.
- Torches (flashlights).
- Blue-light kits and supplies.
- Egg candler.
- X-ray viewing screen.
- Magnifying glasses/hand lenses.
- Magnifying loupe or dissecting microscope.
- Clipboards and record sheets, plus pens and pencils.
- Chalk and crayons.
- Elastic bands and string.
- Tape recorder (preferably voice-activated) and tapes.
- Evidence seals/tape.
- Kits and systems for collecting and preserving delicate crime-scene evidence (see text).
- Computer and appropriate software, e.g. barcode tracking systems for property, evidence and crime-scene reconstruction.
- Hand-held computer.

EQUIPMENT – WHEN WORKING IN THE FIELD

The detailed contents of field kits will depend upon the location and the type of investigations being carried out. A detailed description of a general diagnostic kit, suitable for various types of veterinary work, was provided by Frye *et al.* (2001) and some data from that paper are reproduced here, with permission. Useful tips may also be found in publications about mobile veterinary practice, where equipment that can be readily transported by car is often detailed (Maas, 2006).

The following items are recommended in the field for clinical, *post-mortem* and laboratory diagnostic work, respectively. In each case the list should be supplemented with general items, as above.

Clinical equipment – when live animals have to be examined

- Stethoscope (lightweight).
- Auriscope (otoscope) (lightweight).
- Ophthalmoscope (lightweight).
- Rigid endoscope (battery-operated).
- Pen torch (flashlight).
- Spare bulbs and batteries.
- Syringes and needles (disposable).
- At least one boilable, re-usable syringe and needle.
- Empty drinks cans, labelled 'sharps boxes', for used needles, scalpel blades, etc.
- Disinfectant(s), including ethanol.
- Camping (gas-cylinder-operated) stove – for sterilising, lighting and cooking.
- Pressure cooker for sterilising.
- Selected medicines, including local analgesics, sedatives and agents for euthanasia (plus gun if large animals may need to be killed).
- Cotton wool.
- Dressings.
- Suture materials.
- Basic surgical ('cut-down') set and other instruments as necessary.
- Disposable skin-biopsy punch.
- Cautery (battery-operated).
- Clippers for claws, talons, beaks.
- Ring (band) remover.

- Spring balance(s) or battery-operated scales.
- Cloth bags and other devices for restraining small animals.
- Gloves – surgical and for handling.
- Towel.
- Oesophageal and other tubes.
- Mouth gag/wooden spatulae.
- Aluminium foil.
- Sampling and other equipment for laboratory work (see below).

Post-mortem equipment – when dead animals have to be examined

Standard necropsy items (see also Chapter 7) – portable/folding, lightweight/plastic where appropriate.

- Saw(s).
- Scalpels and blades.
- Knives.
- Forceps.
- Probes – solid and flexible (rubber).
- Scoops for brain, etc.
- Pen torch (flashlight).
- Spare bulbs and batteries.
- Syringes and needles (disposable).
- Empty drinks cans, labelled 'sharps boxes', for used needles, scalpel blades, etc.
- Disinfectant(s), including ethanol/methanol/methylated spirits.
- Camping (gas-cylinder-operated) stove – for sterilising, lighting and cooking.
- Pressure cooker for sterilising.
- Cotton wool.
- Spring balance(s) or battery-operated scales.
- Scalpel handle and disposable sterile blades of several sizes and shapes, dissecting scissors, curved haemostatic forceps, toothed and smooth-jawed fine-pattern thumb forceps and bone forceps.
- Sampling and other equipment for laboratory work (see below).

Laboratory equipment

- Microscope (solar- or battery-operated).
- Immersion oil (or methyl salicylate) with swabs and xylene for cleaning.

- Pre-cleaned, frosted, ground-ended microscope slides and slide box or tray.
- Pencils for marking glass slides.
- Diamond-tipped pen for marking glass slides (if frosted not available).
- Worm-egg counting slide.
- Cover slips.
- Lens tissues.
- Saline, saturated NaCl solution and other reagents for parasitology.
- Transparent polythene strips and methylene blue/malachite green for the KATO method of clearing faecal films for parasites, ova and cysts.
- Fixatives – alcohol, formalin.
- Selected stains for cytology.
- Lightweight (plastic) staining jar or staining rack.
- Urine and blood chemistry test strips.
- Portable centrifuge.
- Polypropylene capillary tubes, some coated with heparin or EDTA, plus commercial haemoglobin and PCV reader.
- Hand-held refractometer.
- Transport media for bacteria, viruses, mycoplasmas and *Trichomonas*.
- Vacuum flask.
- Buffer tablets for use with local water.
- Scalpel, scissors, forceps, artery forceps (haemostats).
- Wash bottles for alcohol, stains, etc., etc.
- Lightweight pots for specimens.
- Disinfectant(s), including ethanol/methanol/methylated spirits.
- Camping (gas-cylinder-operated) stove – for sterilising, lighting and cooking.
- Pressure cooker for sterilising.

Recommended additional items when working overseas in the field

Sharp and other possibly dangerous items should not be placed in hand luggage when travelling by air, or through land or sea security checkpoints.

- Emergency pack containing business cards, letters of authorisation, protocols for snakebite (etc.), medicines and antidotes.

- Multipurpose Swiss Army-type pocket knife.
- Sewing kit with assorted needles, thread.
- Screwdrivers, pliers and an adjustable spanner.
- Elastic bands, string, dental floss, suture material, adhesive tape, insulating tape, duct tape, electrician's tape.
- Spare nylon cable ties for securing lid hasp of case during travel.
- Standard veterinary and other textbooks: where space is limited, the *Merck Veterinary Manual* is recommended (but caution must be exercised in quoting from this in court as it does not include references).
- Phrase books of appropriate languages.
- The *SAS Survival Guide* (Wiseman, 1993), which contains much useful information that can be applied to difficult situations in the field.
- Appropriate clothing, e.g. the shoulders should be covered when working in a Moslem community, a tie is a courtesy in most countries when meeting dignitaries.

ADDITIONAL EQUIPMENT FOR SPECIFIC FORENSIC INVESTIGATIONS

Entomological (invertebrate) collection

In addition to the items discussed in Chapter 9:

- Small ventilated plastic vials, lined with mesh, filled with filter paper (to reduce condensation and subsequent drowning) for holding live ticks or other invertebrates.
- Relevant identification keys and texts.

Blood-sampling live birds and other animals for DNA and other investigative purposes

- Syringes (1 ml, 2 ml, 5 ml, 10 ml) as appropriate.
- Needles (20 g, 22 g, 25 g, 28 g) as appropriate.
- Anti-coagulant serum tubes.
- Cotton wool.
- Frosted-glass slides and box or tray.
- Cover slips.
- Pencils for marking glass slides, plus sharpener.

- Methanol.
- Cards or solutions for blood collection.
- Magnifying glass/hand lens.
- Plastic bags and labels.
- Electronic/spring balance.
- Ruler, tape measure.
- Clipboard, black pen and record sheets.
- Basic clinical equipment.
- Restraining equipment – nets, towels, gloves, hood, bags.

Plus other items from earlier lists, as necessary.

More specialised laboratory investigations in the field

- Vacuum flasks and portable, lightweight, cool-box.
- Normal (isotonic) saline.
- Hypertonic NaCl or sugar (sucrose) solution for flotation/sedimentation examination.
- Tincture of merthiolate for staining faecal protozoa.
- Fixatives for blood and other body fluids, bone marrow and endo- and ectoparasites.
- Rapid-acting stains for blood and other body fluids (sputum, urine, synovial and coelomic, cerebrospinal, bone marrow, etc.) and touch/impression smear cytology.
- Gram, acid-fast and other special stains.
- Lactol-phenol cotton-blue for demonstrating fungi.
- Plastic pipettes.
- Slotted stain jar; lightweight, unbreakable plastic staining jars are preferable to heavy, fragile, glass Coplin jars.
- Mounting media for permanent preparations of blood and bone marrow films.
- Clearing and mounting media for small ectoparasites.
- Lightweight, slide-drying rack.

- Transport media for bacteria, viruses and protozoa (see earlier).
- Microbiological test strips.
- Urine and blood chemistry test strips.
- Rapid diagnostic test strips.
- Cardboard strips, which can be labelled in pencil or waterproof ink, and placed inside specimen containers.
- Safety matches, a small Bunsen burner or disposable butane cigarette lighter.
- Squeeze bottles for methanol, etc.
- Specimen containers, filled with concentrated formaldehyde, for dilution with river or sea water.
- Tongue depressors, wooden applicator sticks, and sterile cotton-tipped applicators; plastic coffee spoons for use as spatulae (see text).
- Non-lubricated condoms as finger covers.
- Plastic film canisters (pots) with labels attached for faecal collection, parasites, etc. They usually can be obtained *gratis* from film dealers or photo-finishing laboratories.
- Sterile disposable venous and urethral catheters; latex or plastic tubing.
- Plastic slide boxes, each pre-filled with polished, frosted-glass microscope slides.

Checklist of battery-operated or solar-powered (direct sun or solar panels) equipment that can be used in isolated locations

- Miniaturised auriscope (otoscope).
- Ophthalmoscope.
- Rigid endoscope.
- Colorimeter.
- Electrocautery.
- Blood-pressure monitoring instrument.
- Minicentrifuge.
- Miniphotometer.
- Respiratory monitor and pulse oximeter.
- Refractometer.

Scientific Names of Species and Taxa of Animals Mentioned in Text, with Notes on Taxonomy

'What's the use of their having names,' the Gnat said, 'if they won't answer to them?'
'No use to them,' said Alice, 'but it's useful to the people that name them, I suppose.'
Lewis Carroll, *Alice Through the Looking-Glass*

The English names below are generally given as they appear in the text, with additions or changes where this may assist the reader.

Some hazardous species, not mentioned below, are to be found in Table 2.2. Likewise, various vertebrates are listed in Chapters 5 and 9, in the context of medical and veterinary forensic entomology. Where plants are referred to in the book, their scientific names are included in the text.

General notes on taxonomy and classification are given at the end of the Appendix.

NOTES ON TAXONOMY AND CLASSIFICATION

Rules and guidance for the naming of animals are issued by the International Commission on Zoological Nomenclature (ICZN) (see Appendix B).

This system follows that promulgated by the Swedish biologist Carl von Linné (Carolus Linnaeus) who devised, in the 18th century, a binomial system for living and extinct animals and plants. Examples of the system, as used today, are given in Table F.3.

Knowing the taxonomic status of an animal or animals is a prerequisite in any legal case. It leads to the collation of information on the biology and natural history of the species – so often important when presenting a report or giving an opinion.

Useful general references to the biology of endothermic animals are *The New Encyclopedia of Mammals* (Macdonald and Norris, 2001) and *A Dictionary of Birds* (Campbell and Lack, 1985). Numerous other texts provide information about reptiles, amphibians, fish and various taxa of invertebrates.

Table F.1 English and scientific names of mammals.

English name	Scientific name	English name	Scientific name
Antelopes	Bovidae	Hamster, golden	*Mesocricetus auratus*
Agouti	*Dasyprocta* sp.	Hare	*Lepus capensis*
Ass	*Equus asinus*	Hedgehog	*Erinaceus europaeus*
Baboon	*Papio* sp.	Howler monkey	*Alouatta* spp
Badger, Eurasian	*Meles meles*	Humpback whale	*Megaptera novaeangliae*
Bats	Rhinolophidae/	Jackal	*Canis aureus*
	Vespertilionidae	Kangaroos	Diprotodontia, Macropodidae and
Bears	Ursidae		Hypsiprymnodontidae
Bighorn sheep	*Ovis canadensis*	Lion	*Panthera leo*
Black rhinoceros	*Diceros bicornis*	Marmoset	*Callithrix* spp
Buffalo, African	*Syncerus caffer*	Mole	*Talpa europaea*
Camel, Arabian	*Camelus dromedarius*	Mongooses	Herpestidae
Caracal	*Felis caracal*	Mountain gorilla	*Gorilla berengei*
Cougar (Puma)	*Felis concolor*	Mouse	*Mus musculus*
Deer, red	*Cervus elaphus*	Opossum	*Didelphis marsupialis*
Dolphin, common	*Delphinus delphis*	Orang-utan	*Pongo* spp
Domestic cat	*Felis catus*	Otter, Eurasian	*Lutra lutra*
Domestic dog	*Canis familiaris*	Peccary	*Tayassu* spp
Domestic goat	*Capra hircus*	Polar bear	*Thalarctos maritimus*
Domestic ox	*Bos taurus/indicus*	Porpoise, harbour	*Phocaena phocaena*
Domestic pig	*Sus scrofa*	Raccoon	*Procyon* spp
Domestic sheep	*Ovis aries*	Rhinoceros	Rhinocerotidae
Donkey	*Equus asinus*	Seal, common	*Phoca vitulina*
Elephant	*Loxodonta/Elephas* sp.	Squirrels	Sciuridae
Ferret	*Mustela putorius furo*	Tibetan antelope	*Pantholops hodgsoni*
Fox	*Vulpes vulpes*	(chiru)	
Fur seal, Antarctic	*Arctocephalus gazella*	Tiger	*Panthera tigris*
Gazelles	Bovidae (various subfamilies)	Warthog	*Phacochoerus aethiopicus*
Giant rat	*Cricetomys gambianus*	Whitetail deer	*Odocoileus virginianus*
Guinea pig	*Cavia porcellus*	Wolf	*Canis lupus*

Table F.2 English and scientific names of birds, reptiles, amphibians, fish and invertebrates.

Class	English name	Scientific name
Aves/Birds	Bald eagle	*Haliaeetus leucocephalus*
	Budgerigar	*Melopsittacus undulatus*
	Canary	*Serinus canaria*
	Cockatoo, sulphur-crested	*Cacatua galerita*
	Cormorant	*Phalacrocorax carbo*
	Domestic duck	*Anas platyrhynchos*
	Domestic fowl	*Gallus domesticus*
	Domestic turkey	*Meleagris gallopavo*
	Eagle, golden	*Aquila chrysaetos*
	Flamingo, lesser	*Phoeniconaias minor*
	Goosander	*Mergus merganser*
	Guinea fowl	*Numida meleagris*
	Gulls	Laridae
	Herons	Ardeidae
	Kereru (New Zealand pigeon)	*Hemiphaga novaeseelandiae*
	Kestrel (European)	*Falco tinnunculus*
	Macaw	*Ara* spp
	Mallard duck	*Anas platyrhynchos*
	Marabou stork	*Leptoptilos crumeniferus*
	Mauritius kestrel	*Falco punctatus*
	Muscovy duck	*Cairina moschata*
	Osprey	*Pandion haliaetus*
	Ostrich	*Struthio camelus*
	Parrot and related birds	Psittaciformes
	Pelican, brown	*Pelecanus occidentalis*
	Peregrine falcon	*Falco peregrinus*
	Philippine eagle	*Pithecophaga jefferyi*
	Pigeon, feral	*Columba livia*
	Shrikes	Laniidae
	Sparrow-hawk	*Accipiter nisus*
	Starling, common	*Sturnus vulgaris*
	Thrush	*Turdus* spp
	Trinidad piping-guan	*Pipile pipile*
	Waterfowl	Anseriformes
Reptilia/Reptiles	Green iguana	*Iguana iguana*
	Nile crocodile	*Crocodylus niloticus*
	Rattlesnake	*Crotalus* spp
	Royal python	*Python regius*
	Spiny-tailed lizard	*Uromastyx aegypticus*
	Tortoise, leopard	*Geochelone pardalis*
	Tortoises, Mediterranean	*Testudo* spp
Amphibia/Amphibians	African clawed toad	*Xenopus laevis*
	Marine (cane) toad	*Bufo marinus*
	Toad, common	*Bufo bufo*
Pisces/Fish	Brotulids	*Bassogigas* spp
	Carp	*Cyprinus carpio*
	Halibut	*Hippoglossus* spp/*Paralichthys* spp

Table F.2 *Continued.*

Class	English name	Scientific name
	Koi	*Cyprinus carpio*
	Lion (Scorpion)	*Pterois volitans*
	Puffer	*Diodin* spp (and other genera)
	Sharks	Selachii
	Sturgeon	*Achipenser* spp
	Trout	*Salmo trutta*
Invertebrata/Invertebrates including Insecta/Insects and other Arthropoda/Arthropods	Bee, honey	*Apis mellifera*
	Beetle, Colorado	*Leptinotarsa decemlineata*
	Beetle, coccinellid (ladybirds)	Coleoptera, Coccinellidae
	Birdwing butterflies	*Ornithoptera* spp
	Blowflies	*Calliphora* spp
	Carrion beetles	*Silpha* spp
	Cinnabar moth	*Callimorpha jacobaeae*
	Grasshoppers	Orthoptera, Acrididae
	Leeches	Hirudinea
	Scarab beetles	Scarabeidae
	Scorpions	Arachnida, Scorpiones
	Scorpion, emperor	*Pandinus imperator*
	Sexton beetles	*Necrophorus* spp
	Stick insects	Phasmida
	Ticks	Arachnida, Acarina

Table F.3 Examples of the classification of animals.

	Domestic dog	*Peregrine falcon*	*Honey bee*
Kingdom	Animalia	Animalia	Animalia
Phylum	Chordata	Chordata	Arthropoda
Class	Mammalia	Aves	Insecta
Order	Carnivora	Falconiformes	Hymenoptera
Family	Canidae	Falconidae	Apidae
Genus	*Canis*	*Falco*	*Apis*
Species	*familiaris*	*peregrinus*	*mellifera*
Binomial	*Canis familiaris*	*Falco peregrinus*	*Apis mellifera*

The CRFP's Code of Practice

The Council for the Registration of Forensic Practitioners (CRFP) has a Code of Practice for those who are registered with it. That Code, reproduced below with permission, provides valuable guidelines for anyone who may be involved in forensic work.

BEING A FORENSIC PRACTITIONER – WHAT WE EXPECT FROM YOU

Registration with CRFP, which is voluntary, carries both privileges and responsibilities. The public will accept your registration as proof of your competence. Your responsibility is, in return, to maintain and develop your professional performance, adhering at all times to the standards in this code.

As a registered forensic practitioner you must:

(1) Recognise that your overriding duty is to the court and to the administration of justice: it is your duty to present your findings and evidence, whether written or oral, in a fair and impartial manner.

(2) Act with honesty, integrity, objectivity and impartiality.

(3) Not discriminate on grounds of race, belief, gender, language, sexual orientation, social status, age, lifestyle or political persuasion.

(4) Comply with the code of conduct of any professional body of which you are a member.

(5) Provide advice and evidence only within the limits of your professional competence and only when fit to do so.

(6) Inform a suitable person or authority, in confidence where appropriate, if you have good grounds for believing there is a situation which may result in a miscarriage of justice.

In all aspects of your work as a provider of forensic advice and evidence you must:

(7) Take all reasonable steps to maintain and develop your professional competence, taking account of material research and development within the relevant field and practising techniques of quality assurance.

(8) Declare to your client, patient, or employer if you have one, any prior involvement or personal interest which gives, or may give, rise to a conflict of interest, real or perceived, and act in such a case only with their explicit written consent.

(9) Take all reasonable steps to ensure access to all available evidential materials which are relevant to the examinations requested; to establish, so far as reasonably practicable, whether any may have been compromised before coming into your possession; are maintained whilst in your possession.

(10) Accept responsibility for all work done under your supervision, direct or indirect.

(11) Conduct all work in accordance with the established principles of your profession,

using methods of proven validity and appropriate equipment and materials.

(12) Make and retain full, contemporaneous, clear and accurate records of the examinations you conduct, your methods and your results in sufficient detail for another forensic practitioner competent in the same area of work to review your work independently.

(13) Report clearly, comprehensively and impartially, setting out or stating:

(a) your terms of reference and the source of your instructions;

(b) the material upon which you based your investigation and conclusion;

(c) summaries of your and your team's work, results and conclusions;

(d) any ways in which your investigations or conclusions were limited by external factors, especially if your access to relevant material was restricted; or if you believe unreasonable limitations on your time, or on the human, physical or financial resources available to you, have significantly compromised the quality of your work;

(e) that you have carried out your work and prepared your report in accordance with this code.

(14) Reconsider and, if necessary, be prepared to change your conclusions, opinions or advice and to reinterpret your findings in the light of new information or new developments in the relevant field; and take the initiative in informing your client or employer promptly of any such change.

(15) Preserve confidentiality unless:

(a) the client or patient explicitly authorises you to disclose something;

(b) a court or tribunal orders disclosure;

(c) the law obliges disclosure; or

(d) your overriding duty to the court and to the administration of justice demands disclosure.

(16) Preserve legal professional privilege: only the client may waive this. It protects communications, oral and written, between professional legal advisers and expert witnesses in connection with the giving of legal advice, or in connection with, or in contemplation of, legal proceedings and for the purposes of those proceedings.

When you register with CRFP, you accept these as the principles that must govern your professional practice. They are the standards against which CRFP would judge any information that called into question your fitness to stay on the register. You must therefore always be prepared to justify, in the light of this code, the actions and decisions you take in the course of your professional work.

In considering a complaint against a registered forensic practitioner, CRFP will be guided primarily by the provisions of the code. But they reserve the right to take action where a practitioner's fitness to practise is questioned for other reasons. This would include circumstances such as a criminal conviction or an allegation of behaviour which, while not specifically addressed in the code, might be regarded as bringing forensic practice into disrepute.

Reproduced with the permission of the CRFP.

References and
Further Reading

This list of references is intended to provide the reader with indications as to where further information may be obtained. It intentionally encompasses a wide range of topics of forensic significance.

References to papers and books in languages other than English are only given in the original language where this is important historically or because no readily available or reliable translations exist. Where there are comprehensive abstracts in English, either in the original or in the searches carried out by CABI (see Appendix B), the publication is anglicised.

In a few references not all of the authors are listed and, instead, the term 'et al.' (and others) is used. This applies to papers with either large numbers of authors or where there are 'contributors' or 'assistants' listed in addition to authors or editors.

Adair, T.W. (1999) Chain of custody in the university setting: considerations for entomologists. *Antenna*, **23** (3), 140–43.

Adams, I.H., Graham, D.I. & Gennarelli, T.A. (1983) Head injury in man and experimental animals: neuropathology. *Acta Neurochiurgica Supplement*, **32**, 15–30.

Adolphsen, J. (2002) The new horse purchase legislation. *Pferdeheilkunde. Hippiatrika*, **18** (3), 294–7 [German].

Adrian, W.J. (1992) *Wildlife Forensic Manual*. Association of Midwest Fish and Game Law Enforcement Officers. Colorado Division of Wildlife, Fort Collins, USA.

Agnew, D.W., Hagey, L. & Shoshani, J. (2005) The elephants of Zoba Gash Barka, Eritrea: Part 4. Cholelithiasis in a wild African elephant (*Loxodonta africana*). *Journal of Zoo and Wildlife Medicine*, **36** (4), 677–83.

Alder, M. & Easton, G. (2005a) Editorial. Working with the medical profession. *Veterinary Record*, **156** (16), 493.

Alder, M. & Easton, G. (2005b) Editorial. Human and veterinary medicine. *British Medical Journal*, **330**, 858–9.

Alexander, K. (2005) Wood decay, insects, palaeoecology and woodland conservation policy and practice – breaking the halter. *Antenna*, **29** (3), 171–8.

Alexander, R. McN. (1984) Optimum strength for bones liable to fatigue and accidental damage. *Journal of Theoretical Biology*, **109**, 621–36.

Allen, E. & Cooper, J.E. (1983) Zoography: the use of animal terms in medicine. *British Medical Journal*, **286**, 14.

Allen, T.A. & Toll, P.W. (1995) Medical implications of fasting and starvation. In: *Kirk's Current Veterinary Therapy XII: Small Animal Practice* (ed. J.D. Bonagura). W.B. Saunders, Philadelphia, USA.

Allison, R.T. & Whittaker, D.K. (1990) Use of benzidine for histological demonstration of haemoglobin in human bite marks. *Journal of Clinical Pathology*, **43**, 600–603.

Amato, G. & Lehn, C. (2002) Biomaterials as an essential component of applied conservation research: in situ and ex situ case studies. *Proceedings American Association of Zoo Veterinarians*, *2002*, p. 279.

Anderson, G.S. & Huitson, N.R. (2004) Myiasis in pet animals in British Columbia: the potential of forensic entomology for determining duration of possible neglect. *Canadian Veterinary Journal*, **45** (12), 993–8.

Anderson, P.K., Cunningham, A.A., Patel, N.G., Morales, F.J., Epstein, P.R. & Daszak, P. (2004) Emerging infectious diseases of plants: pathogen pollution, climate change and agrotechnology drivers. *Trends in Ecology and Evolution*, **19**, 535–44.

Anderson, R. (2004) Forensic toxicology. In: *Crime Scene to Court. The Essentials of Forensic Science*, 2nd edn. (ed. P.C. White). The Royal Society of Chemistry, Cambridge, UK.

André, E. (1904) *A Naturalist in the Guianas.* Smith, Elder & Co, London, UK.

Anita, B.A. (2004) Dolphin harvesting in the Solomon Islands – a clash of cultures. *CVA (Commonwealth Veterinary Association) News*, July, 38–42.

Anon. (2001) *Forging the Link.* Proceedings, One-Day Conference, 22 November 2001, London Intervet Milton Keynes, UK.

Anon. (2002a) *Animal Cruelty: Family Violence.* Scottish SPCA and First Strike, Scotland, UK.

Anon. (2002b) Better information increases the capacity of scientists and healthcare workers in developing countries. *TDR News*, **69**, 11.

Anon. (2003a) RCVS issues guidance on dealing with abuse in animals and humans. *Veterinary Record*, **152** (15), 446.

Anon. (2003b) Student training on recognizing animal abuse. *Veterinary Record*, **152**, 151.

Anon. (2003c) Brains network via the web. *Animal Health News*, CSIRO, Australia, October 2003.

Anon. (2004) Dealing with death in man and animals. *Veterinary Record*, **154**, 250–51.

Anon. (2005a) Delhi struggles to rope in stray cattle as deadline looms. *The Gulf Times*, Qatar, 5 May 2005.

Anon. (2005b) Tackling MRSA in animals and humans. *Veterinary Record*, **157**, 671–2.

Anon. (2005c) One medicine? Editorial. *Veterinary Record*, **157**, 669.

Anon. (2005d) Increase in alleged cruelty complaints. *Veterinary Record*, **157**, 100.

Anon. (2005e) How to catch a holy cow – with bare hands, rope and a prayer. *Khaleej Times*, 6 May 2005.

Anon. (2005f) Concern over US 'wildlife rescuers'. *Legal Eagle*, **45**, 10.

Anon. (2005g) DNA badger bank. *Legal Eagle*, **44**, 9.

Anon. (2005h) Shambles in North Yorkshire trapping case. *Legal Eagle*, **44**, 6.

Anon. (2005i) Frozen in time, protest over display of child mummies. *Guardian Weekly*, September 30– October 6, 4.

Anon. (2005j) *Proceedings of the Veterinary Association for Arbitration & Jurisprudence*, **2** (1).

Anon. (undated) *Inside Wildlife Crime.* Carlton Television, London, UK.

Archer, C.B. & Robertson, S.J. (1995) *Black and White Skin Diseases.* Blackwell, Oxford, UK.

Archer, M.S. (2004) Rainfall and temperature effects on the decomposition rate of exposed neonatal remains. *Science and Justice*, **44** (1), 35–41.

Arendt, W., Faaborg, J., Wallace, G. & Garrido, O. (2004) Biometrics of birds throughout the Greater Caribbean Basin. *Proceedings of the Western Foundation of Vertebrate Zoology*, **8** (1).

Arkow, P. (1992) The correlations between cruelty to animals and child abuse and the implications for veterinary medicine. *Canadian Veterinary Journal*, **33** (8), 518–21.

Arkow, P. (1994) Child abuse, animal abuse, and the veterinarian. *Journal of the American Veterinary Medical Association*, **204** (7), 1004–7.

Arkow, P. (2003) *Breaking the Cycles of Violence: A Guide to Multi-Disciplinary Interventions. A Handbook for Child Protection, Domestic Violence and Animal Protection Agencies.* Latham Foundation, Almeda, USA.

Arkow, P. (2004) The veterinarian's roles in preventing family violence: the experience of the human medical profession. *Protecting Children*, **19** (1), 4–12.

Arkow, P. & Munro, H. (2006) The veterinary profession's roles in recognizing and preventing family violence: the experiences of the human medicine field and the development of diagnostic indicators of non-accidental (injury). In: *International Handbook on Cruelty to Animals* (ed. F. R. Ascione). Purdue University Press, West Lafayette, USA.

Arluke, A. & Luke, C. (1997) Physical cruelty towards animals in Massachusetts, 1975–1996. *Society & Animals*, **5** (3), 195–204.

Ascione, F.R. & Arkow, P. (eds) (1999) *Animal Abuse, Child Abuse and Domestic Violence: Linking the Circles of Compassion for Prevention and Intervention.* Purdue University Press, West Lafayette, Indiana, USA.

Asher, R. (1951) Munchausen's syndrome. *Lancet*, **1**, 339–41.

Ashley, E.P. & Robinson, J.T. (1996) Road mortality of amphibians, reptiles, and other wildlife on the Long Point Causeway, Lake Erie, Ontario. *Canadian Field-Naturalist*, **110**, 403–12.

Atkinson, D. & Moloney, T. (2005) *Blackstone's Guide to the Criminal Procedure Rules.* Oxford University Press, UK.

Aughey, E. & Frye, F.L. (2001) *Comparative Veterinary Histology with Clinical Correlates.* Manson Publications, London, UK.

Averill, D.C. (ed.) (1991) *Manual of Forensic Odontology.* American Society of Forensic Odontology, American Academy of Forensic Sciences, Colorado, USA.

AWI (1990) *Animals and their Legal Rights*, 4th edn. Animal Welfare Institute, Washington, D.C., USA.

Badger Trust (2005) Barbaric 17th century activity. *Badger News*, **22**, 7.

Bailey, T.A., Samour, J.H., Naldo, J.L., Cooper, J.E. & Nicholls, P.K. (1997) The establishment of a biomedical reference collection for a captive-breeding and restoration programme. *International Zoo Yearbook*, **35**, 337–42.

Baker, J.R. & Brothwell, D.R. (1980) *Animal Diseases in Archaeology*. Academic Press, London, UK.

Balding, D.J. (2005) *Weight-of-Evidence for DNA Profiles*. Wiley, London, UK.

Ball, S. & Bell, S. (1991) *Environmental Law. The Law and Policy Relating to the Protection of the Environment*, 3rd edn. Blackstone Press, UK.

Barker, D. & Padfield, C. (2002) *Law*. Made Simple Books, Oxford, UK.

Barnes, J. (2005) *Arthur and George*. Jonathan Cape, London, UK.

Baron, D.N. (ed.) (1994) *Units, Symbols and Abbreviations*, 5th edn. Royal Society of Medicine Press, London, UK.

Barrand, K. (2006) Beginner's guide to going digital. *In Practice*, **28**, 41–6.

Barsley, R.E. (1993) Forensic and legal issues in oral diagnosis (Review). *Dental Clinics of North America*, **37**, 133–56.

Barsley, R.E., West, M.H. & Fair, J.A. (1990) Forensic photography. Ultraviolet imaging of wounds on skin. *American Journal of Forensic Medicine & Pathology*, **11**, 300–8.

Bartges, J.W. & Osborne, C.A. (1995) Influence of fasting and eating on laboratory values. In: *Current Veterinary Therapy XII: Small Animal Practice*. W.B. Saunders, Philadelphia, USA.

BASC (2001) *Trapping Pest Birds: A Code of Practice*. British Association for Shooting and Conservation, Wrexham, UK.

Bayvel, A.C.D. (2005a) Animals in science and agriculture – a global perspective. *Biologist*, **52** (6), 339–44.

Bayvel, A.C.D. (2005b) Animal welfare – an international perspective. *Journal of the Commonwealth Veterinary Association*, pp 10–14.

Bayvel, A.C.D., Rahman, S.A. & Gavinelli, A. (eds) (2005) Animal Welfare: Global Issues, Trends and Challenges. *O.I.E. Scientific and Technical Review*, **24** (2). Paris, France.

BCT (undated) *Bats and the Law. What to do when the Law is Broken*. Bat Conservation Trust, London, UK.

Bean, M.J. & Rowland, M.J. (1997) *The Evolution of Wildlife Law*, 3rd edn. Greenwood Press, USA.

Beck, C.A. & Baros, N.B. (1991) The impact of debris on the Florida manatee. *Marine Pollution Bulletin*, **22** (10), 508–10.

Becker, D.B., Needleman, H.L. & Kotelchuck, M. (1978) Child abuse and dentistry, orofacial trauma and recognition by dentists. *Journal of the British Dental Association*, **97**, 24–8.

Bedford, P.G.C. (1974) Toad venom toxicity and its clinical occurrence in small animals in the United Kingdom. *Veterinary Record*, **94**, 613–14.

Belcher, T. & Newell, D.G. (2005) Crossing the boundaries. *Veterinary Record*, **157**, 682–4.

Bell, S. and McGillivray, D. (2000) *Environmental Law. The Law and Policy Relating to the Protection of the Environment*, 5th edn. Blackstone Press, London, UK.

Bello, S. & Soligo, C. (2005) A new method for the quantitative analysis of cut-mark micromorphology. Abstract, Winter Meeting of Primate Society of Great Britain, London, December 9, 2005. *Primate Eye*, **87**, 28–9.

Belveze, H. (2003) The precautionary principle and its legal implications in the area of food safety. (Veterinary services: organisation, quality assurance, evaluation.) *Revue Scientifique et Technique – Office International des Epizooties*, **22** (2), 387–96. [French]

Bemmann, K. (2004) Veterinary purchase examination of horses: the radiographic class II in the viewpoint of the law. *Praktische Tierarzt*, **85** (12), 898–902. [German]

Bender, J.B., Torres, S.M.F., Gilbert, S.M., Olsen, K.E. & LeDell, K.H. (2005) Isolation of methicillin-resistant *Staphylococcus aureus* from a non-healing abscess in a cat. *Veterinary Record*, **157**, 388–9.

Benecke, M. & Lessig, R. (2001) Child neglect and forensic entomology. *Forensic Science International*, **120** (1/2), 155–9.

Berger, M.A. (2005) What has a decade of Daubert wrought? *American Journal of Public Health*, **95**: Supplement 1, S59–65. Washington, USA.

Bergsma, D. (ed.) (1982) *Birth Defects Compendium*, 2nd edn. The National Foundation – March of Dimes, Alan R. Liss, New York, USA.

Bevel, T. & Gardner, R.M. (2002) *Bloodstain Pattern Analysis: with an Introduction to Crime Scene Reconstruction*, 2nd edn. CRC Press, Florida, USA/London, UK.

Beveridge, A. (1998) *Forensic Investigation of Explosions*. Taylor & Francis, London, UK.

Beyer, J.C. (1962) (ed.) *Wound Ballistics*. Office of the Surgeon General, Department of the Army: Washington DC Library of Congress. Cat. No. 62-60002, p. 883. USA.

BFSS (undated) *Code of Welfare and Husbandry of Birds of Prey and Owls*. British Field Sports Society, London, UK.

Blanchard, W. (1781) *The Proceedings at Large on the Trial of John Donellan, Esq. For the Wilful Murder (by Poison) of Sir the Edward Allesley Boughton, Bart., Late of Lawford-Hall, in the County of Warwick Tried before*

Mr. Justice Buller of the Assizes at Warwick, on Friday the 30th day of March, 1781. Printed for J. Almon and J. Debrett, London, UK.

Blau, S. & Skinner, M. (2005) The use of forensic archaeology in the investigation of human rights abuse: unearthing the past in east Timor. *The International Journal of Human Rights*, 9, 449–63.

Blood, D.C. (1985) *Veterinary Law: Ethics, Etiquette and Convention.* The Law Book Company, New South Wales, Australia.

Blood, D.C. & Studdert, V.P. (1988) *Baillière's Comprehensive Veterinary Dictionary.* Baillière Tindall, London, UK.

Bloom, B.S., Retbi, A., Dahan, S. & Jonsson, E. (2000) Evaluation of randomized controlled trials on complementary and alternative medicine. *International Journal for the Assessment of Health Care*, 16, 13–21.

Blowey, R. (2005) Factors associated with lameness in dairy cattle. *In Practice*, 27, 154–62.

BMA (2001) *The Medical Profession and Human Rights: A Handbook for a Changing Agenda.* British Medical Association, London, UK.

Bohan, T.L. & Heels, E.J. (1995) The case against *Daubert*: The new scientific evidence 'standard' and the standards of the several states. *Journal of Forensic Sciences*, 40 (6), 1030–44.

Bonagura, J.D. (ed.) (1995) *Kirk's Current Veterinary Therapy XII: Small Animal Practice.* W.B. Saunders, Philadelphia, USA.

Bond, C., Solon, M. & Harper, P. (1999) *The Expert Witness in Court. A Practical Guide*, 2nd edn. Shaw & Sons, Crayford, Kent, UK.

Bonner, J. (2001) Vets could do more to stop abuse. *Veterinary Times*, 31 (44), 1.

Boroda, A. & Gray, W. (2005) Hair analysis for drugs in child abuse. *Journal of the Royal Society of Medicine*, 98, 318–19.

Borucinska, J., Kohler, N., Natanson, L. & Skomal, G. (2002) Pathology associated with retained fishing hooks in blue sharks, *Prionace glauca* (L.), with implications for their conservation. *Journal of Fish Diseases*, 25, 515–21.

Bourel, B., Hubert, N., Hedouin, V. & Gosset, D. (2000) Forensic entomology applied to a mummified corpse. *Annales de la Société Entomologique de France. Société Entomologique de France, Paris*, 36 (3), 287–90. [French]

Bowers, M.C. (2004) *Forensic Dental Evidence. An Investigator's Handbook.* Elsevier, Oxford, UK.

Boyd, D.K., Forbes, S.H., Pletscher, D.H. & Allendorf, F.W. (2001) Identification of Rocky Mountain gray wolves. *Wildlife Society Bulletin*, 29 (l), 78–85.

Bradley, M.T. (ed.) (1996) *Wildlife Crime.* The Stationery Office. London, UK,

Brahams, D. (1995) The medicolegal implications of teleconsulting in the UK. *Journal of Telemedicine and Telecare*, 1, 916–201.

Brandt, A. (2001) A fascination for flies. *Bulletin of the Royal Entomological Society, Antenna*, 28, 181–2.

Brandwood, A., Jayes, A.S. & Alexander, R. McN. (1986) Incidence of healed fracture in the skeletons of birds, molluscs and primates. *Journal of Zoology, London*, 208, 55–62.

Branicki, W. & Kupiec, T. (1999) Species identification using mitochondrial DNA analysis. *Proceedings of the International Association of Forensic Sciences, 75th Triennial Meeting August 22–28, 1999, Los Angeles, California, USA.*

Branthwaite, M. & Beresford, N. (2003) *Law for Doctors: Principles and Practicalities.* The Royal Society of Medicine, London, UK.

Brearley, M.J., Cooper, J.E. & Sullivan, M. (eds) (1991) *Color Atlas of Small Animal Endoscopy.* Mosby, St. Louis, USA.

Breeze, R.G. & Wheeldon, E.B. (1979) Pneumoconiosis. In: *Spontaneous Animal Models of Human Disease* (eds E.J. Andrews, B.C. Ward and N.H. Altmos), Vol. II. Academic Press, New York, USA.

Brodbelt, D., Breavley, J., Young, L., Wood, J. & Pfeiffer, D. (2005) Anaesthetic-related mortality risks in small animals in the UK. *Proceedings of the Association of Veterinary Anaesthetists*, Rimini.

Brodbelt, D.C., Hammond, R., Tuminaro, D., Pfeiffer, D.U. & Wood, J.L.N. (2006) Risk factors for anaesthetic related death in referred dogs. *Veterinary Record*, 158, 563–4.

Brogdon, B.G. (1998) *Forensic Radiology.* CRC Press, Boca Raton, USA.

Brooks, L. & Anderson, H.F. (1998) Dental anomalies in bottlenose dolphins, *Tursiops truncatus*, from the West Coast of Florida. *Marine Mammal Science*, 14 (4), 849–53.

Broom, D.M. (1996) Animal welfare defined in terms of attempts to cope with the environment. *Acta Agriculturae Scandinavica. Section A. Animal Science, Supplementation* 27, 22–8.

Broom, D.M. (2001) Evolution of pain. In: *Pain: its Nature and Management in Man and Animals* (eds Lord Soulsby and D. Morton.). Royal Society of Medicine International Congress Symposium Series, 246, 17–25.

Broom, D.M. (2003) *The Evolution of Morality and Religion.* Cambridge University Press, UK.

Broom, D.M. & Johnson, K.G. (1993) *Stress and Animal Welfare*. Chapman & Hall, London, UK.

Brooman, S. & Legge, D. (1997) *Law Relating to Animals*. Cavendish Publishing, London, Sydney.

Broughton, J.M., Rampton, D. & Holanda, K. (2002) A test of an osteologically based age determination technique in the Double-crested Cormorant *Phalacrocorax aritus*. *Ibis*, **144**, 143–6.

Brown, K., Townsend, G. & Winning, T. (2005) Forensic applications of dental and oral anatomy. In: *Oral and Maxillofacial Anatomy, Histology and Embryology* (ed. S.R. Prabhu). Oxford University Press, UK.

Buck, C., Llopis, A., Najera, E. & Terris, M. (1988) *The Challenge of Epidemiology*. Pan American Health Organization, Washington, D.C., USA.

Bucknall, T.E. & Ellis, H. (eds) (1984) *Wound Healing for Surgeons*. Baillière Tindall, London, UK.

Bugarsky, A. (2004a) Selected chapters from forensic veterinary medicine. Part 3. *Informany Spracodjca*, **13** (8), 19–22. [Slovakian]

Bugarsky, A. (2004b) Selected chapters from forensic veterinary medicine, Part 2. *Informany Spracodjca*, **13** (7), 23–9. [Slovakian]

Buitkamp, J., Antes, R. & Wagner, V. (1999) DNA profiling in veterinary medicine. In: *DNA Profiling and DNA Fingerprinting* (eds J.T. Eppler and T. Lubjuhn). Birkhäuser Verlag, Basel, Switzerland.

Burton, J. & Rutty, G. (eds) (2001) *The Hospital Autopsy*, 2nd edn. Arnold, London, UK.

Busuttil, A. & Keeling, J. (eds) (2005) *Paediatric Forensic Medicine and Pathology*. Oxford University Press, Oxford, UK.

Butler, J.M. (2001) *Forensic DNA Typing*. Academic Press, San Diego, USA.

Butler-Sloss, E. & Hall, A. (2002) Expert witnesses, courts and the law. *Journal of the Royal Society of Medicine*, **95**, 431–4.

Butterworth, A., Goodship, A.E. & Preece, A.W. (1987) A carbon chamber for vital microscopy of bone healing. *Acta Orthopaedica Scandinavica*, **58**, 545–8.

Bux, R.C. & McDowell, J.D. (1992) Death due to attack from chow dog. *American Journal of Forensic Medicine and Pathology*, **13**, 305–308.

BVA (1990) *Dangerous Wild Animals Act 1976. A Guide to Veterinary Surgeons Concerned with Inspections under this Act*. BVA Publications, London.

BVA (2000) *Code of Practice on Medicines*. British Veterinary Association, London, UK.

BWRC (1989) *Ethics and Legal Aspects of Treatment and Rehabilitation of Wild Animal Casualties*. British Wildlife Rehabilitation Council, London, UK.

Byrd, J.H. & Castner, J.L. (2000) *Forensic Entomology: The Utility of Arthropods in Legal Investigations*. CRC Press, Florida, USA/London, UK.

Caddy, B. (2001) *Forensic Examination of Glass and Paint*. Taylor & Francis, London, UK.

Caddy, B. & Cobb, P. (2004) Forensic science. In: *Crime Scene to Court. The Essentials of Forensic Science*, 2nd edn (ed. P.C. White). The Royal Society of Chemistry, Cambridge, UK.

Callaghan, P.R. (1996) Court testimony and the expert witness. *Proceedings of the 11th International Conference of Racing Analysts and Veterinarians, Queensland, Australia*.

Calvert, I. (2004) Nutrition. In: *Manual of Reptiles*, 2nd edn (eds S.J. Girling and P. Raiti). British Small Animal Veterinary Association, Gloucester, UK.

Cameron, J.M. & Sims, B.E. (1973) *Forensic Dentistry*. Churchill Livingstone, London, UK.

Campbell, B. & Lack, E. (eds) (1985) *A Dictionary of Birds*. T. & A.D. Poyser, Calton, UK.

Camps, F.E. & Cameron, J.M. (1971) *Practical Forensic Medicine*. Hutchinson, London, UK.

Cannings, P. (2000) An investigator's approach to forensic evidence in wildlife cases. *One Day Meeting on Veterinary and Comparative Forensic Medicine, St. George's Hospital, London, UK*.

Carlstead, K. (1996) Effects of captivity on the behaviour of wild mammals. In: *Wild Mammals in Captivity* (eds D.E. Kleiman, M.E. Allen, K.V. Thompson & S. Lumpkin). The University of Chicago Press, USA.

Carvalho, L.M.L., Thyssen, P.J., Linhares, A.X. & Palhares, F.A.B. (2000) A checklist of arthropods associated with pig carrion and human corpses in southeastern Brazil. *Memorias do Instituto Oswaldo Cruz*, **95** (1), 135–8.

Catling, C. & Grayson, J. (1982) *Identification of Vegetable Fibres*. Chapman and Hall, London, UK.

Cattle, J.A., Way, C.P., Fuller, S., Low, G. & Vaughan, G.T. (2004) Identification and matching of environmental samples for regulatory purposes: a systematic approach. *Environmental Forensics*, **5** (4), 185–94.

Catts, E.P. (1992) Problems in estimating the post-mortem interval in death investigations. *Journal of Agricultural Entomology*, **9** (4), 245–55.

Cavendish Law Cards (2002) *Evidence*, 2nd edn. Cavendish Publishing, London, Sydney.

CAWC (2003) *The Welfare of Non-domesticated Animals kept for Companionship*. Companion Animal Welfare Council, London, UK.

Cerling, T.E., *et al.* (2006) Stable isotopes in elephant hair document migration patterns and diet changes. *Proceed-*

ings of the National Academy of Sciences, **103** (2), 371–3.

Chaplin, R.E. (1971) *The Study of Animal Bones from Archaeological Sites.* Seminar Press, London, UK.

Cherry, S. (2005) A clean bill of health: practice hygiene. *In Practice*, **27**, 548–51.

Chesebro, B. (2003) Introduction to the transmissible spongiform encephalopathies or prion diseases. *British Medical Bulletin*, **66**, 1–20.

Chitty, J. (2006) The injured bird of prey. Part 1: Legal and logistical issues. *Small Animal Exotics, UK Vet*, **11** (3), 88–94.

Cina, S. (1994) Flow cytometric evaluation of DNA degradation: A predictor of postmortem interval? *The American Journal of Forensic Medicine and Pathology*, **15** (4), 300–2.

Civil Justice Council (2005) *Protocol for the Instruction of Experts to give Evidence in Civil Claims* (www.dca.gov.uk).

Clark, A. (2005) More animal health, welfare standards go global. *Journal of the American Veterinary Medical Association*, **227**, 207–8.

Clark, A. & Kahler, S.C. (2005) Humans receive skilled care at veterinary school hospital. *Journal of the American Veterinary Medical Association*, **227**, 1382–4.

Clark, D.H. (1994) An analysis of the value of forensic odontology in ten mass disasters. *International Dental Journal*, **44**, 241–50.

Clarke, K.W. & Hall, L.W. (1990) A survey of anaesthesia in small animal practice: AVA/BSAVA report. *Journal of the Association of Veterinary Anaesthetists*, **17**, 4–10.

Clayton Jones, D.G. (2006) Quality of digital X-ray images. *Veterinary Record*, **158**, 31–2.

Clements, R. (2002) *Medical Evidence: A Handbook for Doctors.* RSM, London, UK.

Coburn, H.L., Snary, E.L., Kelly, L.A. & Wooldridge, M. (2005) Qualitative risk assessment of the hazards and risks from wild game. *Veterinary Record*, **157**, 321–2.

Cockcroft, P.D. & Holmes, M.A. (2003) *Handbook of Evidence-based Veterinary Medicine.* Blackwell Publishing, Oxford, UK.

Cocquyt, G., Driessen, B. & Simoens, P. (2005) Variability in the eruption of the permanent incisor teeth in sheep. *Veterinary Record*, **157**, 619–23.

Collar, N.J., Fisher, C.T. & Feare, C.J. (eds) (2003) Why museums matter: avian archives in an age of extinction. *Bulletin of the British Ornithologists' Club Supplement*, 123A; 1–60.

Convention on International Trade in Endangered Species of Wild Fauna and Flora (1980) *Guidelines for Transport and Preparation for Shipment of Live Wild Animals and Plants.* International Union for Conservation of Nature, Gland, Switzerland.

Cooper, J.E. (1967) An unusual case of snakebite. *British Journal of Herpetology*, **4**, 17–18.

Cooper, J.E. (1976) Pets in hospitals. *British Medical Journal*, **1**, 698–700.

Cooper, J.E. (1981) The role and responsibility of zoos: An animal protection viewpoint. *International Journal for the Study of Animal Problems*, **2** (6), 299–304.

Cooper, J.E. (1982) Some aspects of John Hunter's work on the diseases of birds of prey. *Annals of the Royal College of Surgeons of England*, **64**, 345–7.

Cooper, J.E. (1985a) Cats, dogs and caterpillars. *Veterinary Record*, **117**, 135–6.

Cooper, J.E. (1985b) Medico-veterinary collaboration. A review of its importance and relevance, especially in the tropics. *Tropical Doctor*, **15**, 187–91.

Cooper, J.E. (1986) Animals in schools. *Journal of Small Animal Practice*, **27**, 839–50.

Cooper, J.E. (1987) Euthanasia of captive reptiles and amphibians: report of UFAW/WSPA Working Party. *Proceedings of Symposium.* Universities Federation for Animal Welfare, Potter's Bar, UK.

Cooper, J.E. (1989) The Guiding Hand. Foundations of Lower Vertebrate Pathology – The First Edward Elkan Memorial Lecture. *Herpetopathologia*, **1** (1), 1–4.

Cooper, J.E. (1990a) Birds and zoonoses. *Ibis*, **132**, 181–91.

Cooper, J.E. (1990b) A tenderness towards all creatures: paradoxes and portents in wildlife rehabilitation. *Proceedings of the International Wildlife Rehabilitation Council Conference, Washington, D.C.*, pp 4–10.

Cooper, J.E. (1990c) A veterinary approach to leeches. *Veterinary Record*, **127**, 226–8.

Cooper, J.E. (1990d) Euthanasia of invertebrates. *Codes of Practice for the Care of Invertebrates in Captivity*, IWG 2. National Federation of Zoological Gardens of Great Britain and Ireland, London, UK.

Cooper, J.E. (1990e) Invertebrates – an introduction. In: *The Management and Welfare of Invertebrates in Captivity* (ed. N.M. Collins). National Federation of Zoological Gardens of Great Britain and Ireland, London, UK.

Cooper, J.E. (1990f) On the origin of 'veterinary surgeon'. *Journal of the American Veterinary Medical Association*, **197**, 1112.

Cooper, J.E. (1995a) Docking and other practices. *Veterinary Record*, **137**, 51.

Cooper, J.E. (ed) (1995b) Wildlife species for sustainable food production. Special Issue. *Biodiversity and Conservation* **4** (3).

Cooper, J.E. (1995c) Permit problems. *New Scientist*, **149**, 53.

Cooper, J.E. (1996a) Physical injury. In: *Non-infectious Diseases of Wildlife*, 2nd edn (eds A. Fairbrother, L.N. Locke & G.L. Hoff). Iowa State University Press, Ames, Iowa.

Cooper, J.E. (1996b) Parasites and pathogens of non-human primates. *Veterinary Record*, **139**, 48.

Cooper, J.E. (1998a) What is forensic veterinary medicine? Its relevance to the modern exotic animal practice. *Forensic Veterinary Medicine, Seminars in Avian and Exotic Pet Medicine*, 7 (4), 161–5.

Cooper, J.E. (1998b) Minimally invasive health monitoring of wildlife. *Animal Welfare*, 7, 35–44.

Cooper, J.E. (1999a) Avian microbiology. In: *Laboratory Medicine Avian and Exotic Pets* (ed. Alan M. Fudge). W.B. Saunders, Philadelphia and London.

Cooper, J.E. (1999b) Reptilian microbiology. In: *Laboratory Medicine Avian and Exotic Pets* (ed. Alan M. Fudge). W.B. Saunders, Philadelphia and London.

Cooper, J.E. (1999c) Emergency care of invertebrates. *Veterinary Clinics of North America: Exotic Animal Practice*, **1** (1), 251–64.

Cooper, J.E. (2001) Invertebrate anesthesia. *Veterinary Clinics of North America: Exotic Animal Practice*, **4** (1), 57–67.

Cooper, J.E. (2002) *Birds of Prey: Health & Disease*. Blackwell Science, Oxford, UK.

Cooper, J.E. (2003) *Captive Birds in Health and Disease*. World Pheasant Association, Fordingbridge, UK/ Hancock Publishing, Canada.

Cooper, J.E. (2003a) Pathology of exotic species. *Journal of the Caribbean Veterinary Medical Association*, **3** (1), 7–12.

Cooper, J.E. (2003b) Principles of clinical pathology and post-mortem examinations. In: *Manual of Wildlife Casualties* (eds E. Mullineaux, D. Best & J. E. Cooper). British Small Animal Veterinary Association, Gloucester, UK.

Cooper, J.E. (2004a) Information from dead and dying birds. In: *Bird Ecology and Conservation* (eds W.J. Sutherland, I. Newton & R.E. Green). Oxford University Press, UK.

Cooper, J.E. (2004b) Searching the literature. *Veterinary Record*, **155**, 375.

Cooper, J.E. (2004c) The need for portable field kits in improved veterinary diagnosis in the Neotropics. *Proceedings of Third Seminar on Appropriate Medical Technology for Developing Countries*. IEE, London, UK.

Cooper, J.E. (2005) The microbiology of animal bites. *The Bulletin of The Royal College of Pathologists*, **130**, 67.

Cooper, J.E. & Anwar, M.A. (2001) Blood parasites of birds: a plea for more cautious terminology. *Ibis*, **143**, 149–50.

Cooper, J.E. & Cooper, M.E. (1981) The use of animals in films: a veterinary and legal viewpoint. *British Kinematograph Sound and Television Society*, **63**, 544–6.

Cooper, J.E. & Cooper, M.E. (1986) Is this eagle legal? A veterinary approach to litigation involving birds. *Proceedings Forensic Zoology Discussion Group*. Zootechnology, London, UK.

Cooper, J.E. & Cooper, M.E. (1991) Legal cases involving birds: the role of the veterinary surgeon. *Veterinary Record*, **129**, 505–7.

Cooper, J.E. & Cooper, M.E. (1996) Veterinary and legal implications of the use of snakes in traditional dancing in East Africa. *British Herpetological Society Bulletin*, **55**, 29–34.

Cooper, J.E. & Cooper, M.E. (1997) Avian forensic work: guidelines for practitioners. *Proceedings of the European Committee of the Association of Avian Veterinarians (EAAV)*. London, England.

Cooper, J.E. & Cooper, M.E. (eds) (1998) Forensic veterinary medicine. *Seminars in Avian and Exotic Pet Medicine* 7, 4.

Cooper, J.E. & Cooper, M.E. (1999) Forensic studies on wildlife and 'exotic' animals – an overseas perspective. *Proceedings of the International Association of Forensic Sciences, 75th Triennial Meeting August 22–28, 1999, Los Angeles, California, USA*.

Cooper, J.E. & Cooper, M.E. (2001) Legal and ethical aspects of working with wildlife, with particular reference to Africa. *ANZCART News*, **14** (4), 4–5.

Cooper, J.E. & Cooper, M.E. (2004) Veterinary science. In: *Forensic Practice in Criminal Cases* (eds L. Townley and R. Ede). The Law Society, London, UK.

Cooper, J.E. & Cooper, M.E. (2006) Ethical and legal implications of treating casualty wild animals. *In Practice*, **28** (1), 2–6.

Cooper, J.E. & Cunningham, A.A. (1991) Pathological investigation of captive invertebrates. *International Zoo Yearbook*, **30**, 137–43.

Cooper, J.E., Brearley, M.J. & Sullivan, M. (eds) (1991) *Color Atlas of Small Animal Endoscopy*. Mosby Year Book, USA.

Cooper, J.E. & Jackson, O.F. (eds) (1981) *Diseases of the Reptilia*. Academic Press, London, UK.

Cooper, J.E. & Jones, C.G. (1986) A reference collection of endangered Mascarene specimens. *The Linnean*, **2** (3), 32–7.

Cooper, J.E. & Laurie, A. (1987) Investigation of deaths in marine iguanas (*Amblyrhynchus cristatus*) on

Galapagos. *Journal of Comparative Pathology,* **97,** 129–36.

Cooper, J.E. & Samour, J.H. (1997) Portable and field equipment for avian veterinary work. *Proceedings European Committee of AAV (Association of Avian Veterinarians).* London, UK.

Cooper, J.E. & West, C.D. (1988) Radiological studies on endangered Mascarene fauna. *Oryx,* **22,** 18–24.

Cooper, J.E. & Williams, D.L. (1995) Veterinary perspectives and techniques in husbandry and research. In: *Health and Welfare of Captive Reptiles* (eds C. Warwick, F.L. Frye and J.B. Murphy). Chapman and Hall, London, UK.

Cooper, J.E., Dutton, C.J. & Allchurch, A.F. (1998) Reference collections: their importance and relevance to modern zoo management and conservation biology. *Dodo,* **34,** 159–66.

Cooper, J.E., Ewbank, R., Platt, C. & Warwick, C. (eds) (1989a) *Euthanasia of Amphibians and Reptiles.* Report of a Joint UFAW/WSPA Working Party. Universities Federation for Animal Welfare, Potter's Bar and World Society for the Protection of Animals, London, UK.

Cooper, J.E., Gschmeissner, S. & Ion, F. (1989b) The laboratory investigation of feathers. *Proceedings of Second European Symposium on Avian Medicine and Surgery.* University of Utrecht, the Netherlands March 8–11, 1989 (Dutch translation in *Dier en Arts Wetenschappelijke Praktijkgenekte Informatie*), **4,** 102–10.

Cooper, M.E. (1987) *An Introduction to Animal Law.* Academic Press, London, UK.

Cooper, M.E. (1991) British mammals and the law. In: *The Handbook of British Mammals* (eds G.B. Corbet and S. Harris). Blackwell Scientific, Oxford, UK.

Cooper, M.E. (1996) Community responsibility and legal issues. *Seminars in Avian and Exotic Pet Medicine,* **5,** 37–45.

Cooper, M.E. (1998) Birds, exotic animals, and the law. *Seminars in Avian and Exotic Pet Medicine,* **7** (4).

Cooper, M.E. (2002) Legislation. In: *Manual of Exotic Pets* (eds A. Meredith & S. Redrobe). BSAVA Publications, Gloucester, UK.

Cooper, M.E. (2003a) Zoo legislation. *International Zoo Year Book,* **38,** 81–93.

Cooper, M.E. (2003b) The law affecting British wildlife casualties. In: *Manual of Wildlife Casualties* (eds E. Mullineaux, D. Best & J.E. Cooper). British Small Animal Veterinary Association, Gloucester, UK.

Cooper, M.E. & Cooper, J.E. (1988) Legal and ethical provisions. In: *Animals in Science Teaching: A Directory of Audio Visual Alternatives.* British Universities Film and Video Council, London and Universities Federation for Animal Welfare, Potters Bar, UK.

Cooper, M.E. & Cooper, J.E. (1999) Animal law for forensic wildlife work. *Proceedings of the International Association of Forensic Sciences, 75th Triennial Meeting, August 22–28, 1999, Los Angeles, California, USA.*

Cooper, M.E. & Sinclair, D.A. (1990) Wildlife rehabilitation and the law: an introduction. In*: The Proceedings of the Third Symposium of the British Wildlife Rehabilitation Council.* Stoneleigh (1990) (ed. T. Thomas), pp 63–5. British Wildlife Rehabilitation Council, London, UK.

Cooper, T. (2005) Sins of omission and commission. *Proceedings of the Veterinary Association for Arbitration and Jurisprudence* **2** (1), 49–54.

Cork, S.C. & Halliwell, R.W. (2002) *The Veterinary Laboratory and Field Manual: A Guide for Veterinary Laboratory Technicians and Animal Health Advisors.* Nottingham University Press, UK.

Cornelius, E.H. (1978) John Hunter as an expert witness. *Annals of the Royal College of Surgeons of England,* **60** (5), 412–18.

Cornelius, E.H. & Harding Rains, A.J. (1976) *Letters from the Past from John Hunter to Edward Jenner.* The Royal College of Surgeons of England, London, UK.

Corradi, A., Luppi, A., Biagi, G., Signorini, G. & Pittioni, E. (2000) Medico-legal expertise and expert post-mortem examination. *Obiettivi e Documenti Veterinari,* **21** (4), 23–30. [Italian]

Corradi, A., Luppi, A. & Pittioni, E. (2001) Veterinary forensic medicine and firearm lesions: characterization and diagnosis. *Annali della Facoltà di Medicina Veterinaria, Università di Parma,* **21** (3). [Italian]

Cottone, J.A. & Standish, S.M. (eds) (1982) *Outline of Forensic Dentistry.* Yearbook Medical Publishing, Chicago, USA.

Cox, M. (2003) A multidisciplinary approach to the investigation of crimes against humanity, war crimes and genocide: the Inforce Foundation. *Science & Justice,* **43** (4), 225–7.

Cox, M. & Mays, S. (2000) *Human Osteology in Archaeology and Forensic Science.* Greenwich Medical Media, London, UK.

Coyle, H.M. (ed.) (2004) *Forensic Botany: Principles and Applications to Criminal Casework.* CRC Press, Florida, USA/London, UK.

Cramers, T., Mikkelsen, K.B., Enevoldsen, C., Jensen, H.E. & Andersen, P. (2005) New types of foreign bodies and the effect of magnets in traumatic reticulitis in cows. *Veterinary Record,* **157,** 287–9.

Cray, C., Roskos, J. & Zielezienski-Roberts, K. (2005) Detection of cotinine, a nicotine metabolite, in the plasma of birds exposed to second-hand smoke. *Journal of Avian Medicine and Surgery,* **19,** 277–9.

Cross, D. (2005) The expert witness system is coping rather well. *Biologist*, **52** (5), 265.

Crossley, D.A. & Penman, S. (eds) (1995) *Manual of Small Animal Dentistry*. British Small Animal Veterinary Association, Gloucester, UK.

Curnett, J. (2000) *Animals and the Law. A Dictionary*. ABL-CLIO, Santa Barbara, California, USA.

Cyrus, A.C. (1989) *A Clinical and Pathological Atlas: the Records of a Surgeon in St. Vincent, The West Indies*. Dr. A. Cecil Cyrus, St. Vincent, The West Indies.

Cyrus, C. (2005) The Dr Cecil Cyrus Museum: public attitudes to tissue donation for display in St. Vincent. *The Bulletin of The Royal College of Pathologists*, **131**, 44–7.

Dabas, Y.P.S. & Saxena, O.P. (1994) *Veterinary Jurisprudence and Post-mortem*. International Book Distributing, Lucknow, India.

Daéid, N.N. (2003) *Fire Investigation*. Taylor & Francis, London, UK.

Danbury, T.C., Weeks, C.A., Chambers, J.P., Waterman-Pearson, A.E. & Kestin, S.C. (2000) Self-selection of the analgesic drug carprofen by lame broiler chickens. *Veterinary Record*, **146**, 307–11.

David, E.R. (ed.) (1979) *Manchester Museum Mummy Project*. Manchester Museum: Manchester University Press, UK.

David, T.J. (1986) Adjunctive use of scanning electron microscopy in bite mark analysis: a three dimensional study. *Forensic Science*, **31**, 1126–34.

David, T.J. (2005) Child abuse and paediatrics. *Journal of the Royal Society of Medicine*, **98**, 229–31.

Davies, E.B. (1989) The veterinary surgeon as a law enforcement officer. *Veterinary Record*, **124**, 101–2.

Davies, K. (2001) *Understanding European Union Law*. Cavendish Publishing, London, UK.

Davis, B.T. (1974) George Edward Male, MD – The father of English medical jurisprudence. *Proceedings of the Royal Society of Medicine*, **67**, 117–20.

Davis, S.J.M. (1987) *The Archaeology of Animals*. B.T. Batsford, London, UK.

Davison, A.M. (2004) The incised wound. In: *Essentials of Autopsy Practice* (ed. G.N. Rutty). Springer-Verlag, London, UK.

Day, M.G. (1966) Identification of hair and feather remains in the gut and faeces of stoats and weasels. *Journal of Zoology, London*, **148**, 201–17.

Day, R. & Reader, J.A. (2003) *Health, Safety and Environment Legislation*. The Royal Society of Chemistry, London, UK.

DCMS (2003) *Guidance on the Care of Remains in Museums*. Department for Culture, Media and Sport, London, UK.

DEFRA (2003 and continuing) *Zoos Forum Handbook*. Department for Environment, Food and Rural Affairs, Bristol, UK.

DEFRA (2004) *Secretary of State's Standards of Modern Zoo Practice*. Department for Environment, Food and Rural Affairs, London, UK.

de Keuster, T. (2005) Dogbite prevention – how can a blue dog help. *European Journal of Companion Animal Practice*, **15** (2), 136–9.

de Klemm, C. & Shine, C. (1993) *Biological Diversity Conservation and the Law*. IUCN Environmental Policy and the Law, Paper No. 29. IUCN – the World Conservation Union, Gland, Switzerland and Cambridge, UK.

Dennis, T., Start, R.D. & Cross, S.S. (2005) The use of digital imaging, video conferencing, and telepathology in histopathology: a national survey. *Journal of Clinical Pathology*, **58**, 254–8.

Department for Environment, Food and Rural Affairs (various dates,a) Information Sheets (on aspects of the Wildlife and Countryside Act). Department for Environment, Food and Rural Affairs, Bristol, UK.

Department for Environment, Food and Rural Affairs (various dates,b) Guidance Notes (on aspects of the CITES Regulations). Department for Environment, Food and Rural Affairs, Bristol, UK.

Department of Health, Chief Medical Officer, Department for Education and Employment & Home Office (2001) *The Removal, Retention and Use of Human Organs and Tissue from Post-Mortem Examination: Advice from the Chief Medical Officer*. Stationery Office, London, UK.

Department of the Environment (1996) *Wildlife Crime: A Guide to Wildlife Law Enforcement in the UK*. The Stationery Office, London, UK.

Department of the Environment (1997) *Wildlife Crime: Using DNA Forensic Evidence*. London, UK.

Department of the Environment (1998) *Proceedings of the EU Wildlife Law Enforcement Workshop*. The Stationery Office, London, UK.

Department of the Environment (2004) *Wildlife Crime: Proceedings of the Wildlife Inspectors' Seminar*. Redwood Lodge, Bristol.

De Vore, D.T. (1977) Radiology and photography in forensic dentistry. *Dental Clinics of North America*, **21**, 69–83.

Dhammika, V.S. (1993) *The Edicts of King Ashoka*. Bhuddist Publication Society, Kandy, Sri Lanka.

Dhammika, V.S. (1994) *The Edicts of King Ashoka*. DharmaNet edn. DharmaNet International http://www.cs.colostate.edu/~malaiya/ashoka.html. Also available as (Dhammika, 1993) above.

Diaz, D. (ed.) (2005) *The Mycotoxin Blue Book*. Nottingham University Press, UK.

Dierauf, L.A. & Gulland, F.M.D. (eds) (2001) *CRC Handbook of Marine Mammal Medicine*, 2nd edn. CRC Press, Florida, USA/London, UK.

DiMaio, V.J.M. (1999) *Gunshot Wounds: Practical Aspects of Firearms, Ballistics, and ForensicTechniques*, 2nd edn. CRC Press, Florida, USA/London, UK.

DiMaio, V.J.M. & DiMaio, D.J. (2001) *Forensic Pathology*, 2nd edn. CRC Press, Florida, USA/London, UK.

Dinkel, E.H. & Captain, M.S. (1976) The use of bite mark evidence as an investigative aid. *Journal of Forensic Science*, **19** (3), 535–46.

Disney, H. (2002) Fraudulent forensic scientists. *Journal de Médecine Légale Droit Médical*, **45**, 230.

Disney, H. (2006) The expert witness system. *Biologist*, **53**, 9–10.

Dix, J. (2000) *Color Atlas of Forensic Pathology*. CRC Press, Florida, USA/London, UK.

Doherr, M.E. (2003) Bovine spongiform encephalopathy (BSE) – infectious, contagious, zoonotic or production disease? *Acta Veterinaria Scandinavica*, Supplement 98, 33–42.

Dolente, B.A., Beech, J., Lindborg, S. & Smith, G. (2005) Evaluation of risk. Factors for development of catheter-associated jugular thrombophlebitis in horses: 50 cases (1993–1998). *Journal of the American Veterinary Medical Association*, **227** (7), 1134–41.

Dolinak, D., Matshes, E. & Lew, E.O. (2005) *Forensic Pathology. Principles and Practice*. Elsevier, Oxford, UK.

Dorion, R.B.J. (1987) Transillumination in bite mark evidence. *Forensic Science*, **32**, 690–97.

Dorland, W.A.N. (2000) *Dorland's Illustrated Medical Dictionary*. W.B. Saunders, Philadelphia, USA.

Draper, G., Vincent, T., Kroll, M.E. & Swanson, J. (2005) Childhood cancer in relation to distance from high voltage power lines in England and Wales: a case-control study. *British Medical Journal*, **330**, 1290–3.

Drobatz, K.J. & Smith, G. (2003) Evaluation of risk factors for bite wounds inflicted on caregivers by dogs and cats in a veterinary teaching hospital. *Journal of the American Veterinary Medical Association*, **223**, 312–16.

Dubner, R. (1994) Methods of assessing pain in animals. In: *Textbook of Pain*, 3rd edn (eds P.D. Wall & R. Melsack). Churchill-Livingstone, Edinburgh, UK.

Duff, J.P. & Hunt, B.W. (1995) Courtship and mortality in foxes (*Vulpes vulpes*). *Veterinary Record*, **136**, 367.

Duhig, C. (2003) Non-forensic remains: the use of forensic archaeology, anthropology and burial taphonomy. *Science & Justice*, **43** (4), 211–14.

Durnford, T. (2005) What the Trading Standards Office expects of its witnesses. *Proceedings of the Veterinary Association for Arbitration and Jurisprudence*, **2** (1), 9–10.

Durrant, G.R. (2002) Bioterrorism: the current threat. *Journal of the Royal Society of Medicine*, **95**, 609–11.

Durrell, G. (1982) *The Amateur Naturalist*. Hamish Hamilton, London, UK.

Dye, J.A. & Costa, D.L. (1995) A brief guide to indoor air pollutants and relevance to small animals. In: *Kirk's Current Veterinary Therapy XII: Small Animal Practice*. W.B. Saunders, Philadelphia, USA.

Echols, S. (ed.) (2003) Practical gross necropsy of exotic animal species. *Seminars in Avian and Exotic Pet Medicine*, **12** (2).

Edmondson, P. (2002) Advice on writing expert reports. *Veterinary Times*, 16 September 2002, 28–30.

Edworthy, S.M. (2001) Telemedicine in developing countries. *British Medical Journal*, **323** (7312), 524–5.

Elkan, E. (1981) Pathology and histopathological techniques. In: *Diseases of the Reptilia* (eds J.E. Cooper & O.F. Jackson). Academic Press, London, UK.

Ellen, D. (1997) *The Scientific Examination of Documents*. Taylor & Francis, London, UK.

Elliott, O. & Scott, J.P. (1961) The development of emotional distress reactions to separation in puppies. *Journal of Genetic Psychology*, **99**, 3–22.

Ellison, G.T.H. (1990) The effect of scavenger mutilation on insect succession of impala carcasses in southern Africa. *Journal of Zoology, London*, **220**, 679–88.

Emes, A. & Price, C. (2004) Bloodstain pattern analysis. In: *Crime Scene to Court. The Essentials of Forensic Science* (ed. P.C. White), 2nd edn. The Royal Society of Chemistry, Cambridge, UK.

Ennion, E.A.R. & Tinbergen, N. (1967) *Tracks*. Oxford University Press, UK.

Eppler, J.T. & Lubjuhn, T. (eds) (1999) *DNA Profiling and DNA Fingerprinting*. Birkhaüser Verlag, Basel, Switzerland.

Epstein, R. (undated) *Religious Thought about Animals*. http://online.sfsu.edu/~rone/Religion/religionanimals.html

Erb, E., Shaughnessy, P.D. & Norman, R. J. de B. (1996) Dental and mandibular injury in an Antarctic fur seal, *Arctocephalus gazelle*, at Heard Island, Southern Ocean. *Journal of Wildlife Diseases*, **32** (2), 376–80.

Errol, J. (1971) *Moon on a Rainbow Shawl*. Faber, London, UK.

Erwin, J.M. & Hof, P.R. (eds) (2002) *Aging in Nonhuman Primates*. Karger, Basel, Switzerland.

Erzinclioglu, Z. (1998) British forensic science in the dock. *Nature*, **392**, 859–60.

Erzinclioglu, Z. (2000a) Q&A. *Antenna*, **24**, 276–7.

Erzinclioglu, Z. (2000b) *Maggots, Murder and Men: Memories and Reflections of a Forensic Entomologist*. Harley Books, Colchester, UK.

EU (1997a) *Treaty of Amsterdam Amending the Treaty on European Union, the Treaties Establishing The European Communities and Related Acts*. Official Journal C340, 10 November 1997 (http://europa.eu/eur-lex/en/treaties/dat/amsterdam.html).

EU (1997b) *Protocol on Protection and Welfare of Animals*. http://europa.eu/eur-lex/en/treaties/dat/amsterdam.html#0110010013 and http://www.eurotreaties.com/amsterdamprotocols.pdf, p. 17.

European Commission (2000) *Preliminary Opinion. Oral Exposure of Humans to the BSE Agent: Infective Dose and Species Barrier*. EC Steering Committee, Brussels, Belgium.

EWI (2004) Expert across Europe. *Your Witness*, Issue 36. J S Publications, Newmarket, UK.

Fackler, M.L. (1988) Ballistic injury. *Annals of Emergency Medicine*, **15**, 1451–5.

Fain, S. & LeMay, J. (1995) DNA analysis and wildlife forensic genetics: Identifying species, gender and individuals. In: *Forensic DNA Technology* (eds M. Farley & I. Kobilinsky). American Chemical Society, Washington, D.C., USA.

Fang ShengGuo & Wan QuiHong (2002) A genetic fingerprinting test for identifying carcasses of protected deer species in China. *Biological Conservation*, **103** (3), 371–3.

Farr, S. (1788) *Elements of Medical Jurisprudence*. London, UK.

Farrel, W.L., Rawson, R.D., Steffens, R.S. & Stephens, D. (1987) Computerised axial tomography as an aid in bite mark analysis: a case report. *Forensic Science*, **32**, 266–72.

Fatjó, J., Stub, C. & Manteca, X. (2002) Four cases of aggression and hypothyroidism in dogs. *Veterinary Record*, **151**, 547–8.

Favre, D.S. & Loring, M. (1983) *Animal Law*. Quorum Books, Connecticut, London.

FAWC (2001) *Interim Report on the Animal Welfare Implications of Farm Assurance Schemes*. Farm Animal Welfare Council, London, UK.

Fearon, R. (2006) Profession faces ugly truth. *Veterinary Times*, 26 June 2006, **36**.

Feder, H.A. (1991) *Succeeding as an Expert Witness*. Van Nostrand Reinhold, New York, USA.

Fedun, I. (1995) Fatal light attraction. *Journal of Wildlife Rehabilitation*, **18** (3), 10–11.

Feineis, E.F. (2002) *Manuel de la Protection des Animaux*. Protection Suisse des Animaux. Switzerland. http://www.protection-animaux.com/publikationen/diverse/infothek/texte/handbuch.pdf

Felthous, A.R. (1980) Aggression against cats, dogs and people. *Child Psychiatry and Human Development*, **10** (3), 169–77.

Felthous, A.R. (1981) Childhood cruelty to cats, dogs and other animals. *Bulletin of the American Academy of Psychiatric Law*, **8** (2), 48–53.

Felthous, A.R. & Bernard, H. (1979) Firesetting and cruelty to animals: The significance of two thirds of this triad. *Forensic Sciences*, **29** (1), 240–6.

Fenner, P.I., Williamson, J.A. & Skinner, R.A. (1989) Fatal and non-fatal stingray envenomation. *Medical Journal of Australia*, **151**, 621–25.

Fergusson, R. (2004) Human–crocodile conflicts. *Newsletter of the IUCN, SSC, Crocodile Specialist Group* **23** (4), 20–3.

Ferlini, R. (2003) The development of human rights investigations since 1945. *Science & Justice*, **43** (4), 219–24.

Fernando, P., Wikramanayake, E., Weerakoon, D., Jayasinghe, L.K.A., Gunawardere, M. & Janaka, H.K. (2005) Perceptions and patterns of human–elephant conflict in old and new settlements in Sri Lanka: insights for mitigation and management. *Biodiversity and Conservation*, **14**, 2465–81.

Ferner, R.E., Norman, E. & Rawlins, M.D. (1996) *Forensic Pharmacology: Medicines, Mayhem, and Malpractice*. Oxford University Press, Oxford, UK.

Field-Fisher, T.G. (1964) *Animals and the Law*. The Universities Federation for Animal Welfare (UFAW), London, UK.

Filer, J. (1995) *Disease*. Egyptian Bookshelf. BM Press, London, UK.

Finnie, J.W. & Blumbergs, P.C. (2002) Animal models: traumatic brain injury. *Veterinary Pathology*, **39**, 679–89.

Flaherty, D. & Musk, G. (2005) Anaesthetic monitoring equipment for small animals. *In Practice*, **27** (10), 512–21.

Flemming, D.D. (2004) Dog bites veterinarian: the legal issue. *Journal of the American Veterinary Medical Association*, **225** (5), 695–7.

Flemming, D.D. & Scott, J.F. (2004) The informed consent doctrine: what veterinarians should tell their clients. *Vet Med Today: Veterinary Medicine and the Law*, *JAVMA*, **224** (9), 1436.

Florence, L. & Reilly, P. (2003) Assessing the Strasser method: the perspective of two farriers at referral veterinary hospitals. *Journal of Equine Veterinary Science*, **23** (11), 502–5.

Floro, C.D., Samways, M.J. & Armstrong, B. (2004) Taxonomic patterns of bleaching within a South African coral assemblage. *Biodiversity and Conservation*, **13**, 1175–94.

Flower, M. (2005) What the RSPCA expects of its witnesses. *Proceedings of the Veterinary Association for Arbitration and Jurisprudence*, **2** (1), 11–12.

Forbes, N. (2004) An exacting science: the veterinary surgeon as expert witness. *In Practice*, **26**, 503–6.

Forbes, N.A. (1998) Clinical examination of the avian forensic case. *Seminars in Avian and Exotic Pet Medicine*, 7, 4.

Forbes, T. (1981) Early forensic medicine in England: the Angus murder trial. *Journal of the History of Medicine and Allied Sciences*, **36** (3), 296–309.

Foreman, D.M. & Farsides, C. (1993) Ethical use of covert videoing techniques in detecting Munchausen syndrome by proxy. *British Medical Journal*, **370**, 611–13.

Forrest, R. (2001) Reform of the Criminal Justice System in England and Wales. *Science & Justice*, **41** (4), 237.

Forrest, R. (2004) Whither academic forensic science? *Science & Justice*, **44** (1), 105.

Fowler, M.E. (1978) *Restraint and Handling of Wild and Domestic Animals.* Iowa State University Press, Ames, USA.

Fox, H. (1923) *Disease in Captive Wild Mammals.* J.B. Lippincott, Philadelphia, USA.

Fox, M.W. (2001) *Bringing Life to Ethics: Global Bioethics for a Humane Society.* State University of New York Press, USA.

Fox, M.W. & Mickley, L.D. (eds) (1986/87) *Advances in Animal Welfare Science.* Humane Society of the United States.

Fox, N., Blay, N., Greenwood, A.G., Wise, D. & Potapov, E. (2005) Wounding rates in shooting foxes (*Vulpes vulpes*). *Animal Welfare*, **14**, 93–102.

Francione, G.L. (1995) *Animals, Property and the Law.* Temple University Press, USA.

Franklin, C.J. (1999) *Law for the Expert Witness*, 2nd edn. Taylor and Francis Group, New York, USA.

Fraser, A.F. & Broom, D.M. (1990) *Farm Animal Behaviour and Welfare.* Baillière Tindall, London, UK.

French, M.C., Haines, C.W. & Cooper, J. (1987) Investigation into the effects of ingestion of zinc shot by mallard ducks (*Anas platyrhynchos*). *Environmental Pollution*, **47**, 305–14.

Froede, R.C. (1997) *The Scientific Witness in Court. Principles and Guidelines.* AACC Press, Washington, D.C., USA.

Frye, F.L. (1999) Establishing the time of death in reptiles and amphibians. *Proceedings of the Association of Reptilian and Amphibian Veterinarians*, pp 23–5.

Frye, F.L., Cooper, J.E. & Keymer, I.F. (2001) Outfitting and employing a compact field laboratory. *The Bulletin of the British Veterinary Zoological Society*, **1** (2).

Gallop, A. & Stockdale, R. (2004) Trace and contact evidence. In: *Crime Scene to Court. The Essentials of Forensic Science* (ed. P.C. White), 2nd edn. The Royal Society of Chemistry, Cambridge, UK.

George, I. (2005) If only fireworks were silent. *Veterinary Times*, 21 November 2005, pp 10–11.

Geraci, J.R. & Lounsbury, V.J. (2005) *Marine Mammals Ashore: A Field Guide for Strandings.* National Aquarium, Baltimore, MD, USA.

Gerhards, A.U. (2002) Eye examination in the scope of horse purchase examination: proposal for a standardised examination protocol. *Pferdeheilkunde*, **18**, 297–8. [German]

Gibbs, E.P.J. (2005) Emerging zoonotic epidemics in the interconnected global community. *Veterinary Record*, **157**, 673–9.

Gilbert-Barness, E. & Debich-Spicer, D.E. (2004) *Handbook of Pediatric Autopsy Pathology.* Humana Press, USA.

Giles, A. (2004) The forensic examination of documents. In: *Crime Scene to Court. The Essentials of Forensic Science* (ed. P.C. White), 2nd edn. The Royal Society of Chemistry, Cambridge, UK.

Giles, N. & Simmons, J.R. (1975) Electrocution of pigs. *Veterinary Record*, **97**, 305–6.

Gillett, K.E. & Blake, B.H. (1985) Chipmunks. In: *Manual of Exotic Pets* (eds J.E. Cooper & M.F. Hutchison). British Small Animal Veterinary Association, Gloucester, UK.

Gilligan, B. (2002) *Practical Horse Law. A Guide for Owners and Riders.* Blackwell, Oxford, UK.

Gilpin, A. (2000) *Dictionary of Environmental Law.* Edward Elgar, Cheltenham, UK.

Gippoliti, S. (2005) Historical museology meets tropical biodiversity conservation. *Biodiversity and Conservation*, **14**, 3127–34.

Glaser, C.A., Angulo, F.J. & Roosey, J.A. (1994) Animal-associated opportunistic infections among persons infected with the human immunodeficiency virus. *Clinical Infection and Disease*, **18**, 14–24.

Glass, R.T., Jordan, F.B. & Andrews, E.E. (1975) Multiple animal bite wounds: a case report. *Forensic Science*, **62**, 305–14.

Glatz, P.C. (ed.) (2005) *Poultry Welfare Issues: Beak Trimming.* Nottingham University Press, UK.

Gloor, K.T., Winget, G.D. & Swanson, W.F. (2005) Conservation science in a terrorist age: the impact of airport security screening on viability and DNA integrity of frozen felid spermatozoa. *Proceedings of AAZW, AAWV and AZA/NAG Joint Conference 2005*, pp 238–9.

Goff, M.L. (2000) *A Fly for the Prosecution: How Insect Evidence Helps Solve Crimes.* Harvard College, USA.

Goff, M.L., Omori, A.I. & Goodbrod, J.R. (1989) Effects of cocaine in tissues on the development rate of *Boettcherisca peregrine* (Diptera: Sancophagidae). *Journal of Medical Entomology*, **26**, 91–3.

Gomes, L., Zuben, C.J. & von Govone, J.S. (2002) Behaviour of postfeeding radial larval dispersion in blowflies of genus Chrysomya (Diptera: Calliphoridae): search for new food resources. *Entomologia y Vectores*, **9** (1), 115–32. [Portuguese]

Gonczi, G. (2003) The story of a veterinary malpractice lawsuit. *KisallatPraxis. BetuVet, Budapest, Hungary*, **4** (4), 204–9. [Hungarian]

Gorrel, C. (2004) *Veterinary Dentistry for the General Practitioner.* W.B. Saunders, Philadelphia, USA.

Gosler, A. (2004) Birds in the hand. In: *Bird Ecology and Conservation* (eds W.J. Sutherland, I. Newton & R.E. Green). Oxford University Press, UK.

Gotch, A.F. (1979) *Mammals – Their Latin Names Explained.* Blandford Press, Poole, UK.

Graham, D.I. & Gennarelli, T.A. (2000) Pathology of brain damage after injury. In: *Head Injury*, 4th edn (eds P.R. Cooper & J.G. Golfinos). McGraw-Hill, NY, USA.

Graham, S. (1996) Issues of surplus animals. In: *Wild Mammals in Captivity* (eds D.E. Kleiman, M.E. Allen, K.V. Thompson & S. Lumpkin). University of Chicago Press, USA.

Green, P.D. (1979) Protocols in medicolegal veterinary medicine 1. Identification of cases and preparation for court. *Canadian Veterinary Journal*, **20**, 8–12.

Green, P.C. & Gullone, E. (2005) Knowledge and attitudes of Australian veterinarians to animal abuse and human inter-personal violence. *Australian Veterinary Journal*, **83** (10), 619–25.

Green, S.L., Moorhead, R.C. & Bouley, D.M. (2003) Thermal shock in a colony of South African clawed frogs (*Xenopus laevis*). *Veterinary Record*, **152**, 336–7.

Greenberg, B. (1991) Flies as forensic indicators. *Journal of Medical Entomology*, **28**, 565–77.

Gregory, N. (2004) *Physiology and Behaviour of Animal Suffering.* UFAW/Blackwell, Oxford, UK.

Gregory, N.E., Gepp, M.J. & Babidge, P.J. (2005) Method for checking label accuracy in barn and free range eggs. *Journal of the Science of Food and Agriculture*, **85**, 1421–6.

Gregory, N.G. & Constantine, E. (1996) Hyperthermia in dogs left in cars. *Veterinary Record*, **139**, 349–50.

Gregory, S. (2005) How good is your hand hygiene? *In Practice*, **27**, 178–80.

Gresham, G.A. (1975) *A Colour Atlas of Forensic Pathology.* Wolfe, the Netherlands.

Griffiths, C.S. & Bates, J.M. (2002) Morphology, genetics and the value of voucher specimens: an example with *Cathartes* vultures. *Journal of Raptor Research*, **36** (3), 183–7.

Griffiths, I. (2005) Postmortem examination of cattle and sheep. *In Practice*, **27**, 458–65.

Grove, N. & Raymer, S. (1981) Wild cargo: the business of smuggling animals. *National Geographic*, **159** (3), 286–315.

Grove, W.R. (1943) Rex V. Donellan, Warwick Assizes 1781. *The Medico-legal and Criminological Review*, **2**, 314–39.

Grubb, T.G. & Bowerman, W.W. (1997) Variations in breeding bald eagle responses to nets, light planes and helicopters. *Journal of Raptor Research*, **31**, 213–22.

Gunn, A. (2006) *Essential Forensic Biology.* John Wiley & Sons, Bognor Regis, UK.

Guthrie, M. (1989) *Animals of the Surface Film.* The Company of Biologists, Cambridge, UK.

Guy, R.J. (2004) Shell shock. *Journal of the Royal Society of Medicine*, **97**, 255.

Hadlow, W.J. (1997) Dubbing animal diseases with color. *Veterinary Pathology*, **34**, 74–8.

Haglund, W.D. & Sorg, M.H. (1996) *Forensic Taphonomy.* CRC Press, Florida, USA.

Hailey, A. (2000) Assessing body mass condition in the tortoise *Testudo hermanni. Herpetological Journal*, **10**, 57–61.

Hale, A. (1978) The admissibility of bite mark evidence. *Southern California Law Review*, **51**, 309–34.

Halinen, K., Kullula, M., Alitalo, I. & Sukura, A. (2002) What is veterinary forensic medicine? *Suomen Elainlaakarilehti. Suomen Elainlaakariliitto*, **108** (5), 273–7. [Finnish]

Hall, D.M.B. (2006) The future of child protection. *Journal of the Royal Society of Medicine*, **99**, 6–9.

Hall, J.G. (1992) *The Expert Witness.* Barry Rose Law Publishers, Chichester, UK.

Hall, M. & Donovan, S. (2001) What can maggots tell us about murders? *Biologist*, **48** (6).

Hamilton, A.C. (2004) Medicinal plants, conservation and livelihoods. *Biodiversity and Conservation*, **13**, 1477–1517.

Hansen, P.J. (1990) Effects of coat colour on physiological responses to solar radiation in Holsteins. *Veterinary Record*, **127**, 333–4.

Harbison, S.A., Hamilton, J.F. & Walsh, S.J. (2001) The New Zealand DNA databank: its development and significance as a crime solving tool. *Science & Justice*, **41** (1), 33–7.

Harcourt, R.A. (1971) The palaeopathology of animal skeletal remains. *Veterinary Record*, **89**, 267–72.

Harris, D. & Haboudi, N. (2005) Malnutrition screening in the elderly population. *Journal of the Royal Society of Medicine*, **98**, 411–14.

Harris, J.M. (1997) Court appearances: expert witness, defendant, plaintiff. *Proceedings of the Association of Avian Veterinarians, Australian Committee, Perth, Australia.*

Harris, J.M. (1998) The role of the practicing veterinarian as an expert witness. *Seminars in Avian and Exotic Pet Medicine*, **7** (4), 176–81.

Harvey, C.E. (1985) *Veterinary Dentistry*. W.B. Saunders, Philadelphia, USA.

Harwood, D. (2004) Alimentary tract perforation in cattle caused by tyre wire. *Veterinary Record*, **154**, 574–5.

Haughey, K.G. (1973) Cold injury in newborn lambs. *Australian Veterinary Journal*, **49**, 554–63.

Havard, J.D.J. (1960) *The Detection of Secret Homicide.* Macmillan, London, UK.

Havel, D.A. (1985) The role of photography in the presentation of bite mark evidence. *Biological Photography*, **53**, 59–62.

Hayes, A. (2005) Safe use of anticancer chemotherapy in small animal practice. *In Practice*, **27**, 118–27.

Hayward, J. (2004) National Theft Register. *Annual Report of the British and Irish Association of Zoos and Aquariums 2004*, p. 19.

Health and Safety Commission (1985) *Zoos – Safety, Health and Welfare Standards for Employers and Persons at Work.* Approved Code of Practice and Guidance Notes. HMSO, London, UK.

Heath, S. (2005) Why do dogs bite? *European Journal of Companion Animal Practice*, **15** (2), 129–32.

Heath, S.E. (1999) *Animal Management in Disasters.* Mosby, St. Louis, USA.

Heidenreich, M. (1997) *Birds of Prey – Medicine and Management.* Blackwell, Oxford, UK.

Heisler, M., Moreno, A., DeMonner, S., Keller, A. & Iacopino, V. (2003) Assessment of torture and ill treatment of detainees in Mexico: attitudes and experiences of forensic physicians. *Journal of the American Medical Association*, **289** (16), 2135–43.

Hektoen, L. (2005) Review of the current involvement of homeopathy in veterinary practice and research. *Veterinary Record*, **157**, 224–9.

Hellebrekers, L.J. (ed.) (2000) *Animal Pain.* Van der Vees, Utrecht, the Netherlands.

Hellman, D.S. & Blackman, N. (1966) Enuresis, firesetting and cruelty to animals: A triad predictive of adult crime. *American Journal of Psychiatry*, **122**, 1431–5.

Henry, J. (2004) Computer based media. In: *Crime Scene to Court. The Essentials of Forensic Science* (ed. P.C. White), 2nd edn. The Royal Society of Chemistry, Cambridge, UK.

Henssge, C., Knight, B., Krompecher, T., Madea, B. & Nokes, L. (2002) *The Estimation of the Time Since Death In the Early Post Mortem Period*, 2nd edn. Arnold, London, UK.

Hertsch, B. (2004) Influences of clinical and radiological findings on the total evaluation of a horse in a pre-purchase examination. *Praktische Tierarzt*, **85** (6), 410–16. [German]

Hesse, B. & Wapnish, P. (1985) *Animal Bone Archaeology.* Taraxacum, Washington, D.C., USA.

Heyer, W.R., Donnelly, M.A., McDiarmid, R.W., Hayek, L-A.C. & Foster, M.S. (eds) (1994) *Measuring and Monitoring Biological Diversity. Standard Methods for Amphibians.* Smithsonian Institution Press, Washington, USA/London, UK.

Hilbeck, A. & Andow, D. (eds) (2005) *Environmental Risk Assessment of Genetically Modified Organisms. Volume I: A Case Study of Bt Maize in Kenya.* CABI Publishing, Oxfordshire, UK.

Hirsch, S.R. & Harris, J. (eds) (1988) *Consent and the Incompetent Patient: Ethics, Law, and Medicine.* Gaskell (The Royal College of Psychiatrists), London, UK.

Hladik, G. & Mosing, M. (2002) Purchase examination and horse buying in Austria. *Pferdeheilkunde. Hippiatrika*, **18** (3), 292–4. [German]

Hodgkinson, T. (1990) *Expert Evidence: Law and Practice.* Sweet & Maxwell, London, UK.

Hodgkinson, T. & James, M. (2006) *Expert Evidence: Law and Practice.* Sweet & Maxwell, London, UK.

Holden, J. (1998) *By Hook or by Crook – a Reference Manual on Illegal Wildlife Trade and Prosecutions in the United Kingdom.* Elphick Colour Print, Bedford, UK.

Holmes, M. & Cockcroft, P. (2004) Evidence-based veterinary medicine 3. Appraising the evidence. *In Practice*, **26**, 154–64.

Holmstrom, S.E. (2000) *Veterinary Dentistry for the Technician & Office Staff.* W.B. Saunders, Philadelphia, USA.

Holmstrom, S.E., Frost, P. & Gammon, R.L. (1992) *Veterinary Dental Techniques for the Small Animal Practitioner.* W.B. Saunders, Philadelphia, USA.

Holt, J.K. (1980) Identification from bitemarks. *Journal of the Forensic Science Society*, **20**, 247–50.

Holton, L.L., Scott, E.M., Nolan, A.M., Reid, J., Welsh, E. & Flaherty, D. (1998) Comparison of three methods of pain scoring used to assess clinical pain in dogs.

Journal of the American Veterinary Association, **212**, 61–5.

Holton, L., Reid, J., Scott, E.M., Pawson, P. & Nolan, A.M. (2001) Development of a behaviour-based scale to measure acute pain in dogs. *Veterinary Record*, **148**, 525–31.

Horsnell, M. (2004) I lied over murder on safari trip, pathologist tells inquest. *The Times*, 27 April.

Horswell, J. (2003) *The Practice of Crime Scene Investigation*. Taylor & Francis, London, UK.

House of Commons Science and Technology Committee (2005) *Forensic Science on Trial*. House of Commons Science and Technology Committee 7th Report, Session 2004/2005. http://www.publications.parliament.uk/pa/cm200405/cmselect/cmsctech/96/96i.pdf

Huber, R.A. & Headrick, A.M. (1999) *Handwriting Identification: Facts and Fundamentals*. CRC Press, Florida, USA/London, UK.

Hue, S. (2005) Methods of assessing the well-being of laboratory fish. *Resource, Canadian Council on Animal Care*, **28** (1), 7.

Hulsenbusch, M. (2005) Consequences of the judgment of the Federal Constitutional Court on dangerous dogs (special issue: Animal Welfare). *Deutsche Tierärztliche Wochenschrift*, **12** (3), 98–9. [German]

Hume, C.W. (1951) *The Religious Attitude towards Animals*. Paper read at the World Congress of Faiths, 1951. The Universities Federation for Animal Welfare, London, UK.

Humphrey, J.H. & Hutchinson, D.L. (2001) Characteristics of hacking trauma. *Forensic Science*, **46** (920), 228–33.

Hunter, J. (undated,a) *Cases and Dissections*. Manuscript number 59. Clift Transcripts. Vol. V:133–6. Royal College of Surgeons of England Library, London, UK.

Hunter, J. (undated,b) *Dissections of Morbid Bodies*. Manuscript number 33. Clift Transcripts. Vol. 111.211. Royal College of Surgeons of England Library, London, UK.

Hunter, J. (1794) *A Treatise on the Blood, Inflammation and Gun Shot Wounds*. G. Nicholl, London, UK.

Hunter, W. (1783) *On the Uncertainty of the Signs of Murder in the Case of Bastard Children*. London, UK.

IATA (Annual) *Live Animals Regulations*. International Air Transport Association, Geneva, Switzerland and Montreal, Canada.

Iburg, U. (2000) Practical problems concerning the criminal law of prevention of cruelty to animals. *Deutsche Tierärztliche Wochenschrift*, **107** (3), 88–91. [German]

ICAZ (2000) *Veterinary Palaeopathology Working Group Second Meeting Timetable, Abstracts and Information*. University of Sheffield, June 2000.

Ide, R. (2004) Fire investigation. In: *Crime Scene to Court. The Essentials of Forensic Science*, 2nd edn (ed. P.C. White). The Royal Society of Chemistry, Cambridge, UK.

IFAW (2005) *Caught in the Web: Wildlife Trade on the Internet*. International Fund for Animal Welfare, London, UK.

Iggo, A. (1984) *Pain in Animals*. UFAW, Potters Bar, UK.

Ikram, S. & Dodson, A. (1998) *The Mummy in Ancient Egypt: Equipping the Dead for Eternity*. Thames and Hudson, UK.

Imrie, F. & Lord, J. (1998) Biologists in the witness box. *Biologist*, **45**, 62–6.

Inman, K. & Rudin, N. (2001) *Principles and Practice of Criminalistics. The Profession of Forensic Science*. CRC Press, Florida, USA/London/UK.

Institute of Biology (2004) *Code of Conduct & Guide on Ethical Practice*. Institute of Biology, London, UK.

Irwin, M. (2005) An inspector calls – checking up on health and safety. *In Practice*, **27**, 337–79.

Isitor, G.N. & Cooper, J.E. (2004) Observations on the nuclear chromatin pattern in cells of a case of canine circumanal gland adenoma in Trinidad. *Journal of the Caribbean Veterinary Medical Association*, **4** (2), 3–10.

Ivanusa, T. & Pogacnik, M. (2001) Radiological diagnostics and forensic of canine hip dysplasia. *Slovenian Veterinary Research*, **38** (4), 305–18.

Jack, D.C. (2000) Horns of dilemma: the vetri-legal implications of animal abuse. *Canadian Veterinary Journal*, **41** (9), 715–20.

Jack, D.C. (2005) North American view – ownership v guardianship and other matters. *Proceedings of the Veterinary Association for Arbitration and Jurisprudence*, **2** (1), 69–72.

Jackson, O.F. (1980) Weight and measurement data on tortoises (*Testudo graeca* and *Testudo hermanni*) and their relationship to health. *Journal of Small Animal Practice*, **21**, 409–16.

James, S.H. & Eckert, W.G. (1998) *Interpretation of Bloodstain Evidence at Crime Scenes*, 2nd edn. CRC Press, Florida, USA/London, UK.

James, S.H. & Nordby, J.J. (2002) *Forensic Science – An Introduction to Scientific and Investigative Techniques*. CRC Press, Florida, USA/London, UK.

Jarrette, Z.D. (2005) Pelican fever. Wardens pounce on poachers in Icacos. *Trinidad Guardian*, Tuesday, April 26.

Jarvie, J.K. (1976) The preparation of models of teeth and bite-marks in food and on bodies. In: *Dental Identifica-*

tion and Forensic Odontology (ed. W. Harvey). Kimpton, London, UK.

Jeffree, R.A., Markich, S.J. & Tucker, A.D. (2005) Patterns of metal accumulation in osteoderms of the Australian freshwater crocodile *Crocodylus johnstoni*. *Science of the Total Environment*, **336**, 71–80.

Jepson, P.D., Bennett, P.M., Deaville, R., Allchin, C.R., Baker, J.R. & Law, R.J. (2005) Relationships between polychlorinated biphenyls and health status in harbor porpoises (*Phocoena phocoena*) stranded in the United Kingdom. *Environmental Toxicology and Chemistry*, **24**, 238–48.

Johnson, B.J. (2001) Handling forensic necropsy cases (Toxicology). *Veterinary Clinics of North America, Equine Practice*, **17** (3), 411–18.

Jones, D.M. (ed.) (2002) *Human Bones from Archaeological Sites*. Centre for Archaeology Guidelines for Producing Assessment Documents and Analytical Reports, English Heritage, London, UK.

Jones, L. & Marshall, M. (2004) Explosions. In: *Crime Scene to Court. The Essentials of Forensic Science*, 2nd edn (ed. P.C. White). The Royal Society of Chemistry, Cambridge, UK.

Jukic, D., Patel, A.A. & BT.cich, M.J. (2005) The digital future of histopathology: where we are today and where we are heading. *The Bulletin of The Royal College of Pathologists*, **131**, 27–31.

Jung, K., Ha, S.-K., Chung, H.-K., *et al.* (2003) Archival PCR-based diagnosis of *Clostridium difficile* in piglets. *Veterinary Record*, **153**, 466–7.

Kahler, S.C. & Clark, A. (2005) Animal welfare, state advocacy initiating approved. *Journal of the American Veterinary Medical Association*, **226**, 1623–7.

Kahn, A., Bauche, P. & Lamoureux, J. (2003) Child victims of dog bites treated in emergency departments: a prospective survey. *European Journal of Pediatrics*, **162**, 254–8.

Kaiser, L., Heleski, C.R., Siegford, J. & Smith, K.A. (2006) Stress-related behaviors among horses used in a therapeutic riding program. *Journal of the American Veterinary Medical Association*, **228**, 39–45.

Karstad, L.H. & Sileo, L. (1971) Causes of death in captive wild waterfowl in the Kortright Waterfowl Park, 1969–1970. *Journal of Wildlife Diseases*, 7, 236–41.

Kavaliers, M. (1989) Evolutionary aspects of the neuromodulation of nociceptive behaviors. *American Zoologist*, **29**, 1345–53.

Keane, A. (2005) *The Modern Law of Evidence*, 6th edn. Butterworth, London, UK.

Kearney, K.P. (2003) Welfare perspectives of large-scale animal welfare disasters. *Proceedings of the Third Pan Commonwealth Conference*. Vet Learn Publication 231, Wellington, New Zealand.

Keele, C.A. & Smith, R. (1962) *The Assessment of Pain in Man and Animals*. UFAW, London, UK/E. & S. Livingstone, Edinburgh and London, UK.

Kellert, S. (1979) American attitudes toward and knowledge of animals: An update. *International Journal for the Study of Animal Problems*, **2**, 87–119.

Kellert, S. (1988) Human–animal interaction: a review of American attitudes to wild and domestic animals in the twentieth century. *Animals and People Sharing the World* (ed. A.M. Rowan). University Press of New England, New Hampshire, USA.

Kellert, S.R. & Felthous, A.R. (1985) Childhood cruelty toward animals among criminals and noncriminals. *Human Relations*, **38** (12), 1113–29.

Kelly, N. & Wills, J. (eds) (1994) *Manual of Companion Animal Nutrition & Feeding*. British Small Animal Veterinary Association, Gloucester, UK.

Kempe, C.H., Silverman, F.N., Steele, B.F., Droegemuller, W. & Silver, H.K. (1962) The battered-child syndrome. *Journal of the American Medical Association*, **181**, 17–24.

Kennedy, I. & Grubb, A. (1998) *Principles of Medical Law*. Oxford University Press, UK.

Keymer, I.F., Malcolm, H.M., Hunt, A. & Horsley, D.T. (2001) Health evaluation of penguins (Sphenisciformes) following mortality in the Falklands (South Atlantic). *Diseases of Aquatic Organisms*, **45**, 159–69.

Kiely, T.F. (2001) *Forensic Evidence. Science and the Criminal Law*. CRC Press, Florida, USA/London, UK.

Kienzler, J.M. *et al.* (1984) Temperature-based estimation for the time of death in white-tailed deer. *Biometrics*, **40**, 849–54.

King, J.M., Roth Johnson, L., Dodd, D.C. & Newson, M.E. (2005) *The Necropsy Book*. Charles Louis Davis, DVM, Foundation, USA.

King, L.W. (undated) *Hammurabi's Code of Laws*. Translation. http://eawc.evansville.edu/anthology/hammurabi.htm

King, R. (2005) Insurance legislation: what does it mean to be authorised? *In Practice*, **27**, 380–83.

Kingston, S.K., Dussault, C.A., Zaidlicz, R.S., *et al.* (2005) Evaluation of two methods for mass euthanasia of poultry in disease outbreaks. *Journal of the American Veterinary Medical Association*, **227** (5), 730–8.

Kirk, K. (2000) The state veterinary service inspection. *Cattle Practice*, **8** (2), 155–7.

Kirkwood, J.K. & Soulsby, Professor Lord (2005) Quality of life. *Veterinary Record*, **157** (24), 783.

Kirkwood, J.K., Sainsbury, A.W. & Bennett, P.W. (1994) The welfare of free-living wild animals: methods of assessment. *Animal Welfare*, **3**, 257–73.

Klepinger, L.L. (2006) *Fundamentals of Forensic Anthropology*. John Wiley & Sons, Bognor Regis, UK.

Klés, V., Martin, S. & Poul, J.M. (2000) Médicaments vétérinaires injectables par la voie intra-musculaire dans l'espèce porcine. *Revue Médicine Vétérinaire*, **151** (1), 51–6. [French]

Knight, B. (1975) The dynamics of stab wounds. *Forensic Science*, **6**, 249–55.

Knight, B. (1992) *Legal Aspects of Medical Practice*, 5th edn. Churchill Livingstone, Edinburgh, UK.

Knight, B. (1996) *Forensic Pathology*, 2nd edn. Arnold, London, UK.

Knight, B. (1997) *Simpson's Forensic Medicine*, 11th edn. Oxford University Press, UK.

Knight, C.M., Gutzke, W.H.N. & Quesnel, V.C. (2004) Shedding light on the luminous lizard (*Proctoporus shrevei*) of Trinidad: a brief natural history. *Caribbean Journal of Science*, **40**, 422–6.

Knight, M. (1948) The study of bird pellets as a subject of interest and instruction to amateur naturalists. *South-Eastern Naturalist and Antiquary*, 1–8.

Knight, M. (1968) *Be a Nature Detective*. Frederick Warne & Co, London, UK.

Knightsbridge, R. (2004) An ecological challenge. *Solicitors Journal, Expert Witness Supplement*, Winter 04, pp 9–11.

Korbel, R.T. & Sturm, K. (2005) Individual identification of various bird species using a digital scanning ophthalmoscopy technique. *Proceedings of the Association of Avian Veterinarians, August 9–11, Monterey, California, USA.*

Korim, P., Bugarsky, A., Tacacova, D. & Korimova, J. (1999) Forensic veterinary medicine – official veterinary autopsy. *Slovensky Veterinary Casopis*, **24** (6), 319–21. [Slovakian]

Kraus, T.C. (1985) The forensic science use of reflective ultraviolet photography. *Forensic Science*, **30**, 262–8.

Krenger, B. & Straub, R. (2002) Legal aspect of purchase examination of horses in Switzerland. *Pferdeheilkunde. Hippiatrika*, **18** (3), 291–2. [German]

Krogman, W. & Iscan, M.Y. (1986) *The Skeleton in Forensic Medicine*, 2nd edn. Charles C. Thomas, Springfield, USA.

Kuiken, T. & Hartman, M.G. (1992) Cetacean pathology: dissection techniques and tissue sampling. *Proceedings of the European Cetacean Society Workshop*. Leiden, the Netherlands.

Kuiken, T. *et al.* (1994) Mass mortality of common dolphins (*Delphinus delphis*) in southwest England due to incidental capture in fishing gear. *Veterinary Record*, **134**, 81–9.

Kumar, S. *et al.* (2005) Cervical spine injuries in 64 attempted suicidal hangings in India. *Tropical Doctor*, **35**, 198–200.

Lacroix, C.A. (2004a) Legal-ethical dilemmas in shelter medicine (Parts I and II): Small animal and exotics. Book two: pain management-zoonosis. *Proceedings of the North American Veterinary Conference. Volume 18.* Florida, USA.

Lacroix, C.A. (2004b) Negligence in equine practice in a nutshell. Large animal. *Proceedings of the North American Veterinary Conference*. Florida, USA.

Lagoni, L., Butler, C. & Hetts, S. (1994) *The Human–Animal Bond and Grief*. W.B. Saunders, Philadelphia, USA.

Lakestani, N.N., Waran, N., Verga, M. & Phillips, C. (2005) Dog bites in children. *European Journal of Companion Animal Practice*, **15** (2), 133–5.

Lane, J. (1990) Eighteenth-century medical practice: a case study of Bradford Wilmer, Surgeon of Coventry, 1737–1813. *Social History of Medicine*, **3**, 369–86.

Langbein, J., Putman, R. & Hooton, D. (2004) National deer-vehicle collisions database – an update. *Veterinary Record*, **154** (24), 767–8.

Langdon-Down, G. (2004) Trial by expert: are you sure about your evidence? *The Times*, November, London, UK.

Langlois, N.E.I. & Gresham, G.A. (1991) The ageing of bruises: a review and study of the colour changes with time. *Forensic Science International*, **50**, 227–38.

Larsen, B.H. & Holm, C.N. (1996) Microscopical examination of bronchial fluid from harbour porpoises (*Phocoena phocoena* L) for the presence of marine flora and fauna and mineral grains as a possible method to diagnose by-catch. In: *Diagnosis of By-Catch in Cetaceans, Proceedings of the Second European Cetacean Society Workshop on Cetacean Pathology*. Montpellier, France.

Laurence, C. & Newman, R. (2000) Acting as a material witness. *In Practice*, **22** (8), 491–4.

Lavocat, R. (ed.) (1966) *Faunes et Flores Préhistoriques de L'Europe Occidentale*. Boubée, Paris, France.

Lawton, M.E. & Sutton, J.G. (1982) Species identification of deer blood by isoelectric focusing. *Journal of Forensic Science*, **22**, 361–6.

Le Fanu, J. (2005) Wrongful diagnosis of child abuse – a master theory. *Journal of the Royal Society of Medicine*, **98**, 249–54.

Leadbeatter, S. (1996) *Limitations of Expert Evidence*. Royal College of Physicians, London, UK.

Leclercq, M. (1978) *Entomologie et Médecine Légale Datation de la Mort*. Masson, Paris, France. [French]

Leclercq, M. (1999) Entomology and forensic medicine: importance of phorid flies on human corpses. *Annales de la Société Entomologique de France*, **35** (Supplement), 566–8. [French]

Leclercq, M. & Tinant-Dubois, J. (1973) Entomologie et médecine légale: observations inédites. *Bulletin Médecine Légale Toxicologie*, **16**, 251–67. [French]

Leclercq, M. & Watrin, P. (1973) Entomologie et médecine légale: Acariens et insects trouvés sur un cadavre humain, en décembre 1971. *Bulletin et Annales da la Société Royale Entomologique de Belgique*, **109**, 195–201.

Leestma, J.E. (1988) *Forensic Neuropathology*. Raven Press, New York, USA.

Legood, G. (2002) *Veterinary Ethics: an Introduction*. Continuum Publishing, London.

Lemos-Espinal, J.A. & Ballinger, R.E. (1992) Observations on the tolerance to freezing of the lizard, *Sceloporus grammicus*, from Iztaccihuati Volcano, México. *Herpetological Review*, **23**, 8–9.

Lever, C. (1977) *The Naturalised Animals of the British Isles*. Hutchinson, London, UK.

Levins, R. (1998) Environmental assessment: by whom, for whom, and to what ends? In: *Ecosystem Health* (eds D. Rapport, P.R. Costanza, C. Epstein, C. Gaudet & R. Levins). Blackwell, Oxford, UK.

Levinson, J. & Granot, H. (2002) *Transportation Disaster Response Handbook*. Elsevier, Oxford, UK.

Lewbart, G.A. (2006) *Invertebrate Medicine*. Blackwell, Ames, USA.

Lightsey, J.D., Rommel, S.A., Costidis, A.M. & Pitchford, T.D. (2006) Methods used during gross necropsy to determine watercraft related mortality in the Florida manatee (*Trichechus manatus latirostris*). *Journal of Zoo and Wildlife Medicine*, **37** (3), 262–75.

Lilleyman, J. (2006) Being open. *Bulletin of The Royal College of Pathologists*, **133**, 27–8.

Lincoln, R. & Rainbow, P. (2003) *Specimens. The Spirit of Zoology*. The Natural History Museum, London, UK.

Linnaeus, C. (1788) *Systema Naturae, Per Regna Tria Naturae, Secundum Classes, Ordines, Genera, Species, Cum Charateribus, Differentiis, Synonymis, Locis*. Lepizig, Germany.

Local Government Association (1998) *The Pet Animals Act 1951 Model Standards for Pet Shop Licence Conditions*. Local Government Association, London.

Lopatenok, A.A., Boiko, L.P. & Budjakov, O.S. (1964) Forensic significance of observations about the fauna of dead human bodies. *Sudebno-meditsinskaya ékspertisa*, 7, 47–50. [Russian]

Lord, W.D. & Burger, J.F. (1983) Collection and preservation of forensically important entomological materials. *Journal of Forensic Sciences*, **28**, 936–44.

Lord, W.D. & Burger, J.F. (1984) Arthropods associated with harbour seal (*Phoca vitulina*) carcasses stranded on islands along the New England coast. *International Journal of Entomology*, **26**, 282–5.

Lorenz, K. (1952) *King Solomon's Ring. New Light on Animal Ways* (Translated from the German by Marjorie Kerr Wilson). Methuen & Co., London, UK.

Lorton, R. (2000) *A–Z of Countryside Law*. The Stationery Office, Norwich.

Lothe, F. (1964) The use of larva infestation in determining the time of death. *Medicine Science and the Law*, **4**, 113–15.

Loue, S. (1999) *Forensic Epidemiology: A Comprehensive Guide for Legal and Epidemiology Professionals*. Southern Illinois University Press, USA.

Lovell, N.C. (1990) *Patterns of Injury and Illness in Great Apes. A Skeletal Analysis*. Smithsonian Institution Press, Washington, USA.

Lundrigan, B. (1996) Standard methods for measuring mammals. In: *Wild Mammals in Captivity* (eds D.E. Kleiman, M.E. Allen, K.V. Thompson & S. Lumpkin). The University of Chicago Press, USA.

Lundt, H. (1964) Ecological observations about the invasion of insects into carcasses buried in soil. *Pedobiologia*, **4**, 158–80.

Lyster, S. (1985) *International Wildlife Law. An Analysis of International Treaties Concerned with the Conservation of Wildlife*. Grotius Publications, UK.

Maas, A.K. (2006 The mobile exotic animal practice. *Journal of Exotic Pet Medicine*, **15**, 122–31.

Macdonald, A.A. & Charlton, N. (2000) *A Bibliography of References to Husbandry and Veterinary Guidelines for Animals in Zoological Collections*. The Federation of Zoological Gardens of Great Britain and Northern Ireland, London, UK.

Macdonald, D. & Norris, S. (eds) (2001) *The New Encyclopedia of Mammals*. Oxford University Press, UK.

MacDonell, H.L. (1993) *Bloodstain Patterns*. Laboratory of Forensic Science, New York, USA.

Mackenzie, J. (2001) *Horse Law*. J. A. Allen, London, UK.

Mackness, B.S. & Sutton, R.H. (2000) Possible evidence for intraspecific aggression in a Pliocene crocodile from north Queensland. *Alcheringa*, **24**, 55–62.

Magana, C. (2001) Forensic entomology and its application in legal medicine. Data of death. *Boletin de la S. E.A., Sociedad Entomologica Aragonesa*, **28**, 49–57. [Spanish]

Male, G.E. (1816) *Epitome of Juridical or Forensic Medicine for the Use of Medical Men, Coroners and Barristers.* Birmingham, UK.

Maniere, C.A., Rhinehart, H.L., Barros, N.B., Byrd, L. & Cunningham-Smith, P. (2004) An approach to the rehabilitation of *Kogia* spp. *Aquatic Mammals*, **30** (2), 257–70.

Mann, M.J. *et al.* (1994) Shot pellets: An overview. *Journal of the Association of Firearms and Tool Examiners*, **26**, 223–41.

Manning, D.P., Cooper, J.E., Stirling, I., Jones, C.M., Bruce, M. & McCausland, P.C. (1985) Studies on the footpads of the polar bear (*Ursus maritimus*) and their possible relevance to accident prevention. *Journal of Hand Surgery*, **10** (13), 303–7.

Manning, D.P., Cooper, J.E., Jones, C. & Bruce, M. (1990) Slip-shod or safely shod: the bighorn sheep as a natural model for research. *Journal of the Royal Society of Medicine*, **83**, 686–9.

Markwell, P.J. & Edney, A.T.B. (1994) The obese animal. In: *Manual of Companion Animal Nutrition & Feeding* (eds N. Kelly & J. Wills). British Small Animal Veterinary Association, Gloucester, UK.

Martin, J. & Turner, C. (2002) *European Law*. Hodder & Stoughton, London, UK.

Mason, I.L. (1984) *Evolution of Domesticated Animals*. Longman, London, UK.

Mason, J.K. (ed.) (1989) *Paediatric Forensic Medicine and Pathology*. Chapman and Hall, London, UK.

Mason, J.K. & Purdue, B.N. (eds) (2000) *The Pathology of Trauma*, 3rd edn. London, Arnold.

Mason, G. & Rushen, J. (eds) (2006) *Stereotypic Animal Behaviour: Fundamentals and Applications to Welfare*, 2nd edn. CABI, Wallingford UK.

Matson, J.V. (2004) *Effective Expert Witnessing*, 4th edn. Taylor and Francis Group, New York, USA.

Maxwell, A. (2005) Expert evidence and the role of the expert witness – a practical guide. *Fish Veterinary Journal*, **8**, 93–100.

Mayer, C.B. (1998) *Expert Witnessing: Explaining the Science*. Taylor and Francis Group, New York, USA.

Mayer, J. (2004) CITES and other regulations regarding reptiles and amphibians in the United States. *Proceedings of the Association of Reptilian and Amphibian Veterinarians*. Ed. C.K. Baer. May 8–1, Naples, Florida.

Mayer, J. (2005) Comparison of different methods applicable for the reptilian urolith analysis. *Journal of Herpetological Medicine and Surgery*, **15** (2), 31.

Mazet, J.A.K., Hunt, T.D., Ziccardi, M.H. *et al.* (2004) *Assessment of the Risk of Zoonotic Disease Transmission to Marine Mammal Workers and the Public. Survey of Occu-* pational Risks. Report prepared for the United States Marine Mammal Commission, Wildlife Health Center, School of Veterinary Medicine, University of California, Davis, USA.

McCall Smith, A. (1998) *The No. 1 Ladies Detective Agency*. Abacus, London, UK.

McEwan, S.A., Wilson, T.M., Ashford, D.A., Heegaard, E.D., Kuiken, T. & Kournikakis, B. (2006) Microbe forensics for natural and intentional incidents of infectious disease involving animals. *Office International Epizooties Scientific and Technical Review*, **25** (1), 329–39.

McGarity, T.O. (2005) Daubert and the proper role for the courts in health, safety and environmental regulation. *American Journal of Public Health*, **95** (Suppl. 1), S92–8. Washington, USA.

McGavin, M.D. & Zachary, J.F. (eds) (2007) *Pathologic Basis of Veterinary Disease*. Mosby Elsevier, Missouri, USA.

McGuinness, K., Allen, M. & Jones, B.R. (2005) Non-accidental injuries in companion animals in the Republic of Ireland. *Irish Veterinary Journal*, **58**, 392–6.

McKeating, F. (2005) The professional indemnity of witnesses. *Proceedings of the Veterinary Association for Arbitration and Jurisprudence*, **2** (1), 13.

McKnight, B.E. (1981) *The Washing Away of Wrongs: Forensic Medicine in Thirteenth-Century China*. University of Michigan, Ann Arbor, USA. [Translated]

McLean, I., Anderson, M. & White, C. (2003) The accuracy of guestimates. *Journal of the Royal Society of Medicine*, **96** (10), 497–8.

Meadow, R. (1997) Munchausen syndrome by proxy. In: *ABC of Child Abuse* (ed. R. Meadow). British Medical Journal Publishing Group, London, UK.

Mégnin, P. (1894) *La Faune des Cadavres. Encyclopédie Scientifique des Aide-Memoire*. G. Masson, Gauthier-Villars et Fils, Paris, France. [French]

Mench, J.A. & Kreger, M.D. (1996) Ethical and welfare issues associated with keeping wild mammals in captivity. In: *Wild Mammals in Captivity* (eds D.E. Kleiman, M.E. Allen, K.V. Thompson & S. Lumpkin). University of Chicago Press, USA.

Menotti-Raymond, M., David, V.A. & O'Brien, S.J. (1997) Pet cat hair implicates murder suspect. *Nature*, **386**, 774.

Merck, M.D. (2004) Veterinary forensics: animal CSI. Small animal and exotics. Book one: alternative medicine – orthopedics. *Proceedings of the North American Veterinary Conference, Volume 18*. Orlando, Florida, USA.

Mertens, P.A. (2002) Canine aggression. In: *Manual of Canine and Feline Behavioural Medicine* (eds D.F.

Horwitz, D.S. Mills and S. Heath). British Small Animal Veterinary Association, Gloucester, UK.

Michell, A.R. (1985) What is shock? *Journal of Small Animal Practice*, **26**, 719–38.

Michell, A.R. (2002) Revalidation and virtual patients: a vision for the future. *In Practice*, **24**, 221–3.

Michell, A.R. (2005) The Shipman reports: lessons and warnings. *Veterinary Record*, **156**, 153.

Michell, A.R. & Ewbank, R. (1998) *Ethics, Welfare, Law and Market Forces: The Veterinary Interface*. Universities Federation for Animal Welfare, Herts, UK.

Mikhailov, K.E. (1997) *Avian Eggshells: An Atlas of Scanning Electron Micrographs*. British Ornithologists Club, Tring, UK.

Mildred, R.H. (1982) *The Expert Witness*. George Goodwin, London, UK.

Miles, A.E.W. & Grigson, C. (1990) *Colyer's Variations and Diseases of the Teeth of Animals*, revised edn. Cambridge University Press, Cambridge, UK.

Miles, P.M. (1952) *The Entomology of Bird Pellets*. Leaflet No. 24, The Amateur Entomologists' Society, London, UK.

Miller, E., Ragsdale, B.D. & Ortner, D.J. (1996) Accuracy in dry bone diagnosis: a comment on palaeopathological methods. *International Journal of Esteoarchaeology*, **6**, 221–9

Miller, H. (2000) *Secrets of the Dead*. Channel 4 Books, London, UK.

Millichamp, R.I. (1987) *Anglers' Law*. A & C Black, London, UK.

Millington, P. (1974) Histological studies on skin carrying bite marks. *Forensic Science*, **14**, 239–40.

Mills, D.S. & Nicol, C.J. (1990) Tonic immobility in spent hens after catching and transport. *Veterinary Record*, **126**, 210–12.

Moberg, G.P. (ed.) (1985) *Animal Stress*. American Physiological Society, Bethesda, USA.

Moberg, G.P. & Mench, J.A. (2000) *The Biology of Animal Stress*. CABI, UK.

Moberly, R.L., White, P.L.C. & Harris, S. (2004) Mortality due to fox predation in free-range poultry flocks in Britain. *Veterinary Record*, **155**, 48–52.

Moe, R.O. & Bakken, M. (1998) Anxiolytic drugs inhibit hyperthermia induced by handling in farmed silver foxes (*Vulpes vulpes*). *Animal Welfare*, **7,** 97–100.

Molyneux, J. (2005) Vets on track: working as a greyhound vet. *In Practice*, **27**, 277–9.

Monies, B. (2004) Alimentary tract perforation in cattle caused by tyre wire. *Veterinary Record*, **154**, 735.

Moore, G.E., Frana, T.S., Guptill, L.F., Ward, M.P., Lewis, H.B. & Glickman, L.T. (2005) Postmarketing surveillance for dog and cat vaccines: new resources in changing times. *Journal of the American Veterinary Medical Association*, **227** (7), 1066–8.

Moore, M.K., Bemiss, J.A., Ball, R.M. & Woodley, C.M. (1999) Identification of suspected sea turtle evidence using mtDNA analyses. *Proceedings of the International Association of Forensic Sciences, 75th Triennial Meeting, August 22–28, 1999, Los Angeles, California, USA*.

Moore, T.D. *et al.* (1974) Identification of dorsal guard hairs of some mammals of Wyoming. *Wyoming Game and Fish Department Bulletin*, **14**, 1–177.

Moore, W. (2005) *The Knife Man*. Bantam Press, London, UK.

Morgan, M. (2004) The microbiology of animal bites. *The Bulletin of The Royal College of Pathologists*, **28**, 16–19.

Morgan, M.S. (1999) Tiger bites. *Journal of the Royal Society of Medicine*, **92**, 545.

Morrison, R.D. (1999) *Environmental Forensics: Principles and Applications*. CRC, Florida, USA.

Morrow, A.N. & Sewell, M.M.H. (1990) Equine anhidrosis. In: *Animal Diseases in the Tropics* (eds M.M.H. Sewell & D.W. Brocklesby). Baillière Tindall, London, UK.

Morse, D.R., Esposito, J.V., Kessler, H.P. & Gorin, R. (1994) Age estimation using dental periapical radiographic parameters. A review and comparative study of clinically based and regression models with the Operation Desert Storm victims. *The American Journal of Forensic Medicine and Pathology*, **15** (4), 303–18.

Morton, D.B. & Griffiths, P.H.B. (1985) Guidelines on the recognition of pain, distress and discomfort in experimental animals and an hypothesis for assessment. *Veterinary Record*, **116**, 432–6.

Muir, R. (1924) *Text-book of Pathology*. Edward Arnold, London, UK.

Mullan, S. (2006) Everyday ethics. *In Practice*, **28**, 52.

Mullineaux, E., Best, D. & Cooper, J.E. (eds) (2003) *Manual of Wildlife Casualties*. British Small Animal Veterinary Association, Gloucester, UK.

Munger, L.L. & McGavin, M.D. (1972) Sequential postmortem changes in chicken liver at 4, 20 or 37°C. *Avian Diseases*, **16**, 587–605.

Munro, H.M.C. (1996) Battered pets. *Veterinary Record*, **138**, 576.

Munro, H.M.C. & Thrusfield, M.V. (2001a) 'Battered pets': features that raise suspicion of non-accidental injury. *Journal of Small Animal Practice*, **42**, 218–26.

Munro, H.M.C. & Thrusfield, M.V. (2001b) 'Battered pets': non-accidental physical injuries found in dogs and cats. *Journal of Small Animal Practice*, **42**, 279–90.

Munro, H.M.C. & Thrusfield, M.V. (2001c) 'Battered pets': sexual abuse. *Journal of Small Animal Practice*, **42**, 333–7.

Munro, H.M.C. & Thrusfield, M.V. (2001d) 'Battered pets': Munchausen syndrome by proxy (factitious illness by proxy). *Journal of Small Animal Practice*, **42**, 385–9.

Munro, R. (1998) Forensic necropsy. *Seminars in Avian and Exotic Pet Medicine*, 7 (4).

Munson, L. (2002) The living dead: keeping wildlife alive through scientific use of biomaterials. *Proceedings, American Association of Zoo Veterinarians, 2002*, pp 269–71.

Murphy, B.L. & Morrison, R.D. (2002) *Introduction to Environmental Forensics*. Academic Press, New York, USA.

Murphy, E.M. (2005) Animal palaeopathology in prehistoric and historic Ireland: A review of the evidence. In: *Diet and Health in Past Animal Populations* (eds J. Davies, M. Fabis, I Mainland, M. Richards & R. Thomas). Oxbow, Oxford, UK.

Murphy, P. (1990) *Evidence & Advocacy*, 5th edn. Blackstone Press, London, UK.

Murphy, P. (2005) *Murphy on Evidence*, 9th edn. Oxford University Press, UK.

Murray, R. & Mair, T. (2005) Use of magnetic resonance imaging in lameness diagnosis in the horse. *In Practice*, **27**, 138–46.

Murrey, G.J. (2000) *The Forensic Evaluation of Traumatic Brain Injury. A Handbook for Clinicians and Attorneys*. CRC Press, Florida, USA/London, UK.

Myskowiak, J.B., Chauvet, B., Pasquerault, T., Rocheteau, C. & Vian, J.M. (1999) A summary of six years of forensic entomology field work. The role of necrophagous insects in forensic science. *Annales de la Société Entomologique de France*, **35**, 569–72. [French]

Nakkazi, E. (2005) Bwindi National Park gets first telecentre service. *The Monitor* (Uganda).

Nambiar, P. & Nadesan, K. (2004) Application of dental science in forensic investigations. In: *Textbook of Oral Medicine* (ed. S.R. Prabhu). Oxford University Press, UK.

Napley, D. (1991) *The Technique of Persuasion*, 4th edn. Sweet and Maxwell, London, UK.

Naru, A. & Dykes, E. (1996) The use of digital imaging technique to aid bite mark analysis. *Science & Justice*, **36**, 47–50.

Nash, C.E. (ed.) (1991) *Production of Aquatic Animals. Crustaceans, Molluscs, Amphibians and Reptiles*. Elsevier, Amsterdam, Netherlands.

Needham, C., Wilkinson, C. & Knüsel, C.J. (2003) Reconstructing visual manifestations of disease from archaeological human remains. *Journal of Audiovisual Media in Medicine*, **26** (3), 103–7.

Neff, R.A. & Goldman, L.R. (2005) Regulatory parallels to Daubert: stakeholder influence, 'sound science', and the delayed adoption of health-protective standards. *American Journal of Public Health*, **95** (Suppl. 1), S81–91. Washington, USA.

Nelson, W. (1753) *The Laws Concerning Game*, 5th edn. T Waller, London, UK.

Newbery, S. (2006) Forensic sketching. *Newsletter of the VAAJ*, **4**, 6–9.

Newman, R. (2004a) How to avoid getting sued – lessons from the lawyer who sues veterinarians. Large animal. *Proceedings of the North American Veterinary Conference, 17–24 January 2004, Orlando, Florida, USA*.

Newman, R. (2004b) Veterinary malpractice – how to protect your practice and cover your assets. Small animal and exctics. Book two: pain management – zoonosis. *Proceedings of the North American Veterinary Conference, 17–24 January 2004, Orlando, Florida, USA*.

Newman, R. (2004c) Veterinary malpractice – how to protect your practice and cover your assets. Large animal. *Proceedings of the North American Veterinary Conference, 17–24 January 2004, Orlando, Florida, USA*.

Neumann, N. (1979) *Untersuchungen über das Vorkommen von netzmagen-fremdkörpen bei Schlachtrindern in Bayern*. Dissertation, Faculty of Veterinary Medicine, University of Munich, Germany.

Newton, J. (2005a) Negligence case is harsh reminder for professicn. *Veterinary Times*, 15 August.

Newton, J. (2005b) Cruelty survey prompts fresh airgun ban calls. *Veterinary Times*, 7 November.

Newton, J. (2006) Vets urged to face taboo of animal sexual abuse. *Veterinary Times*, 28 August.

NFBG (2000) *Badgers and the Law*. National Federation of Badger Groups, London, UK.

Nightingale, F. (1860) *Notes on Nursing*. Harrison and Sons, London, UK.

Nind, F. (2005) Keeping track of adverse reactions to microchips. *Journal of Small Animal Practice*, **46**, 361–2.

Nolen, R.S. (2003) LSU laboratory vandalized: animal extremist group claims responsibility. *Journal of the American Veterinary Medical Association*, **223** (9), 1239–40.

Nolte, I. (2002) Malpractice in small animals. *Tierärztliche Praxis. Ausgabe K, Kleintiere/Heimtiere*, **30** (3), 158–63. [German]

North, P.M. (1972) *The Modern Law of Animals*. Butterworths, London, UK.

Nozdryn-Potnicki, Z., Liston, P., Opuszynski, W. & Debiak, P. (2005) Section investigation of animals wounded from fire arms: some remarks. *Medycyna Weterynaryjna. Polskiego Towarzystwa Nauk Wetery-naryjnych*, **61** (8), 887–9. [Polish]

Nuffield Council (2005) *The Ethics of Research Involving Animals*. Nuffield Council on BioEthics, London, UK.

Nunn, J.F. & Tapp, E. (2000) Tropical diseases in ancient Egypt. *Transactions of the Royal Society of Tropical Medicine and Hygiene*, **94**, 147–53.

Nuorteva, P. (1977) Sarcosaprophagous insects as forensic indicators. *Forensic Medicine, a Study in Trauma and Environmental Hazards. Vol. II Physical Trauma* (eds C.G. Tedeschi, W.G. Eckert & L.G.Tedeschi). W.B. Saunders, Philadelphia, USA.

O'Callaghan, P.T., Jones, M.D., James, D.S., Leadbetter, S., Holt, C.A. & Nokes, L.D. (1999) Dynamics of stab wounds: force required for penetration of various cadaveric human tissues. *Forensic Science*, **104**, 173–5.

O'Connor, T. (2000) *The Archaeology of Animal Bones*. Sutton Publishing, Stroud, UK.

O'Hare, J. & Browne, K. (2003) *Civil Litigation*, 11th edn. Sweet and Maxwell, London, UK.

Oaks, J.L. *et al.* (2004) Diclofenac residues as the cause of vulture population decline in Pakistan. *Nature*, **10**, 1038.

Oates, D. (1992) Time of death. In: *Wildlife Forensic Field Manual* (ed. W.J. Adrian). Colorado Division of Wildlife, Fort Collins, USA.

Oates, D.W. *et al.* (1984) *A Guide to the Time of Death in Selected Wildlife Species*. Nebraska Technical Series No. 14. Lincoln, N.E., Nebraska Game and Parks Commission, USA.

Oexmann, B. (2002) Forensic problems of veterinary liability in the horse. *Tierärztliche Praxis*, **30** (5), 344–9. [German]

Ogle, R.R. & Fox, M.J. (1999) *Atlas of Human Hair: Microscopic Characteristics*. CRC Press, Florida, USA/ London, UK.

OIE (2004) *Handbook on Import Risk Analysis for Animal and Animal Products*. Organisation Internationale des Epizooties, Paris, France.

Olpin, S.E. & Evans, M.J. (2004) The investigation of inherited metabolic diseases after death. In: *Essentials of Autopsy Practice. Recent Advances, Topics and Developments* (ed. G.N. Rutty). Springer-Verlag, London, UK.

Olson, P. (ed.) (1998) *Recognizing & Reporting Animal Abuse*. American Humane Association, Colorado, USA.

Olumbe, A.K., Dada, M.A. & McQuoid-Mason, J.D. (undated) *Handbook of Forensic Medicine and Medical Law in Kenya*. The Independent Medico Legal Unit (IMLU), Nairobi, Kenya.

Ormerod, E.J., Edney, A.T.B., Foster, S.J. & Whyham, M. C. (2005) Therapeutic applications of the human–companion animal bond. *Veterinary Record*, **157**, 689–91.

Ouro-Bang'na Maman, A.F. *et al.* (2005) Deaths associated with anaesthesia in Togo, West Africa. *Tropical Doctor*, **35**, 220–22.

Overgaauw, P.A.M. & Kirpensteijn, J. (2006) Application of honey in the treatment of skin wounds. *European Journal of Companion Animal Practice*, **10**, 17–19 (originally published in *Tijdschrift voor Diergeneeskunde* (2005) **130**, 115–16).

Packer, C., Ikanda, D., Kissui, B. & Kushnir, H. (2005) Lion attacks on humans in Tanzania. *Nature*, **436**, 927–8.

PAHO (2005) Epidemiological calendar 2006. *Epidemiological Bulletin. Pan American Health Organization*, **26** (2), 16.

Palmer, J. (2001) *Animal Law*, 3rd edn. Shaw & Sons, London, UK.

Palmer, R. & Wetherill, D. (eds) (2004) *Medicine for Lawyers*. The Royal Society of Medicine, London, UK.

Pankaj Kulshrestha and Satpathy, D.K. (2001) Use of beetles in forensic entomology. *Forensic Science International*, **120** (1/2), 15–17.

Parkes, C. & Thornley, J. (1997) *Fair Game: The Law of Country Sports and the Protection of Wildlife*. Pelham, UK.

Parkes, C. & Thornley, J. (2000) *Deer: Law and Liabilities*. Swan Hill Press, Shrewsbury, UK.

Parliamentary Office of Science and Technology (2005) Science in Court. *Postnote*, October, Number 248.

Parsons, P.A. (1992) Fluctuating asymmetry! A biological monitor of environmental and genomic stress. *Heredity*, **68**, 361–4.

Paul, E.S. & Podberscek, A.L. (2000) Veterinary education and students' attitudes towards animal welfare. *Veterinary Record*, **146**, 269–72.

Pavletic, M.M. (1986a) Gunshot wounds in veterinary medicine: Projectile ballistics – Part I. *Compendium on Continuing Education*, **8**, 47–61.

Pavletic, M.M. (1986b) Gunshot wounds in veterinary medicine: Projectile ballistics – Part II. *Compendium on Continuing Education* **8**, 125–34.

PAW (2005) *Wildlife Crime: A Guide to the Use of Forensic and Specialist Techniques in the Investigation of Wildlife Crime*. DEFRA, Bristol, UK.

Payne-James, J. *et al.* (eds) (2005) *Encyclopedia of Forensic and Legal Medicine*. Elsevier, London, UK.

Penell, J.C., Egenvall, A., Bonnett, B.N., Olson, P. & Pringle, J. (2005) Specific causes of morbidity among

Swedish horses insured for veterinary care between 1997 and 2000. *Veterinary Record*, **157**, 470–7.

Penketh, A. (2005) Bear's killing prompts court to reconstruct crime scene. *The Independent*, Wednesday, 9 November.

Pepper, I.K. (2005) *Crime Scene Investigation. Methods and Procedures*. McGraw-Hill, UK.

Perednia, D.A. & Allen, A. (1995) Telemedicine technology and clinical applications. *Journal of the American Medical Association*, **273** (6), 483–8.

Peschel, R.E. & Peschel, E. (1989) What physicians have in common with Sherlock Holmes: discussion paper. *Journal of the Royal Society of Medicine*, **82**.

Petraco, N. (1987) A microscopic method to aid in the identification of animal hair. *Microscope*, **35**, 83–92.

Pezza, F. (2003) The horse and the law. *Summa. Edizioni Veterinarie & Agrozootechniche*, Milano, Italy. **20** (3), 9. [Italian]

Phillips, J.H. (1996) Foreword. In: *Forensic Medicine and the Law: An Introduction* (D. Ranson). Melbourne University Press, Victoria, Australia.

Pidancier, N., Miquel, C. & Miaud, C. (2003) Buccal swabs as a non-destructive tissue sampling method for DNA analysis in amphibians. *Herpetological Journal*, **13**, 175–8.

Plant, C. (1999) *Blackstone's Guide to the Civil Procedure Rules*. Oxford University Press, UK.

Platt, S. (2005) Evaluation and treatment of the head trauma patient. *In Practice*, **27**, 31–5.

Plewa, D. (2002a) Guiding principle from the jurisdiction on the purchase inspection of a horse. *Pferdeheilkunde. Hippiatrika*, **18** (3), 289–90. [German]

Plewa, D. (2002b) Purchase inspection of the horse from a legal aspect. *Pferdeheilkunde. Hippiatrika* **18** (3), 284–8. [German]

Plewa, D. (2002c) Veterinary liability in equine practice. *Pferdeheilkunde. Hippiatrika* **18** (2), 173–8. [German]

Poppenga, R.H. (1995) Risks associated with herbal remedies. In: *Kirk's Current Veterinary Therapy XII: Small Animal Practice*. W.B. Saunders, Philadelphia, USA.

Porter, A.R.W. (1971) The veterinary surgeon as a witness. *Veterinary Record*, **89**, 505–9.

Porter, V. (1989) *Animal Rescue*. Ashford, Southampton, UK.

Prabhu, S.R. (ed.) (2004) *Textbook of Oral Medicine*. Oxford University Press, UK.

Pretty, I.A. & Addy, L.D. (2002) Associated postmortem dental findings as an aid to personal identification. *Science and Justice*, **42** (2), 65–74.

Pye, K. & Croft, D.J. (2004) *Forensic Geoscience: Principles, Techniques and Applications*. Forensic Science Service, Geological Society, London, UK.

Quadros, J. & Monteiro-Filho, E.I. (1998) Effects of digestion, putrefaction, and taxidermy processes on *Didelphis albiventris* hair morphology. *Journal of Zoology*, **244**, 331–4.

Qui-Hong Wan & Sheng-Guo Fang (2003) Application of species-specific polymerase chain reaction in the forensic identification of tiger species. *Forensic Science International*, **131** (1), 75–8.

Radford, M. (2001) *Animal Welfare Law in Britain: Regulation and Responsibility*. Oxford University Press, UK.

Ralston, R.M. (1999) Investigation of a source of blunt force trauma in cattle egrets. *Proceedings of the International Association of Forensic Sciences, 75th Triennial Meeting August 22–28, 1999, Los Angeles, California, USA*.

Ranson, D. (1996) *Forensic Medicine and the Law, an Introduction*. Melbourne University Press, Victoria, Australia.

Rapport, D., Costanza, P.R. & Epstein, C. (eds) (1998) *Ecosystem Health*. Blackwell, Oxford, UK.

Rawson, A.J., Anderson, H.F., Patton, G.W. & Beecher, T. (1991) Anthracosis in the Atlantic bottlenose dolphin (*Tursiops truncatus*). *Marine Mammal Science*, 7 (4), 413–16.

Rawson, R.D., Bell, A. & Kinard, J.G. (1979) Radiographic interpretation of contrast media-enhanced bite marks. *Forensic Science*, **24**, 898–901.

RCVS (2000) *Guide to Professional Conduct*. RCVS, London, UK.

Read, A.J. & Murray, K.T. (2000) Gross evidence of human-induced mortality in small cetaceans. US Department of Commerce, National Oceanic and Atmospheric Administration, National Marine Fisheries Service, *NOAA Technical Memorandum NMFS – OPR – 15*, USA.

Redman, D (2005) Helping clients in times of loss. *In Practice*, **27** (10), 554.

Redmond, A.D. (2005) ABC of conflict and disaster. Needs assessment of humanitarian crises. *British Medical Journal*, **330**, 1320–2.

Redsicker, D.R. (2000) *The Practical Methodology of Forensic Photography*, 2nd edn. CRC Press.

Redsicker, D.R. & O'Connor, J.J. (1997) *Practical Fire and Arson Investigation*, 2nd edn. CRC Press, Florida, USA/London, UK.

Rees, P. (2002) *Urban Environments and Wildlife Law*. Blackwell, Oxford, UK.

Reeve, R. (2002) *Policing International Trade in Endangered Species. The CITES Treaty and Compliance*. Earthscan Publications, London, UK.

Reisman, A.B. & Stevens, D.L. (2002) *Telephone Medicine: A Guide for the Practising Physician*. The Royal Society of Medicine, London, UK.

Reneau, J.K., Seykora, A.J., Heins, B.J., Endres, M.I., Farnsworth, R.J. & Bey, F.F. (2005) Association between hygiene scores and somatic cell scores in dairy cattle. *Journal of the American Veterinary Medical Association*, **227** (8), 1297–1301.

Report (2001) The Royal Liverpool Children's Inquiry. Alder Hey Children's Hospital. Stationery Office, London, UK.

Restian, A. (1990) Informational stress: discussion paper. *Journal of the Royal Society of Medicine*, **83** (6), 380–2.

Richardson, D.H.S. (1992) *Pollution Monitoring with Lichens*. The Company of Biologists, Cambridge, UK.

Rideout, B.A. (2002) Creating and maintaining a post-mortem biomaterials archive: why you should do it and what's in it for you. *Proceedings, American Association of Zoo Veterinarians, 2002*, pp 272–4.

Rigdon, J.D. & Tapia, F. (1977) Children who are cruel to animals – a follow-up study. *Journal of Operative Psychiatry*, **8** (1), 27–36.

Robbins, S.L., Cotran, R.S., Kumar, V. & Collins, T. (1999) *Robbins Pathologic Basis of Disease*, 6th edn. W. B. Saunders, Philadelphia, USA.

Roberts, C. & Manchester, K. (2005) *The Archaeology of Disease*, 3rd edn. Sutton, UK.

Roberts, D.H. (1986) Determination of predators responsible for killing small livestock. *South African Journal of Wildlife Research*, **16**, 150–2.

Robertson, J. (1999a) *The Forensic Examination of Human Hair*. Taylor & Francis, London, UK.

Robertson, J. (1999b) *The Forensic Examination of Fibres*. Taylor & Francis, London, UK.

Robinson, P. (1982) *Bird Detective*. Elm Tree Books, London, UK.

Robinson, R. (1990) *Genetics for Dog Breeders*, 2nd edn. Pergamon Press, Oxford, UK.

Robinson, S.P. (1996) *Principles of Forensic Medicine*. Oxford University Press, UK.

Rochlitz, I., Podberscek, A.L. & Broom, D.M. (1998) Welfare of cats in a quarantine cattery. *Veterinary Record*, **143**, 35–9.

Rogers, W.V.H. (2002) *Winfield and Jolowicz on Tort*. Sweet and Maxwell, London, UK.

Rollins, C.E. & Spencer, D.E. (1995) A fatality and the American mountain lion: bite mark analysis and profile of the offending lion. *Journal of Forensic Science*, **40**, 486–9.

Rose, P. (2002) *Forensic Speaker Identification*. Taylor & Francis, London, UK.

Rose, W., Sime, S. & French, D. (2005) *Blackstone's Civil Practice*. Oxford University Press, UK.

Rosel, P. (1999) Identification of multiple whale species in canned meat using DNA sequence analysis. *Proceedings of the International Association of Forensic Sciences, 75th Triennial Meeting August 22–28, 1999, Los Angeles, California, USA.*

Ross, H.M. & Wilson, B. (1996) Violent interactions between bottlenose dolphins and harbour porpoises. *Proceedings of the Royal Society of London B*, **263**, 283–6.

Ross, J.M. (1925) *Post-Mortem Appearances*, 4th edn. Oxford University Press, UK.

Rothschild, B.M. & Martin, L. (1993) *Palaeopathology: Disease in the Fossil Record*. CRC, London, UK.

Rothschild, B.M. & Panza, R.K. (2005) Epidemiologic assessment of trauma-independent skeletal pathology in non-passerine birds from museum collections. *Avian Pathology*, **34** (3), 212–19.

Rothschild, M.A. & Schneider, V. (1997) On the temporal onset of post-mortem animal scavenging. 'Motivation' of the animal. *Forensic Science International*, **89**, 57–84.

Rothwell, B.R. (1995) Bite marks in forensic dentistry: a review of legal, scientific issues. *American Dental Association*, **126**, 223–32.

Rothwell, T. (2004) Presentation of expert forensic evidence. In: *Crime Scene to Court. The Essentials of Forensic Science* (ed. P.C. White), 2nd edn. The Royal Society of Chemistry, Cambridge, UK.

Rotstein, D.S., Pabst, D.A. & McLellan, W.A. (2006) Surf and turf: approaching single and multiple die-offs of free-living species. *Journal of Exotic Pet Medicine*, **15** (1), 40–8.

Rowcliffe, J.M., de Merode, E. & Cowlishaw, E. (2004) Do wildlife laws work? Species protection and the application of a prey choice model to poaching decisions. *Proceedings of the Royal Society of London B.*, **271**, 2631–6.

Rowley, I. (1970) Lamb predation in Australia: incidence, predisposing conditions, and the identification of wounds. *CSIRO Wildlife Research*, **15**, 79–123.

Royal College of Obstetricians and Gynaecologists & Royal College of Pathologists (2001) *Fetal and Perinatal Pathology*, Royal College of Pathologists, London, UK.

Royal College of Veterinary Surgeons (2000) *Guide to Professional Conduct. Mutilation of Animals.* Report of Working Party established by RCVS Council to Consider the Mutilation of Animals, June 1986/February 1987.

RSPB (1998) *Wild Birds and the Law* (booklet). Royal Society for the Protection of Birds, Sandy, Bedfordshire, UK. Also on RSPB website.

RSPB (1999) *Birdcrime: Offences against Wild Bird Legislation in 1999*. The Royal Society for the Protection of Birds, Sandy, UK.

RSPB (2005) *Bird Crime 2004*. The Royal Society for the Protection of Birds, Sandy, UK.

RSPCA (1999) *Principal UK Animal Welfare Legislation; a Summary* (booklet). Royal Society for the Prevention of Cruelty to Animals, Horsham, UK.

Ruddick, R.F. (1987) Ultraviolet photography in the detection of abuse. *Criminologist*, **2**, 68–73.

Rudin, N. & Inman, K. (2002) *An Introduction to Forensic DNA Analysis*, 2nd edn. CRC Press, Florida, USA.

Rutherford, K.M.D. (2002) Assessing pain in animals. *Animal Welfare*, **11**, 31–53.

Rutty, G.N. (ed.) (2001) *Essentials of Autopsy Practice Volume 1*. Springer-Verlag, London, UK.

Rutty, G.N. (2004) The pathology of shock versus postmortem change. In: *Essentials of Autopsy Practice. Recent Advances, Topics and Developments* (ed. G.N. Rutty). Springer-Verlag, London, UK.

Ryder, O.A. (2002) Evaluating the importance of biomaterials banking: converging interests and diversifying opportunities for conservation efforts. *Proceedings, American Association of Zoo Veterinarians, 2002*.

Sadler, T.W. (2005) *Longman's Essential Medical Embryology*. Lippincott, Williams & Wilkins, Philadelphia, USA.

Salisbury, J. (2005) Voice recognition in histopathology: a personal experience and appraisal. *The Bulletin of The Royal College of Pathologists*, **131**, 18–19.

Sands, P. (2003) *Principles of International Environmental Law*, 2nd edn. Cambridge University Press, Cambridge, UK.

Sarre, S. (2001) Genetic sampling. *Proceedings of the Seminar Wildlife Health in Conservation*, 11–13 July 2000. Publication No. 204. Veterinary Continuing Education. Massey University, New Zealand.

Saukko, P. & Knight, B. (2004) *Knight's Forensic Pathology*, 3rd edn. Oxford University Press, UK.

Saxena, C.B., Rai, P. & Shrivastara, V.P. (1998) *Veterinary Post-mortem Examination – A Laboratory Manual*. Vikas Publishing House, New Delhi, India.

Saxton, G.N. & Engel, B. (2005) A survey of soil sample handling procedures of state pesticide regulatory agencies. *Environmental Forensics*, **6** (2), 105–8.

Schryver, H.F., Hintz, H.F., Lowe, U.E., Hintz, R.L., Harper, B.B. & Reid, J.T. (1974) Mineral composition of the whole body, liver and bone of young horses. *Journal of Nutrition*, **104**, 126–32.

Schwabe, C.W. (1984) *Veterinary Medicine and Human Health*. Williams & Wilkins, Baltimore, USA.

Schwär, T.G., Olivier, J.A. & Loubser, J.D. (1988) *The Forensic ABC in Medical Practice*. Education Publishers, Pretoria, South Africa.

Schwoeble, A.J. & Exline, D. (2000) *Current Methods in Forensic Gunshot Residue Analysis*. CRC Press, Florida, USA/London, UK.

Seaman, W.J. (1987) *Postmortem Change in the Rat: A Histologic Characterization*. Iowa State University Press, USA.

Sedley, S. (2005) DNA and the Courts. *Science & Justice*, **45** (2), 59–60.

Selye, H. (1950) *The Physiology and Pathology of Exposure to Stress*. Acta Montreal, Canada.

Selye, H. (1974) *Stress without Distress*. Lippincott, New York, USA.

Sen Gupta, B.K. (1999) *Modern Foraminifera*. Kluwer, Dordrecht, the Netherlands.

Shafer, J. & Fain, S.R. (1999) Diverse analytical approaches for determining species of bear parts. *Proceedings of the International Association of Forensic Sciences, Acta, Montreal Canada. 75th Triennial Meeting August 22–28, 1999, Los Angeles, California, USA*.

Shah-Kazemi, R. (1998) *Avicenna*. Robin Hood, London, UK.

Sharpe, R.T. & Livesey, C.T. (2005) Surveillance of suspect animal toxicoses with potential food safety implications in England and Wales between 1990 and 2002. *Veterinary Record*, **157**, 465–9.

Shaw, S.E. (2004) Editorial. Dogs, cats and methicillin-resistant *Staphylococcus aureus*. *Journal of Small Animal Practice*, **45**, 587–8.

Shepherd, R. (2003) *Simpson's Forensic Medicine*, 12th edn. Arnold, London, UK.

Sherwin, C.M. (2001) Can invertebrates suffer? Or, how robust is argument by analogy? *Animal Welfare*, **10**, 103–18.

Short, C.E. & Van Poznak, A. (eds) (1992) *Animal Pain*. Churchill-Livingstone, New York, USA/Edinburgh, UK.

Siegel, J., Saukko, P. & Knupfer, G. (2000) *Encyclopedia of Forensic Sciences*. Harcourt Publishers Ltd, UK.

Signorini, G., Biagi, G., Luchette, E., Cardini, G. & Bernocchi, R. (2004) Veterinary case history: forensic and medical legal aspects. *Veterinary Research Communications, Netherlands*, **28** (Suppl. 1), 381–4.

Sillis, M. (2003) Disposal of veterinary sharps. *Veterinary Record*, **152**, 116.

Silverman, M.E., Murray, T.J. & Bryan, C.S. (eds) (2003) *The Quotable Osler*. American College of Physicians, Philadelphia, USA.

Sime, S. (2002) *A Practical Approach to Civil Procedure*. Oxford University Press, Oxford, UK.

Simmons, V.C.G. & Sohan, L. (2001) A retrospective study of the treatment of toad poisoning in dogs in Trinidad. *Journal of the Caribbean Veterinary Medical Association*, **1** (1), 23–8.

Simpson, V. (2006) Postmortem identification of swans. *Veterinary Record*, **158**, 604.

Simpson, V., Stirling, D. & Britton, R. (2006) Investigation of otter *(Lutra lutra)* deaths using forensic techniques. *British Veterinary Zoological Society Proceedings May 2006* (ed. Victoria Roberts). Luton, UK.

Simpson, V.R. (2006) Patterns and significance of bite wounds in Eurasian otters (*Lutra lutra*) in southern and south-west England. *Veterinary Record*, **158**, 113–19.

Sims, C. (1999) Comparative morphology of the hand and foot bones of American black bear and human. *Proceedings of the International Association of Forensic Sciences, 75th Triennial Meeting August 22–28, 1999, Los Angeles, California, USA.*

Skilton, D. & Thompson, J. (2005) Needlestick injuries. *Veterinary Record*, **156**, 522.

Smith, D.A., Barker, I.K. & Allen, B.O. (1988) The effect of ambient temperature on healing cutaneous wounds in the common garter snake (*Thamnophis sirtalis*). *Canadian Journal of Veterinary Research*, **52**, 120–8.

Smith, E.L., Evans, J.E. & Párraga, C.A. (2005) Myoclonus induced by cathode ray tube screens and low-frequency lighting in the European starling (*Sturnus vulgaris*). *Veterinary Record*, **157**, 148–50.

Smith, F.H. (1951) *The Influence of Religions on Man's Attitude towards Animals*. The Universities Federation for Animal Welfare, London, UK.

Smith, K.C., Parkinson, T.J., Pearson, G.R., Sylvester, L. & Long, S.E. (2003) Morphological, histological and histochemical studies of the gonads of ovine freemartins. *Veterinary Record*, **152**, 164–9.

Smith, K.V. (1986) *A Manual of Forensic Entomology*. British Museum of Natural History, London, UK.

Smith, R.M. & Giannoudis, P.V. (1998) Trauma and the immune response. *Journal of the Royal Society of Medicine*, **91** (8), 417–20.

Soave, O.A. (2000) *Animals, The Law and Veterinary Medicine: a Guide To Veterinary Law*. Austin & Winfield, Lanham, MD, USA.

Sommerville, B.A. & Broom, D.M. (1998) Olfactory awareness. *Applied Animal Behaviour Science*, **57**, 269–86.

Sopher, I.M. (1976) *Forensic Dentistry*. Charles C. Thomas, Bannerstone House, Illinois, USA.

Sornogyi, E. & Tedeschi, C.G. (1977) Injury by electrical force. In: *Forensic Medicine* (eds C.G. Tedeschi, W.G. Eckert & L.G. Tedeschi). W.B. Saunders, Philadelphia, USA.

Spedding, C. (2005) The Animal Welfare Bill. *Biologist*, **52**, 6, 337–8.

Sperber, N.D. (1989) Bite marks, oral and facial injuries – harbingers of severe child abuse? *Pediatrician*, **16**, 207–11.

Spratt, D. (1993) Gin'll fix it. *Institute of Medical Laboratory Sciences Gazette*, **29** (1), 26–7.

Sprayson, T. (2006) Taking the lead: veterinary intervention in disaster relief. *In Practice*, **28**, 48–51.

Spring, G. (1996) Principles of forensic photography: The photographer and the law. *Journal of Biological Photography*, **64**, 33–9.

Spurlock, S.L. & Spurlock, G.H. (1990) Risk factors of catheter-related complications. *Compendium Continuing Education for the Practicing Veterinarian*, **12**, 214–45.

Squier, W. (2005) Neuropathology and the new laws: will we survive. *The Bulletin of The Royal College of Pathologists*, **131**, 32–5.

Stashak, T.S. (1987) *Adams' Lameness in Horses*, 4th edn. Williams & Wilkins, Baltimore, USA.

Stephenson, T. & Bialas, Y. (1996) Estimation of the age of bruising. *Archives of Diseases of Children*, **74**, 53–5.

Stevens, P.M.C. & McAlister, E. (2003) Ethics in zoos. *International Zoo Yearbook (2003)*, **38**, 94–101.

Stiff, R.E., Morris-Stiff, G.J. & Torkington, J. (2003) Hypothermia and acute pancreatitis: myth or reality? *Journal of the Royal Society of Medicine*, **96**, 228–9.

Stone, E. & Johnson, H. (1987) *Forensic Medicine*. The Criminal Law Library – No. 3. Waterloo Publishers, Oyez House, London, UK.

Storey, K.B. & Storey, J.M. (1988) Freeze tolerance in animals. *Physiological Review*, **68**, 27–84.

Storey, K.B., Storey, J.M., Brooks, S.P.J., Churchill, T.A. & Brooks, R.J. (1988) Hatchling turtles survive freezing during winter hibernation. *Proceedings of the National Academy of Sciences* **85**, 8350–4.

Stoskopf, M.F., Spelman, L.H., Sumner, P.W., Redmond, D.P., Jochem, W.J. & Levine, J.F. (1997) The impact of water temperature on core body temperature of North American River Otters (*Lutra canadensis*) during simulated oil spill recovery washing protocols. *Journal of Zoo and Wildlife Medicine*, **28** (4), 407–12.

Strafuss, A.C. (1988) *Necropsy: Procedures and Basic Diagnostic Methods for Practicing Veterinarians*. Charles C. Thomas, Springfield, Illinois, USA.

Strickland, G.T. (1991) *Hunter's Tropical Medicine*, 7th edn. W.B. Saunders Company, Philadelphia, USA.

Stroud, R.K. (1995) Wildlife forensics: A new and challenging role for the comparative pathologist. *Comparative Pathology Bulletin*, **27**, 1–2.

Stroud, R.K. (1998) Wildlife forensics and the veterinary practitioner. *Seminars in Avian and Exotic Pet Medicine*, 7 (4).

Stroud, R.K. & Adrian, W.J. (1996) Forensic investigational techniques for wildlife law enforcement investigations. In: *Non-Infectious Diseases of Wildlife* (eds A. Fairbrother, L.N. Locke & G.L. Hoff). Iowa State University Press, USA.

Stroud, R.K., Ralston, R.M. & Kirms, M. (1999) Investigating wildlife poisoning cases in the United States: eight years of experience. *Proceedings of the International Association of Forensic Sciences, 75th Triennial Meeting August 22–28, 1999, Los Angeles, California, USA.*

Stuart, C. & Stuart, T. (1994) *A Field Guide to the Tracks and Signs of Southern and East African Wildlife.* Southern Book Publishers, Halfway House, South Africa.

Stub, C., Mitskes-Hoitinga, M., Thon, R., Hanser, C.K. & Hanser, A.K. (2001) Fluctuating asymmetry in mice and rats: evaluation of the method. *Laboratory Animals*, 36, 193–9.

Suliman, H.B., Bkhiet, H.A. & Fagari, I. (1989) A clinical syndrome in imported cows subjected to environmental stress in Sudan. *Veterinary Record*, 125, 240.

Surosky, A.E. (1993) *The Expert Witness Guide for Scientists and Engineers.* Krieger Publishing, Malabar, Florida, USA.

Surpure, J. (1982) Heat-related illness and the automobile. *Annals of Emergency Medicine*, 11, 263–5.

Sutherland, W.J., Newton, I. & Green, R.E. (eds) (2004) *Bird Ecology and Conservation.* Oxford University Press, UK.

Sutton, P.G. (2005) Conservation law: food for thought. *Antenna*, 29, 50–3.

Swallow, J. *et al.* (2005) Guidance on the Transport of Laboratory Animals. Report of the Working Group, Laboratory Animal Science Association (LASA). *Laboratory Animals*, 39, 1–39.

Symmers, W.S. (1984) *Exotica.* Oxford University Press, Oxford, UK.

Tapia, F. (1971) Children who are cruel to animals. *Clinical Psychiatry and Human Development*, 2 (2), 70–1.

Tapper, C. (2003) *Cross and Tapper on Evidence*, 10th edn. Butterworth, London, UK.

ten Duis, H.J. *et al.* (1987) Superficial lightning injuries – their 'fractal' shape and origin. *Burns*, 13, 141–6.

Thompson, P. (1922) Bird pellets and their evidence as to the food of birds. *Essex Naturalist*, 115–42.

Thompson, S.W. & Luna, L.G. (1978) *An Atlas of Artifacts Encountered in the Preparation of Microscopic Tissue Sections.* Charles Louis Davis, DVM, Foundation, USA.

Thompson, T. (2001) Legal and ethical considerations of forensic anthropological research. *Science & Justice*, 41 (4), 261–70.

Thornley, R.G. (1978) *General Pathology.* W.B. Saunders, Philadelphia, USA/London, UK.

Thrusfield, M. (1997) *Veterinary Epidemiology.* Blackwell, Oxford, UK.

Tibi, S. (2006) Al-Razi and Islamic medicine in the 9th century. *Journal of the Royal Society of Medicine*, 99, 207–8.

Tilstone, W.J. & Lothridge, K.J. (2003) *Crime Laboratory Management.* Taylor & Francis, London, UK.

Tobias, P.V.T. & Cooper, J.E. (2003) The mountain gorilla: a little known chapter of pioneering studies. *Transactions of the Royal Society of South Africa*, 58 (1), 75–7.

Townley, L. & Ede, R. (2004) *Forensic Practice in Criminal Cases.* The Law Society, London, UK.

Tsokos, M. (ed.) (2004) *Forensic Pathology Reviews*, 1–3. Humana Press New Jersey, USA.

Tucker, B.K. *et al.* (2001) Characteristics of microscopic hacking trauma on bone. *Forensic Science*, 46 (2), 234–40.

Turk, J.L., Allen, E. & Cooper, J.E. (2000) The legacy of John Hunter, pioneer in comparative pathology. *European Journal of Veterinary Pathology*, 6 (1), 11–18.

Urquhart, K.A. & McKendrick, I.J. (2003) Survey of permanent wound tracts in the carcases of culled wild red deer in Scotland. *Veterinary Record*, 152, 497.

Urquhart, K.A. & McKendrick, I.J. (2006) Prevalence of 'head shooting' and the characteristics of the wounds in culled wild Scottish red deer. *Veterinary Record*, 159, 75–9.

U.S. Department of Justice (1998) *Forensic Laboratories: Handbook for Facility Planning, Design, Construction and Moving.* National Criminal Justice Reference Service, Maryland, USA.

Valkiunas, G. (2004) *Avian Malaria Parasites and other Haemosporidia.* CRC Press, Florida, USA.

Van Gelder, J.J. & Strijbosch, H. (1996) Marking amphibians: effects of toe-clipping on *Bufo bufo* (Anura: Bufonidae). *Amphibia-Reptilia*, 17, 169–74.

Van Kirk, D.J. (2001) *Vehicular Accident Investigation and Reconstruction.* CRC Press, Florida, USA/London, UK.

Veterinary Medicines Directorate (1998) *Guidance to the Veterinary Profession.* Animal Medicines European Licensing Information and Advice *Guidance Notes 8 (AMELIA 8).* Veterinary Medicines Directorate, Addlestone, UK.

Viner, B. (2005) Clinical audit in veterinary practice – the story so far. *In Practice*, 27, 215–18.

Viner, B.P. & Jenner, C.S. (2005) Clinical audit – learning from the medical profession. *Veterinary Record*, **157** (2), 695–6.

von den Driesch, A. (1976) *Das vermesser von Tierknochen as vor und Frühgeschichtlichen siedlungen*. Institute for Palaeoanatomy, University of Munich, Germany (English translation: *A Guide to the Measurement of Animal Bones from Archaeological Sites*. Peabody Museum Bulletin I, Harvard University Massachusetts, USA.)

Wagner, W. (2005) The perils of relying on interested parties to evaluate scientific quality. *American Journal of Public Health*, **95** (Suppl. 1), S99–106.

Walcott, H.E. (2004) Foiling bioterrorists attacks in zoos; risk assessment and wildlife forensic approaches. *Proceedings AAZV, AAWV, WDA Joint Conference*, USA.

Walker, C. (1996) *Signs of the Wild*. Struik, Cape Town, South Africa.

Wall, J. & Hamilton, I. (2000) *Handbook for Expert Witnesses in Children Act Cases*. Jordan Publishing, Bristol, UK.

Wall, P.D. & Melzack, R. (eds) (1994) *Textbook of Pain*, 3rd edn. Churchill-Livingstone, Edinburgh, UK.

Wallace, C. (2005) Can I get a witness? *Biologist*, **52** (4), 200.

Wallace, J. & Beavis, V. (2004) Firearms. In: *Crime Scene to Court. The Essentials of Forensic Science*, 2nd edn (ed. P.C. White). The Royal Society of Chemistry, Cambridge, UK.

Wallman, J.F. (2001) A key to the adults of species of blowflies in southern Australia known or suspected to breed in carrion. *Medical and Veterinary Entomology*, **15** (4), 433–7.

Walsh, A.L. & Morgan, D. (2005) Identifying hazards, assessing the risks. *Veterinary Record*, **157**, 684–7.

Wan, Q-H. & Fang, S-G. (2003) Application of species – specific polymerase chain reaction in the forensic identification of tiger species. *Forensic Science International*, **131** (1), 75–8.

Wander, P.A. & Gordon, P.D. (1987) *Dental Photography*. British Dental Association, London, UK.

Ware, S. (2005) Professional conduct in court. *Proceedings of the Veterinary Association for Arbitration and Jurisprudence*, **2** (1), 5–7.

Warlow, T.A. (1996) *Firearms, the Law and Forensic Ballistics*. Taylor & Francis, London, UK.

Warnick, A.J., Biedrzycki, L. & Russanow, G. (1987) Not all bite marks are associated with abuse, sexual activities or homicides: a case study of a self-inflicted bite mark. *Forensic Science*, **32**, 788–92.

Warriss, P.D., Pope, S.J., Brown, S.N., Wilkins, L.J. & Knowles, T.G. (2006) Estimating the body temperature

of groups of pigs by thermal imaging. *Veterinary Record*, **158**, 331–4.

Watkins, J., Drury, L. & Bray, S. (1996) *The Future of the UK Professional Associations*. Cheltenham Strategic Publications, Cheltenham, UK.

Watson, A.A. (1989) *Forensic Medicine – A Handbook for Professionals*. Gower Aldershot, Brookfield, USA.

Watson, N. (2004) The analysis of body fluids. In: *Crime Scene to Court. The Essentials of Forensic Science* (ed. P.C. White), 2nd edn. The Royal Society of Chemistry, Cambridge, UK.

Wax, D.E. & Haddox, V.G. (1974) Enuresis, firesetting and animal cruelty in male adolescent delinquents: a triad predictive of violent behavior. *Journal of Psychiatric Law*, **2** (1), 45–72.

WCS (undated) *Wildlife Health Sciences*. Wildlife Conservation Society, New York, USA.

Weatherley, A.H. & Gill, H.S. (1987) *The Biology of Fish Growth*. Academic Press, London, UK.

Webb, A.A., Jeffery, N.D., Olby, N.J. & Muir, G.D. (2004) Behavioural analysis of the efficacy of treatments for injuries to the spinal cord in animals. *Veterinary Record*, **155**, 225–30.

Webster, J. (1994) *Animal Welfare – A Cool Eye towards Eden*. Blackwell Science, Oxford, UK.

Webster, J. (2005) *Animal Welfare – Limping towards Eden*. Blackwell, Oxford, UK.

Wells, A. & Wilesmith, J.W. (2004) Bovine spongiform encephalopathy and related diseases. *Prion Biology and Diseases* (ed. S.B. Prusiner). CSHL Press, New York, USA.

Wensley, S. (2005) From Darwin to Dawkins. *Off the Record*, BVA News Monthly **4** (5), 1–2.

Wessum, R. van. (2001) The veterinary statement as evidence and the role of veterinarians in legal procedures. *Tijdschrift voor Diergeneeskunde. Koninklijke Nederlandse Maatschappij voor Diergeneeskunde*, **126** (5), 130–32. [Dutch]

West, M.H. & Friar, J. (1989) The use of videotape to demonstrate the dynamics of bite marks. *Forensic Science*, **34**, 88–95.

Weston, N. (2004) The crime scene. In: *Crime Scene to Court. The Essentials of Forensic Science* (ed. P.C. White), 2nd edn. The Royal Society of Chemistry, Cambridge, UK.

Westwell, M. (2005) Public perceptions of pathology- survey results. *Bulletin of The Royal College of Pathologists*, **131**, 68–9.

White, E., Hunter, J., Dubetz, C., *et al.* (2000) Microsatellite markers for individual tree genotyping: application in forest crime prosecutions. *Journal of Chemical Technology & Biotechnology*, **75** (10), 923–6.

White, P.C. (ed.) (2004) *Crime Scene to Court. The Essentials of Forensic Science*, 2nd edn. The Royal Society of Chemistry, Cambridge, UK.

White, T. & Folkens, P.A. (2005) *The Human Bone Manual*. Elsevier, Oxford, UK.

Whittaker, D.K. (1989) The dentist's role in non-accidental injury cases. In: *Paediatric Forensic Medicine and Pathology* (ed. J.K. Mason). Chapman & Hall, London, UK.

Whittaker, D.K. (1990) Principles of forensic dentistry: 2 Nonaccidental injury, bite marks and archaeology. *Dental Update*, **17**, 386–90.

Whittaker, D.K. & MacDonald, D.G. (1989) *Colour Atlas of Forensic Dentistry*. Wolfe Medical Publications, London, UK.

Whitwell, H. (ed.) (2005) *Forensic Neuropathology*. Oxford University Press, Oxford, UK.

WHO (2005) *Landmark Study on Domestic Violence*. News Release WHO/62, 24 November 2005. World Health Organization, Geneva, Switzerland.

WHO/IAEA/UNDP (2005) *Chernobyl: The True Scale of the Accident*. Joint News Release WHO/IAEA/UNDP/39, 5 September 2005. World Health Organization, Geneva, Switzerland.

Wiegers, A.L. (2004) Laboratory quality considerations for veterinary practitioners. *Journal of the American Veterinary Medical Association*, **225**, 1386–90.

Wiepkema, P.R. & Koolhaas, J.M. (1993) Stress and animal welfare. *Animal Welfare*, **2**, 195–218.

Wijnstekers, W. (2005) *The Evolution of CITES*, 8th edn. CITES Secretariat, Lausanne. Also available as e-book at http://www.cites.org/eng/resources/publications.shtml.

Wilkins, L.J., Brown, S.N., Zimmerman, P.H., Leeb, C. & Nicol, C.J. (2004) Investigation of palpation as a method for determining the prevalence of keel and furculum damage in laying hens. *Veterinary Record*, **155**, 547–9.

Willemser, R.E. & Hailey, A. (2002) Body mass condition in Greek tortoises: regional and interspecific variation. *Herpetological Journal*, **12**, 105–14.

William, O.M. & John, W. (2001) Immunological differentiation of camel meat from other mammalian meats. *Journal of Camel Practice and Research*, **8** (1), 1–6.

Williams, D.J., Ansford, A.J., Priday, D.S. & Forrest, A.S. (1998) *Forensic Pathology*. Churchill Livingstone, Edinburgh and London, UK.

Williams, G. & Smith, A.T.H. (2002) *Learning the Law*, 12th edn. Sweet & Maxwell, UK.

Willams, V. (2005) *Civil Procedure Handbook*, 2nd edn. Oxford University Press, Oxford, UK.

Wilson, B. (2005) Obituary. Robin Cook. *Guardian Weekly*, August 12–18, 2005.

Wilson, C.A., Bonner, A.K. & Rutty, G.N. (2004) Radiological investigations in autopsy practice. In: *Essentials of Autopsy Practice* (ed. G.N. Rutty). Springer-Verlag, London, UK.

Wilson, D.F. & Brown, K.A. (1993) Forensic odontology. In: *Oral Diseases in the Tropics*. (eds S.R. Prabhu, D.F. Wilson, D.K. Daftary & N.W. Johnson). Oxford University Press, UK.

Wilson, E.O. (1988) *Biodiversity*. National Academy of Sciences, Smithsonian Institution, Washington, D.C., USA.

Wilson, G.H. (ed.) (2004) Wound healing and management. *Veterinary Clinics of North America: Exotic Animal Practice*, 7, 1.

Wilson, J.F. (1988) *Law and Ethics of the Veterinary Profession*. Priority Press, Yardley, Philadelphia, USA.

Wilson, S. (2005) Principles of certification. *Proceedings of the Veterinary Association for Arbitration and Jurisprudence*, **2** (1), 43–7.

Windsor, P.A., Bush, R., Links, I. & Epplestone, J. (2005) Injury caused by self-inoculation with a vaccine of a Freund's complete adjuvant nature (GudairTM) used for control of ovine paratuberculosis. *Australian Veterinary Journal*, **83**, 216–20.

Wiseman, J. (1993) *SAS Survival Guide*. Harper Collins, Glasgow, UK.

Withler, R.E., Candy, J.R., Beacham, T.D. & Miller, K.M. (2004) Forensic DNA analysis of Pacific salmonid samples for species and stock identification. *Environmental Biology of Fishes*, **69**, 275–85.

Wobeser, G. (1996) Forensic (medico-legal) necropsy of wildlife. *Journal of Wildlife Diseases*, **32** (2), 240–9.

Wolf, C., Rentsch, J. & Hübner, P. (1999) PCR-RFLP analysis of mitochondrial DNA: a reliable method for species identification. *Journal of Agricultural and Food Chemistry*, **47**, 1350–5.

Wolfes, R., Mathe, J. & Seitz, A. (1991) Forensics of birds of prey by DNA fingerprinting with P-labelled oligonucleotide probes. *Electrophoresis*, **12**, 175–80.

Wood, V.J.W., Milner, G.R., Harpending, H., Weiss, K.M. (1992) The osteological paradox. Problems of inferring prehistoric health from skeletal samples. *Current Anthropology*, **33**, 343–70.

Woodbine, N. (2005) Vets report increase in doped-up domestic pets. *Veterinary Times*, 28 November.

Woolf, Lord (1996) *Access to Justice. Final Report to the Lord Chancellor on the Civil Justice System in England and Wales*, http://www.dca.gov.uk/civil/final/

Wootton, R. (2002) *Teledermatology*. The Royal Society of Medicine, London, UK.

Wootton, R. (2003) *Telepsychiatry and e-Mental Health.* The Royal Society of Medicine, London, UK.

Wootton, R. (2004) *Telepediatrics: Telemedicine and Child Health.* The Royal Society of Medicine, London, UK.

Wootton, R. & Craig, J. (1999) *Introduction to Telemedicine.* The Royal Society of Medicine, London, UK.

Wyllie, I. (1993) *Guide to Age and Sex in British Birds of Prey.* Institute of Terrestrial Ecology, Monkswood, England.

Wyllie, I. & Newton, I. (1999) Use of carcasses to estimate the proportions of female Sparrowhawks and Kestrels which bred in their first year of life. *Ibis*, **141**, 489–506.

Yagi, Y. & Gilbertson, J.R. (2005) Digital imaging in pathology: the case for standardization. *Journal of Telemedicine and Telecare*, **11** (3), 109–16.

Yalden, D.W. (1977) *The Identification of Remains in Owl Pellets.* An Occasional Publication of the Mammal Society, Reading, UK.

Yarrow, R. (2005) The tsunami and its aftermath. *Veterinary Record*, **156**, 687.

Yates, B. (1999) The morphology of secondary guard hairs. *Proceedings of the International Association of Forensic Sciences, 75th Triennial Meeting August 22–28, 1999, Los Angeles, California, USA.*

Young, R. (2003) *Environmental Enrichment for Captive Animals.* UFAW/Blackwell, Oxford, UK.

Youngner, S.J., Arnold, R.M. & Schapiro, R. (eds) (1999) *The Definition of Death: Contemporary Controversies.* Johns Hopkins University Press, USA.

Yovanovitch, P. (1888) *Entomologie Appliquée à la Médicine Légale.* Ollier-Henrey, Paris, France.

Zeitler-Feicht, M.H. (2004) *Horse Behaviour Explained. Origins, Treatment and Prevention of Problems.* Manson, London, UK.

Zhang, Y. *et al.* (2002) Genetic diversity and conservation of endangered animal species. *Pure and Applied Chemistry*, **74** (4), 575–84.

ZSL (2002) *Bushmeat & Forests.* Conservation Programmes. Zoological Society of London, UK.

Zumwalt, R.E., Petty, C.S. & Holman, W. (1976) Temperature in closed automobiles in hot weather. *Forensic Science Gazette*, 7, 7–8.

Zwart, P., de Vries, H.R. & Cooper, J.E. (1989) Het correct doden van vissen, amfibieën, reptielen en vogels. *Tijdschrift voor Diergeneeskunde*, **114** (10), 557–65. [Dutch]

Index

Abbreviations used throughout the book are listed on page xvi. For Glossary of Terms, some of which do not appear in this Index, see Appendix C. For scientific names of species and taxa of animals, see Appendix F. Figures designated with a letter (A, B, C…) are to be found in the relevant Appendices in the book.